The Health Professional's Guide to

Popular Dietary Supplements

Third Edition

Allison Sarubin Fragakis, MS, RD
With Cynthia Thomson, PhD, RD

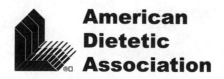

American Dietetic Association

Diana Faulhaber, Publisher
Pamela Woolf, Development Editor
Elizabeth Nishiura, Production Manager

10 9 8 7 6 5 4 3 2 1

Library of Congress Cataloging-in-Publication Data

Sarubin Fragakis, Allison.
     The health professional's guide to popular dietary supplements / Allison Sarubin Fragakis, with Cynthia Thomson. — 3rd ed.
          p. ; cm.
     Includes bibliographical references and index.
     ISBN-13: 978-0-88091-363-8
     1. Dietary supplements—Handbooks, manuals, etc. I. Thomson, Cynthia, 1957–
     II. American Dietetic Association. III. Title.
     [DNLM: 1. Dietary Supplements—Handbooks. QU 39 S251h 2007]

     RM258.5.S27 2007
     613.2'8—dc22
                                                                                            2006025874

ABOUT THE AUTHORS

Allison Sarubin Fragakis, MS, RD, is a dietitian and freelance writer based in the San Francisco Bay area. Her articles have been published in *Prevention, Self, Weight Watchers,* and several other publications. She is a contributing editor to *Prevention* magazine and reviews the magazine's supplement advertisements for safety. Allison was on the task force to help write the American Dietetic Association's "Guidelines Regarding the Recommendation and Sale of Dietary Supplements" and has coauthored a chapter on vitamins in *Medical Nutrition and Disease,* third edition. Currently, she is a contributing author for a book on the health benefits of native diets from around the world. Allison completed her undergraduate degree at University of Pennsylvania and received her master's in clinical nutrition from New York University.

Cynthia Thomson, PhD, RD, is a registered dietitian who earned her PhD in Nutritional Sciences from the University of Arizona in 1998, after which she completed postdoctoral training at the Arizona Cancer Center through funding from the National Cancer Institute. She currently holds the position of assistant professor in Nutritional Sciences, Medicine, and Public Health at the University of Arizona. Her research is focused on the areas of diet and women's cancers. As cancer patients frequently consume dietary supplements, Cyndi developed a professional interest in dietary supplementation well over a decade ago in an effort to better serve the needs of her patients who had been diagnosed with cancer.

REVIEWERS

Jeffrey Blumberg, PhD, FACN, CNS
Director, Antioxidants Research
  Laboratory
Jean Mayer USDA Human Nutrition
  Research Center on Aging
Professor, Friedman School of Nutrition
  Science and Policy
Tufts University

Sarah L. Booth, PhD
Jean Mayer USDA Human Nutrition
  Research Center on Aging
Tufts University

Sarah Harding Laidlaw, MS, RD, MPA
Nutrition Services Director
Mesa View Regional Hospital, Mesquite,
  NV
Editor, Nutrition in Complementary Care
  DPG newsletter

Tara Newton, MS
Consultant
University of Arizona

Jennifer Salguero
Scientist, United States Pharmacopeia

Tamara Schryver, PhD, RD
Senior Nutrition Scientist
General Mills
Bell Institute of Health and Nutrition

Reviewers for the Second Edition

Annette Dickinson, PhD; Norman R.
Farnsworth, PhD; Tracy A. Fox, MPH,
RD; Kristin A. Franco; Barbara F. Harland,
PhD, RD, FADA; Harold Holler, RD; Amy
B. Howell, PhD; Cathy Kapica, PhD, RD,
CFCS; Sharon L. Miller, PhD; Sylvia
Moore, PhD, RD, FADA; Michael W.
Pariza, PhD; Carol Seaborn, PhD, RD;
Cynthia Thomson, PhD, RD; John
Westerdahl, PhD, MPH, RD; Pamela
Williams, MPH, RD

Reviewers for the First Edition

Martha A. Belury, PhD; Jeffrey Blumberg,
PhD, FACN; Mary A. Carey, PhD, RD;
Kathryn Carroll, PhD; Ellen Coleman,
MA, MPH, RD; John R. Crouse III, MD;
Norman R. Farnsworth, PhD; Lisa K.
Fieber, MS, RD; John Finley PhD; Jane W.
Folkman, MS, RD; Tracy Fox, MPH, RD;
Constance J. Geiger, PhD, RD; William
Harris, PhD; Steve Hertzler, PhD, RD;
Cathy Kapica, PhD, RD, CFCS; Todd R.
Klaenhammer, PhD; Mindy Kurzer, PhD;
Alice J. Lenihan, MPH, RD, Joel Mason,
MD; Sylvia Moore, PhD, RD; Forrest
Nielson, PhD; Donna Porter, PhD, RD;
Susan M. Potter, PhD; Bruce D. Rengers,
PhD, RD; Dennis Savaino, PhD; Carol
Seaborn, PhD, RD; V. Srini Srinivasan,
PhD; Cynthia Thomson, PhD, RD; Connie
M. Weaver, PhD; John Westerdahl, PhD,
MPH, RD; Pamela Williams, MPH, RD;
Steven Zeisel, MD, PhD

CONTENTS

Preface ix

Acknowledgments xi

Introduction xiii

Frequently Used Abbreviations xxii

Alphabetical Guide to Dietary Supplements

Acidophilus /*Lactobacillus*
   Acidophilus (LA) 2
Alanine 10
Aloe Vera 14
Alpha-Lipoic Acid (ALA) 18
Androstenedione and Androstenediol 23
Arginine (L-arginine) 26
Aspartic Acid/Asparagine 36
Bee Pollen 39
Bitter Melon (*Momordica charantia*) 42
Black Cohosh (*Cimicifuga racemosa*) 46
Boron 52
Branched Chain Amino Acids (BCAA) 57
Bromelain 63
Calcium 69
Carnitine (L-Carnitine) 81
Cat's Claw (*Uncaria tomentosa*) 92
Chitosan 96
Chondroitin Sulfate 101
Chromium 105
Coenzyme Q_{10} 115
Colostrum/Bovine Colostrum 123
Conjugated Linoleic Acid 129
Cranberry Extract 136
Creatine 140
Dehydroepiandrosterone (DHEA) 148
Dong quai (*Angelica sinensis*) 157
Echinacea 160
Fenugreek (*Trigonella foenum-graecum*) 166
Feverfew (*Tanacetum parthenium*) 169

Fish Oil 172
Flaxseed 188
Folate/Folic Acid 195
Fructo-oligosaccharides (FOS) 205
Gamma-Linolenic Acid 210
Gamma-Oryzanol 219
Garlic 222
Ginger (*Zingiber officinale*) 232
Ginkgo Biloba 236
Ginseng 245
Glucosamine 254
Glutamine 262
Glycerol 267
Goldenseal (*Hydrastis canadensis*) 271
Grape Seed Extract 275
Green Tea Extract 278
Guarana 287
Guggul/Guggulipids 289
Hawthorn 292
Horse Chestnut 295
5-Hydroxy-Tryptophan (5-HTP) 298
β-Hydroxy β-Methylbutyrate (HMB) 303
Hydroxycitric Acid (*Garcinia cambogia*) 307
Indole-3-carbinol (I-3C) 311
Iron 315
Kava 320
Lecithin/Choline 325
Licorice Root 330
Lutein 335
Lycopene 340

Lysine	344	Selenium	462
Magnesium	349	Senna	472
Ma Huang *(Ephedra sinica)*	360	Shark Cartilage	474
Melatonin	366	Sodium Bicarbonate	479
Methylsulfonylmethane (MSM)	375	Soy Protein and Isoflavones	482
Milk Thistle *(Silybum marianum)*	377	Spirulina/Blue-Green Algae	499
N-Acetylcysteine (NAC)	382	Turmeric *(Curcuma longa)*	505
Noni Juice	388	Valerian *(Valeriana officinalis)*	508
Pancreatin	390	Vanadium	514
Pantothenic Acid	395	Vitamin A/Beta Carotene	518
Pau d'arco	398	Vitamin B-1 (Thiamin)	534
Phosphatidylserine	400	Vitamin B-2 (Riboflavin)	540
Phytosterols	404	Vitamin B-3 (Niacin)	543
Policosanol	408	Vitamin B-6 (Pyridoxine)	550
Potassium	414	Vitamin B-12 (Cobalamin)	558
Pygeum	419	Vitamin C	566
Pyruvate	422	Vitamin D	578
Red Clover	428	Vitamin E	588
Red Yeast Rice	432	Vitamin K	608
Resveratrol	435	Wheat Grass and Barley Grass	612
Royal Jelly	438	Whey Protein	615
S-adenosylmethionine (SAM-e)	442	Wild Yam *(Dioscorea villosa)*	620
St John's Wort *(Hypericum perforatum)*	451	Yohimbine/Yohimbe	622
Saw Palmetto *(Serenoa repens)*	459	Zinc	626

Appendixes

Appendix A: Government Regulation of Dietary Supplements 639

Appendix B: Ethical Issues and Dietary Supplements 649

Appendix C: Dietary Intake Tables 652

Appendix D: Additional Resources 658

Appendix E: Dietary Supplement Intake Assessment: Questions to Ask Clients 662

Index 665

PREFACE

The seed for this book was first planted by SCAN (the Sports, Cardiovascular, and Wellness Nutritionists Dietetic Practice Group of the American Dietetic Association). In 1996, the editors at SCAN asked me (Allison) to summarize research on sports supplements for their annual *Guide*. Realizing there was a need for a large-scale version of SCAN's publication, I began working with the American Dietetic Association on the first edition of the *Health Professional's Guide to Popular Dietary Supplements*. An advisory panel of dietitians and experts was formed to provide professional input during the development process.

As more research becomes available, there is a need to update the content of the book. The second edition (published in 2003) added the new Dietary Reference Intakes (DRIs) for several vitamins and minerals that were released by the Institute of Medicine's Food and Nutrition Board. Now, in the third edition, we have included 29 new entries on additional dietary supplements and have updated and expanded analysis of the safety and efficacy of the dietary supplements covered in the previous edition. The third edition includes 107 entries, summarizes more than 450 new studies, and is indexed for the first time.

The public, along with the medical community, is becoming more "supplement-savvy," and consumers are demanding evidence that dietary supplements are safe, effective, and reliable. This book uses an evidence-based approach and aims to provide the reader with objective and practical information for use in clinical practice. Despite this goal, the content of the book was met with a mixed reception during the peer-review process. For instance, reviewers often had differing opinions about whether there was enough evidence to rate a supplement as effective or ineffective. Some noted that the book seemed biased toward using supplements; others suggested that the book was too conservative; still others suggested that more decisive recommendations were needed. For certain, the reader can be assured that the opinions and comments of more than 30 expert reviewers have been incorporated into this edition and that those involved in the book's development were united in their opinion that dietetics professionals need this information.

The bottom line is that, regardless of whether you work with these products, it is important to be aware of their potential beneficial or harmful effects. No matter what your opinion about dietary supplementation, our aim is that you find this book helpful in making sense of the marketing claims, the scientific evidence in support of those claims (or the lack of such evidence), and the safety issues surrounding a select sampling of the more commonly used dietary supplements on the market.

Allison Sarubin Fragakis, MS, RD
Cynthia Thomson, PhD, RD

ACKNOWLEDGMENTS

Many thanks go to the numerous people involved in the final development of the *Health Professional's Guide to Popular Dietary Supplements*. A number of people were integral to the development of this third edition. Thank you to Pamela Woolf, ADA development editor, for organizing the revision process with such skill that it appeared easy (even though it was hard work). Also, a special heart-felt thank you to the reviewers who spent hours editing the manuscript pages, including Dr. Jeffrey Blumberg, Jennifer Salguero, Dr. Tamara Schryver, Dr. Sarah L. Booth, and Sarah Harding Laidlaw. Many thanks as well to Leila G. Saldanha, PhD, RD, who revised Appendix A for this edition, and Lisa K. Fieber, MS, RD, Samuel L. Fieber, JD, and Nancy Cotugna, DrPH, RD, for their work on Appendix B. Thank you to Elizabeth Nishiura; her attention to detail while overseeing production is a skill so important to the final product. We would also like to extend sincere gratitude to Tara Newton and Nicole Bergier for the endless hours they spent collecting the research for development of this third edition.

We are ever-grateful to those who contributed to the first and second editions and who initiated this ongoing effort to educate health care providers about dietary supplementation. We offer a special thank you to June Zaragoza, MPH, RD, Kathryn Carroll, Beth Birnham, Lisa Fieber, MS, RD, Samuel Fieber, JD, Ruth DeBusk, PhD, Laura Brown, Judith Clayton, Cathy Kapica, PhD, RD, Barbara Harland PhD, RD, and the Nutrition in Complementary Care (NCC) Dietetic Practice Group.

I, Allison, would like to thank Chris, my dear husband, for his ongoing support, encouragement, and bright smile. Thank you to my beautiful children, my marvelous parents, and my entire family for all of their love.

I, Cyndi, am indebted to my husband, Rob, and my sons, Daniel James and Patrick Cary Thomson, for their unending patience during the writing process. They have stood by me through the "bumps in the road," and this book was no exception. I love each of you and appreciate your sacrifice.

INTRODUCTION

National surveys show that more than 50% of Americans take some form of dietary supplement (1). The US Food and Drug Administration (FDA) estimates that more than 29,000 supplement products are on the market, supplied by approximately 500 to 850 manufacturers. According to *Nutrition Business Journal* (NBJ), supplement sales have been steadily increasing (2). Table 1 summarizes components of these sales figures. NBJ projects that supplement sales will grow 4% between 2005 and 2013 (2).

Table 1   US Supplement Industry in Consumer Sales* from All Retail Channels, Direct Sales, Multilevel Marketing, Mail Order, and Practitioner Sales

Products	1998	1999	2000	2001	2002	2003	2004
Vitamins	5,732	5,864	5,972	6,025	6,177	6,648	6,891
Botanicals/herbs	4,002	4,110	4,260	4,397	4,276	4,178	4,301
Sports nutrition	1,340	1,450	1,590	1,729	1,829	1,979	2,097
Minerals	1,140	1,290	1,351	1,396	1,527	1,765	1,738
Meal supplements	1,840	1,909	2,070	2,305	2,571	2,522	2,520
Specialty/other	1,453	1,785	2,052	2,222	2,368	2,711	2,977
Total Sales	**$15,507**	**$16,408**	**$17,295**	**$18,074**	**$18,748**	**$19,803**	**$20,524**

Figures are in millions of dollars.
Source: Data are from reference 2.

Health professionals should fully understand the beneficial and harmful effects of dietary supplements marketed to the public. Most Western-educated health professionals have had little, if any, training in this area. To stay abreast of the latest supplement trends, in order to advise patients or clients appropriately, it is important to research the literature and evaluate studies.

The *Health Professional's Guide to Popular Dietary Supplements, Third Edition,* is designed to inform health professionals about 107 dietary supplements. The science behind dietary supplements is constantly evolving; thus, the information presented in this book is not exhaustive but aims rather to familiarize readers with the scope and types of currently available research. Because in many cases the state of the research is rapidly changing, it is important to also check other resources, such as Medline and the new database made available by the National Institutes of Health (NIH) Office of Dietary

Supplements, to keep up to date on new studies and safety issues (see Appendix D for Additional Resources).

How To Use This Book

There are many ways to use this book. Practitioners can scan for information to answer a patient's or colleague's question, to prepare for a presentation or television interview, to use as background for writing consumer nutrition articles, or simply to become better educated about today's supplement market.

Supplements are presented alphabetically with information provided in an easy-to-read bullet format for quick access. In cases where a supplement is known by more than one name, cross-references appear within the text and in the index. For example, a reader looking under "Beta Carotene" is advised to "see Vitamin A."

The content of each entry is organized in the same sequence:

◆ A brief overview of the dietary supplement
◆ A table summarizing media and marketing claims and efficacy
◆ Safety information
◆ Drug/supplement interactions
◆ Key points about the supplement
◆ Food sources
◆ Dosage information and bioavailability
◆ Relevant research
◆ References

Media and Marketing Claims

The media and marketing claims listed for each supplement were gathered from Web sites, product literature, magazine articles and advertisements, books and newsletters promoting supplement use, and health food stores. The claims are *not* based on scientific facts. Many of the media and marketing claims listed in this section—for example, "Lowers cholesterol"—would not be considered legal if printed on supplement labels or in promotional materials. However, the claims illustrate how many books, magazine articles, and some practitioners refer to the benefits of the supplement. (Refer to Appendix A, "Government Regulation of Dietary Supplements" for more details about allowable health claims for dietary supplements.)

Efficacy

In the Efficacy column of the table, a coding system indicates whether available scientific evidence supports the media and marketing claims. Table 2 presents the symbols used to indicate efficacy.

Table 2 Key to Efficacy Symbols

↑	Evidence from several controlled trials in humans (in vivo) supports efficacy claims.
↑?	Preliminary evidence from a few controlled trials in humans supports efficacy claims, but more research is needed. (Research that is positive and has only been performed in vitro is so designated in the column.)
↔	Evidence from conflicting controlled research in humans is equivocal.
↓	Research in humans does not support efficacy claims.
↓?	Preliminary evidence from a few controlled trials in humans does not support efficacy claims, but more research is needed. (Research that is negative and has only been performed in vitro is so designated in the column.)
NR	Not enough research in humans is available to evaluate the efficacy of the claims, or the quality of research is poor.

Safety

Safety is the most important factor when deciding to use supplements, and yet in many cases this is difficult to assess given the dearth of supporting data. There is often very little human research regarding food-herbal, drug-herbal, or multiple herbal interactions. The Safety subsection lists reported information about toxicity, known drug interactions, or adverse events associated with supplementation. It also discusses whether any long-term studies have been completed.

Note: Pregnant or lactating women should not use *any* dietary supplement without the advice of their physician. This population should clearly avoid supplements that are associated with serious adverse effects, including those listed in the Safety subsection. However, routine supplementation during pregnancy should include a prenatal multivita min and mineral supplement with particular attention to the nutrients folic acid, iron, and calcium in healthy populations (3).

If an adverse effect occurs in association with a dietary supplement, it should be reported to MedWatch, the FDA's Medical Products Reporting Program. MedWatch is a postmarket surveillance program designed to educate health professionals about the critical importance of being aware of, monitoring, and reporting adverse events and product problems to the FDA and/or manufacturer. Health professionals may report a problem by calling the MedWatch hotline at 800/FDA-1088 (800/332-1088) or by using its Web site (http://www.fda.gov/medwatch/report/hcp.htm). Consumers may also report an adverse effect by calling the hotline or using a separate Web site (http://www.fda.gov/medwatch/report/consumer/consumer.htm).

Drug/Supplement Interactions

This section provides a list of possible or known interactions between the supplement and any drug or other supplement. This information was derived from a variety of sources including a Medline search of original research and the following resources:

- Ang-Lee MK, Moss J, Yuan CS. Herbal medicines and perioperative care. *JAMA*. 2000;286:208–216.

- Basch EM, Servoss JC, Tedrow UB. Safety assurances for dietary supplements policy issues and new research paradigms. *J Herb Phramacother*. 2005;5:3–15.

- Blumenthal M. Interactions between herbs and conventional drugs: introductory considerations. *HerbalGram*. 2000;49:52–63.

- Boullata J. Natural health product interactions with medication. *Nutr Clin Pract*. 2005;20:33–51.

- Brinker F. *Herb Contraindications and Drug Interactions*. 2nd ed. Sandy, Ore: Eclectic Medical Publications; 1998.

- Cupp MJ. Herbal remedies: adverse effects and drug interactions. *Am Fam Phys*. 1999;59:1239–1244.

- Fugh-Berman A. Herb-drug interactions. *Lancet*. 2000;355:134–138.

- Jellin JM, Gregory P, Batz F, et al. *Pharmacist's Letter/Prescriber's Letter Natural Medicines Comprehensive Database*. 3rd ed. Stockton, Calif: Therapeutic Research Faculty; 2000.

- Jellin JM, Gregory P, Batz F, et al. *Pharmacist's Letter/Prescriber's Letter Natural Medicines Comprehensive Database*. 5th ed. Stockton, Calif: Therapeutic Research Faculty; 2003.

- Miller L. Herbal medicinals: selected clinical considerations focusing on known or potential drug-herb interactions. *Arch Intern Med*. 1998;158:2200–2211.

- Miller SC. Safety concerns regarding ephedrine-type alkaloid containing dietary supplements. *Mil Med*. 2004;169:87–93.

- Phillips GC. Medicolegal issues and ergogenic aids: trade, tragedy, and public safety, the example of ephedra and the Dietary Supplement Health and Education Act. *Curr Sports Med Rep*. 2004;3:224–228.

- Pittler MH, Schmidt K, Ernst E. Adverse events of herbal food supplements for body weight reduction: systematic review. *Obes Rev*. 2005;6:93–111.

- Schilter B, Andersson C, Anton R, et al. Guidance for the safety assessment of botanicals and botanical preparations for use in food and food supplements. *Food Chem Toxicol*. 2003;41:1625–1649.

- Willett KL, Roth RA, Walker L. Workshop overview: hepatotoxicity assessment for botanical dietary supplements. *Toxicol Sci*. 2004;79:4–9.

Key Points

This section gives a general summary of the supplement. Each key point specifically addresses whether available scientific evidence supports the media and marketing claims for a particular supplement. The conclusions should be considered a snapshot in time, which can potentially change as science emerges. Refer to the Key Points when time is short and a brief overview is needed.

Food Sources

This section lists food sources of a particular supplement (if applicable). Because the science and safety of ingesting isolated nutrients in supplement form is still relatively understudied and because foods contain a wide array of known and unknown nutrients and health-promoting constituents, food sources are recommended as a first choice whenever possible. Dietary supplements should be viewed as "supplemental" to a healthy diet. Not only may food sources of a particular nutrient or phytochemical contain additional nutrients and health benefits, but they are also often less expensive than supplement forms. However, in some instances, one would have to consume an excessive amount of food to get the desired quantity of a certain nutrient, and supplementation is therefore appropriate. Use this section to encourage individuals to make appropriate food selections within the context of a balanced eating plan.

Note: Unless otherwise indicated, the serving sizes noted in Food Sources tables are for cooked foods.

Dosage Information/Bioavailability

This section reports the range of doses suggested on supplement labels and the doses used in clinical trials. It indicates whether supplements are available in tablet, capsule, tincture, or powder form and whether products are voluntarily standardized. The Dosage Information/Bioavailability section also notes the various chemical compounds found in different products (eg, chromium is available as chromium picolinate or chromium chloride supplements). If there are data on bioavailability and absorption, they are also included under this heading.

The following are definitions for terms used in this section (4–6):

- **Extract:** A concentrated preparation of liquid or dry consistency made from dried plant materials.

- **Liquid extract:** A preparation created by dissolving dried extract in alcohol or water or by soaking or percolating dried plant material with solvent and evaporating it to produce a specified ratio of dry matter to solvent. Usually the solvent is evaporated to produce a ratio of 1:1 of dry plant material to solvent.

- **Dried extract:** A preparation created by evaporating all of the liquid solvent from the liquid extract. The powdered material can then be processed into tablets, capsules, or lozenges.

- **Standardized extract:** A preparation created by adjusting extract to a consistent strength. Standardization may be done by dilution with inert materials or by mixing several different strengths to achieve desired levels.

- **Tincture:** A preparation created by steeping dried or fresh plant material with a mixture of water and alcohol to extract the plant material at room temperature. (If glycerol is used as the solvent, the preparation is referred to as a *glycerite*.) Tinctures are often made into strengths with ratios of 1:5 or 1:10 of plant to solvent and are not as concentrated as liquid extracts. Tinctures frequently contain alcohol.

- **Infusion/"Tea":** A preparation created by pouring boiling water over chopped plant material and straining after steeping.
- **Decoction:** A preparation created by adding cold water to chopped plant material, bringing it to a boil, then simmering before cooling and straining.
- **Strength:** The ratio of plant material to solvent.

When reviewing information in this section, it is important to keep in mind certain issues facing consumers and the supplement industry (see also Appendix A, "Government Regulation of Dietary Supplements"). For example:

- The FDA does not have the resources, nor is it the agency's duty, to monitor and ensure the reliability and safety of every supplement on the market.
- The activity and content of herbs vary depending on manufacturer, harvest time, climate, soil, portion of plant used (eg, root or leaves), method of extraction, formulation, and storage.
- Even when an herbal product states that it is standardized to contain a certain amount of an "active" ingredient, the constituents that are biologically active may not be known. In many cases, there may be several compounds that are potentially bioactive. Therefore, standardizing a product to one ingredient does not always ensure a superior product. This is an area of research that is sure to remain controversial and inconclusive for some time.
- Studies have documented inaccuracies in dietary supplement labels. It is not uncommon for the level of ingredients analyzed from individual pills or capsules to differ from the amount stated on the label (even though such deviations are not legally permissible).

Relevant Research

The Relevant Research discussion is usually the largest part of each supplement's entry. Studies, review articles from peer-reviewed journals, and meta-analyses are briefly summarized and listed by relevant category (eg, diabetes, cardiovascular disease, weight loss, exercise performance, etc). The entries are brief overviews and are not intended to be indepth analyses of the literature. When a study is reported as having a "significant" result, this is stated as a statistical significance at a *P* value of .05 or less. In general, only journal articles in English are included. With few exceptions, this book does not cover research about supplement use during pregnancy, lactation, infancy, or childhood. More information on a particular study can be found by checking the reference list at the end of the dietary supplement entry.

Some of the studies listed under this heading have important limitations, and these are generally identified for the reader. When flawed studies are included, it is because some supplement manufacturers may cite small or uncontrolled studies to promote their products. Thus, the descriptions help to point out the scientific nature of the supporting research. In a few cases, published abstracts are described and noted as such.

Criteria for Evaluating Research

No study is perfect. It is imperative to critically review research designs. Because research on dietary supplements is emerging so rapidly, readers are encouraged to be proactive in developing critical appraisals of the validity and significance of study results. Even though a trial may report a *statistically* significant result, it does not necessarily equate with *biological or clinical* significance. Nor does it follow that the research was methodologically sound. Because scientific discovery emerges through often-contradictory findings, it is important to consider the totality of evidence rather than the results of one study. When reviewing research articles, readers should consider the following questions:

- Was the study double-blinded and placebo-controlled?
- Were the subjects randomly assigned to treatment and control groups?
- What was the sample size? (Results from randomized trials with fewer than 80 subjects or crossover studies with fewer than 40 subjects should be viewed as preliminary.)
- What is the population being studied? To whom do the results apply?
- Do the subjects represent the population to whom the supplements are marketed?
- How long did the study last? Was there ample time to assess biological effects?
- Were important variables controlled (age, weight, diet, fitness level, medication)?
- What endpoint biomarker(s) was used? A subjective measure, such as perceived pain, or a biological marker of health status, such as serum cholesterol level?
- Could there have been a publication bias (ie, were only positive papers printed)?
- Is the journal peer-reviewed? (Check *Ulrich International Periodicals Directory* or contact the journal's publisher directly.)

Types of Research Design

The following terms are frequently used to describe research design (7,8):

- **Case-control study:** A retrospective observational study in which the subjects are selected based on whether they have a disease or condition. Subjects with the disease are the "cases" and subjects without are the "controls." Case-control studies explore associations only, not causality (eg, a study of the history of the use of vitamin C supplements by subjects with breast cancer compared with subjects without breast cancer.)
- **Cross-sectional study:** A cross-sectional assessment of exposure to possible risk factors and prevalence of disease or health problems in a population at one point or period of time (eg, National Food Consumption Surveys). Cross-sectional studies do not provide information on the etiology of the disease or condition being studied.
- **Prospective cohort study:** An epidemiological study that follows a group of subjects for a certain period of time to observe the effect of certain variables on outcome variables such as disease incidence or mortality.
- **Relative risk:** A statistical formula used in a cohort study/cross-sectional epidemiological study. It is calculated by dividing the cumulative incidence of disease among

those exposed to the variable by the cumulative incidence of the disease among those not exposed.

- **Retrospective cohort study:** An epidemiological study that requires subjects to recall past behaviors or examines previously recorded information to determine the effect of certain variables on disease incidence. This study design is inferior to prospective research because of errors in recall and the likelihood that behaviors change after diagnosis.

Terminology Used in Controlled Clinical Research

The following terms are frequently used to describe controlled clinical research studies:

- **Controlled study:** An interventional study where a comparable group of subjects is also examined but does not receive the treatment. A *placebo-controlled study* is an interventional study where subjects receive either treatment or a placebo (inert or inactive substance). The gold standard in clinical research is a study that is randomized, double-blinded, and placebo-controlled.

- **Crossover-design study:** A controlled study comparing two or more treatments whereby subjects complete one course of treatment and then are switched to the other. Typically, assignment to the first treatment is randomized. Well-designed crossover studies include a washout period between treatments to avoid the possibility of run-over effects.

- **Double-blind study:** Through the use of a "blinded" or masked coding system, neither the researchers nor the subjects know which subjects are in the treatment and control groups until after the study. This process is only effective when the intervention used is easily masked.

- **Meta-analysis:** A statistical technique in which the results of many studies are pooled to make overall conclusions. Meta-analyses must select studies that are well-designed and have similar protocols. However, if studies chosen for grouped analysis are flawed, or if a publication bias exists, meta-analyses will not provide accurate information.

- **Randomization:** The process of assigning subjects randomly to a treatment or control group so that each subject has an equal chance of being assigned to either group.

Appendixes

In addition to the Alphabetical Guide to Dietary Supplements, this book includes five appendixes:

- **Appendix A: Government Regulation of Dietary Supplements** explains how the supplement industry is regulated and discusses the Dietary Supplement Health and Education Act (DSHEA) of 1994, the proper labeling of dietary supplements, quality control, and how to choose quality dietary supplements. This appendix was revised for the third edition by Leila G. Saldanha, PhD, RD.

♦ **Appendix B: Ethical Issues and Dietary Supplements** discusses the ethical and legal considerations that arise with widespread use of dietary supplements. This appendix was authored by Lisa K. Fieber, MS, RD, and Samuel L. Fieber, JD, and revised for the third edition by Nancy Cotugna, DrPH, RD.

♦ **Appendix C: Dietary Intake Tables** summarizes current Dietary Reference Intakes (DRIs)for vitamins and elements.

♦ **Appendix D: Additional Resources** provides information about relevant organizations, publications, Web sites, and books.

♦ **Appendix E: Dietary Supplement Intake Assessment** offers a number of questions for practitioners to ask patients and clients in order to assess their use of supplements.

References

1. Radimer K, Bindewald B, Hughes J, et al. Dietary supplement use by US adults: data from the National Health and Nutrition Examination Survey, 1999-2000. *Am J Epidemiol.* 2004;60:339-349.
2. Supplement business report. *Nutrition Business Journal.* October 2005.
3. American Dietetic Association. Position of the American Dietetic Association: food fortification and dietary supplements. *J Am Diet Assoc.* 2001;101:115-125.
4. Blumethal M, ed. *The Complete German Commission E Monographs Therapeutic Guide to Herbal Medicines.* Boston, Mass: Integrative Medicine Communications; 1998.
5. Schulz V, Hansel R, Tyler VE. *Rational Phytotherapy: A Physician's Guide to Herbal Medicine.* 3rd ed. Berlin, Germany: Springer-Verlag; 1998.
6. Ody P. *The Complete Medicinal Herbal.* New York, NY: Dorling Kindersley; 1993.
7. Monsen ER, ed. *Research: Successful Approaches.* 2nd ed. Chicago, Ill: American Dietetic Association; 2003.
8. Fennick JH. *Studies Show: A Popular Guide to Understanding Scientific Studies.* Amherst, NY: Prometheus Books; 1997.

FREQUENTLY USED ABBREVIATIONS

AI	Adequate Intake
AIDS	acquired immunodeficiency syndrome
BMI	body mass index
CDC	Centers for Disease Control and Prevention
CI	confidence interval
CNS	central nervous system
CVD	cardiovascular disease
DRI	Dietary Reference Intake
FDA	Food and Drug Administration
GRAS	Generally Recognized As Safe
HDL	high-density lipoprotein
HIV	human immunodeficiency virus
HR	hazards ratio
IV	intravenous
LDL	low-density lipoprotein
NIH	National Institutes of Health
NSAID	nonsteroidal anti-inflammatory drug
OR	odds ratio
PMS	premenstrual syndrome
RDA	Recommended Dietary Allowance
RR	relative risk
UL	Tolerable Upper Intake Level
VLDL	very low-density lipoprotein

Alphabetical Guide to Dietary Supplements

Acidophilus/*Lactobacillus Acidophilus* (LA)

Lactobacillus acidophilus (LA) is the scientific name for a heterogeneous group of lactic acid bacteria including gram-positive rods and cocci that use carbohydrates for energy and in the process produce lactic acid, hydrogen peroxide, enzymes, and B vitamins via fermentation of food and dairy products. These bacteria normally colonize the gut. LA is one of many strains of lactic acid bacteria, found in the human gastrointestinal tract, that seems to play a role in stimulating the immune response and in combating intestinal and foodborne pathogens. Within the LA species, there also exist individual strains, each with differing actions. After being ingested, LA withstands the stomach pH and travels to the lower intestine. Some portion of a bacterial load may adhere to the epithelium and thus potentially help defend the host against harmful bacteria. Antibiotics, oral contraceptives, physical stress, and malnutrition may affect the delicate balance of microflora in the intestine. Some researchers suggest that recolonizing the gut with LA and other *Lactobacillus* bacteria (via food or supplements) will create a healthy microflora and reduce gastrointestinal symptoms and vaginal infections associated with harmful bacteria overgrowth (1–3).

Media and Marketing Claims	Efficacy
Reduces lactose intolerance	NR
Prevents or reduces length of vaginal yeast infections	↔ (LA yogurt)
	NR (LA supplements)
Helps control rotaviral diarrhea (LA GG)	↑
Prevents antibiotic-associated diarrhea and traveler's diarrhea	↔
Controls irritable bowel symptoms	↓
Reduces cholesterol	↔
Prevents cancer	NR
Prevents or reduces severity of atopic disease (allergies, eczema, etc)	NR

Safety

- There have been no reports of any adverse effects in human studies supplementing LA at dose levels of 10^{10} or 10^{11} colony-forming units/day. In addition, various LA products (milk, yogurt, sweet acidophilus milk) have been on the market for decades with no reports of bacteremic infections (4).

- Two case reports have been published of LA sepsis related to probiotic therapy among immunocompromised children, indicating a need to further monitor use of LA supplements (5). In addition, some authors suggest that immunosuppressed patients should avoid use of LA (or other probiotic) supplements (6).

- Short-bowel syndrome may predispose an individual to pathogenic infection; use LA supplements with caution.

Drug/Supplement Interactions

+ LA may have a positive effect on gut flora when administered with antibiotics.
+ Separate ingestion of LA and antibiotics by at least 2 hours to avoid possibility of decreasing the effectiveness of LA.

Caution

Some products may contain little or no LA, and some may contain other strains of lactobacilli or contaminants.

Key Points

+ There is conflicting evidence as to whether LA-cultured dairy products may improve absorption of lactose and reduce symptoms such as cramps and diarrhea in individuals with lactose intolerance. Currently, different strains of LA are being tested for their relative effectiveness.
+ There is preliminary evidence that LA-cultured yogurt (2 cups/day) may reduce episodes of vaginal infections. Evidence does not support that LA supplements either prevent antibiotic use–related vaginitis or bacterial vaginitis. However, one study demonstrated the effectiveness of yogurt cultured with LA in reducing the recurrence of bacterial vaginosis (7). Women with vaginitis may wish to try LA-cultured dairy products, not only for their potential ability to improve the infection, but also because they are good sources of calcium, which is important for women's health in general.
+ As discussed in several review articles, LA and other probiotic bacteria administered in dairy products or supplements (particularly LA plantarum) may reduce diarrhea associated with antibiotic use and *Clostridium difficile* and other pathogens. Oral LA GG can prevent traveler's diarrhea, but efficacy varies depending on the country of exposure. Diarrheal events in children, including rotaviral diarrhea, seem particularly responsive to oral LA GG supplementation.
+ In general, studies have not found that LA supplementation reduces symptoms associated with irritable bowel syndrome. However, in one preliminary study, *Bifidobacteria* (another probiotic often included in LA supplements) did show some benefit in people with IBS. Better controlled research in larger samples is needed before recommendations can be made.
+ There is preliminary evidence that dairy products fermented with LA may reduce cholesterol levels in subjects with and without hyperlipidemia. Larger controlled trials testing LA foods and supplements are needed to verify this lipid-lowering effect.
+ There is no clear evidence that LA plays a role in cancer prevention; however, theoretically maintaining a healthy gut microflora may be important to optimal immune function and gut integrity, both important to reducing cancer risk. No clinical studies have specifically tested the influence of LA dairy products or supplements on biomarkers of

cancer in humans. Preliminary evidence suggests that LA supplementation may reduce *Helicobacter pylori* viral load and thus indirectly reduce risk for gastric cancer—further research is warranted.

◆ Preliminary research has found that the use of *lactobacillus rhamnosus* GG strain by women during late pregnancy and early lactation may reduce inflammatory biomarkers present in the breastmilk and the incidence of atopic eczema in newborns with a family history of these illnesses.

◆ Conflicting data regarding efficacy of LA may be a result of differing experimental designs, differing *Lactobacillus* strains, variations in preparation and storage of LA, and the use of nonviable bacteria in studies (8). The strongest evidence to date is related to the use of LA GG strain.

Food Sources

Yogurt containing live LA cultures, kefir, and acidophilus milk

Dosage Information/Bioavailability

LA supplements are sold in powders, tablets, or capsules, often with other *Lactobacilli (L casei, L delbruekii)* or *Bifidobacteria (B adolescentis, B bifidum, B longum, B infantis)*. Dosages are expressed in millions or billions of viable bacteria. Most manufacturers recommend taking 1 billion to 10 billion viable LA cells daily, but up to 100 billion live bacteria daily has been safely administered to children with diarrhea, and lower doses are sometimes ineffective. LA supplements must be used by the expiration date (usually 1 year for freeze-dried) and some require refrigeration to maintain viability.

Relevant Research

LA and Lactose Intolerance

◆ During fermentation of yogurt and acidophilus milk, *Lactobacilli* produce lactase, which hydrolyzes milk lactose to glucose and galactose. Thus, up to 50% of lactose in acidophilus milk and yogurt is predigested by lactase during the fermentation process, which potentially reduces symptoms associated with lactose ingestion in intolerant individuals (9).

◆ Several studies have demonstrated that fermented dairy products (acidophilus milk, yogurt [not pasteurized or heated]) are absorbed better (as measured by breath hydrogen) and are associated with fewer intestinal symptoms than nonfermented dairy foods (2,9).

LA and Intestinal Infections

◆ Possible mechanisms for the protective role of LA against intestinal and vaginal disorders include (*a*) LA forms antimicrobial compounds such as lactic acid; acetic acid;

hydrogen peroxide; broad-range, antibiotic-like compounds, and bacteriocins that inhibit the growth of pathogenic bacteria; (*b*) LA byproducts such as short-chain fatty acids reduce pH and inhibit pathogenic organisms; and (*c*) LA competes with pathogenic bacteria for nutrients and adhesion sites (1,9).

◆ A detailed review in *JAMA* evaluated all available placebo-controlled, human studies of supplementation with biotherapeutic agents (*L acidophilus, Bifidobacterium longum, Lactobacillus casei GG*, and other selected microorganisms) from 1966 to 1995. The authors concluded that these studies "have shown that biotherapeutic agents have been used successfully to prevent antibiotic-associated diarrhea, to prevent acute infantile diarrhea, to treat recurrent *Clostridium difficile* disease, and to treat various other diarrheal illnesses." The authors noted that many of the studies included small numbers of subjects (10).

◆ In a double-blind, placebo-controlled study, 820 Finnish subjects traveling to southern Turkey to two destinations (Marmaris or Alayna) were randomly assigned to receive 2×10^9 LA GG (a new *Lactobacillus* strain isolated from human intestine) powder or placebo twice daily before departure and continuing during the trip. A total of 756 subjects completed the study, with equal representation from the two groups. No significant difference was shown overall ($P = .065$), but there was a destination effect, with travelers to Alayna demonstrating protection against diarrhea with supplementation (11).

◆ Three meta-analyses have been conducted investigating the role of LA in prevention or treatment of diarrhea. The first included 29 papers wherein intake of LA GG consistently reduced number of days with diarrhea in the setting of rotavirus (12), but did not prevent viral or bacterial diarrhea. The second analysis, focused on prevention of antibiotic-associated diarrhea in children, showed a 66% reduction in risk with supplementation (13). The third included nine studies, all of which were randomized and placebo-controlled. This analysis supported a reduction in the duration of diarrhea by a mean of 0.7 days and a mean reduction in stool frequency of 1.6 stools/day (14).

◆ There may be a differential effect of LA supplementation for diarrheal episodes in children vs adults. A multicenter European study showed that supplementation with LA GG (with oral rehydration therapy) significantly reduced duration of diarrhea, risk of a protracted course, and length of hospital stay among infants (N = 287) (15). This is supported by research from Chandra et al, a placebo-controlled intervention with LA in children (16).

◆ However, in a study of adults (N = 302) given LA GG or placebo, there was no significant difference in occurrence of diarrhea after antibiotic therapy (17).

LA and Irritable Bowel Syndrome

◆ To date, studies investigating the role of LA supplementation to reduce diarrheal symptoms associated with irritable bowel syndrome generally have been negative. In a study of 12 subjects receiving LA plantarum 299V or placebo for 4 weeks in a crossover design, there was no significant difference in colonic fermentation or symptoms with supplementation (18). Using a similar study design in 25 subjects with IBS, no significant differences in pain, urgency, or bloating were shown between *Lactobacillus casei* strain GG and placebo (19).

- In a larger study, 77 subjects with IBS (mean age 44.3 years) were randomly assigned to (*a*) LA *salvarius* UCC4331, (*b*) *Bifidobacterium infantis* 35624, or (*c*) placebo for 8 weeks, with 4 weeks of follow up. There were more smokers in the group taking LA (smoking has been associated with reduced symptoms of IBS). Efficacy was assessed using both self-report of gastrointestinal symptoms and cytokine expression. Cytokine levels were compared over time and with age- and gender-matched healthy control subjects. Results showed that the bifidobacterium significantly improved symptoms and improved cytokine profiles toward reduced inflammatory response. The group taking LA had no significant improvement in IBS symptoms or cytokine profile (20).

- In a randomized, double-blind study, 64 children with IBS (12 males and 52 females; mean age 12 years) were randomly assigned to a 6-week intervention using LA GG or placebo. Twenty five children in each group completed the intervention. There was no difference between the two groups in self-reported disease-related symptoms at the start of the intervention (21). Children enrolled met Rome II criteria for IBS and completed a standardized Gastrointestinal Symptom Rating Scale to measure efficacy of the intervention. At the end of 6 weeks, 11 "responders" were identified within the intervention group and 10 within the control group, indicating no statistical difference across the two groups. However, among those with the highest abdominal pain scores at baseline, there was a significantly greater likelihood of improvement over time. This may be related to regression to the mean, as this was apparent regardless of group assignment. No objective measures of disease severity were reported. The sample size was small, given the wide range of symptoms reported, and subjects were not switched to the alternate treatment.

- In a double-blind study, 54 subjects with IBS were randomly assigned to LA *reuteri* ATCC 55730 or placebo. Efficacy was evaluated through self-report of gastrointestinal symptoms (Francis Severity score and IBS quality of life score). At the end of the 6-month intervention, there was no significant difference between groups (22). Fifteen subjects dropped out of the study, which makes interpretation of the results difficult.

LA and Vaginal Yeast Infections

- A randomized, placebo-controlled, double-blind, factorial 2 × 2 study sought to test the hypothesis that oral or vaginal LA can reduce vulvovaginitis after antibiotic treatment. Two hundred thirty-five of 278 women completed the study. Women took LA orally, vaginally, or both from the start of antibiotics through 4 days after antibiotic therapy. No protective effect was shown regardless of administration route(s) (23).

- A crossover trial of six subjects assigned to one of two groups, receiving 150 mL of either pasteurized yogurt or yogurt containing live LA, studied the effectiveness of the

LA to reduce candidal yeast infections or bacterial vaginosis. Those women who received the LA-containing yogurt exhibited an increased colonization of favorable bacteria in the rectum and vagina and a decreased incidence of bacterial vaginosis (7).

LA and Cholesterol

◆ Several hypotheses have been offered to explain how LA might help reduce serum cholesterol. For example, LA may (*a*) inhibit 3-hydroxy-3-methylglutaryl CoA reductase, a rate-limiting enzyme in endogenous cholesterol synthesis; or (*b*) bind with cholesterol in the intestinal lumen, thus reducing absorption into the blood (1,9).

◆ According to two review articles of more than 25 animal and in vitro studies, isolated LA and lactic acid bacteria found in fermented dairy products were associated with hypocholesterolemic effects (1,9).

◆ In a double-blind, placebo-controlled crossover study, 40 subjects with hypercholesterolemia were randomly assigned to receive 200 mL yogurt containing live cultures of LA or placebo daily for 4 weeks each, with a 2-week washout. LA yogurt (strain L-1) was associated with a significant 2.9% reduction of serum cholesterol (24).

◆ In a double-blind, placebo-controlled crossover trial, 30 healthy male subjects with borderline elevated cholesterol levels were randomly assigned to receive 125 mL yogurt fermented with LA and added fructooligosaccharides (2.5%) or a traditional yogurt fermented only with yogurt strains. Subjects consumed 3 × 125 mL yogurt daily for 3 weeks, each with a 1-week washout period. Blood samples were taken before the study and at the end of both treatments. Compared with the control product, LA yogurt resulted in significantly lower values for serum total cholesterol, LDL cholesterol, and the LDL-to-HDL ratio (values were decreased by 4.4%, 5.4%, and 5.3%, respectively). Serum HDL cholesterol, triglycerides, and blood glucose levels were unaffected (25). In a separate crossover design study using control yogurt and yogurt supplemented with LA 145 and *B longum* 913, 29 women with (N = 15) or without (N = 14) elevated serum cholesterol consumed the assigned yogurt for 7 weeks each. Total and LDL cholesterol did not change, but HDL cholesterol increased by a mean of 0.3 mmol/L in the LA-supplemented group, and the ratio of LDL to HDL decreased from 3.24 to 2.48 (26). In a study of 78 healthy adults with normal or borderline serum cholesterol levels, LA strain L-1 in the form of yogurt (or control yogurt) for 2 weeks did not alter lipid levels. However, 2 weeks of intervention may be inadequate, and it is less likely that normolipidemic individuals would respond (27).

LA and Cancer

◆ Several possible mechanisms of the potential anticarcinogenic action of LA have been hypothesized. These include the production of compounds that inhibit tumor cell growth, antagonistic action against organisms that convert procarcinogens into carcinogens, and degradation of carcinogens (1) or immunomodulation (28).

◆ Observational studies have suggested that consumption of fermented dairy products is correlated with a lower prevalence of colon cancer (1).

♦ According to a review article of several animal studies, orally administered LA (fermented dairy products and single preparations) may slow tumor development in animals. However, the researchers stressed that there is currently no proof in humans that *Lactobacilli* or their fermented products can prevent cancer (9).

♦ A study of mice with induced mammary tumors showed that neither the initiation nor the promotion phase of cancer was affected by supplementation of LA, *bifidobacteria,* or fermented yogurt powder (29).

LA and Atopic Disease

♦ Among infants at risk for atopic disease (asthma, allergic rhinitis, eczema) due to family history, there is preliminary evidence that supplementation with LA GG in the final weeks of pregnancy and 3 to 6 months postpartum can reduce disease in the newborn (administered via breastmilk or in formula). A blinded Finnish study was conducted among 159 pregnant women with a family history of atopic disease. Compared with placebo, daily administration of LA GG (2×10^{10} colony forming units during the final 4 weeks of pregnancy and during the first 3 months of lactation significantly reduced inflammatory biomarkers profile (increased TGF-ß2 anti-inflammatory growth factor) in the infants. Infants with elevated cord blood IgE were most responsive to the LA GG supplementation (30). In a follow up analysis, LA GG or placebo was given to the infants for 6 months after birth. Eczema incidence at age 2 years was shown to be 23% in for the LA GG group vs 46% for the control group, indicating that risk of eczema was significantly reduced with supplementation (31).

References

1. Mital BK, Garg SK. Anticarcinogenic, hypocholesterolemic, and antagonistic activities of Lactobacillus acidophilus. *Crit Rev Microbiol.* 1995;21:175–214.
2. Canganella F, Paganini S, Ovidi M, et al. A microbiology investigation on probiotic pharmaceutical products used for human health. *Microbiol Res.* 1997;152:171–179.
3. Salminen S, Deighton M. Lactic acid bacteria in the gut in normal and disordered states. *Dig Dis.* 1992;10:227–238.
4. Salminen S. Functional dairy foods with *Lactobacillus* strain GG. *Nutr Rev.* 1996;54 (11 pt 2):S99-S101.
5. Land MH, Rouster-Stevens K, Woods CR, et al. Lactobacillus sepsis associated with probiotic therapy. *Pediatrics.* 2005;115:178–181.
6. MacGregor G, Smith AJ, Thakker B, et al. Yoghurt biotherapy: contraindicated in immunosuppressed patients? *Postgrad Med J.* 2002;78:366–367.
7. Shalev E, Battino S, Weiner E, et al. Ingestion of yogurt containing Lactobacillus acidophilus compared with pasteurized yogurt as prophylaxis for recurrent candidal vaginitis and bacterial vaginosis. *Arch Fam Med.* 1996;5:593–596.
8. Reid G, Bruce AW, McGroarty JA, et al. Is the re a role for lactobacilli in prevention of urogenital and intestinal infections? *Clin Microbiol Rev.* 1990;3:335–344.
9. Gorbach SL. Lactic acid bacteria and human health. *Ann Med.* 1990;22:37–41.

10. Elmer GW, Surawicz CM, McFarland LV. Biotherapeutic agents. A neglected modality for the treatment and prevention of selected intestinal and vaginal infections. *JAMA.* 1996;275:870–876.

11. Oksanen PJ, Salminen S, Saxelin M, et al. Prevention of traveller's diarrhea by *Lactobacillus* GG. *Ann Med.* 1990;22:53–56.

12. deRoos NM, Katan MB. Effects of probiotic bacteria on diarrhea, lipid metabolism, and carcinogenesis: a review of papers published between 1988 and 1998. *Am J Clin Nutr.* 2000;71:405–411.

13. D'Souza AL, Rajkumar C, Cooke J, et al. Probiotics in prevention of antibiotic associated diarrhoea: meta-analysis. *BMJ.* 2002;324:1361.

14. Van Niel CW, Feudtner C, Garrison MM, et al. Lactobacillus therapy for acute infectious diarrhea in children: a meta-analysis. *Pediatrics.* 2002;109:678–684.

15. Guandalini S, Pensabene L, Zikri MA, et al. Lactobacillus GG administered in oral rehydration solution to children with acute diarrhea: a multicenter European trial. *J Pediatr Gastroenterol Nutr.* 2000;30:54.

16. Chandra RK. Effect of Lactobacillus on the incidence and severity of acute rotavirus diarrhoea in infants. A prospective placebo-controlled double-blind study. *Nut Res.* 2001;22:65–69.

17. Thomas MR, Litin SC, Osmon DR, et al. Lack of effect of Lactobacillus GG on antibiotic-associated diarrhea: a randomized, placebo-controlled trial. *Mayo Clin Proc.* 2001;76:883–889.

18. Sen S, Mullan MM, Parker TJ, et al. Effect of Lactobacillus plantarum 299v on colonic fermentation and symptoms of irritable bowel syndrome. *Dig Dis Sci.* 2002;47: 2615–2620.

19. O'Sullivan MA, O'Morain CA. Bacterial supplementation in the irritable bowel syndrome. A randomized double-blind placebo-controlled crossover study. *Dig Liver Dis.* 2000;32:294–301.

20. O'Mahony L, McCarthy J, Kelly P, et al. Lactobacillus and bifidobacterium in irritable bowel syndrome: symptom responses and relationship to cytokine profiles. *Gastroenterology.* 2005;128:541–545.

21. Bausserman M, Michail S. The use of lactobacillus GG in irritable bowel syndrome in children: a double-blind randomized control trial. *J Pediatr.* 2002;147:197–201.

22. Niv E, Naftali T, Hallak R, et al. The efficacy of lactobacillus reuteri ATCC 55730 in the treatment of patients with irritable bowel syndrome—double-blind, placebo controlled, randomized study. *Clin Nutr.* 2005;24:925–931.

23. Pirotta M, Gunn J, Chondros P, et al. Effect of lactobacillus in preventing post-antibiotic vulvovaginal candidiasis: a randomized, controlled trial. *BMJ.* 2004;329:548.

24. Anderson JW, Gilliland SE. Effect of fermented milk (yogurt) containing *Lactobacillus acidophilus* L1 on serum cholesterol in hypercholesterolemic humans. *J Am Coll Nutr.* 1999;18:43–50.

25. Schaafsma G, Meuling WJ, van Dokkum W, et al. Effects of a milk product, fermented by *Lactobacillus acidophilus* and with fructo-oligosaccharides added, on blood lipids in male volunteers. *Eur J Clin Nutr.* 1998;52:436–440.

26. Kiessling G, Schneider J, Jahreis G. Long term consumption of fermented dairy products over 6 months increases HDL cholesterol. *Eur J Clin Nutr.* 2002;56:843–849.

27. de Roos NM, Schouten G, Katan MB. Yoghurt enriched with Lacto bacillus acidophilus does not lower blood lipids in healthy men and women with normal to borderline high serum cholesterol levels. *Eur J Clin Nutr.* 1999;53:277–280.

28. Lee JW, Shin JG, Kim EH, et al. Immunomodulatory and antitumor effects in vivo by the cytoplasmic fraction of Lactobacillus casei and Bifidobacterium longum. *J Vet Sci.* 2004;5:41–48.

29. Rice LJ, Chai YJ, Conti CJ, et al. The effects of dietary fermented milk products and lactic acid bacteria on the initiation and promotion stages of mammary carcinogenesis. *Nutr Cancer.* 1995;24:99–109.

30. Rautava S, Kalliomaki M, Isolauri E. Probiotics during pregnancy and breast-feeding might confer immunomodulatory protection against atopic disease in the infant. *J Allergy Clin Immunol.* 2002;109:119–121.

31. Kalliomaki M, Salminen S, Arvilommi H, et al. Probiotics in primary prevention of atopic disease: a randomized placebo-controlled trial. *Lancet.* 2001;357:1076–1079.

Alanine

L-alanine is a nonessential amino acid involved in glucose metabolism when the exogenous glucose supply is low. In the process known as the alanine cycle, pyruvate from glucose oxidation in skeletal muscle is aminated to form alanine, which is transported to the liver, deaminated, and converted to glucose. Alanine also carries nitrogen from peripheral tissues to the liver for excretion (1).

Media and Marketing Claims	Efficacy
Stabilizes blood glucose in hypoglycemia	↔
Protects the liver	NR
Spares muscle during intense exercise or training	NR

Safety

◆ In limited studies with small numbers of subjects, alanine seems to be safe in the doses administered (20 to 40 g). However, there are no studies testing the long-term safety of alanine supplementation at those dosages.

Drug/Supplement Interactions

Alanine may potentially interact with drugs used to reduce blood glucose.

Key Points

◆ Animal studies support a role for alanine in inducing insulin release by beta cells (2,3).

◆ There is preliminary evidence that high doses of alanine (20 to 40 g) in solution with 10 g glucose may prevent or treat nocturnal hypoglycemia in individuals with type 1 diabetes. Larger, controlled studies are needed to further explore the effects of alanine on hypoglycemia. Until more information is available, self-supplementation with alanine is not recommended in this population without the monitoring of a physician because of possible adverse effects on glycemic control.

◆ There is preliminary evidence in animal studies that alanine has a protective effect on hepatocyte function and regeneration. However, there are no human studies testing alanine in individuals with liver disease. At this time, alanine supplements are not recommended for this population because the safety and efficacy have not been determined in controlled clinical trials.

◆ Although alanine is a glucogenic amino acid and plasma levels increase during exercise (4), there is currently no evidence that supplemental alanine spares muscle during exercise or enhances exercise performance.

Food Sources

Alanine is found in protein-rich foods such as egg, dairy, meat, fish, and poultry.

Food	Alanine, g/serving
Beef, lean (3 oz)	1.498
Chicken, meat only (3 oz)	1.455
Salmon (3 oz)	1.025
Egg (1 large)	0.348
Beans, kidney (½ cup)	0.322
Milk (1 cup)	0.276

Source: Data are from reference 5.

Dosage Information/Bioavailability

Alanine is found in single preparations of 450-mg capsules or as a powder. It is also found in supplements with a variety of amino acids and in some sport beverages. There is no dietary requirement for alanine because it is synthesized in vivo in humans.

Relevant Research

Alanine and Hypoglycemia

◆ In a controlled, crossover (not blinded) study, 15 subjects with type 1 diabetes were given the same individualized dose of NPH insulin at 10 PM on four occasions, separated by 2 weeks, completed in random order: (*a*) NPH with no treatment (control); (*b*) 200-kcal snack (2% milk and toast); (*c*) 40 g alanine plus 10 g glucose (200 kcal);

and (*d*) 5 mg terbutaline (stimulates the B_2-adrenergic actions of epinephrine that increase plasma glucose). During the first half of the night, plasma glucose concentrations were significantly higher after the snack, alanine and glucose, or terbutaline compared with the control. During the second half of the night, mean plasma glucose levels were not different from control after the snack but tended to be higher after alanine (did not reach statistical significance) and were significantly higher after terbutaline. Nocturnal hypoglycemia, ie, plasma glucose levels of 40 mg/dL or less, occurred on 13 occasions in 7 subjects in the control arm and 10 occasions in 6 subjects in the snack arm (not statistically significant). There was only one occasion in the alanine plus glucose arm (significant compared with control) and the terbutaline arm. The authors concluded that an evening dose of NPH insulin with a conventional snack exerts an inconsistent glycemic effect during the first half of the night, and bedtime ingestion of alanine prevents nocturnal hypoglycemia more effectively than a snack. The authors note that alanine must be taken in solution and this has an unpleasant taste (6).

- Hypoglycemia was artificially induced by subcutaneous insulin injection in nine subjects with type 1 diabetes mellitus and eight normal control subjects. During hypoglycemia, subjects with diabetes were given (in random order): (*a*) 10 and 20 g glucose, (*b*) glucagon injection, (*c*) 40 g alanine, (*d*) oral terbutaline, (*e*) terbutaline injection, or (*f*) a placebo. All subjects with diabetes participated in the placebo arm; six participated in the two oral glucose arms and the glucagon arm; and six participated in the oral and subcutaneous terbutaline arms and alanine arm of the study. Subjects without diabetes only participated in the placebo arm. In subjects with diabetes, oral alanine increased glucose levels within 30 minutes, with a gradual increase over practical hours, when compared with placebo. Oral terbutaline had a similar effect as alanine. Glucose and glucagon initially increased plasma glucose, but the effects were short-term. The authors concluded that alanine produced sustained glucose recovery from hypoglycemia in diabetes and is potentially useful for the treatment and prevention of mild or moderate iatrogenic hypoglycemia when food intake is not possible for several hours (7).

- A study by the same researchers with a similar protocol found that alanine supplementation (20 and 40 g) increased plasma glucagon and insulin, with no significant changes in blood glucose in six subjects without diabetes. In six subjects with type 1 diabetes, alanine increased glucagon and plasma glucose but had no effect on insulin levels (8).

- Alanine infusion during induction of hypoglycemia in seven healthy men showed that the brain can preferentially use alanine to support cognitive function directly or via increased availability of lactate when glucose levels are low (9).

Alanine and Liver Function

- Rats with induced acute liver failure from a lethal dose of D-galactosamine were given alanine or a placebo. Liver function parameters improved in alanine-treated rats, and the hepatic ATP content was significantly greater in treated rats than in control rats. The authors concluded that "alanine is effective for the treatment of experimental acute liver failure, probably caused by the promotion of ATP synthesis. Alanine may be a good candidate for clinical application because of its preventative effect on hepatocyte necrosis and its promotive effect on liver regeneration" (10).

◆ Other animal studies reported a protective effect of alanine on damaged liver cells (11–13).

Alanine and Exercise

◆ In a small study of six males, supplementation with 1 g/kg during prolonged, low workload exercise resulted in positive nitrogen balance of 8.5 ± 0.3 g. However, no placebo group was included (14). Therefore, the results of this study should be viewed with caution.

References

1. Matthews DE. Proteins and amino acids. In: Shils ME, Olson JA, Shike M, Ross AC, eds. *Modern Nutrition in Health and Disease*. 9th ed. Baltimore, Md: Williams & Wilkins; 1999:11–48.
2. Dixon G, Nolan J, McClenaghan N, et al. A comparative study of amino acid consumption by rat islet cells and the clonal beta-cell line BRIN-BD11-the functional significance of L-alanine. *J Endocrinol*. 2003;179:447–454.
3. Sener A, Malaisse WJ. The stimulus—secretion coupling of amino acid induced insulin release. Insulinotropic action of L-alanine. *Biochim Biophys Acta*. 2002;1573:100–104.
4. Williams BD, Chinkes DL, Wolfe RR. Alanine and glutamine kinetics at rest and during exercise in humans. *Med Sci Sports Exerc*. 1998;30:1053–1058.
5. USDA Nutrient Database. Available at: http://www.nal.usda.gov/fnic. Accessed April 17, 2005.
6. Saleh TY, Cryer PE. Alanine and terbutaline in the prevention of nocturnal hypoglycemia in IDDM. *Diabetes Care*. 1997;20:1231–1236.
7. Wiethop BV, Cryer PE. Alanine and terbutaline in treatment of hypoglycemia in IDDM. *Diabetes Care*. 1993;16:1131–1136.
8. Wiethop BV, Cryer PE. Glycemic actions of alanine and terbutaline in IDDM. *Diabetes Care*. 1993;16:1124–1130.
9. Evans ML, Hopkins D, Macdonald IA, et al. Alanine infusion during hypoglycaemia partly supports cognitive performance in healthy human subject. *Diabet Med*. 2004;21:440–446
10. Maezono K, Mawatari K, Kjiwara K, et al. Effect of alanine on D-galactosamine-induced acute liver failure in rats. *Hepatology*. 1996;24:1211–1216.
11. Moriyama M, Makiyama I, Shiota M, et al. Decreased ureagenesis from alanine, but not from ammonia and glutamine, in the perfused rat liver after partial hepatectomy. *Hepatology*. 1996;23:1584–1590.
12. Maezono K, Kajiwara K, Mawatari K, et al. Alanine protects liver from injury caused by F-galactosamine and CC14. *Hepatology*. 1996;24:185–191.

13. Tanaka T, Ando M, Yamashita T, et al. Effects of alanine and glutamine administration on the inhibition of liver regeneration by acute ethanol treatment. *Alcohol Suppl.* 1993;1B:41–45.
14. Korach-Andre M, Burelle Y, Peronnet F, et al. Differential metabolic fate of the carbon skeleton and amino-N of [13C] alanine and [15N] alanine ingested during prolonged exercise. *J Appl Physiol.* 2002;93:499–504.

Aloe Vera

Aloe vera is a succulent perennial plant belonging to the lily family. Aloe vera gel, produced from the inner portion of the plant leaves, has been used topically for centuries to promote wound healing and restore healthy skin. Because topical use is not considered a dietary supplement, it will only be discussed briefly. Aloe vera may also be taken orally in the latex form known as aloe juice. The latex form of aloe is derived from a bitter yellow "juice" found beneath the outer skin of the leaves. The latex has a strong laxative effect and is rarely recommended. Because of the risk of hypokalemia and renal damage, aloe has been removed from the market as a laxative product.

Media and Marketing Claims	Efficacy
Reduces symptoms of gastrointestinal disorders, including ulcerative colitis and radiation-related mucositis	NR
Helps control blood cholesterol	NR
Helps reduce blood glucose	NR
Topical application helps heal skin damage related to radiation therapy, wounds, psoriasis	↔
Reduces constipation (latex)	Safety concern

Safety

- As with all stimulant laxatives in large doses and with excessive use, aloe vera latex may cause potassium depletion, and prolonged use can lead to nephritis and acute kidney failure (1).

- Due to suspected genotoxic effects of anthroquinones, the FDA required manufacturers to remove or reformulate all over-the-counter (OTC) laxative products containing aloe from the US market starting Nov 5, 2002. The anthroquinones in aloe, including aloe-emodin, do not seem to be well-absorbed. Aloe itself can still be sold as a dietary supplement (2).

- Topical use is well-tolerated; there are no reports of adverse events.

Drug/Supplement Interaction

Although data are sparse, concomitant use of aloe gel (orally) with hypoglycemic agents may have an additive effect in reducing blood glucose. Monitor blood glucose in individuals with diabetes.

Key Points

- Preliminary data that suggests that aloe vera gel may be beneficial in the treatment of active ulcerative colitis (UC) (3). Oral aloe vera taken for 1 month produced a clinical response more often than placebo. Further research is needed to determine the potential significance of this treatment.

- Although data are limited, oral aloe vera taken daily was associated with reduced total and LDL cholesterol as reported in a systematic review of the literature (4). Further research is needed to develop clinical recommendations.

- Preliminary evidence in rats suggests that aloe vera gel may reduce blood glucose levels, but the mechanism of action has not been clearly elicited, so clinical use for this application is not recommended until more is known.

- Although topical aloe vera is commonly used to promote wound healing, its efficacy seems to be related to superficial cuts and abrasions rather than deep surgical wounds or pressure ulcers. In a pilot study conducted among 21 women with postoperative gynecological incisions, aloe wound gel was associated with a significant delay in healing time as compared with standard wound care without aloe vera (5).

- Research assessing topical aloe gel as a treatment of acute radiation dermatitis is sparse. A review article indicates that aloe gel is not harmful but the reviewed randomized trials using aloe vera did not find efficacy (6). More clinical trials are warranted to determine the effectiveness of topical aloe gel in the treatment of radiation dermatitis.

- Aloe latex (not to be confused with aloe vera) is an effective laxative because it increases motility and reduces transit time through the colon within 8 hours of the first dose. As with all stimulant laxatives, excessive habitual use creates a dependency and a need to increase the dosage to maintain a laxative effect. Continual use at high doses may lead to hypokalemia and paralysis of the intestinal muscles (1).

Food Sources

None

Dosage Information/Bioavailability

Dosages used to treat ulcerative colitis are in the range of 100 mL of a 50% oral solution taken twice daily for 4 weeks (3). For reducing blood glucose, a dosage of 15 mL of aloe gel taken orally has been used (4).

Aloe vera gel for skin-related clinical conditions is usually applied at a dose of 0.5% aloe extract cream two or three times per day (7). However, many of the active ingredients of the gel tend to deteriorate over time, and therefore efficacy of preparations may vary greatly.

Relevant Research

Aloe Vera Gel and Intestinal Health

- In a double-blind, randomized, placebo-controlled trial, 44 subjects with mild to moderate active UC were randomly assigned to take 100 mL aloe vera orally or placebo twice per day for 4 weeks in an outpatient setting. There were 30 subjects in the aloe vera group and 14 were assigned to the placebo. Six subjects from the aloe vera group and three from the placebo group were dropped from study because of disease severity. Withdrawals were determined by blinded physician monitoring of clinical condition of all patients. Outcomes include clinical remission, sigmoidoscopic remission (no lesions/ulceration on repeat visual sigmoid examination), or histologic remission (collected tissue from biopsy showed no disease present). Secondary outcomes included subjective assessments and laboratory studies. Clinical remission (Simple Clinical Colitis Activity Index) and clinical improvement were shown in 30% of subjects given aloe vera compared with 7% in subjects given placebo. Histological measures were also improved in the aloe vera group compared with the placebo group. However, there was no significant difference between the groups for sigmoidoscopic evaluation or laboratory values such as hemoglobin, platelet count, erythrocyte sedimentation rate, or C-reactive protein. Furthermore, the physician's global assessment and the Inflammatory Bowel Disease Questionnaire failed to detect any significant change during treatment (8). This study provides preliminary evidence for a role of aloe vera in UC; however, the small sample size and inability to modulate sigmoidoscopy or histological scores limits clinical application at this time.

- In a double-blind, randomized, placebo-controlled trial, 58 subjects with primary head-and-neck cancers undergoing radiation therapy received either 20 mL swish-and-swallow aloe vera gel solution or placebo four times daily during treatment (mean length of treatment = 46 days in the aloe vera group and 61 days in the placebo group) to assess whether aloe vera could reduce the incidence of radiation-induced mucositis. All subjects completed the trial; however, the sample size was too small to measure statistical significance. Analysis of 28 subjects in the treatment arm and 30 in the placebo arm found that aloe vera gel solution did not reduce mucositis severity or duration, quality of life, body weight, use of pain medications, or rates of oral infections (9). Studies with larger sample sizes are needed before recommendations can be made.

Aloe Vera and Blood Lipid Control

- A systematic review of the clinical effectiveness of aloe vera was published in 1999 (4). The paper suggests that, "oral administration of aloe vera (gel) might be a useful adjunct for reducing blood lipid levels in patients with hyperlipidemia." However, specifics of study design in the trials reviewed are not presented in this article and thus its conclusions about efficacy cannot be evaluated. Well-designed clinical trials are needed.

Aloe Vera Gel and Diabetes

- The safety of aloe vera leaf gel and pulp extract taken orally was investigated in healthy rats and rats rendered diabetic by exposure to streptozotocin. Aloe vera gel and the diabetic medication glibenclamide both reduced levels of nonenzymatic glycosylation, whereas aloe pulp increased glycosylation. Aloe vera pulp reduced lipid peroxidation similar to glibenclamide. Diabetic rats exhibited liver damage compared with control rats. This liver damage was reduced by treatment with aloe vera gel (10).

- Using a rat model, investigators tested the capacity of aloe vera leaf gel to modulate blood glucose control among rats with experimentally induced diabetes. Four groups of 10 rats were used: (*a*) control, (*b*) diabetic control rats, (*c*) diabetic rats given 300 mg/kg aloe vera leaf gel extract via intragastric tube for 21 days, and (*d*) rats given 600 µg/kg glibenclamide via intragastric tube for 21 days. Rats given aloe vera had blood glucose levels 60% less than levels of untreated diabetic rats and 20% less than that of diabetic rats receiving glibenclamide (11). Glycated hemoglobin levels were also significantly less in aloe vera–treated rats compared with diabetic control rats and slightly less than that of glibenclamide-treated rats (6.5 vs 6.9, respectively).

Aloe Vera (Topical) and Wound Healing

- In a clinical trial with 21 women with postoperative gynecological incisions that were not healing on follow-up evaluation (approximately 2 to 4 weeks post-surgery), healing averaged 53 days with standard care and 83 days with aloe vera—a statistically significant difference (5). Wound healing was defined by clinician assessment; no specific biomarkers were measured. All wounds were associated with cesarean section or laparotomy; however, it is unclear whether the analysis was controlled for wound "severity" or whether aloe vera in addition to standard wound therapy would provide clinical benefit.

- In a double-blind, randomized, Phase III study of 225 women receiving radiation therapy for breast cancer, topical aloe vera gel did not significantly reduce radiation-induced skin irritation. Surprisingly, aqueous placebo cream was significantly more efficacious than aloe vera gel at reduction of pain and dry desquamation. Supplementation was provided 3 times daily for the 6 weeks of radiation therapy and 2 additional weeks after radiation therapy. Skin irritation was common (and not significantly different) in both groups; it was more common in women with larger breast size, smokers, and those with lymph node involvement (12).

- A review of several therapies for treatment of radiation dermatitis's included two randomized studies specific to aloe vera use (6). In both of these studies, aloe vera use was not significantly associated with prevention of radiation dermatitis.

References

1. Bisset NG, Wichtl MW, eds. *Herbal Drugs and Phytopharmaceuticals*. Stuttgart, Germany: Medpharm GmbH Scientific Publishers; 1994.
2. Natural Standard Web site. Available at: http://naturalstandard.com. Accessed July 31, 2005.
3. Langmead L, Feakins RM, Goldthorpe S, et al. Randomized, double-blind, placebo-controlled trial of oral aloe vera gel for ulcerative colitis. *Aliment Pharmacol Ther.* 2004;19:739–747.
4. Vogler BK, Ernst E. Aloe vera: a systematic review of its clinical effectiveness. *Br J Gen Pract.* 1999:49:823–828.
5. Schmidt JM, Greenspoon JS. Aloe vera dermal wound gel is associated with a delay in wound healing. *Obstet Gynecol.* 1991;78:115–117.
6. Wickline NM. Prevention and treatment of acute radiation dermatitis: a literature review. *Oncol Nurs Forum.* 2004;31:237–247.
7. Syed TA, Ahmad SA, Holt AH, et al. Management of psoriasis with aloe vera extract in a hydrophilic cream: a placebo-controlled, double-blind study. *Trop Med Int Health.* 1996;1:505–509.
8. Langmead L, Makins RJ, Rampton DS. Anti-inflammatory effects of aloe vera gel in human colorectal mucosa in vitro. *Ailment Pharmacol Ther.* 2004;19:521–527.
9. Su CK, Mehta V, Ravikumar L, et al. Phase II double-blind randomized study comparing oral aloe vera versus placebo to prevent radiation-related mucositis in patients with head-and-neck neoplasms. *Int J Radiat Oncol Biol Phys.* 2004;60:171–177.
10. Can A, Akan N, Ozsoy N, et al. Effect of aloe vera leaf gel and pulp extracts on the liver of type II diabetic rat models. *Biol Pharm Bull.* 2004;27:694–698.
11. Rajasekaran S, Sivagnanam K, Subramanian S. Antioxidant effect of *Aloe vera* gel extract in streptozotocin-induced diabetes in rats. *Pharmacol Rep.* 2005;57:90–96.
12. Heggie S, Bryant GP, Tripcony L, et al. A phase III study on the efficacy of topical aloe vera gel on irradiated breast tissue. *Cancer Nurs.* 2002;25:442–451.

Alpha-Lipoic Acid (ALA)

Alpha-lipoic (thioctic) acid (ALA) is classified as a nonessential vitamin-like compound or coenzyme. Synthesized in the mitochondria, ALA is involved in intermediary cell metabolism leading to ATP production and is believed to possess antioxidant activity both intracellularly and extracellularly. ALA absorbed from the diet crosses the blood—brain barrier and is taken into brain cells and tissues. It functions in the pyruvate dehydrogenase complex, where it promotes the conversion of thiamin to form acetyl CoA. It is both fat- and water-soluble and has been demonstrated to regenerate endogenous vitamins C and E and glutathione. Because of its potential antioxidant properties, ALA has been investigated for its protective role in conditions believed to be related to oxidative stress, including diabetes, cataracts, HIV, neuropathy, and radiation injury (1,2).

Media and Marketing Claims	Efficacy
Normalizes blood glucose	NR
Improves peripheral neuropathy in diabetes	↑?
Inhibits HIV infection	NR
Improves cardiovascular health	NR
Slows dementia	NR
Supports healthy liver	NR

Safety

♦ ALA in dosages up to 2,000 mg/day have been well-tolerated with few reported adverse effects in studies from several months to 2 years.

♦ Reported adverse effects include allergic skin reactions and possible hypoglycemia as a consequence of improved glucose utilization (1).

♦ Because one study showed ALA had lethal effects on rats that were severely thiamin-deficient, researchers recommend that individuals who may be thiamin-deficient (eg, individuals with alcoholism) should take thiamin supplements while taking ALA (2).

♦ The lethal dose of ALA in animals is 400 to 500 mg/kg body weight.

♦ Some in vitro data indicate that a metabolic breakdown product of ALA (dihydrolipoate) may exert a prooxidant effect in the presence of iron. The physiological consequences are not known, but researchers think that this does not occur in vivo (2).

♦ ALA may reduce blood glucose levels. This should be monitored by physician.

Drug/Supplement Interactions

♦ Potential additive effect on reducing blood glucose if taken with medications or herbs with hypoglycemic potential.

♦ Potential interference with drugs used to treat hyper- or hypothyroid conditions. Monitor use.

Key Points

♦ More research is needed on the effect of oral ALA supplementation on blood glucose control. Although there is evidence from in vitro and animal trials that ALA may play a beneficial role in conditions related to diabetes (cataracts, glucose utilization, oxidative stress), controlled clinical trials in humans are needed before recommendations can be made. To date, most of the research in diabetes has focused on the effects of ALA supplements and diabetic neuropathy.

- ◆ ALA generally seems to improve symptoms of peripheral neuropathy associated with diabetes, but additional research is warranted to determine optimal dosage.

- ◆ There is preliminary evidence that ALA may play a role in slowing HIV replication in vitro; however, no human studies have tested whether ALA affects morbidity or mortality in individuals with HIV. According to one study, ALA did not improve HIV-associated dementia.

- ◆ Evidence that ALA may reduce risk for cardiovascular disease or improve cardiovascular health is generally lacking; additional research is needed.

- ◆ There is also preliminary evidence from in vitro and animal studies that ALA may aid treatment of neurodegenerative diseases. A recent Cochrane database has reported that there are no controlled trials from which conclusions could be drawn (3).

- ◆ Only limited and poorly designed studies regarding the role of ALA in liver disease are available at this time. More well-designed trials are needed.

Food Sources

Yeast and liver (4)

Dosage Information/Bioavailability

Manufacturers provide ALA in pills and capsules in doses ranging from 50 mg to 300 mg. Most studies have used 100 mg/day to 800 mg/day. It is estimated that only 30% of supplemental ALA is absorbed, and it is rapidly reduced to dihydrolipoic acid (DHLA) in tissue (5). A sustained-release capsule has also been developed (6) as well as a 5% topical cream (7).

Relevant Research

ALA and Diabetes

- ◆ In a double-blind, placebo-controlled trial, 73 subjects with type 2 diabetes and cardiac autonomic neuropathy (CAN) were randomly assigned to receive 800 mg/day ALA or a placebo for 4 months. Seventeen subjects dropped out of the study for various reasons (noncompliance, relocation, lack of efficacy). Parameters of heart rate variability at rest using an electrocardiogram included coefficient of variation (CV); root mean square successive difference (RMSSD); and spectral power in the low- and high-frequency (LF and HF). Cardiovascular autonomic symptoms were also assessed. There were no significant differences in symptoms, mean blood pressure, and A1C levels between groups at baseline and during the study. There was a significant improvement in two out of four parameters of heart rate variability (CV and RMSSD) in the ALA group compared with the placebo. The authors concluded that ALA may slightly improve CAN in patients with type 2 diabetes and "long-term studies of oral treatment with alpha-lipoic acid are now needed to confirm the observed improvement in CAN and to address the following questions: Can it be applied to IDDM [type 1 diabetes] patients? Can it be accompanied by effects on clinical endpoints?" (8).

- In a double-blind, placebo-controlled multicenter study, 509 subjects with type 2 diabetes with polyneuropathy were randomly assigned to receive one of three treatments: (*a*) 600 mg IV ALA daily for 3 weeks, followed by 1,800 mg oral ALA daily for 6 months; (*b*) 600 mg IV ALA daily for 3 weeks, followed by oral placebo daily for 6 months; or (*c*) placebo IV followed by oral placebo for 6 months. Outcome measures included the Total Symptom Score (TSS) for neuropathic symptoms (pain, burning, paresthesias, and numbness) in the feet and the Neuropathy Impairment Score (NIS). At the end of the study, ALA had no effect on neuropathic symptoms (TSS) compared with placebo. The authors suggested that this may have been a result of intercenter variability in symptom scoring. Subjects administered IV ALA did have significantly improved NIS scores after 3 weeks, but not after 6 months of oral treatment compared with subjects receiving placebo (9).

- In a double-blind, placebo-controlled trial, 328 subjects with type 2 diabetes and diabetic neuropathy were randomly assigned to receive treatment with IV infusion of ALA (1,200 mg, 600 mg, or 100 mg) daily or a placebo for 3 weeks. Neuropathic symptoms were scored at the baseline and throughout the study. The Hamburg Pain Adjective List and the Neuropathy Symptom and Disability Scores were assessed at baseline and at day 19. The TSS in the feet was significantly decreased in subjects taking ALA compared with those receiving the placebo. There was a significant improvement in the response rates after 19 days (defined as improvement of at least 30% in TSS) and in the Pain Adjective List with ALA supplementation compared with placebo (10).

- In a placebo-controlled pilot study, 74 individuals with type 2 diabetes were randomly assigned to receive either placebo or 600 mg, 1,200 mg, or 1,800 mg ALA daily for 4 weeks. Subjects underwent an isoglycemic glucose-clamp at the beginning and end of the study. When compared with subjects receiving the placebo, subjects receiving ALA supplementation had an increase in insulin-stimulated glucose disposal at the study's end. There was no difference in effect among the three different dosages of ALA (11).

- The SYDNEY trial recruited 120 subjects with diabetic sensorimotor polyneuropathy, and they were randomly assigned to receive either 600 mg ALA or placebo IV 5 days per week for 14 treatments. TSS was significantly improved in the ALA group ($P < .001$). No long-term follow-up was provided, and IV supplementation may not be practical for most individuals (12).

- A meta-analysis combining data from the ALADIN I, ALADIN III, SYDNEY, and NATHAN II trials providing 600 mg ALA IV for 3 weeks (N = 1258, ALA = 716, placebo = 542) showed a 24.1% reduction in TSS (particularly pain, burning, and numbness) and a 16% reduction in NIS (13).

ALA and HIV

- In a randomized, double-blind, placebo-controlled trial using a parallel group 2 × 2 factorial design, 36 subjects with HIV-associated cognitive impairment received deprenyl (a monoamine oxidase B inhibitor and putative antiapoptic agent), ALA, or placebo. There was no improvement in cognitive function in subjects supplemented with ALA compared with a placebo, whereas deprenyl resulted in significant improvement (14).

- In vitro studies have shown that ALA inhibits nuclear factor kappa B (NF-kappa B), which is believed to play an important role in the activation of HIV (17,18), and T-cell lines infected with HIV and supplemented with ALA demonstrated a 90% reduction in reverse transcriptase activity. Reverse transcriptase is an indicator of viral replication (15).

ALA and Cardiovascular Disease

- Theoretical benefits have been postulated (16). In a crossover-design study, a single dose of 600 mg oral ALA or placebo was given 1 week apart to healthy middle-aged men. ALA supplementation did not change central blood pressure, indexes of arterial stiffness, forearm blood flow, or plasma oxidative stress biomarkers (17). However, the single dose, the small sample size, and the selection of healthy subjects may have contributed to the negative outcomes. Further research is warranted.

ALA and Cognition/Dementia

- A Cochrane Database review published in 2004 describes the biological basis for ALA's potential role in improving cognitive function (3). However, the review of the literature in the same article reported that no randomized, placebo-controlled trials had been published and thus a meta-analysis was not possible.

ALA and Liver Disease

- One review reported that no well-controlled research supports the use of ALA in the treatment of alcoholic liver disease. Most studies that showed a benefit were flawed, and one double-blind, placebo-controlled, long-term study showed no effect (1).

References

1. Packer L, Tritschler HJ, Wessel K. Neuroprotection by the metabolic antioxidant alpha-lipoic acid. *Free Radic Biol Med.* 1997;22:359–378.
2. Packer L, Witt EH, Tritschler HJ. Alpha-lipoic acid as a biological antioxidant. *Free Radic Biol Med.* 1995;19:227–250.
3. Sauer J, Tabet N, Howard R. Alpha lipoic acid for dementia. *Cochrane Database Syst Rev.* 2004;(1):CD004244.
4. Linder MC. Nutrition and metabolism of vitamins. In: Linder MC, ed. *Nutritional Biochemistry and Metabolism with Clinical Applications.* 2nd ed. Norwalk, Conn: Appleton & Lange; 1991:112–122.

5. Teicher J, Kern J, Tritschler HJ, et al. Investigations on the pharmacokinetics of alpha-lipoic acid in healthy volunteers. *Int J Clin Phamacol Ther.* 1998;36:625–628.
6. Bernkop-Schnurch A, Reich-Rohrwig E, Marschutz M, et al. Development of a sustained release dosage form for alpha-lipoic acid. II. Evaluation in human volunteers. *Drug Dev Ind Pharm.* 2004;30:35–42.
7. Beitner H. Randomized, placebo-controlled, double blind study on the clinical efficacy of a cream containing 5% alpha lipoic acid related to photageing of facial skin. *Br J Derm.* 2003;149:841–849.
8. Ziegler D, Schatz H, Conrad F, et al. Effects of treatment with the antioxidant alpha-lipoic acid on cardiac autonomic neuropathy in NIDDM patients. A 4-month randomized controlled multicenter trial (DEKAN Study). *Diabetes Care.* 1997;20:369–373.
9. Ziegler D, Hanefeld M, Ruhnau KJ, et al. Treatment of symptomatic diabetic polyneuropathy with the antioxidant alpha-lipoic acid: a 7 month multicenter randomized controlled trial (ALADIN III Study). ALADIN III Study Group. Alpha-lipoic Acid in Diabetic Neuropathy. *Diabetes Care.* 1999;22:1296–1301.
10. Jacob S, Henriksen EJ, Schiemann AL, et al. Enhancement of glucose disposal in patients with type 2 diabetes by alpha-lipoic acid. *Arzneimittelforschung.* 1995;45:872–874.
11. Jacob S, Ruus P, Hermann R, et al. Oral administration of RAC-alpha-lipoic acid modulates sensitivity in patients with type-2 diabetes mellitus: a placebo-controlled pilot trial. *Free Radic Biol Med.* 1999;27:309–314.
12. Ametov AS, Barinov A, Dyck PJ, et al. The sensory symptoms of diabetic polyneuropathy are improved with alpha-lipoic acid. *Diabetes Care.* 2003;26:770–776.
13. Ziegler D, Nowak H, Kemplert P, et al. Treatment of symptomatic diabetic polyneuropathy with the antioxidant alpha-lipoic acid: A meta-analysis. *Diabet Med.* 2004;21:114–121.
14. A randomized, double-blind, placebo-controlled trial of deprenyl and thioctic acid in human immunodeficiency virus-associated cognitive impairment. Dana Consortium of the Therapy of HIV Dementia and Related Cognitive Disorders. *Neurology.* 1998;50:645–651.
15. Baur A, Harrer T, Peukert M, et al. Alpha-lipoic acid is an effective inhibitor of human immuno-deficiency virus (HIV-1) replication. *Klin Wochenschr.* 1991;69:722–724.
16. Wollin SD, Jones PJ. Alpha-lipoic acid and cardiovascular disease. *J Nutr.* 2003;133:3327–3330.
17. Sharman JE, Gunaruwan P, Knez WL, et al. Alpha-lipoic acid does not acutely affect resistance and conduit artery function or oxidative stress in healthy men. *Br J Clin Pharmacol.* 2004;58:243–248.

Androstenedione and Androstenediol

Androstenedione (4-Androstene-3ß,17ß-dione) is one of the primary androgens secreted by the human adrenal glands as well as ovaries and testes. Androgens are steroid hormones that increase male characteristics. Androstenedione has weak androgenic activity; however, it can be converted into the active steroids testosterone and dihydrotestosterone (1). Andro-stenediol (4 or 5-Androstene-3ß,17ß-diol), a metabolite of dehydroepiandrosterone (DHEA), is also an androgen, but possesses weak activity. Androstenedione and androstene-diol are banned by the US Olympic Committee, the National Collegiate Athletic Association, and the National Football League (2).

Note

Effective January 2005, androstenedione was reclassified from a dietary supplement to an anabolic steroid (a schedule III controlled substance) in the United States by the Anabolic Steroid Control Act of 2004.

Media and Marketing Claims	Efficacy
Increases testosterone production	⟷
Increases muscle mass and strength	NR
Enhances recovery from exercise	NR
Improves libido	NR

Safety

- Due to the known dangers, androstenedione supplements are illegal.
- The FDA considers dietary supplements that contain androstenedione to be adulterated under the Federal Food, Drug, and Cosmetic Act (FD&C Act). Supplements containing new dietary ingredients have to meet certain requirements, and because these requirements have not been met for androstenedione, supplements containing the ingredient cannot be marketed legally. In March 2004, FDA sent warning letters to 23 companies, asking them to stop distributing dietary supplements that contain androstenedione and warning them that they could face enforcement actions if they do not take appropriate actions (3). Despite the FDA efforts and the Anabolic Steroid Control Act of 2004, some androstenedione supplements are still being sold "under the table."
- Because women with severe major depression demonstrate elevated endogenous testosterone levels, there is concern that androstenedione may worsen depressive symptoms (4).
- In older men, increased androgen levels could result in cancerous growth of the prostate, increase of blood lipids, and acceleration of male-pattern baldness (2).
- Tumor growth was stimulated by high levels of androstenedione in rats transplanted with human prostate tumor (PC-82) (1).
- Increased androgen levels caused by supplementation could stimulate hormone-sensitive cancers and conditions (breast, uterine, ovarian, prostate, endometriosis, and uterine fibroids).

- Androstenedione may induce premature labor when taken orally during pregnancy.
- Androstenedione may cause premature closure of bone growth plates when taken orally by children.
- Androstenedione may promote masculinizing hormonal effects in women and feminizing hormonal effects in men.
- Adverse liver effects are possible. Avoid use with existing liver disease; consider monitoring liver function tests in healthy individuals.

Drug/Supplement Interactions

- No reported adverse interactions.
- Possible interaction with androgenic and estrogenic drugs.

Key Points

- Most of the research has not found that androstenedione/androstenediol supplements increase testosterone levels in men. However, two studies have reported increases in testosterone levels, as well as increases in the hormones estradiol and estrone.
- Androgen supplements do not seem to affect muscle size or strength or body composition in athletically trained or untrained males. No research has been done in women.
- There is no evidence published in peer-reviewed journals to support the claims that androstenedione or androstenediol enhances recovery from exercise.
- There is no evidence that androstenedione improves mood or libido.

Food Sources

None

Dosage Information/Bioavailability

Androstenedione was sold in capsules with labels suggesting dosages of 100 to 600 mg per day. Androstenediol was sold in 200-mg capsules.

Relevant Research

In general, there is limited evidence that androstenedione improves muscle mass or muscle strength (5–11).

References

1. van Weerden WM, van Kreuningen A, Elissen NMJ, et al. Effects of adrenal androgens on the transplantable human prostate tumor PC-82. *Endocrinology.* 1992;131:2909–2913.

2. Gwartney DL, Stout JR. Androstenedione: physical and ethical considerations relative to its use as an ergogenic aid. *Strength Cond.* 1999;21:65–66.
3. Crackdown on Andro products. *FDA Consumer Magazine.* May-June 2004. Available at: http://www.fda.gov/fdac/features/2004/304_andro.html. Accessed May 3, 2006.
4. Weber B, Lewicka S, Deuschle M, et al. Testosterone, androstenedione and dihydrotestosterone concentrations are elevated in female patients with major depression. *Psychoneuroendocrinology.* 2000;25:765–771.
5. King DS, Sharp RL, Vukovich MD, et al. Effect of oral androstenedione on serum testosterone and adaptations to resistance training in young men: a randomized controlled trial. *JAMA.* 1999;281:2020–2028.
6. Ballantyne CS, Phillips SM, MacDonald JR, et al. The acute effects of androstenedione supplementation in healthy young males. *Can J Appl Physiol.* 2000;25:68–78.
7. Wallace MB, Lim J, Cutler A, et al. Effects of dehydroepiandrosterone vs androstenedione supplementation in men. *Med Sci Sport Exerc.* 1999;31:1788–1792.
8. Dorgan JF, Stanczyk FZ, Longcope C, et al. Relationship of serum dehydroepiandrosterone (DHEA), DHEA sulfate, and 5-androstene-3ß,17ß-diol to risk of breast cancer in postmenopausal women. *Cancer Epidemiol Biomark Prev.* 1997;6:177–181.
9. Broeder CE, Quindry J, Brittingham K, et al. The Andro Project: physiological and hormonal influences of androstenedione supplementation in men 35 to 65 years old participating in a high-intensity resistance training program. *Arch Intern Med.* 2000;160:3093–3104.
10. Leder BZ, Longcope C, Catlin DH, et al. Oral androstenedione administration and serum testosterone concentrations in young men. *JAMA.* 2000;283:779–782.
11. Green GA, Catlin DH, Starcevic B. Analysis of over-the-counter dietary supplements. *Clin J Sport Med.* 2001;11:254–259.

Arginine (L-arginine)

Arginine and its precursors, ornithine and citrulline, are nonessential amino acids involved in the synthesis of urea in the liver. Arginine becomes essential during growth and catabolic states because it is thought to stimulate anabolic hormone secretion (human growth hormone [GH] and insulin) (1). Arginine is also precursor to nitric oxide, which has potent vasodilating properties in endothelial cells. There is a large body of literature on the role of nitric oxide in hypertension, myocardial dysfunction, inflammation, cell death, and protection against oxidative damage (2). Nitric oxide synthesis or activity may contribute to the initiation and progression of atherosclerosis (3). Because arginine is a substrate for nitric oxide, the potential role of L-arginine supplements has been examined in cardiovascular disease, cancer, and immune function (2,4).

Media and Marketing Claims	Efficacy
Builds muscle	↔
Improves angina pain	↔
Reduces risk for heart disease	↓
Improves immunity, particularly for cancer patients	↔
Improves overall nutritional status in elderly	NR
Promotes wound healing	↑?
Assists repletion of lean body mass in HIV/AIDS wasting	↑?
Reduces severity of necrotizing enterocolitis in premature infants	NR
Treats erectile dysfunction	NR

Safety

- Arginine supplements (3 to 9 g/day) were associated with an increased risk of death in patients recovering from heart attack.

- There are no human studies testing the safety of long-term supplementation of arginine, ornithine, or citrulline, but, in general, arginine supplements have been well-tolerated. Possible detrimental effects of supplements include greater loss of sodium and water and reduced plasma-free lysine concentrations (5).

- High intakes of any one amino acid may interfere with the metabolism of other amino acids (5).

- Arginine is required for the herpes simplex virus to replicate, whereas the amino acid lysine has an inhibitory effect on replication. Patients with herpes simplex virus may be adversely affected by taking arginine supplements (6,7).

- If, as hypothesized, arginine increases growth hormone levels, then long-term supplementation could theoretically negatively affect pituitary regulation of growth hormone.

Key Points

- Research done with small numbers of subjects conflicts regarding the acute effect of arginine in increasing basal growth hormone secretion. The claim that arginine and other amino acids "build muscle" is unsubstantiated at this time.

- Preliminary studies in small numbers of subjects have suggested that arginine supplements may reduce cell adhesion (a marker of inflammation), improve blood flow, and enhance exercise function. However, a study published in 2006 in the *Journal of the American Medical Association* reported that, compared with placebo, arginine supplements taken after subjects had a heart attack actually *increased* their risk of dying. Given these recent findings, arginine supplements should not be used by patients with cardiovascular disease (specifically post–heart attack) until more research is done to determine safety.

◆ Preliminary studies of high doses of arginine (30 g) before chemotherapy treatment improved some immune parameters in individuals with breast cancer or colon cancer. However, until more information is available, people with cancer should not use arginine supplements without physician approval. Additional controlled research is needed before recommendations can be made.

◆ Preliminary studies suggest arginine/ornithine supplements may improve nutritional status in the elderly. However, because protein intake was not controlled in these studies, improvements may be due to the additional protein in the diet and not specifically to ornithine. Arginine supplements enhanced wound healing and immune function in one study of older adults.

◆ Preliminary evidence in humans suggests that arginine supplements enhance wound healing and immune response. Studies in animals have also reported improved healing with arginine supplementation.

◆ A combination of L-arginine, hydroxymethylbutyrate, and glutamine increased body weight and lean body mass (LBM) in individuals with HIV/AIDS wasting syndrome.

◆ Enteral supplementation using L-arginine—enriched beverages, orally or via feeding tube, seems to enhance postsurgical recovery and slightly reduce length of hospital stay.

◆ One of the most promising uses for L-arginine relates to modulation of necrotizing enterocolitis in premature infants; however, research is limited.

◆ Preliminary studies have found that L-arginine may help treat erectile dysfunction if given at adequate dosing levels (5 g/day).

Food Sources

The average American diet provides approximately 5.5 g arginine daily, mainly from meat and fish (4). Arginine, citrulline, and ornithine are found in protein-rich foods and also in nuts, whole grains, and chocolate.

Food	Arginine, mg
Beef, ground (3.5 oz)	1437
Beans, garbanzo (1 cup)	1369
Salmon, Atlantic (3 oz)	1124
Peanuts, roasted (1 oz)	803
Soy milk (1 cup)	514
Rice, brown (1 cup)	382
Egg (1)	378
Milk, nonfat (1 cup)	301
Cheese, cheddar (1 oz)	267
Baking chocolate (1 oz)	163
Shredded wheat cereal (1 oz)	160

Source: Data are from reference 8.

Dosage Information/Bioavailability

Arginine, citrulline, and ornithine are found in tablets, capsules, drinks, and protein powders in various doses (500 mg, 2 to 3 g, 25 g). They are also available in products with several other amino acid combinations and in creatine monohydrate supplements. In addition, specialized enteral feeding formulas have been developed to increase L-arginine intake (along with eicosapentanoic acid [EPA] and RNA) in postoperative or critically ill patients.

Relevant Research

Effects of Arginine and Ornithine on Exercise Hormones

- In a double-blind, placebo-controlled, crossover study, 16 male subjects (mean age 22 years) completed four trials in random order with 1-week washout periods: (*a*) placebo followed by resistance exercise session; (*b*) 1,500 mg L-arginine and 1,500 mg L-lysine, immediately followed by exercise; (*c*) the same amino acids with no exercise; or (*d*) a placebo and no exercise. Dietary protein intake was not controlled nor assessed. All subjects were tested to ensure normal growth hormone metabolism. Growth hormone levels were higher during the exercise trials (*a* and *b*) compared with the resting trials (*c* and *d*). There was no effect of arginine and lysine on GH during the exercise trials. However, a small but significant increase in GH was seen during resting conditions 60 minutes after amino acid ingestion compared with the placebo (9).

- In a double-blind, placebo-controlled study, 22 untrained male subjects (mean age 37 years) participating in a 5-week progressive strength-training program were randomly assigned to receive 1 g each of L-arginine and L-ornithine or a placebo. At the end of the study, subjects were tested for total strength on a series of weight machines, LBM, and urinary hydroxyproline (a marker of exercise-induced soreness and tissue damage). Dietary protein intake was neither controlled nor assessed. Compared with the placebo group, the arginine–ornithine supplemented subjects scored higher on total strength and LBM measures and lower in hydroxyproline excretion. The results of this study should be viewed with caution because subjects were not matched to control subjects and not pretested for strength and body mass (10).

Arginine and Cardiovascular Disease

- In a double-blind, placebo-controlled study, 153 patients who had just had a myocardial infarction were randomized to receive L-arginine (goal dose 3 g, 3 times/day) or matching placebo for 6 months. Half the patients were older than 60 years. There were no differences in baseline characteristics, vascular stiffness measurements, or left ventricular function between groups. At the end of 6 months, there were still no differences in those parameters in either of the two groups, including those 60 years or older and the entire study group. However, six subjects (8.6%) in the L-arginine group died during the study vs none in the placebo group ($P = .01$). The study was terminated due to concerns with the safety of arginine. The authors concluded: "L-Arginine, when added to standard postinfarction therapies, does not improve vascular stiffness measurements or ejection fraction and may be associated with higher postinfarction mortality. L-Arginine should not be recommended following acute myocardial infarction" (11).

- In a double-blind, placebo-controlled study, 41 subjects with intermittent claudication were randomly assigned to one of three groups for 2 weeks: (*a*) two HeartBars (6.6 g L-arginine); (*b*) one HeartBar (3.3 g L-arginine) and one placebo bar; or (*c*) two placebo bars. Pain-free and total walking distances were measured by treadmill exercise testing, and quality of life was assessed by the Medical Outcome Survey. There were no differences in walking distances at baseline. After 2 weeks, the pain-free walking distance in the 6.6-g L-arginine group was significantly (66%) greater and the total walking distance was significantly increased by 23%. These effects were not seen in the lower-dose arginine or placebo groups. Likewise, there was a significant benefit in perceived general, emotional, and social function in the 6.6 g L-arginine group, but not in the other treatments (12).

- In a double-blind comparative study, 39 subjects with intermittent claudication were randomly assigned to receive one of three treatments for 3 weeks: (*a*) 16 g L-arginine/day in two doses, (*b*) 80 g prostaglandin E_1 (PGE_1)/day in two doses, or (*c*) control (no active treatment). The pain-free and absolute walking distances were assessed on a treadmill, and nitric oxide–mediated, flow-induced vasodilation of the femoral artery was assessed by ultrasonography at baseline; at weeks 1, 2, and 3 of therapy; and 6 weeks after the end of treatment. Urinary nitrate and cyclic guanosine-3', 5'-monophosphate (GMP) were assessed as indexes of endogenous nitric oxide production. Arginine treatment, but not PGE_1 treatment, increased urinary nitrate and cyclic GMP excretion rates, indicating normalized endogenous nitric oxide formation. Arginine supplements significantly improved pain-free walking distance by 230% ± 63% and absolute walking distance by 155% ± 48%. PGE_1 also resulted in significant improvements, whereas control subjects experienced no significant change. In both the arginine group and the PGE_1 group, there was a significant improvement in subjective assessment of pain on a visual analog scale (13).

- In a double-blind, placebo-controlled trial, 22 subjects with stable angina pectoris and healed myocardial infarction were randomly assigned to receive 6 g L-arginine divided into three doses or placebo for 3 days. Blood samples were obtained and performance on an exercise test was determined before and after treatment. Blood pressure and an electrocardiogram were recorded during exercise. Exercise capacity improved in the arginine-supplemented group compared with the placebo group (significant increase in maximum workload and mean exercise time to maximal ST-depression on an electrocardiogram). The authors hypothesized that supplements possibly improve an inefficient L-arginine/nitric oxide system that contributes to impaired heart muscle perfusion and/or poor vasodilation during exercise (14). Similar positive findings were demonstrated in a placebo-controlled trial in 36 subjects with stable angina. Arginine, provided as HeartBar, was associated with a significant increase in flow-mediated vasodilation, increased treadmill time, and quality of life (15).

♦ In a double-blind, placebo-controlled, crossover design trial, 15 subjects with heart failure were given L-arginine chloride (5.6 g arginine/day to 12.6 g/day) for 6 weeks and 6 weeks of placebo capsules in random sequence. Forearm blood flow during exercise was significantly increased during arginine supplementation compared with placebo. Functional status (distance in a 6-minute walk test) along with scores on the Living with Heart Failure Questionnaire were significantly better during arginine supplementation, as was arterial compliance (16).

♦ In a prospective, double-blind, placebo-controlled, crossover study, 10 men (mean age 41 years) with coronary atherosclerosis (confirmed by angiogram) were randomly assigned to receive either 21 g L-arginine or placebo, divided into three doses per day, for 3 days, followed by a 10-day washout period and crossover to the alternate treatment. After arginine treatment, there was a significant improvement in endothelium-dependent dilation of the brachial artery. No changes were observed in endothelium-independent dilation of the brachial artery, blood pressure, heart rate, or fasting lipid levels. Monocyte adhesion to endothelial cells was significantly reduced with arginine compared with placebo (17).

♦ In a double-blind, placebo-controlled, crossover study, 27 individuals (age 19 to 40 years) with hypercholesterolemia, known endothelial dysfunction, and mean LDL cholesterol levels of 238 mg/dL, were assigned in random order to receive 21 g L-arginine or placebo (divided into three daily doses) for 4 weeks each, with a 4-week washout period. Dietary intake was not controlled. Brachial artery diameter was measured at rest, during increased flow (causing endothelium-dependent dilation [EDD]) and after sublingual glyceryl trinitrate (causing endothelium-independent dilation). After arginine supplementation, there was a statistically significant increased in plasma arginine levels and a significant improvement in brachial artery diameter measured during increased flow (EDD). There were no significant changes in response to glyceryl trinitrate. Lipid levels did not change in either group (18).

♦ In a double-blind, placebo-controlled crossover study, 10 healthy postmenopausal women received (in random order) 9 g L-arginine or a placebo each day for 1 month (separated by a month washout period). Serum nitric oxide levels, brachial artery EDD responses, and cell adhesion molecules (markers of inflammation in blood) were measured at the end of each treatment period. L-arginine levels were increased in all women during L-arginine administration. However, there was no change in serum nitric oxide levels nor an effect on EDD during hyperemia compared with the placebo. There was also no effect of L-arginine on cell adhesion molecules compared with placebo (19).

♦ Acute intravenous infusion of L-arginine significantly improved brachial artery flow-mediated dilation in subjects with hypercholesterolemia (n = 9) and subjects who smoked (n = 9), but had no effect on subjects with type 1 diabetes (n = 9) or healthy control subjects (n = 9) (20).

Arginine and Cancer

- In a double-blind, placebo-controlled study, 96 subjects with breast cancer were randomly assigned to receive 30 g L-arginine or a placebo for 3 days prior to each of six chemotherapy (treatments every 21 days). There was no difference in the overall response rate between groups. However, in subjects with tumors smaller than 6 cm in initial diameter, histopathologic responses were significantly improved in the group receiving L-arginine supplements (88% responded) compared with the placebo group (52% responded) (21).

- A smaller study with a similar protocol found 30 g L-arginine administered to 10 subjects with breast cancer (ages 42 to 73 years) before chemotherapy delayed the onset and severity of immunosuppression compared with subjects not taking arginine (n = 6) before chemotherapy. Arginine supplementation also stimulated natural killer and lymphokine-activated killer cell activity (22).

- In a randomized, controlled (not blinded) study, 18 subjects with colorectal cancer received either a standard diet (60 g protein/3.2 g arginine) or the same standard diet supplemented with 30 g of L-arginine for 3 days before surgery. Tumor biopsies and blood samples were taken during surgery. Arginine supplementation resulted in significant alterations in tumor-infiltrating lymphocytes (believed to be involved in regulating tumor growth). Specifically, there was a significant increase in the number of cells expressing characteristics of natural killer and lymphokine-activated killer cells. However, there was no change in the number of T and B cells, T-helper and T-suppresser cells. The authors concluded: "These findings confirm the potentially powerful therapeutic effects of dietary manipulation and have important implications for the immunotherapeutic treatment of malignant disease in humans" (23).

Arginine and Ornithine for the Elderly

- In a placebo-controlled, double-blind study, 45 healthy elderly subjects were given 17 g free arginine as arginine-aspartate (n = 30) or a placebo (n = 15) for 2 weeks. Dietary intake was not controlled. Arginine supplementation resulted in a significant increase in serum insulin-like growth factor and improved nitrogen balance compared with the placebo. Arginine supplementation also was associated with reduced total cholesterol without a decrease in HDL cholesterol (24).

- In a double-blind, placebo-controlled trial, 194 elderly subjects (mean age 74 years) recovering from acute illness were randomly assigned to receive 10 g ornithine oxoglutarate (containing 1.3 g nitrogen) or a placebo (isocaloric maltodextrin) for 2 months. One-hundred-eighty-five subjects completed the study (93 in the ornithine group, 92 in the placebo group). After 30 and 60 days of supplementation, the ornithine group had significantly improved appetite, body weight, and independence compared with the placebo group. Two months after treatment, there was still an improvement in the quality-of-life index and the medical-cost index (overall cost savings of 37%). The authors hypothesized that the benefits may be attributed to the stimulation of insulin and growth hormone (not measured) and by the promotion of anabolism by endogenous production of proteins in the liver and fibroblasts (25).

Arginine and Ornithine for Wound Healing

♦ In a double-blind, placebo-controlled study, 32 elderly nursing home residents with pressure ulcers were randomly assigned to receive one of three enteral formulas daily for 1 month: (*a*) 0 g L-arginine (placebo); (*b*) 8.5 g L-arginine; or (*c*) 17 g L-arginine. Markers of immune function (lymphocyte proliferation to phytohemagglutinin and interleukin-2 production) were measured at baseline and at 4 weeks. Supplemental arginine significantly increased plasma arginine levels and were tolerated by subjects with normal renal function who were adequately hydrated. Markers of immune function (and, thus, healing of pressure sores) were not enhanced by arginine (26).

♦ In a double-blind, placebo-controlled study, 60 healthy elderly men and women (age > 65 years) were randomly assigned to receive 30 g arginine-aspartate (17 g free arginine) or placebo for 2 weeks. A catheter inserted subcutaneously into the right deltoid was used to evaluate fibroblastic wound responses, and a wound on the upper thigh was made to assess epithelialization. The researchers analyzed the mitogenic response of peripheral lymphocytes to concanavalin A, phytohemagglutinin, poke-weed mitogen, and allogeneic stimuli at the baseline and after 2 weeks. Use of the arginine supplement significantly improved wound catheter hydroxyproline (measure of collagen synthesis repair) and total protein content. Arginine did not change the DNA content (measure of cellular infiltration) of the catheters or the rate of epithelialization of the skin defect. The group taking arginine showed significantly greater responses to mitogenic and allogenic stimulation. The authors concluded that the arginine supplementation may improve wound healing and immune responses in the elderly (27).

♦ Plasma fluxes of arginine, citrulline, and ornithine were studied in nine burn subjects. Arginine fluxes were higher in burn subjects than healthy controls, leading the researchers to hypothesize that higher rates of arginine loss from the body after burn injury would need to be balanced by exogenous intake of preformed arginine to maintain protein homeostasis and promote recovery (28).

♦ An L-arginine–enriched enteral formula (which also contains EPA) has been shown to reduce perioperative infections and shorten length of stay in surgical patients (29).

Arginine and AIDS

♦ In a randomized, double-blind, placebo-controlled study, 55 outpatient subjects with HIV received a daily nutritional supplement (606 kcal) or the nutritional supplement plus 7.4 g arginine and 1.7 g n-3 fatty acids for 6 months. The arginine and n-3 supplement had no effect on body weight or immunologic parameters (CD4 and CD8 lymphocyte counts, tumor necrosis factor soluble receptors, viremia) (30).

♦ A randomized, controlled, double-blind, placebo-controlled study using arginine combined with betahydroxybutyrate and glutamine in 68 subjects with HIV-wasting syndrome showed a significant mean 3.0 kg weight gain at the 8-week time point in the 22 subjects on the combined therapy compared with the 21 subjects receiving placebo. Of the weight gained in the subjects on combined therapy, 2.6 kg was associated with increased lean body mass. CD3 and CD8 cell counts also improved with the combined supplement as compared with placebo (31). No follow up studies in this cohort or additional HIV patients using this combination of suppplements have been published.

Arginine and Necrotizing Enterocolitis in Newborns

+ One hundred fifty-two premature infants at risk for necrotizing enterocolitis (NEC) were randomly assigned to receive arginine or placebo with oral/parenteral feedings for 28 days postpartum. NEC developed in five infants receiving L-arginine and 21 on placebo ($P < .001$). Thus, arginine supplementation at 1.5 mmol/kg/day seems to significantly reduce NEC incidence in at-risk premature infants (32).

Arginine and Erectile Dysfunction

+ Preliminary evidence from a randomized controlled study of 5 g arginine supplementation for 6 weeks among 50 men with organic erectile dysfunction showed significant improvements in self-reported sexual function among those receiving arginine only *if* subjects demonstrated low baseline nitric oxide levels; those with normal nitric oxide levels at baseline showed no benefit of arginine supplementation in terms of erectile function (33). Further research is needed because studies using lower doses have not shown efficacy.

References

1. Cynober L. Can arginine and ornithine support gut functions? *Gut.* 1994;35(1 Suppl):S42-S45.
2. Abcouwer SF, Souba WW. Glutamine and arginine. In: Shils ME, Olson JA, Shike M, Ross AC, eds. *Modern Nutrition in Health and Disease.* 9th ed. Baltimore, Md: Williams & Wilkins; 1999:559–569.
3. Cooke JP. Is atherosclerosis an arginine deficiency disease? *J Investig Med.* 1998;46:377–380.
4. Tenenbaum A, Fisman EZ, Motro M. L-arginine: rediscovery in progress. *Cardiology.* 1998;90:153–159.
5. Beaumier L, Castillo L, Ajami AM, et al. Urea cycle intermediate kinetics and nitrate excretion at normal and "therapeutic" intakes of arginine in humans. *Am J Physiol.* 1995;269(5 pt 1):E844-E896.
6. Griffith RD, DeLong DC, Nelson JD. Relation of arginine-lysine antagonism to herpes simplex growth in tissue culture. *Chemotherapy.* 1981;27:209–213.
7. Flodin NW. The metabolic roles, pharmacology, and toxicology of lysine. *J Am Coll Nutr.* 1997;16:7–21.
8. Pennington JAT. *Bowes and Church's Food Values of Portions Commonly Used.* 17th ed. Philadelphia, Pa: Lippincott-Raven Publishers; 1998.
9. Suminski RR, Robertson RJ, Goss FL, et al. Acute effects of amino acid ingestion and resistance exercise on plasma growth hormone concentration in young men. *Int J Sport Nutr.* 1997;7:48–60.
10. Elam RP, Hardin DH, Sutton RA, et al. Effects of arginine and ornithine on strength, lean body mass, and urinary hydroxyproline in adult males. *J Sports Med.* 1989;29:52–56.

11. Schulman SP, Becker LC, Kass DA, et al. L-arginine therapy in acute myocardial infarction. *JAMA*. 2006;295:58–64.
12. Boger RH, Bode-Boger SM, Thiele W, et al. Restoring vascular nitric oxide formation by L-arginine improves the symptoms of intermittent claudication in patients with peripheral arterial occlusive disease. *J Am Coll Cardiol*. 1998;32:1336–1344.
13. Maxwell AJ, Anderson BE, Cooke JP. Nutritional therapy for peripheral arterial disease: a double-blind, placebo-controlled, randomized trial of HeartBar. *Vasc Med*. 2000;5:11–19.
14. Ceremuzynski L, Chamiec T, Herbaczynska-Cedro K. Effect of supplemental oral L-arginine on exercise capacity in patients with stable angina pectoris. *Am J Cardiol*. 1997;80:331–333.
15. Maxwell AJ, Zapien MP, Pearce GL, et al. Randomized trial of a medical food for the dietary management of chronic, stable angina. *J Am Coll Cardiol*. 2002;39:37–45.
16. Rector TS, Bank AJ, Mullen KA, et al. Randomized, double-blind, placebo-controlled study of supplemental oral L-arginine in patients with heart failure. *Circulation*. 1996;93:2135–2141.
17. Adams MR, McCredie R, Jessup W, et al. Oral L-arginine improves endothelium-dependent dilatation and reduces monocyte adhesion to endothelial cells in young men with coronary artery disease. *Atherosclerosis*. 1997;129:261–269.
18. Clarkson P, Adams MR, Powe AJ, et al. Oral L-arginine improves endothelium-dependent dilation in hypercholesterolemic young adults. *J Clin Invest*. 1996;97:1989–1994.
19. Blum A, Hathaway L, Mincemoyer R, et al. Effects of oral L-arginine on endothelium-dependent vasodilation and markers of inflammation in healthy post-menopausal women. *J Am Coll Cardiol*. 2001;35:271–276.
20. Thorne S, Mullen MJ, Clarkson P, et al. Early endothelial dysfunction in adults at risk from atherosclerosis: different responses to L-arginine. *J Am Coll Cardiol*. 1998;32:110–116.
21. Heys S, Ogston K, Miller I, et al. Potentiation of the response to chemotherapy in patients with breast cancer by dietary supplementation with L-arginine: results of a randomized controlled trial. *Int J Oncol*. 1998;12:221–225.
22. Brittendon J, Heys SD, Ross J, et al. Natural cytotoxicity in breast cancer patients receiving neoadjuvant chemotherapy: effects of L-arginine supplementation. *Eur J Surg Oncol*. 1994;20:467–472.
23. Heys SD, Segar A, Payne S, et al. Dietary supplementation with L-arginine: modulation of tumor-infiltrating lymphocytes in patients with colorectal cancer. *Br J Surg*. 1997;84:238–241.
24. Hurson M, Regan MC, Kirk SJ, et al. Metabolic effects of arginine in a healthy elderly population. *JPEN*. 1995;19:227–230.
25. Brocker P, Vellas B, Albarede JL, et al. A two-center, randomized, double-blind trial of ornithine oxoglutarate in 194 elderly, ambulatory, convalescent subjects. *Age Ageing*. 1994;23:303–306.
26. Langkamp-Henken B, Herrlinger-Garcia KA, Stechmiller JK, et al. Arginine supplementation is well tolerated but does not enhance mitogen-induced lymphocyte proliferation in elderly nursing home residents with pressure ulcers. *JPEN J Parenter Enteral Nutr*. 2000;24:280–287.

27. Kirk SJ, Hurson M, Regan MC, et al. Arginine stimulates wound healing and immune function in elderly human beings. *Surgery.* 1993;114:155–159.
28. Yu YM, Ryan CM, Burke JF, et al. Relations among arginine, citrulline, ornithine, and leucine kinetics in adult burn patients. *Am J Clin Nutr.* 1995;62:960–968.
29. Tepaske R, Velthuis H, Oudemans-van Straaten HM, et al. Effect of preoperative oral immune-enhancing nutritional supplement on patients at high risk of infection after cardiac surgery: a randomised placebo-controlled trial. *Lancet.* 2004;358:696–701.
30. Pichard C, Sudre P, Karsegard V, et al. A randomized double-blind controlled study of 6 months of oral nutritional supplementation with arginine and omega-3 fatty acids in HIV-infected patients. Swiss HIV cohort study. *AIDS.* 1998;12:53–63.
31. Clark RH, Feleke G, Din M, et al. Nutritional treatment for acquired immunodeficiency virus-associated wasting using beta-hydroxy beta-methylbutyrate, glutamine, and arginine: a randomized, double-blind, placebo-controlled study. *JPEN J Parenter Enteral Nutr.* 2000;24:133–139.
32. Amin HJ, Zamora SA, McMillan DD, et al. Arginine supplementation prevents necrotizing enterocolitis in the premature infant. *J Pediatr.* 2002;140:425–431.
33. Chen J, Wollman Y, Chernichovsky T, et al. Effect of oral administration of high-dose nitric oxide donor L-arginine in men with organic erectile dysfunction: results of a double-blind, randomized, placebo-controlled study. *BJU Int.* 1999;83:269–273.

Aspartic Acid/Asparagine

Aspartic acid (aspartate) is a nonessential amino acid involved in urea synthesis and is a glucogenic and pyrimidine precursor. In the tricarboxylic acid (Krebs) cycle, aspartic acid and oxaloacetic acid are interconvertible. Asparagine is also a nonessential amino acid that can be hydrolyzed into aspartic acid. Asparagine acts as a reservoir of amino groups throughout the body. It has been hypothesized that aspartate salts enhance athletic performance. The proposed mechanism of action is that aspartate spares glycogen by increasing the availability of free fatty acids (FFAs) for fuel and potentially reduces exercise fatigue by clearing excess ammonia from the blood through urea synthesis (1).

Media and Marketing Claims	Efficacy
Reduces fatigue, increases energy for athletic performance	NR
Improves cognition in those with liver disease (encephalopathy)	NR

Safety

♦ There are no long-term studies testing the safety of aspartic acid or asparagine. Acute ingestion (5 to 10 g aspartate) was not associated with adverse effects in human studies.

♦ It is not known whether high doses of aspartic acid or asparagine negatively affect absorption and metabolism of other amino acids.

Drug/Supplement Interactions

♦ No reported negative interactions; however, it is not known whether high doses of aspartic acid or asparagine negatively affect absorption and metabolism of other amino acids.

Key Points

♦ The ergogenic effect of aspartate salts on exercise performance is controversial. None of the studies evaluated serum aspartate levels. In addition, the small number of subjects makes interpretation of the data difficult. Aspartate salts do not seem to reduce accumulation of ammonia in plasma. Most studies do not show a benefit, and until additional controlled trials with larger sample sizes are conducted, supplementation is not warranted.

♦ Aspartate is metabolized by resting muscle and does not enhance mineral absorption as has been suggested among those using it to improve athletic performance.

♦ In individuals with hepatic encephalopathy and intrahepatic shunts, preliminary evidence suggest that aspartate may help improve cognition; however, additional research using well-designed studies is needed before clinical recommendations can be formulated.

Food Sources

Aspartic acid and asparagine are found in protein-rich animal foods. The sugar-free sweetener aspartame is a combination of aspartic acid and phenylalanine (40% aspartic acid).

Food	Aspartic Acid, g/serving
Beef, ground (3 oz)	6.683
Chicken breast (½)	2.377
Flour, whole wheat (1 cup)	0.844
Egg (1 large)	0.627
Corn (1 ear)	0.194

Source: Data are from reference 2.

Dosage Information/Bioavailability

L-aspartic acid is available in single or mixed amino acid preparations providing 500 to 1,200 mg as potassium, calcium, or magnesium aspartate. L-asparagine is usually only found in mixed amino acid supplements in 60-mg doses.

Relevant Research

Aspartic Acid and Asparagine for Exercise

- In a double-blind, comparative crossover trial, 12 male weight trainers were randomly assigned to receive aspartate salts (150 mg/kg) or vitamin C (150 mg/kg) over a 2-hour period, 5 hours before a resistance workout. Trials were separated by 1 week. Vitamin C was chosen as the placebo because it has no known effects on ammonia production or clearance. There were no significant differences in plasma ammonia levels or bench-press tests between treatments (3).

- In a double-blind, crossover study, seven trained subjects were given 10 g potassium and magnesium aspartic salts providing 5 g aspartate or a placebo 24 hours prior to an exercise-to-exhaustion on a cycle ergometer, separated by a 1-week washout. Following aspartate ingestion, there was a significant increase in time to exhaustion and postexercise FFA levels. There was a significant decrease in lactate concentrations. Blood ammonia levels were significantly lower throughout exercise during the aspartate supplementation compared with the placebo. The researchers hypothesized that the ergogenic benefit of aspartate was attributable to improved ammonia clearance (4).

- In a double-blind, placebo-controlled, crossover study, eight young male subjects received 6 g aspartic acid salts (as magnesium-potassium aspartate) or a placebo over a 24-hour period before exercising to exhaustion on a cycle ergometer (75% maximum oxygen uptake), with a 1-week washout period. There were no differences in blood glucose, lactate, ammonia, or plasma FFA levels between treatments groups during or after exercise. There was also no effect on respiratory exchange ratio. The authors concluded: "These results show no beneficial effect of oral aspartate administration on work capacity in man and also suggest that the metabolic processes that occur during exercise are not influenced by this treatment" (5).

L-Aspartate and Hepatic Encephalopathy

- In a double-blind study of subjects with cirrhosis, eight without intrahepatic shunts and seven with shunts, were administered glutamine (to induce clinical elevation in ammonia levels) with 5 g IV L-ornithinine plus L-aspartate or placebo. In subjects without shunts, ammonia levels increased to 36 mmol/L with L-ornithinine/L-aspartate and to 62 mmol/L with placebo, indicating a significant therapeutic benefit of supplementation in subjects without shunts (6). No benefit was seen in those without shunts. Studies with larger sample sizes and orally administered supplementation are warranted.

References

1. Abcouwer SF, Souba WW. Glutamine and arginine. In: Shils ME, Olson JA, Shike M, Ross AC, eds. *Modern Nutrition in Health and Disease*. 9th ed. Baltimore, Md: Williams & Wilkins; 1999:561.

2. USDA Nutrient Database. Available at: http://www.nal.usda.gov/fnic. Accessed April 17, 2005.

3. Tuttle JL, Potteiger JA, Evans BW, et al. Effect of acute potassium-magnesium aspartate supplementation on ammonia concentrations during and after resistance training. *Int J Sport Nutr.* 1995;5:102–109.

4. Wesson M, McNaughton L, Davies P, et al. Effects of oral administration of aspartic acid salts on the endurance capacity of trained athletes. *Res Q Exerc Sport.* 1988;59:234–239.

5. Maughan RJ, Sadler DJ. The effects of oral administration of salts of aspartic acid on the metabolic response to prolonged exhausting exercise in man. *Int J Sports Med.* 1983;4:119–123.

6. Rees C, Oppong K, Mardini H, et al. Effect of L-ornithine-L-aspartate on patients with and without TIPS undergoing glutamine challenge: a double blind, placebo controlled trial. *Gut.* 2000;47:571–574.

Barley Grass. *See* Wheat Grass and Barley Grass.

BCAA. *See* Branched Chain Amino Acids (BCAA).

Bee Pollen

Bee pollen has been extensively used as a dietary supplement in Europe and Asia because of purported nutritional benefits (1). Bee pollen is a powder form of nonairborne pollen collected by bees from male seed flowers. The pollen mixes with secretions from the bee and forms into granules for the bee to carry back to the hive on its hind legs. Bees store pollen in the hive as food for larvae.

Considerable variation in the nutritional content of pollen exists (ie, protein content varies from 7% to 40%) (2). In one study, the composition of two types of bee pollen from western Australia were estimated to contain 57% carbohydrate, 1% fat, and 20% to 28% protein (2). Analysis of the mineral composition of these pollens showed that potassium, phosphorus, calcium, and sodium were present in the highest concentration (no analysis of vitamin content) (2). However, when calculated to determine the amounts found in a typical dose of a commercial bee pollen supplement (7 g), the actual quantities of these nutrients are relatively insignificant (4 to 8 mg calcium, 33 mg potassium, 0.31 to 0.46 mg zinc, 6 mg magnesium, 1.8 g protein, 4 mg carbohydrates, and less than 1 g fat).

Media and Marketing Claims	Efficacy
Enhances memory	NR
Reduces symptoms of premenstrual syndrome	NR
Reduces symptoms of chronic prostatitis	NR
Enhances well-being; "nature's perfect food"	↓

Safety

- Evidence supports safe use of 1 teaspoon/day for up to 30 days.

- Although relatively rare, an anaphylactic reaction can occur in some sensitive individuals. Accordingly, bee pollen is contraindicated for people with asthma or allergies to honey or bee stings. There have been reports of anaphylactic reactions to bee pollen in individuals with a sensitivity to bee stings and honey allergies (3,4). However, not all individuals who had allergic reactions to bee pollen had prior allergic reactions to bee stings (1).

- Individuals with liver disease should avoid using bee pollen.

- General herbal reference texts recommend that pregnant women avoid bee pollen supplements due to potential uterine stimulatory effects.

Drug/Supplement Interactions

No reported adverse interactions

Key Points

- The typical dose of bee pollen (½ to 1 teaspoon) provides insignificant quantities of protein, carbohydrate, fat, and most vitamins and minerals.

- Currently, there is no scientific evidence to substantiate the claims about bee pollen supplementation. A regular multivitamin/mineral supplement is less costly and more efficient than bee pollen, and also a safer alternative given the possibility of an allergic reaction.

Food Sources

Small amounts are found in honey.

Dosage Information/Bioavailability

Bee pollen is sold in powder, granules, or capsule forms. Some manufacturers suggest taking ½ to 1 teaspoon (approximately 3 to 7 g) pure bee pollen powder or 1,000 to 1,500 mg in capsule form daily. Bee pollen is also a popular ingredient added to fruit "smoothies" and certain multivitamin/mineral supplements. In one study, the digestibility of the protein in two different bee pollens ranged from 52% to 59%, compared with 89% for casein. The authors of this study noted, "Their relatively low digestibility will be a limiting factor in their usefulness as a food for humans" (2). In addition, the amounts of protein consumed from supplements contribute minimally to overall protein intake.

Relevant Research

Bee Pollen and Memory

- ◆ In general, research on bee pollen is scant, though some studies, mostly using experimental animals, have been published in Chinese and Russian journals.

- ◆ A double-blind, placebo-controlled, crossover trial of 100 elderly Danish subjects with self-reported memory deterioration tested the effects of a traditional Chinese mixture known as NaO Li Su containing bee pollen and a variety of Chinese herbs. There were no improvements in memory functions between groups as assessed by a battery of psychological and biochemical tests. There was a statistically significant increase in red blood cell count and serum creatinine concentration in subjects taking supplements (5). Because bee pollen was administered as part of a mixture of herbs, the pharmacological effect of bee pollen cannot be determined from this study.

Bee Pollen and Premenstrual Syndrome

- ◆ In a randomized, placebo-controlled, double blind, crossover study testing the effects of a mixed herbal supplement containing bee pollen on premenstrual symptoms, women showed a significant improvement in symptoms during the two menstrual cycles in which they took the mixed herbal supplement as compared with the two menstrual cycles when they took placebo. The mixed supplement (Femal) provided 72 mg of bee pollen daily. While the study did randomly assign women to start with the herbal supplement or placebo, the small sample size (15 and 16 per group, respectively) limits the statistical power of the study. The most significant improvement was in premenstrual weight gain, which suggests that some diuretic effect may have contributed to the reported improvement in symptoms. Additional studies are needed (6).

Bee Pollen and Prostatitis

- ◆ Few studies have assessed the role of bee pollen in prostatitis, and the studies available are more than 10 years old. Preliminary evidence from those studies suggests that bee pollen may reduce symptoms of prostatisis, presumably because of the supplement's anti-inflammatory properties. However, study designs have been flawed. In one study, only 15 subjects participated and the study design was open-label and without a placebo control group (7). In a second prospective, treatment-only study (no placebo control), 42% of the 78 subjects with mild to moderate disease (without significant complications such as urethral strictures or sclerosis) reported an improvement in symptoms with treatment (Cernilton N), and 36% reported total alleviation of symptoms (8). In this study, objective measures (those factors that do not rely simply on self-reported improvements) also changed favorably for these subjects, including increased urine flow and decreased incidence of leukocyte presence in the postprostate massage urine. However, only one of the 18 patients with substantial complications related to prostatitis showed any improvement with supplementation. Further research is needed.

References

1. Geyman JP. Anaphylactic reaction after ingestion of bee pollen. *J Am Board Fam Pract.* 1994;7:250–253.
2. Bell RR, Thornber EJ, Seet JL, et al. Composition and protein quality of honeybee-collected pollen of Eucalyptus marginata and Eucalyptus calophylla. *J Nutr.* 1983;113: 2479–2484.
3. Prichard M, Turner KJ. Acute hypersensitivity to ingested processed pollen. *Aust N Z J Med.* 1985;15:346–347.
4. Greenberger PA, Flais MJ. Bee pollen-induced anaphylactic reaction in an unknowingly sensitized subject. *Ann Allergy Asthma Immunol.* 2001;86:239–242.
5. Iversen T, Fiigaard KM, Schriver P, et al. The effect of NaO Li Su on memory functions and blood chemistry in elderly people. *J Ethnopharmacol.* 1997;56:109–116.
6. Winther K, Hedman C. Assessment of the effects of the herbal remedy Femal(R) on the symptoms of premenstrual syndrome: a randomized, double-blind, placebo-controlled study. *Curr Ther Res Clin Exp.* 2002;63:344–353.
7. Buck AC, Rees RW, Ebeling L. Treatment of chronic prostates and prostatodynia with pollen extract. *Br J Urol.* 1989;64:496–499.
8. Rugendorff EW, Weidner W, Ebeling L, et al. Results of treatment with pollen extract (Cernilton N) in chronic prostatitis and prostaodynia. *Br J Urol.* 1993;71:433–438.

Beta Carotene. *See* Vitamin A.

Bitter Melon *(Momordica charantia)*

Chinese bitter melon *(Momordica charantia),* a cucumber-shaped green vegetable, has a high iron content, which increases its value as a preventive medicine. The fruit, which is used most often in Chinese medicinal preparations, tastes extremely bitter. Although the seeds, leaves, and vines of bitter melon have all been used, the fruit is the safest and most prevalent part of the plant used medicinally. Bitter melon has been used for many years to treat an assortment of conditions ranging from common infections to cancer and diabetes. The leaves and fruit have both been used to season soups and make tea and beer.

Media and Marketing Claims	Efficacy
Helps reduce blood glucose in people with type 2 diabetes	NR
Reduces blood lipid levels	NR
Prevents cancer	NR
Improved immune response for individuals with HIV	NR

Safety

- Severe hypoglycemia and hypoglycemic coma in children who consumed bitter melon tea have been reported (1).
- Pregnant women should not take bitter melon. It can cause premature contractions, bleeding, and miscarriage.
- Animal studies suggest a liver toxicity may be induced by bitter melon; no human evidence is available. To be prudent, people with underlying liver disease should not take bitter melon, and those taking bitter melon should have liver function tests monitored during use.

Drug/Supplement Interactions

Monitor blood glucose in individuals with diabetes. Bitter melon may have an additive effect when taken with insulin.

Key Points

- Preliminary studies in animals have shown bitter melon to decrease serum glucose levels. However, the majority of these studies have been weak in methodology and design. Well-designed human studies are needed. Bitter melon has been historically used in some cultures to promote blood glucose control in people with diabetes. However, given its potential hypoglycemic effects, bitter melon should be used only with the guidance of a health professional.
- Evidence that bitter melon improves blood lipid profiles is limited to animal studies, but the findings suggest that further research is warranted in humans. Clinical use would be premature.
- Laboratory studies using cancer cells exposed to bitter melon suggest that bitter melon may reduce cancer risk; however, no human studies have been published.
- Bitter melon contains proteins that have potential to repress the HIV virus (2). However, its effectiveness in humans has not been substantiated by clinical evidence.

Food Sources

Bitter melon is most commonly found in the form of a supplement, but the vegetable can be purchased in specialty stores or Asian markets under the name karela.

Dosage Information/Bioavailability

There is no standard dosage for bitter melon.

Relevant Research

Bitter Melon and Blood Glucose Control

♦ To test the efficacies of various fresh and dried whole fruits in reducing fasting blood glucose in diabetic rats, extracts were prepared and fed to healthy rats and those rendered diabetic by injection of alloxan. For 4 weeks, rats were then fed a control diet or supplemented twice daily with (*a*) 20 mg/kg of methanol extract of bitter melon, (*b*) chloroform extract of bitter melon, or (*c*) water extract of bitter melon. The methanol extract reduced blood glucose by 39% by the fourth week. The aqueous extract had the largest effect in reducing blood glucose, a 50% reduction. Both the methanol and aqueous extracts also reduced blood glucose in nondiabetic rats. Aqueous extract reduced serum triglyceride and VLDL levels similar to the effect of the diabetic medication glibenclamide. Histologic examination did not find damage to the liver of kidneys (3).

♦ In a second study conducted in rats, rats were fed a low-fat or high-fat diet for 6 weeks followed by a 9-week intervention with bitter melon (4). Control rats remained on the assigned diet throughout. Fifty percent of rats assigned to the low-fat diet were also provided 1.5% bitter melon. Rats assigned to the high-fat diet were divided into groups with escalating dosing of bitter melon juice (0.375%, 0.75%, or 1.5% of total energy), also for 9 weeks. In a substudy within this study, male Sprague-Dawley rats were fed a low-fat diet for 5 weeks and then randomly assigned to a high-fat diet or a high-fat diet plus bitter melon at the same escalating doses for an additional 6 weeks. Bitter melon supplementation at a dosage of 0.75% or 1.5% was associated with reduced adiposity in rats on the high-fat diet and was also associated with reduced insulin resistance, improved oral glucose tolerance, and an increase in free fatty acids. From these results, reductions in blood glucose may be related to reduced adiposity associated with consumption of a high-fat diet. Further research is needed.

Bitter Melon and Blood Lipids

♦ An in vitro study investigated the effects of bitter melon on serum lipids. HepG2 liver cells were exposed to control medium or control medium supplemented with various concentrations of extracted bitter melon juice with or without oleate and/or the proteosome inhibitor ALLN. Bitter melon juice decreased secretion of apoB by cultured liver cells when present at the concentration of 1% in the culture medium. Cells exposed to bitter melon juice also secreted fewer triglycerides and expressed less triglyceride transfer protein (5).

◆ To investigate the effects of bitter melon and bitter melon extracts on serum and liver triglycerides, male Sprague-Dawley rats were divided into groups and fed a controlled diet supplemented with 3% bitter melon powder from various varieties of bitter melon for 2 weeks. Rats fed the variety Koimidori bitter melon powder had significantly reduced liver weight compared with controls at the completion of the feeding period. The Koimidori variety reduced hepatic triglycerides. This was especially true for the methanol fraction of Koimidori. Only marginal effects were seen on serum lipids with any of the treatments (6).

◆ A study conducted using Syrian hamsters fed a high- or no-cholesterol diet showed that at increasing doses for 4 weeks, dietary methanol fraction extracted from bitter melon was associated with reduced food intake (at both 0.5% and 1.0% bitter melon concentration). Among hamsters on the high-cholesterol diet, bitter melon supplementation was associated with a reduction in serum triglyceride levels in a dose-dependent manner, whereas no effect was shown for hamsters on the no-cholesterol diet (7). Although total serum cholesterol also decreased in a dose-dependent manner, it did not show statistical significance.

Bitter Melon and Cancer

◆ To investigate the chemopreventive effects of bitter melon oil on large bowel tumorigenesis, groups of male Fischer 344 rats were fed varying amounts of bitter melon oil after exposure to the carcinogen azoxymethane (AOM). No colonic neoplasms occurred in rats not exposed to AOM, and bitter melon oil significantly decreased the incidence of colonic neoplasms induced by AOM. Bitter melon oil reduced the number of tumors at all dietary concentrations tested in this study (8).

Bitter Melon and Immunity in HIV

◆ In a case report published in 1995, a man diagnosed with HIV residing in California self-prescribed bitter melon (10 ounces of the fruit juice per day, increasing to 16 ounces/day and later daily rectal enemas) for a period of 12 months. Significant increase in CD4 and normalization of CD4/CD8 cell count ratio were reported. Because this is a case report that had no controls, this evidence is weak. However, it may offer, along with experimental and animal data, a rationale to pursue hypotheses of this nature in human controlled trials (9).

◆ Anti-HIV activity, as measured by viral core protein production and inhibition of integration of viral DNA into cell lines, has also been demonstrated experimentally for MAP30, a protein within the bitter melon plant. Testing has been done in HIV-1 infected H9 cell line for both MAP30 and recombinant MAP30—an investigational drug (10).

References

1. Basch E, Gabardi S, Ulbricht C. Bitter melon (*Momordica charantia*): a review of efficacy and safety. *Am J Health Syst Pharm.* 2003;60:356–359.
2. Schreiber CA, Wan L, Sun Y, et al. The antiviral agents, MAP30 and GAP31, are not toxic to human spermatozoa and may be useful in preventing the sexual transmission of human immunodeficiency virus type 1. *Fertil Steril.* 1999;72:686–90.
3. Virdi J, Sivakani S, Shahani S, et al. Antihyperglycemic effects of three extracts from Monodica charantia. *J. Ethnopharm.* 2003;88:107–111.
4. Chen Q, Li ET. Reduced adiposity in bitter melon (Momordica charantia) fed rats is associated with lower tissue triglyceride and higher plasma catecholamines. *Br J Nutr.* 2005;93:747–754.
5. Nerurkar PV, Pearson L, Efird JT, et al. Microsomal triglyceride transfer protein gene expression and apoB secretion are inhibited by bitter melon in HepG2 cells. *J Nutr.* 2005;135:702–706.
6. Senanayake GV, Maruyama M, Shibuya K, et al. The effects of bitter melon (Momordica charantia) on serum and liver triglyceride levels in rats. *J Ethnopharm.* 2004;91:257–262.
7. Senanayake GV, Maruyama M, Sakono M, et al. The effects of bitter melon (momordica charantia) extracts on serum and liver lipid parameters in hamsters fed cholesterol-free and cholesterol-enriched diets. *J Nutr Sci Vitaminol.* 2004;50:253–257.
8. Hohno H, Yasui Y, Suzuki R, et al. Dietary seed oil rich in conjugated linolenic acid from bitter melon inhibits azoxymethane-induced rat colon carcinogenesis through elevation of colonic PPARγ expression and alteration of lipid composition. *Int J Cancer.* 2004;110:896–901.
9. Rebultan SP. Bitter melon therapy: an experimental treatment in HIV infection. *AIDS Asia.* 1995;2(4):6–7.
10. Lee-Huang S, Huang PL, Chen HC, et al. Anti-HIV and anti-tumor activities of recombinant MAP30 from bitter melon. *Gene.* 1995;161:151–156.

Black Cohosh *(Cimicifuga racemosa)*

Black cohosh is a member of the buttercup family. Eighteen species grow in Europe, North America, and Asia. "Black" refers to the dark color of the rhizome. "Cohosh" comes from an Algonquian word meaning "rough," referring to the feel of the rhizome. Traditionally, the root of the plant was used for treatment of dysmenorrhea, dyspepsia, and rheumatism. In the 19th century, black cohosh was a main ingredient in Lydia Pinkhams's Vegetable Compound, a popular remedy used for a variety of "female complaints." Black cohosh has been investigated and used in Germany since the 1950s and is approved by the German Commission E (a governmental regulatory agency in Germany) for premenstrual discomfort, dysmennorrhea, or menopausal ailments. Remifemin (Enzymatic Therapy, Inc, Green Bay, WI), the brand name of the standardized extract, has been used in most clinical trials (1–3).

The exact mechanism of action and particular active components of the herb are not fully understood. The biologically active compounds in the herb are thought to be the triterpene glycosides including actein, cimicifugoside, deoxyacetylacteol, and 27-deoxy-actein. Originally, researchers suggested that isoflavones in black cohosh exerted weak estrogenic effects that reduced menopausal symptoms. However, studies have not found the herb to be estrogenic, nor does it contain isoflavones. Black cohosh does not seem to affect several hormones levels, including estradiol, luteinizing hormone (LH) or follicle stimulating hormone (FSH), and prolactin. Although the biological activities of this herb require further study, US women continue to use black cohosh as an alternative to hormone replacement therapy (HRT) for the management of menopausal symptoms (1–3). Women who have had breast cancer are advised against taking black cohosh because animal studies suggest an increase in metastasis with its use, despite preliminary evidence in animals that black cohosh may act as a selective estrogen-receptor modulator (estrogenic in some tissue but not all) as does tamoxifen. Thus, until the exact mechanism of biological activity is identified, women with estrogen-receptor–positive breast cancer or other estrogen-related cancers should avoid black cohosh.

Media and Marketing Claims	Efficacy
Reduces menopausal symptoms	↔
Reduces premenstrual symptoms	NR

Safety

- Black cohosh seems to be safe in studies of up to 6 months in duration.
- Black cohosh should be avoided during pregnancy; it may stimulate uterine contractions.
- Women who are lactating should avoid black cohosh; it may adversely affect the nursing child.
- Black cohosh should be avoided by women with a history of breast cancer or at risk for breast cancer, and by women with existing hormone-sensitive conditions (such as uterine and ovarian cancers, endometriosis, and uterine fibroids). Preliminary data suggest that black cohosh may act as a selective estrogen receptor modulator (4). More research is needed to determine safety for these women.
- Gastrointestinal upset is common (4); black cohosh may also cause rash, headache, dizziness, weight gain, feeling of heaviness in the legs, and cramping.
- Because of a lack of long-term trials, the German Commission E Monographs recommend limiting the use of black cohosh to 6 months (5).
- Experimental studies demonstrate no toxic, mutagenic, or carcinogenic properties with black cohosh (6).

- ◆ Supplements containing black cohosh have been associated with acute hepatitis (7,8). Individuals with existing liver disease should not take it.

- ◆ The National Institutes of Health Workshop on the Safety of Black Cohosh in Clinical Studies was held November 22, 2004 (9). The summary report explains the need for characterizing and standardizing the specific supplements used in clinical research prior to NIH funding. The report also discusses one animal study on the safety of black cohosh in breast cancer that found increased metastatic lesions; this finding requires replication before specific guidelines can be provided. The researchers concluded that black cohosh supplements do not seem to pose a safety issue in healthy women. The potential adverse effects of black cohosh on liver function warrant the on-going monitoring of liver function in study participants (and thus in patients) taking this supplement.

Drug/Supplement Interactions

Black cohosh may increase the risk of liver damage in individuals taking potentially hepatotoxic drugs or supplements.

Key Points

- ◆ A few controlled and several uncontrolled studies conclude that black cohosh relieves menopausal symptoms such as hot flashes, irritability, and anxiety. However, the lack of a control group in most of the studies makes it difficult to evaluate the efficacy.

- ◆ The American College of Obstetricians and Gynecologists suggests that black cohosh may be helpful in reducing vasomotor symptoms of menopause (10).

- ◆ More research is needed to evaluate the role of black cohosh on PMS and dysmenorrhea. Black cohosh contains fukinolic acid, which has an anti-inflammatory effect and may account for its possible efficacy for premenstrual symptoms. The National Institutes of Health, through the National Center for Complementary and Alternative Medicine, are funding phase I and II studies of black cohosh among women with premenstrual syndrome.

Dosage Information/Bioavailability

Black cohosh is most commonly sold in capsules, tablets, tinctures, and teas. In the United States, black cohosh is marketed as Remifemin (Enzymatic Therapy Inc, Green Bay, WI), a standardized black cohosh root and rhizome extract (standardized for triterpene glycosides, calculated as 23-epi-26-deoxyactein). Most studies have used 80 to 160 mg/day of Remifemin (a total of 4 to 8 mg of 23-epi-26-deoxyactein/day). Because of improved extraction processes, the current recommended dosage of Remifemin is 40 mg/day (3). Bioavailability has not been studied.

Relevant Research

Black Cohosh and Menopause

◆ A well-designed randomized, controlled, double-blind, parallel group clinical trial was conducted in 152 peri- and postmenopausal women (149 included in the intent-to-treat analysis at 12 weeks; 116 at 24 weeks) using 39 vs 127 mg of black cohosh daily for a 24-week period. Women ranged in age from 42 to 60 years and demonstrated a baseline Kupperman Menopause Index Score ≥ 20. Significant reductions in menopausal symptoms as measured by Kupperman Menopause Index were shown with both standard dose (39 mg/day) and high-dose (127 mg/day), with approximately 70% of subjects in each group showing a significant response to supplementation. No dose-response was demonstrated; both doses had similar therapeutic efficacy. There was a lack of biological evidence for estrogenic effects either at the tissue (vaginal cytology reports) or the systemic level (estrogen, luteinizing hormone, follical stimulating hormone or sex hormone–binding globulin), suggesting black cohosh supplementation did not promote estrogenic response (11).

◆ In a double-blind, randomized, placebo-controlled study, 97 postmenopausal women were randomly assigned to receive (*a*) 40 mg BNO 1055 black cohosh, (*b*) conjugated estrogen (0.6 mg), or (*c*) placebo daily. Sixty-two women met all inclusion criteria after randomization (BMI < 30; FSH > 25 mU/mL; 17ß-estradiol < 40 pg/mL). BNO 1055 supplementation was shown to be equivalent to estrogen in reducing climacteric complaints without increasing endometrial thickness. This study also demonstrated positive bone health outcomes related to the supplement. The results suggest that black cohosh may act as a selective estrogen receptor modulator, but further trials are needed (4).

◆ In a double-blind, placebo-controlled study, 85 subjects who were diagnosed with breast cancer and who had completed their primary treatment were randomly assigned to receive black cohosh or a placebo, stratified on tamoxifen use. Subjects self-reported menopausal symptoms on a questionnaire at study entry and at 30 and 60 days and kept a hot flash diary throughout the study. FSH and LH levels were measured on the first and final days of the study. Of the 85 subjects, 59 were taking tamoxifen and 26 were not. Both treatment and placebo groups reported decreased number and intensity of hot flashes and improvements in menopausal symptoms. There were no significant differences between groups. FSH and LH did not differ between the two groups. The researchers concluded that black cohosh was not better than the placebo in the treatment of menopausal symptoms in this population of women, most of whom were taking tamoxifen (12).

◆ In a double-blind, placebo-controlled trial, 80 menopausal women received either 0.625 mg of estrogen, 80 mg of a standardized black cohosh extract, or a placebo for 12 weeks. Hot flashes, night sweats, heart palpitations, headaches, nervousness, irritability, insomnia, depressive moods, and changes in vaginal cell proliferation were assessed by the Kupperman Menopausal Index and the Hamilton Anxiety Scale

(13). Altogether 16 women discontinued treatment before the study ended: 13 subjects—12 in the estrogen group, 1 in the placebo group—stopped after 5 to 8 weeks because of inefficacy); two placebo subjects stopped treatment due to side effects; and one subject with varicosis in the black cohosh group stopped treatment due to thrombophlebitis. Subjects taking black cohosh showed significant improvement in both measures. The estrogen proved to be given in too low a dose for reliable comparison (13).

♦ In a double-blind, placebo-controlled study, 60 women younger than age 40, who had at least one ovary removed and complained of climacteric symptoms, were randomly assigned to one of four groups. These four groups of equal number were treated with either (*a*) 1 mg estriol, (*b*) 1.25 mg of conjugated estrogens, (*c*) estrogen-gestagen combination, or (*d*) Remifemin (80 mg/day). The Menopausal Index (with evaluation of the trophic disturbances of the genitals) and FSH and LH serum concentrations were used as the efficacy criteria. In all four groups there was improvement in the profile of complaints of postoperative ovarian functional deficits, a significant decrease in the modified Menopausal Index, and a moderate decrease in the serum gonadotropin concentrations. There was no significant therapeutic difference among the individual medication groups (14).

♦ In a multicenter, open study, 629 menopausal women received 4 mg of a black cohosh extract twice daily for 6 to 8 weeks. Of the total subjects, 367 women were not previously treated, 204 were treated previously with hormones, 35 were treated with psychopharmaceuticals, 11 were treated with a combination of hormones and psychopharmaceuticals, and 12 were lacking specific treatment data. Forty-nine percent of the participants reported a dramatic reduction in hot flashes, sweating, headaches, vertigo, palpitations, and tinnitus attributed to menopause. More than 39% noted a decrease in nervousness, irritability, and depression. However, the study was not blinded, randomized, or placebo-controlled (15).

♦ A review of randomized, controlled trials related to menopausal symptoms and concluded that "black cohosh may be effective for menopausal symptoms, especially hot flashes, but the lack of adequate long-term safety data precludes recommending long-term use" (16).

Black Cohosh and PMS

♦ A review of integrative medicine for PMS indicated that many claims about using black cohosh for PMS are extrapolated from studies of menopausal symptoms. The authors conclude, "Further studies are needed" (17).

References

1. Foster S. Black cohosh: *Cimicifuga racemosa* a literature review. *HerbalGram*. 1999;45: 34–49.
2. Taylor M. Botanicals: medicines and menopause. *Clin Obstet Gynecol*. 2001;44: 853–863.

3. Pepping J. Black cohosh: *Cimicifuga racemosa. Am J Health Syst Pharm.* 1999;56: 1400–1402.
4. Wuttke W, Seidlova-Wuttke D, Gorkow C. The Cimicifuga preparation BNO 1055 vs conjugated estrogens in a double-blind placebo-controlled study: effects on menopause symptoms and bone markers. *Maturitas.* 2003;44:S67-S77.
5. Blumenthal M, ed. *The Complete German Commission E Monographs Therapeutic Guide to Herbal Medicines.* Austin, Texas: American Botanical Council; 1998.
6. Liske E. Therapeutic efficacy and safety of *Cimicifuga racemosa* for gynecologic disorders. *Adv Ther.* 1998;15:45–54.
7. Vitetta L, Thomsen M, Sali A. Black cohosh and other herbal remedies associated with acute hepatitis. *Med J Aust.* 2003;178:411–412.
8. Lontos S, Jones RM, Angus PW, et al. Acute liver failure associated with the use of herbal preparations containing black cohosh. *Med J Aust.* 2003;179:390–391.
9. The National Institutes of Health Workshop on the Safety of Black Cohosh in Clinical Studies. November 22, 2004. Available at: http://nccam.nih.gov/news/pastmeetings/ blackcohosh_mtngsumm/pdf A#summary. Accessed May 25, 2005.
10. American College of Obstetricians and Gynecologists Committee on Practice Bulletins—Gynecology. ACOG Practice Bulletin. Clinical Management Guidelines for Obstetrician-Gynecologists. Use of botanicals for management of menopausal symptoms. *Obstet Gynecol.* 2001;97(Suppl):1–11.
11. Liske E, Hanggi W, Henneicke-von Zepelin HH, et al. Physiological investigation of a unique extract of black cohosh (Cimicifugae racemosae rhizoma): a 6-month clinical study demonstrates no systemic estrogenic effect. *J Womens Health Gend Based Med.* 2002;11:163–174.
12. Jacobson JS, Troxel AB, Evans J. Randomized trial of black cohosh for the treatment of hot flashes among women with a history of breast cancer. *Clin Oncol.* 2001;19:2739–2745.
13. Stoll W. Phytopharmacon influences atrophic vaginal epithelium. Double-blind study: cimicifuga vs estrogenic substances. *Therapeuticum.* 1987;1:23–31.
14. Lehman-Willenbrock E. Reidel H. Clinical and endocrinologic examinations concerning therapy of climacteric symptoms following hysterectomy with remaining ovaries. *Zentralbl Gynakol.* 1998;110:611–618.
15. Stolze H. An alternative to treat menopausal complaints. *Gynecology.* 1982;3:14–16.
16. Kronenberg F, Fugh-Berman A. Complementary and alternative medicine for menopausal symptoms: a review of randomized, controlled trials. *Ann Intern Med.* 2002;137:805–813.
17. Girman A, Lee R, Kliger B. An integrative medicine approach to premenstrual syndrome. *Am J Obstet Gynecol.* 2003;188(5 Suppl):S56–S65.

Black Currant Oil. *See* Gamma-Linolenic Acid.

Borage Oil. *See* Gamma-Linolenic Acid.

Boron

Originally known as essential in plants, boron, an ultratrace mineral, has recently been recognized as essential for some animals and thus is likely to be essential for humans. Boron is distributed throughout the body, with the highest concentration in the bone, fingernails, teeth, hair, spleen, and thyroid. Although the functions of boron in the human body are unclear, more than 20 years of research has shown that boron may be involved in bone formation and maintenance as well as reproduction and development (1,2).

Media and Marketing Claims	Efficacy
Prevents osteoporosis; improves bone health	NR
Prevents and treats osteoarthritis	NR
Increases muscle mass by increasing testosterone levels	NR
Improves memory, cognitive function	NR
Helps prevent cancer	NR

Safety

- No adverse interactions have been reported at doses less than 10 mg/day.

- The Tolerable Upper Intake Level (UL) for adults is 20 mg/day. Do not exceed the UL.

- ULs are 3 mg/day for children ages 1 to 3 years, 6 mg/day for children ages 4 to 8 years, 11 mg/day for children ages 9 to 13 years, and 17 mg/day for adolescents ages 14 years or older. Do not exceed the UL.

- Boron has a low order of toxicity when consumed in amounts normally found in the diet (1,3). Doses more than 50 mg/day are associated with toxicity; fatality has occurred with oral doses of 300 mg/kg. Toxicity signs generally occur when boron intake exceeds 50 mg/day for an extended period of time (exact period of time may vary depending on the individual's baseline status). Symptoms include nausea, vomiting, fatigue, diarrhea, and dermatitis. High doses cause urinary riboflavin excretion (1). High doses can also reduce urinary magnesium excretion, leading to elevated serum levels.

- Boron should be avoided by women with existing hormone-sensitive conditions (such as breast, uterine, and ovarian cancers; endometriosis; and uterine fibroids).

- Boron should be avoided by individuals with kidney disease or impaired kidney function because the kidneys are the major excretion route.
- Boron may reduce serum phosphorus levels.
- Large doses of boron (1,000 mg/kg) have been shown to interfere with gonad development in rats and cause testicular atrophy in dogs (3).

Drug/Supplement Interactions

Theoretical interaction with estrogenic drugs (increase in serum estrogen).

Key Points

- Evidence suggests that boron deprivation can reduce calcium bioavailability through decreased absorption, but no studies clearly demonstrate that boron supplements can prevent or treat osteoporosis.
- Well-controlled, clinical research regarding the role of boron in osteoarthritis is lacking. Large-scale, controlled studies are needed before boron can be recommended to treat people with osteoarthritis.
- Despite the marketing of boron supplements as a way to increase testosterone, the limited research does not suggest that boron affects lean body mass, testosterone levels, or strength in body builders.
- Preliminary evidence has shown that chronically low dietary intake of boron (< 0.25 mg/day for 42 to 63 days) may negatively affect cognitive function. However, doses more than the amount found naturally in the diet do not seem to enhance brain function.
- In general, Americans seem to consume diets adequate in boron. Daily supplementation with less than 10 mg boron seems to be relatively safe, but it is probably not warranted based on the current scientific evidence.
- Several boron-containing compounds (but not boron alone) are being investigated for potential as an adjunct cancer therapy.
- A review of the physiological effects of boron suggests several potential biological roles but provides little clinical trial data (4).

Food Sources

Non-citrus fruits and leafy vegetables are the main dietary sources of boron. Other rich sources include nuts, dried fruit, avocado, legumes, wine, cider, and beer. Dairy and meat products are low in boron. Coffee and milk, although low in boron, are the top two contributors of boron in the American diet because they are consumed in high amounts (5).

Food	Boron, µg/serving
Raisins (½ cup)	1760
Peanuts, roasted (⅓ cup)	833
Wine (3.5 oz)	628
Applesauce (½ cup)	342
Broccoli, boiled (½ cup)	195
Coffee (1 cup)	69
Milk, 2% (1 cup)	44

Source: Data are from reference 5.

Dosage Information/Bioavailability

There is no RDA or AI set for boron; however, researchers suggest daily intakes of approximately 1 mg/day (2,3). The average American diet provides an estimated 0.96 mg to 1.17 mg boron/day (2,5). Most boron supplements in the form of sodium borate, boron chelates (citrate, aspartate, glycinate), and sodium tetraborate decahydrate provide 3 mg doses and are often combined with other minerals such as calcium and magnesium. Absorption of dietary boron is efficient because most of the boron is excreted in the urine after 3 to 7 days (1).

Relevant Research

Boron and Bone Health

- In the first nutritional human study of boron, 12 postmenopausal women initially consumed a boron-deficient diet that provided 0.25 mg boron per 2,000 kcal for 119 days, and then consumed the same diet with a supplement of 3 mg boron (sodium borate) per day for 48 days. Boron supplementation reduced total plasma calcium, altered calcium and magnesium metabolism, and increased serum levels of 17B-estradiol and testosterone. The authors concluded: "Supplementation of a low-boron diet with an amount of boron commonly found in diets high in fruits and vegetables induces changes in postmenopausal women consistent with the prevention of calcium loss and bone demineralization" (6).

- Four men, nine postmenopausal women (five on estrogen therapy), and one premenopausal woman consumed a diet supplying 0.25 mg boron per 2,000 kcal for 63 days while living in a metabolic unit. They then consumed the same diet supplemented with 3 mg boron per day for 49 days. Women on estrogen therapy had significantly higher serum 17B-estradiol and plasma copper levels, specifically during the boron supplementation phase. Boron enhanced the effects of estrogen in women on estrogen therapy and mimicked some of these effects in men and postmenopausal women not taking estrogen. The authors suggested that because estrogen ingestion is beneficial for calcium metabolism, it may be beneficial for boron metabolism as well (7).

- Twenty eight female college athletes and nonathletes participated in a randomized, placebo-controlled clinical trial assessing the role of boron on bone mineralization. Subjects were given 3 mg boron or placebo daily for 10 months. No efficacy was demonstrated, although data suggested that participants with diets inadequate in vitamin D, calcium, and magnesium might potentially benefit from boron supplementation; however, the study did not include enough subjects to statistically test this hypothesis (8).

Boron and Osteoarthritis

- A review article summarizing evidence of a potential beneficial role of boron in arthritis included the following points: Clinical evidence suggests that subjects with arthritis have lower concentrations of boron in bone and synovial fluid than those without osteoarthritis. Epidemiological evidence suggests that osteoarthritis incidence ranges from 20% to 70% in regions of the world where boron intakes are less than 1.0 mg/day, but the incidence of osteoarthritis is 0% to 10% in regions where boron intakes are 3 to 10 mg per day (9).

- In a double-blind, placebo-controlled pilot trial (not randomized), 20 subjects (17 women, mean age 65 years) with radiographically confirmed osteoarthritis were given 6 mg boron/day (in the form of sodium tetraborate decahydrate) or a placebo for 5 weeks. Twenty-five percent of the subjects dropped out of the study. Boron supplementation improved symptoms in 5 of 10 subjects, whereas only 1 of 10 subjects benefited in the placebo group. Statistical analysis was not performed because of small sample size (10). This study is included despite its limitations because it is commonly cited to support claims that boron supplements benefit subjects with arthritis.

Boron and Body Building

- In a placebo-controlled (not blinded) study, 19 male body builders were randomly assigned to receive 2.5 mg boron/day or a placebo for 7 weeks. There were no differences in testosterone levels, strength tests, or body mass between groups, indicating that boron supplementation was not beneficial (11).

Boron and Cognitive Function

- Three placebo-controlled, double-blind randomized trials evaluated the effect of low vs high intakes of boron (0.25 mg vs 3.25 mg boron per 2,000 kcal) on a variety of cognitive and psychomotor tasks in healthy older adults (total n in the three studies = 28 subjects) for a period of 105 to 126 days. Compared with higher boron intake, low intake of dietary boron resulted in significantly poorer performance in manual dexterity, eye-hand coordination, attention, perception, encoding, and short- and long-term memory tests. Electroencephalograms taken during boron depletion showed depressed mental alertness (12).

Boron and Cancer Prevention

- One epidemiological study of the association between dietary boron intake and prostate cancer has been conducted. Otherwise, there are no data in this area other than the ongoing development of chemotherapeutic agents using related boron compounds. The study used data from NHANES III, including 95 subjects with prostate cancer and 8,720 control subjects. Potential confounders included age, race, education, smoking status, BMI, dietary energy, and alcohol intake. There was a mean 54% reduction in risk for prostate cancer among those with the highest intake of dietary boron (P for trend = .0525). The number of cases was small, dietary measurement was limited, and foods rich in boron are also rich in other nutrients that may play a role in cancer prevention, all of which limit application of these results to clinical practice (13).

- Boron supplementation has also been shown to reduce prostate tumor formation in nude mice (a specific mouse model with reduced immune capacity) as well as to modulate insulin-like growth factor 1, which is thought to be a tumor promoter (14).

References

1. Nielsen FH. Ultratrace minerals. In: Shils ME, Olson JA, Shike M, Ross AC, eds. *Modern Nutrition in Health and Disease.* 9th ed. Baltimore, Md: Williams & Wilkins; 1999:283–288.
2. Institute of Medicine. *Dietary Reference Intakes: Vitamin A, Vitamin K, Arsenic, Boron, Chromium, Copper, Iodine, Iron, Manganese, Molybdenum, Nickel, Silicon, Vanadium, and Zinc.* Washington, DC: National Academy Press; 2001.
3. Nielsen FH. Facts and fallacies about boron. *Nutr Today.* 1992;27:6–12.
4. Devirian TA, Volpe SL. The physiological effects of dietary boron. *Crit Rev Food Sci Nutr.* 2003;43:219–231.
5. Rainey CJ, Nyquist LA, Christensen RE, et al. Daily boron intake from the American Diet. *J Am Diet Assoc.* 1999;99:335–340.
6. Nielsen FH, Hunt CD, Mullen LM, et al. Effect of dietary boron on mineral, estrogen, and testosterone metabolism in postmenopausal women. *FASEB J.* 1987;1:394–397.
7. Nielsen FH, Gallagher SK, Johnson LK, et al. Boron enhances and mimics some effects of estrogen therapy in postmenopausal women. *J Trace Elem Exp Med.* 1992;5: 237–246.
8. Volpe SL, Taper LJ, Meacham S. Effects of boron supplementation on bone mineral density and dietary, blood, and urinary calcium, phosphorus, magnesium, and boron in female athletes. *Environ Health Perspect.* 1994;102(Suppl 7):79–82.
9. Newnham RE. Essentiality of boron for healthy bones and joints. *Environ Health Perspect.* 1994;102(Suppl 7):S83-S85.
10. Travers RL, Rennie GC, Newnham RE. Boron and arthritis: the results of a double-blind pilot study. *J Nutr Med.* 1990;1:127–132.
11. Green NR, Ferrando AA. Plasma boron and the effects of boron supplementation in males. *Environ Health Perspect.* 1994;102(Suppl 7):S73–S77.

12. Penland JG. Dietary boron, brain function, and cognitive performance. *Environ Health Perspect.* 1994;102(Suppl 7):S65-S72.

13. Cui Y, Winton MI, Zhang ZF, et al. Dietary boron intake and prostate cancer risk. *Oncol Rep.* 2004;11:887–92.

14. Gallardo-Williams MT, Chapin RE, King P, et al. Boron supplementation inhibits the growth and local expression of IGF-1 in human prostate adenocarcinoma tumors in mice. *Toxicol Pathol.* 2004;32:73–78.

Bovine Colostrum. *See* Colostrum/Bovine Colostrum.

Branched Chain Amino Acids (BCAA)

Branched-chain amino acids (isoleucine, leucine, and valine) are a group of essential amino acids that have been studied for their potential role in delaying central nervous system (CNS) fatigue, specifically in athletes. BCAA as ingested are not readily degraded by the liver but instead circulate and compete brain with the amino acid tryptophan for uptake into the. Tryptophan is a precursor to serotonin (5-hydroxytryptamine), which may depress the CNS and produce symptoms of fatigue. Research has shown that exercise increases the ratio of free tryptophan–to–BCAA, thus increasing serotonin levels in the brain. There is also evidence that plasma BCAA levels decrease during endurance exercise. Some researchers have proposed that supplementing with BCAA will reduce the free tryptophan–to–BCAA ratio and result in improved mental and physical performance, but the studies to date are inconclusive (1–3).

In addition to their purported benefits in athletes, BCAA have also been studied for potential in treating hepatic encephalopathy. In individuals with liver failure, BCAA circulate at unusually low levels compared with levels of the aromatic amino acids (phenylalanine, tyrosine, and tryptophan). Researchers have hypothesized that low levels of BCAA result in preferential brain uptake of the other amino acids, which are precursors to false neurotransmitters and may exacerbate encephalopathy (4). Although this theory has not been proven, BCAA are included in some enteral formulas specifically indicated for people with liver diseases.

Media and Marketing Claims	Efficacy
Builds muscle; reduces abdominal fat	NR
Improves athletic performance	↓
Helps mental function in people with liver disease	↔
Improves appetite in the elderly	NR

Safety

+ No long-term studies have assessed the safety of BCAA supplementation.

+ No adverse effects were reported in healthy individuals in studies lasting for 1 to 2 weeks or for as long as 6 months.

+ Although no cases of toxicity occurred in any of the cited studies, one review article warned that large doses of BCAA (> 20 g) may increase plasma ammonia levels to toxic levels (1). Liver function should be monitored with supplementation for more than 3 months.

+ Individuals with amyotrophic lateral sclerosis, should avoid BCAA supplementation because of possible increased pulmonary failure and mortality.

+ Individuals with branched-chain ketoaciduria (maple syrup urine disease) should avoid BCAA supplementation.

+ Fatigue and loss of motor coordination may result from increased plasma ammonia associated with high dose BCAA supplementation.

+ Large doses of BCAA (> 20 g) may impair water absorption across the gut and cause gastrointestinal pain (1).

Drug/Supplement Interactions

+ BCAA may stimulate insulin release and have an additive effect with medications used to treat high blood glucose.

+ BCAA may decrease effectiveness of levodopa.

+ Use of diazoxide or glucocorticoids may decrease stimulation of protein synthesis by BCAA.

+ Use of glucocorticoids or thyroid hormones may alter metabolism of BCAA.

Key Points

+ BCAA supplementation seems to reduce the plasma free tryptophan–to–BCCA ratio and prevent the decrease in plasma and muscle BCAA associated with exercise. However, ingestion of carbohydrates before, during, and after exercise also seems to have this effect on blood and muscle and is known to enhance exercise performance (1). Therefore, dietary carbohydrates are recommended to prolong exercise endurance because the ergogenic value of BCAA is still unproven.

+ Preliminary studies in small numbers of subjects suggest that BCAA supplementation may attenuate muscle breakdown that occurs with exercise. More controlled research is needed in this area before conclusions can be made. Leucine seems to be the primary amino acid that modulates skeletal muscle synthesis, and efficacy of leucine supplementation may diminish with age, a factor that is seldom controlled for in reported research (5).

- ◆ BCAA may help improve overall function of people with advanced liver disease and hepatic encephalopathy, but data are conflicting.
- ◆ BCAA may improve appetite in malnourished older adults (6). More research is needed.

Food Sources

Leucine, isoleucine, and valine are amino acids found in protein-rich foods such as eggs, meat, poultry, fish, dairy products, and legumes.

Food	Isoleucine, mg	Leucine, mg	Valine, mg
Chicken breast (½)	1409	2002	1324
Beef, ground, regular (3.5 oz)	1022	1797	1106
Shrimp (3 oz)	862	1411	836
Yogurt, nonfat (1 cup)	711	1310	1076
Beans, pinto (1 cup)	676	1222	801
Egg (1)	343	538	384
Oatmeal (1 cup)	248	459	335

Source: Data are from reference 7.

Dosage Information/Bioavailability

BCAA supplements are sold in pill and powder forms with 7 to 20 g BCAA per serving. BCAA are also found in some sport beverages, with doses ranging from 1 to 7 g/L. Subjects with hepatic encephalopathy have been given 240 mg/kg/day without side effects.

Relevant Research

BCAA and Exercise Performance

- ◆ In a placebo-controlled (not blinded) study, 193 experienced runners were randomly assigned to drink a 5% glucose beverage with 16 g BCAA or a placebo 5% glucose drink during a 42.2-km marathon. Running performance, measured as time ratios for specific distances, improved in the marathon for the slower runners (3.05 to 3.30 hours) when BCAA were taken during the race. No improvement was seen in the faster runners (< 3.05 hour). A second part of this study examined the effects of 7.5 g BCAA on mental performance as measured by the Stroop Color and Word Test (CWT). Runners who took BCAA supplements during a 30-km cross-country race showed improved mental performance after the race, as compared with mental performance measured before the race, whereas mental performance for runners who took the placebo did not improve (8).
- ◆ In a double-blind, placebo-controlled, randomized, crossover study, nine well-trained male cyclists were given a glucose solution alone, a glucose solution plus 18 g BCAA, or

a placebo (water) during 100 km of cycling at maximal speed in a laboratory setting. Each trial was separated by 1 week. There was no difference in performance times among the three trials, suggesting that BCAA had no effect on exercise performance in these trained athletes (9).

◆ In a double-blind, crossover design study, seven endurance-trained male cyclists were given a 7-g BCAA solution or a placebo before cycling on a cycle ergometer for 1 hour at 70% maximal power output, followed by 20 minutes of maximal exercise. Every 10 minutes, subjects rated their perceived exertion and mental fatigue on two scales. There were no differences in physical performance between the two trials. However, the ratings of perceived exertion and mental fatigue were significantly lower (7% and 15% lower, respectively) when subjects were supplemented with the BCAA solution (10).

◆ In a double-blind, placebo-controlled, crossover design study, six well-trained female soccer players consumed either 7.5 g BCAA in a carbohydrate solution or a carbohydrate solution alone (placebo) during two soccer games. Mental performance (measured by the Stroop CWT) was assessed 2 hours to 2.5 hours before the game and within 45 minutes after the end of the game. For subjects who drank the BCAA-supplemented beverage, scores of mental performance were better after the game. No effect on mental performance was noted for subjects in the placebo group (11).

◆ In a double-blind, placebo-controlled, crossover design study, 13 male and female subjects cycled at 40% VO_{2max} to exhaustion in the heat (34°C [93°F], relative humidity 39%) while ingesting either a BCAA-supplemented drink (9.4 g BCAA for females, 15.8 g BCAA for males) or a placebo every 30 minutes. BCAA ingestion resulted in significant improvement in cycle time to exhaustion compared with the placebo (153.1 ± 13.3 vs 137 ± 12.2 min). Cardiovascular responses (heart rate, mean arterial pressure) and thermoregulatory responses (skin and core body temperatures, sweat losses) and psychological measures of fatigue (rate of perceived exertion, ratings of perceived thermal sensations) did not differ between treatments (12).

BCAA and Protein Degradation During Exercise

◆ In a placebo-controlled study, 58 male runners consumed 7.5 to 12 g BCAA in a carbohydrate drink or a placebo (carbohydrate drink without BCAA) during endurance races (26 subjects participated in a 30-km [18.6-mile] cross-country race; 32 participated in a marathon [26.2-mile] race). In 17 of the subjects in the cross-country race and in 14 of the marathon runners, muscle biopsies were taken from the quadriceps 1 to 2 hours before the race and within 90 minutes (cross-country) or 50 minutes (marathon) after the completion of the race. Among subjects who took BCAA supplements, plasma and muscle concentrations of tyrosine and phenylalanine increased at slower rates after both races. The authors proposed that an intake of BCAA during exercise may prevent or decrease the net rate of protein breakdown caused by heavy exercise (13).

BCAA and Abdominal Fat

- In a controlled (not blinded) study, 25 competitive French wrestlers were randomly assigned to one of five diets for 19 days: (*a*) normocaloric diet—55% energy from carbohydrate, 12% energy from protein, 33% energy from fat; (*b*) hypocaloric diet— 55% carbohydrate, 12% protein, 33% fat; (*c*) hypocaloric diet enriched with 0.9 g/kg/day BCAA (51.9 g BCCA per 100 g protein)—60% carbohydrate, 20% protein, 20% fat; (*d*) hypocaloric, high-protein diet (6.1 g BCAA/100 g protein)—60% carbohydrate, 25% protein, 15% fat; or (*e*) hypocaloric, low-protein diet—60% carbohydrate, 15% protein, 25% fat. The normocaloric diet provided 40 kcal/kg/day, whereas the other diets were isocaloric, providing a daily energy intake 28 kcal/kg. Activity levels were not controlled during the study. All subjects on the hypocaloric diets demonstrated reductions in body weight and body fat (measured by magnetic resonance imaging and skinfold measurements). However, subjects on hypocaloric diets taking BCAA supplements showed significant losses of abdominal visceral adipose tissue and preservation of lean body mass compared with the other diet groups. There were no differences in aerobic and strength tests among groups (14).

- In a placebo-controlled (not blinded) study, 24 subjects with type 2 diabetes (mean age 45 years) were randomly assigned to one of four groups: (*a*) BCAA capsules providing 0.6 g BCAA/kg/day plus exercise (45 minutes cycling two times/week); (*b*) BCAA supplement without exercise; (*c*) isocaloric placebo and exercise; (*d*) placebo without exercise. All exercises were performed on a cycle ergometer supervised by researchers. After 2 months, BCAA supplementation had no effect on resting metabolic rate, VO_{2peak}. Abdominal fat (measured by magnetic resonance imaging) and glucose metabolism were not altered by BCAA supplementation (15).

BCAA and Hepatic Encephalopathy

- In a double-blind, randomized, placebo-controlled Italian study, 64 subjects with chronic hepatic encephalopathy consumed 0.24 g/day of BCAA or placebo (casein) for 3 months. In subjects who took BCAA, the index of portal-systemic encephalopathy improved significantly as did nitrogen balance and liver function tests (enzymes). Subjects in the casein group, when switched to receive BCAA, also showed similar significant improvements in liver function (16).

- A randomized, placebo-controlled study reported no clinical advantage of BCAA in treating hepatic encephalopathy. In this study, 65 subjects were randomly assigned to received 0.4 g BCAA per kg (with standard amino acids to equal 1.0 g/kg) or isocaloric glucose for a maximum of 16 days. Although negative nitrogen balance reversed in the BCAA group vs the glucose group, overall prognosis was poor and did not differ between groups (17).

- No recent well-designed studies have been conducted to pursue the role of BCAA for hepatic encephalopathy. Some practitioners suggest providing standard amino acids/protein as tolerated and provide a trial of BCAA if the individual cannot tolerate standard formulas.

BCAA and Anorexia in the Elderly

- Elderly subjects on hemodialysis (n = 44; 28 with anorexia and malnutrition, 16 well-nourished) participated in a placebo-controlled, double-blind study and were randomly assigned to 12 g BCAA per day or placebo. To enhance oral intake, subjects received counseling by an RD prior to the study's initiation. After 6 months, subjects were switched to the alternate intervention. The elderly subjects who were malnourished and had anorexia demonstrated a statistically significant increase in appetite, intake, protein status (albumin), and body weight after taking the BCAA supplement and demonstrated a significant reduction in the same parameters while taking the placebo supplement (6).

References

1. Davis JM. Carbohydrates, branched-chain amino acids and endurance: the central fatigue hypothesis. *Int J Sport Nutr.* 1995;5(Suppl):S29-S38.
2. Newsholme EA, Blomstrand E. The plasma level of some amino acids and physical and mental fatigue. *Experientia.* 1996;52:413–415.
3. Davis JM, Bailey SP. Possible mechanisms of central nervous system fatigue during exercise. *Med Sci Sports Exerc.* 1997;29:45–57.
4. Wolf L, Keutsch GT. Nutrition and infection. In: Shils ME, Olson JA, Shike M, Ross AC, eds. *Modern Nutrition in Health and Disease.* 9th ed. Baltimore, Md: Williams & Wilkins; 1999:1569–1588.
5. Kimball SR, Jefferson LS. Control of protein synthesis by amino acid availability. *Curr Opin Clin Nutr Metab.* 2002;5:63–67.
6. Hiroshige K, Sonta T, Suda T, et al. Oral supplementation of branched-chain amino acid improves nutritional status in elderly patients on chronic haemodialysis. *Nephrol Dial Transplant.* 2001;16:1856–1862.
7. Pennington JA. *Bowes & Church's Food Values of Portions Commonly Used.* 17th ed. Philadelphia, Pa: Lippincott-Raven Publishers; 1998.
8. Blomstrand E, Hassmen P, Ekblom B, et al. Administration of branched-chain amino acids during sustained exercise—effects on performance and on plasma concentration of some amino acids. *Eur J Appl Physiol.* 1991;63:83–88.
9. Madsen K, MacLean DA, Kiens B, et al. Effects of glucose, glucose plus branched-chain amino acids, or placebo on bike performance over 100 km. *J Appl Physiol.* 1996;81:2644–2650.
10. Blomstrand E, Hassmen P, Ek S, et al. Influence of ingesting a solution of branched-chain amino acids on perceived exertion during exercise. *Acta Physiol Scand.* 1997;159:41–49.
11. Blomstrand E, Hassmen P, Newsholme EA. Effect of branched-chain amino acid supplementation on mental performance. *Acta Physiol Scand.* 1991;143:225–226.
12. Mittleman KD, Ricci MR, Bailey SP. Branched-chain amino acids prolong exercise during heat stress in men and women. *Med Sci Sports Exerc.* 1998;30:83–91.
13. Blomstrand E, Newsholme EA. Effect of branched-chain amino acid supplementation on the exercise-induced change in aromatic amino acid concentrations in human muscle. *Acta Physiol Scand.* 1992;146:293–298.

14. Mourier A, Bigard AX, de Kerviler E, et al. Combined effects of caloric restriction and branched chain amino acid supplementation on body composition and exercise performance parameters in elite wrestlers. *Int J Sports Med.* 1997;18:47–55.
15. Mourier A, Gautier JF, de Kerviler E, et al. Mobilization of visceral adipose tissue related to the improvement in insulin sensitivity in response to physical training in NIDDM: effect of branched-chain amino acid supplements. *Diabetes Care.* 1997;20: 385–391.
16. Marchesini G, Dioguardi FS, Bianchi GP, et al. Long-term oral branched-chain amino acid treatment in chronic hepatic encephalopathy. A randomized double-blind casein-controlled trial. The Italian Multicenter Study Group. *J Hepatol.* 1990;11:92–101.
17. Vilstrup H, Gluud C, Hardt F, et al. Branched chain enriched amino acid versus glucose treatment of hepatic encephalopathy. A double-blind study of 65 patients with cirrhosis. *J Hepatol.* 1990;10:291–296.

Bromelain

Bromelain refers to proteases extracted from the stem and fruit of pineapple *(Ananas comosus)*. In addition to its proteolytic fraction, bromelain also contains peroxidase, acid phosphatase, protease inhibitors, and calcium. It has been used throughout Japan, Europe, and South America to treat inflammation and edema resulting from burns, trauma, and athletic injuries. Proposed mechanisms of action include direct or indirect effects on inflammatory mediators. Specifically, bromelain breaks down fibrin, an activator of proinflammatory prostaglandins responsible for clot formation and fluid accumulation. It may also stimulate the conversion of plasminogen to plasmin, causing an increase in fibrinolysis (1,2).

Media and Marketing Claims	Efficacy
Reduces allergic response and respiratory infections	↔
Reduces inflammation associated with osteoarthritis, joint pain, sore muscles	NR
Enhances antibiotic activity	NR
Prevents cancer	NR
Digestive aid	NR
Reduces platelet aggregation	NR

Safety

♦ Doses of up to 10 g/kg of bromelain in mice and rats had no teratogenic or carcinogenic effects. Dogs given 750 mg bromelain/kg body weight daily for 6 months showed no toxic effects (2).

Drug/Supplement Interactions

- Bromelain may increase blood levels of antibiotics, such as tetracycline, if administered at the same time (3–5).

- Although preliminary evidence suggests that bromelain may decrease platelet activity (6), there is no evidence that it increases bleeding time (2). Additional research is needed to thoroughly investigate this possibility. However, as a caution, individuals on anticoagulant therapy should not take bromelain supplements without the advice of their physician.

Key Points

- There is preliminary evidence from trials in the 1960s that bromelain has a beneficial effect on some, but not all, symptoms of sinusitis. In addition, some studies have suggested that bromelain may potentiate the action of antibiotics. However, there is not enough quality research to make therapeutic claims. Updated, well-designed clinical trials are needed.

- More research is needed to determine the anti-inflammatory properties of bromelain. The positive results reported in a few human studies from the 1960s need to be replicated in well-designed and adequately controlled trials.

- The ability of bromelain to increase antibiotic efficacy has not been sufficiently studied.

- At this time, there is no evidence from controlled human trials that bromelain prevents or treats cancer. In preliminary in vitro studies, bromelain and pancreatin, in combination with other enzymes, seem to slow tumor growth. These enzymes also seem to improve immune function in healthy individuals. Additional controlled research in humans is needed to verify its potential therapeutic benefit.

- Bromelain contains proteolytic enzymes, like those found in pancreatin, and may be useful in treating pancreatic insufficiency. However, the effect of bromelain on digestive function in healthy individuals has not been tested in controlled clinical trials (*see* Pancreatin).

- Bromelain seems to have antiplatelet aggregation activity, so individuals receiving anticoagulant therapy should be aware of the possible increased blood thinning effects.

Food Sources

Concentrated amounts of bromelain are found in pineapple stems, and smaller amounts are also found in the flesh of the fruit.

Dosage Information/Bioavailability

Bromelain is sold individually or in combination with other enzymes (pancreatin, papain, betaine, lactase, cellulase). Several different designations are used to describe the proteolytic activity of bromelain, but there is no scientific agreement about how to measure the proteolytic activity. Proteases in bromelain are tested to determine how fast they dissolve a protein such as gelatin or casein. Three common measures of activity are Rorer units (ru), gelatin-dissolving units (gdu), and milk-clotting units (mcu). One gram of bromelain standardized to 2,000 mcu activity is approximately equivalent to 1 g with 1,200 gdu of activity or 8 g with 100,000 ru of activity (3). Manufacturers recommend taking from 500 to 2,000 mg/day divided into three or four doses. However, because proteolytic activity is measured differently in various products, it is difficult to obtain a consistent, standard dose. Highly purified bromelain may have no activity (7).

There is limited research on the absorption and bioavailability of bromelain in humans. In one study of healthy male subjects, oral administration of bromelain (3 g) resulted in intestinal absorption as indicated by the presence of bromelain in the serum (8). In addition, the enzymatic activity of bromelain was maintained in the intestinal tract of mice for several hours after administration (9). Enteric-coating may be necessary to reduce the potential for diarrhea. In a rat study, bromelain was absorbed from the gastrointestinal tract after oral administration and was observable in serum 1 hour after ingestion (10).

Relevant Research

Many of the human studies of bromelain were completed in the 1960s and 1970s and lacked proper control, randomization, and appropriate statistical analysis. Some of these poorly designed trials are reported here because they are frequently cited to support media and marketing claims.

Bromelain and Sinusitis/Bronchitis Infections

- In a double-blind, placebo-controlled study completed in 1967, 49 subjects with sinusitis (age range 9 to 74 years) from one physician's private practice were randomly assigned to receive 160 mg bromelain (400,000 ru of proteolytic activity) or a placebo for 6 days. All subjects received standard, prescribed antibiotic medication for 6 days. Severity of symptoms was measured by the physician before and after treatment. There was a significant improvement in sinusitis symptoms (nasal discomfort, breathing difficulty, and pain), the mean duration of standard therapy required by subjects (9.9 vs 16.5 days), and the overall clinical rating among the subjects taking bromelain compared with the placebo. However, there were no statistical differences between groups for the resolution of edema and inflammation of the nasal mucosa or headache relief. There were no reported adverse effects (11).

- In a double-blind, placebo-controlled study completed in 1967, 48 subjects with moderate to severe sinusitis symptoms (ages 9 to 70 years) were given bromelain (400,000 ru of proteolytic activity) or a placebo for 6 days. Randomization of subjects to treatment was not clearly described in the article. All subjects were given standard therapy for sinusitis. Subjects were evaluated by a physician before, during, and at the end of the study. There were no differences between groups in symptoms of nasal discharge, breathing difficulty, headache, or overall clinical rating. However, subjects receiving bromelain (83%) had a significant reduction in nasal mucosal inflammation compared with the placebo (52%). Among subjects not taking antibiotics, there was a significant difference in complete resolution of nasal mucosal inflammation in the bromelain group (85%) compared with the placebo (40%), but no other significant differences were noted in the other parameters measured (12).

Bromelain and Inflammation/Joint Pain

- In a study of 77 healthy adults given either 200 or 400 mg of bromelain per day for 3 months, there was significant reduction in WOMAC knee health index, stiffness, physical function, and psychological well-being from baseline that seemed to be dose-dependent. However, the study was unblinded and not placebo-controlled. Given the improvement in psychological function, it is likely the positive response was related to participation in a clinical trial, during which subjects receive positive attention, rather than the effect of bromelain supplementation (13).

- A second study focused on subjects with pain of the elbow flexors (n = 40) after exercise. Subjects were randomly assigned to either a bromelain, ibuprofen, placebo, or control group. No differences in range of motion, perceived pain, or peak concentric torque measurements were seen across groups at any time point (1, 2, 3, or 4 days after exercise), indicating no clinical benefit of bromelain supplementation at 300 mg/day (14).

- Researchers induced muscle injury in 75 hamsters, after which they were given 10 mg/kg oral bromelain daily or no treatment for 14 days. The degree of muscle injury was evaluated using a measure of functional status—the maximum isometric tetanic force (P_o). The maximal force (P_o) of injured muscles returned to control levels in bromelain-treated hamsters but not in untreated animals. No adverse effects of bromelain were observed in noninjured skeletal muscle. The authors suggested that bromelain may have worked by inhibiting proinflammatory prostaglandins, the inflammatory mediator bradykinin, and oxygen free radicals, but these possibilities were not tested (15).

- In a double-blind, placebo-controlled study completed in 1960, 146 amateur boxers with bruises to the face and hematomas of the eye orbits, lips, ears, chest, and arms received 160 mg bromelain, divided into four doses, or a placebo for 14 days. At day 4, 78% of the subjects receiving bromelain were completely cleared of bruising compared with 15% in the placebo group. Statistical significance was not tested (16). Because statistical analyses were not performed, it is impossible to assess the degree to which the findings were likely attributable to chance alone.

- In a double-blind, controlled study completed in 1966, 154 surgical patients (76 of 154 subjects were children ages 4 to 12 years) were randomly assigned to receive 400 mg bromelain divided into four doses per day (proteolytic activity not specified) or no treatment (control). Bromelain was administered 1 day before and 4 days after facial plastic surgery. The type of surgical procedures and gender and age of adult subjects were not described. Surgeons evaluated postoperative edema/swelling on the first through the fourth postoperative day. There were no significant differences between groups in the number of postoperative infections, hematomas, or other complications that could affect swelling (17).

♦ In a double-blind, placebo-controlled trial completed in 1969, 73 subjects (age range 25 to 70 years) hospitalized for acute thrombophlebitis were randomly assigned to receive eight tablets of enteric-coated bromelain (1 tablet = 50,000 ru of proteolytic activity) or a placebo daily for 8 days in addition to standard medication. Subjects were examined daily and impressions were recorded of the severity of inflammation. Symptoms of inflammation (pain, edema, redness, tenderness, increased skin temperature, and disability) were also evaluated. At the end of the trial, a clinician rated each subject's overall condition. Although there was a trend toward mean improvement in all symptoms of inflammation in the bromelain group, only the symptom of redness reached statistical significance. Reduction of inflammation was better in the bromelain group than the group using the placebo; however, statistical analyses were not reported. No adverse effects were reported (18).

Bromelain and Antibiotic Activity

♦ Some Phase I pharmacokinetic studies (with limited numbers of subjects) have reported that bromelain increases the absorption of antibiotics, as documented by higher medication levels in blood, tissue, or urine (3–5); however, one study failed to show an increase in tetracycline levels with co-administration of bromelain (19).

Bromelain Effects on Platelet Aggregation

♦ No human studies have been published; however, in vitro and animal studies have shown that bromelain decreases platelet aggregation (2,7,20,21).

Bromelain (and Other Proteases) and Cancer

♦ In an ex vivo study, blood samples from healthy volunteers (n = 44) who were given single oral doses of a commercial preparation of combined proteolytic enzymes (33 mg pancreatin, 15 mg bromelain, 20 mg papain [papaya enzyme], 8 mg trypsin, and 0.3 mg chymotrypsin) were assessed. The polyenzyme preparation containing bromelain stimulated the production of tumor necrosis factor-α (TNF-α), interleukin-1ß, and interleukin-6 in peripheral-blood mononuclear cells of healthy donors. TNF-α has been identified as a stimulator of immune defense against tumor cells, but oral ingestion of this cytokine has been associated with toxicity (22).

♦ In a placebo-controlled study (not double-blind or randomized), 28 healthy subjects were given 10 to 20 tablets (dose not specified) of a commercial preparation of proteolytic enzymes (pancreatin, bromelain, papain, trypsin, and chymotrypsin), 8 subjects received placebo, and 16 subjects served as controls. Blood samples were drawn at 0, 2, 4, 6, and 8 hours after treatment. Enzyme treatment resulted in a time-dependent, significant increase in the release of reactive oxygen species (ROS) in polymorphonuclear neutrophils, the functional significance of which is unknown. However, ROS may mediate tumorcidal activity. (Note: ROS may also damage healthy tissues; however, this effect was not tested.) In the placebo and control subjects, there was no increase in ROS production. In an in vitro experiment within the same study, enzymes stimulated the cytotoxic capacity of polymorphonuclear cells against tumor cells (23).

References

1. Taussig SJ, Yokoyama MM, Chinen A, et al. Bromelain: a proteolytic enzyme and its clinical application. A review. *Hiroshima J Med Sci.* 1975;24:185–193.
2. Taussig SJ, Batki S. Bromelain, the enzyme complex of pineapple (Annas comosus) and its clinical application. An update. *J Ethnopharmacol.* 1988;22:191–203.
3. Tinozzi S, Venegoni A. Effect of bromelain on serum and tissue levels of Amoxycillin. *Drugs Exp Clin Res.* 1978;4:39–44.
4. Luerti M, Vignali ML. Influence of bromelain on penetration of antibiotics in uterus, salpinx, and ovary. *Drugs Exp Clin Res.* 1978;4:45–48.
5. Rimoldi R, Ginesu F, Giura R. The use of bromelain in pneumological therapy. *Drugs Exp Clin Res.* 1978;4:55–66.
6. Felton GE. Fibrinolytic and antithrombotic action of bromelain may eliminate thrombosis in heart patients. *Med Hypotheses.* 1980;6:1123–1133.
7. Taussig SJ. The mechanism of the physiological action of bromelain. *Med Hypotheses.* 1980;6:99–104.
8. Castell JV, Friedrich G, Kuhn CS. Intestinal absorption of undegraded proteins in men: presence of bromelain in plasma after oral intake. *Am J Physiol.* 1997;273: G139–G146.
9. Hale LP. Proteolytic activity and immunogenicity of oral bromelain within the gastrointestinal tract of mice. *Int Immunopharmacol.* 2004;4: 255–264.
10. White RR, Crawley EH, Vellini M, et al. Bioavailability of ^{125}I-bromelain after oral administration to rats. *Biopharm Drug Dispos.* 1988;9:397–403.
11. Seltzer AP. Adjunctive use of bromelains in sinusitis: a controlled study. *Eye Ear Nose Throat Mon.* 1967;46:1281–1288.
12. Ryan RE. A double-blind clinical evaluation of bromelains in the treatment of acute sinusitis. *Headache.* 1967;7:13–17.
13. Walker AF, Bundy R, Hicks SM, et al. Bromelain reduces mild acute knee pain and improves well-being in a dose-dependent fashion in an open study of otherwise healthy adults. *Phytomedicine.* 2002;9:681–686.
14. Stone MB, Merrick MA, Ingersoll CD, et al. Preliminary comparison of bromelain and Ibuprofen for delayed onset muscle soreness management. *Clin J Sport Med.* 2002;12: 373–378.
15. Walker JA, Cerny FJ, Cotter JR, et al. Attenuation of contraction-induced skeletal muscle injury by bromelain. *Med Sci Sports Exerc.* 1992;24:20–25.
16. Blonstein JL. Control of swelling in boxing injuries. *Practitioner.* 1964;193:334.
17. Gylling U, Rintala A, Taipale S, et al. The effect of a proteolytic enzyme combinate (bromelain) on the postoperative oedema by oral application. A clinical and experimental study. *Acta Chir Scand.* 1966;131:193–196.
18. Seligman B. Oral bromelains as adjuncts in the treatment of acute thrombophlebitis. *Angiology.* 1969;20:22–26.

19. Bradbrook ID, Morrison PJ, Rogers HJ. The effect of bromelain on the absorption of orally administered tetracycline. *Br J Clin Pharmacol.* 1978;6:552–554.
20. Metzig C, Grabowska E, Eckert K, et al. Bromelain proteases reduce human platelet aggregation *in vitro,* adhesion to bovine endothelial cells, and thrombus formation in rat vessels in vivo. *In Vivo.* 1999;13:7–12.
21. Glaser D, Hilberg T. The influence of bromelain on platelet count and platelet activity in vitro. *Platelets.* 2006;17:37–41.
22. Desser L, Rehberger A, Kokron E, et al. Cytokine synthesis in human peripheral blood mononuclear cells after oral administration of polyenzyme preparations. *Oncology.* 1993;50:403–407.
23. Zavadova E, Desser L, Mohr T. Stimulation of reactive oxygen species production and cytotoxicity in human neutrophils in vitro and after oral administration of a polyenzyme preparation. *Cancer Biother.* 1995;10:147–152.

Calcium

Calcium is well-known for its structural role in bones and teeth. Ninety-nine percent of the calcium in the body is found in the skeleton, with the remaining 1% in the blood, lymph, and other body fluids. As part of every cell, calcium also acts as a messenger directing cell function, hormone action, and nerve impulses. To consistently provide the calcium ions needed for these functions, serum calcium levels are closely regulated by calcitonin, parathyroid hormone, and vitamin D, which affect calcium transport in the intestine, bone, and kidney (1).

Bone density (calcium deposition) increases during the first 25 to 30 years of life and after that gradually decreases with age. In 1993, the FDA reviewed research demonstrating the benefit of supplemental calcium and approved the health claim for food and supplement labels stating that calcium reduces the risk of osteoporosis (2). The Food and Nutrition Board of the National Academy of Sciences (NAS) recently increased calcium recommendations to those set by the National Institutes of Health (NIH) Consensus Development Conference on Optimal Calcium Intake in 1994 (3). According to the new Dietary Reference Intakes (DRIs), the Adequate Intakes (AIs) for calcium for adolescents (ages 9 to 18 years), adults age 19 to 50, and adults older than 50 years are 1,300 mg, 1,000 mg, and 1,200 mg, respectively (4).

Media and Marketing Claims	Efficacy
Prevents osteoporosis; improves bone mineral density; reduces fracture risk	↑
Reduces blood pressure	↑?
Decreases colon cancer risk	↑?
Aids in weight control	↔
Reduces symptoms of PMS	↔

Safety

- The Tolerable Upper Intake level (UL) for calcium for adults is 2,500 mg/day (4). In controlled studies, constipation and bloating have been reported as adverse effects of excessive calcium intake. Doses exceeding 4,000 mg have been associated with increased blood calcium levels, severe renal damage, and ectopic calcium deposition (milk-alkali syndrome) (3).

- Calcium supplementation is not advisable for individuals with absorptive hypercalciuria, primary hyperthyroidism, renal insufficiency, or sarcoidosis (1,3).

- High calcium intakes may promote kidney stone formation in healthy people. However, some research suggests that a dietary calcium restriction could actually increase the risk of stone formation (5). There may be an increased risk of stones from calcium supplements in individuals with absorptive hypercalciuria (6). Calcium citrate has been suggested as the form to be used by individuals at risk for stone formation (7).

- High-calcium diets generally do not interfere with magnesium status in healthy individuals. However, low magnesium levels may occur if high doses of calcium are taken by individuals with poor renal function or conditions of magnesium depletion (diabetes, alcoholism, malabsorption). A calcium supplement providing 100 mg magnesium for every 500 mg calcium has been suggested for these conditions (8).

- In hyper- or hypophosphatemia, serum calcium levels must be balanced with serum phosphorus; use supplements with caution.

- Fiber components, such as phytic acid (wheat bran), oxalic acid (spinach and rhubarb), and uronic acid, can interfere with calcium absorption.

- High sodium intake increases urinary calcium excretion; in postmenopausal women, sodium chloride intake more than 2 g/day requires calcium intake of 1 g/day to prevent bone loss; sodium chloride intake more than 3 g/day requires calcium intake of 1.5 g/day.

Drug/Supplement Interactions

- Calcium may interfere with absorption of the following drugs: salicylates; bisphosphonates; tetracyclines; thyroid hormones (Synthroid, Levothroid); fluoroquinolones (ciprofloxacin); sotalol.

- Calcium competes for absorption with the following nutrients: fluoride, iron, zinc, and magnesium (9).

- The following drugs may interfere with calcium absorption: anticonvulsants; cholestyramine; corticosteroids; fluoroquinolones (ciprofloxacin); tetracyclines; mineral oil; stimulant laxatives.

- Calcium depletion may occur with chronic use of corticosteroids, laxatives (magnesium salts), anticonvulsants, aluminum salts (aluminum-containing antacids) unless used for hyperphosphatemia in chronic renal failure, loop diuretics (furosemide), high doses of levothyroxine (synthroid, levothyroid) used for suppressive therapy.

♦ High dosages of calcium increase the risk of milk alkali syndrome among those who use thiazide diuretics and among individuals with renal dysfunction (8).

Key Points

♦ There is substantial evidence linking calcium supplementation to increased bone mineral density (BMD) in the elderly and among adolescents. This relationship has been recognized by the NIH, National Academy of Science, and FDA. According to one review article, the increase in BMD from calcium supplementation could reduce fracture rates by as much as 50% (10). Among postmenopausal women, supplementation with 1,000 mg during the first year after menopause results in a 50% reduction in the rate (2% vs 1%) of normal bone loss, and 30 years of supplementation after menopause will increase bone density by 10% compared with women who did not take supplements, resulting in a 50% reduced risk of fracture in this age group (11). However, evidence from the Women's Health Initiative showed no significant reduction in fractures among postmenopausal women receiving calcuim supplementation.

♦ Calcium supplementation may cause a small reduction in systolic blood pressure, but not diastolic blood pressure, according to two meta-analyses. Control of systolic blood pressure is known to be the key clinical goal in reducing the morbidity and mortality associated with hypertension. However, a greater blood pressure reduction (systolic and diastolic) occurred in the Dietary Approaches to Stop Hypertension (DASH) study, in which subjects consumed a 25%-fat diet (low in saturated fat) rich in low-fat dairy products, fruits and vegetables, and whole grains. The mean daily dietary calcium intake in the DASH study was 1,265 mg.

♦ There is growing evidence that calcium (dietary and possibly supplemental) reduces the risk for colon cancer. One large study found a reduced risk of developing recurrent adenomas in subjects who took calcium supplements.

♦ Diets rich in low-fat dairy products may reduce risk for obesity or help promote weight loss in overweight subjects; to date, there is less evidence that calcium supplementation will have similar effects on weight loss.

♦ There is preliminary evidence that calcium supplementation may improve symptoms associated with PMS. Although more research is needed, the amount of calcium supplemented in these studies would be beneficial for women's health, regardless of whether it affects PMS.

♦ Individuals should be encouraged to meet their calcium requirements with dietary sources when possible. However, because it can be difficult for some people to consume enough calcium to meet the AI (particularly preadolescent and adolescent girls, the elderly, or those with lactose intolerance), supplements may be needed.

Food Sources

Food	Calcium, mg/serving
Milk, nonfat (1 cup)	302
Juice, orange (calcium-fortified) (6 oz)	200
Milk, whole (1 cup)	291
Yogurt, low-fat (1 cup)	314
Cheese, mozzarella, part skim (1 oz)	183
Tofu, raw (calcium-precipitated) (½ cup)	130
Almonds, dry-roasted (1 oz)	80
Kale, (½ cup)	47
Beans, garbanzo (½ cup)	40
Broccoli, (½ cup)	36
Beans, kidney (½ cup)	25
Egg (1)	25

Source: Data are from reference 12.

Dosage Information/Bioavailability

Calcium supplements are available in multivitamin/mineral supplements or in single preparations. Calcium is found in the form of calcium carbonate (the form used in antacids), citrate, citrate malate, phosphate, gluconate, lactate, calcium from dolomite (calcium magnesium carbonate), or bone meal. In 1981, the FDA issued a warning against using dolomite, bone meal, or oyster-shell calcium because of high levels of lead (13). Current DRIs suggest intake should not exceed 2,500 mg/day. Supplements typically provide 250 mg to 1,000 mg elemental calcium, often with added vitamin D and magnesium. If labels do not express calcium as "elemental," assume the elemental calcium is 40%, 21%, 13%, and 9% from carbonate, citrate, lactate, and gluconate, respectively (2) (ie, a label that states it supplies 1,000 mg calcium carbonate actually contains 400 mg elemental calcium).

In one study, subjects with achlorhydria absorbed calcium citrate more efficiently than carbonate supplements when taken on an empty stomach, but both types of supplement were equally absorbed when taken with a meal (14). Similarly, in healthy women, calcium citrate supplements were more bioavailable than carbonate when taken on an empty stomach (7,15). The NIH Consensus Statement reported that calcium absorption is most efficient at individual doses of 500 mg or less and when taken between meals in the form of calcium citrate (4). Homebound, institutionalized, or other individuals who lack exposure to the sun may require supplemental vitamin D to ensure adequate calcium absorption (3).

Calcium absorption can be affected by a variety of food factors. Foods high in oxalates (spinach) or phytates (wheat bran) have less available calcium than foods without these constituents (1). High-protein and/or high-sodium diets increase urinary calcium excretion (for each 50-g increment in dietary protein, 60 mg calcium is excreted in urine) but whether this results in reduced calcium nutriture has not been determined (1).

Relevant Research

Calcium and Bone Mineral Density/Osteoporosis

- In the Women's Health Initiative, a randomized, placebo-controlled clinical trial conducted among 36,282 postmenopausal women, daily supplementation with 100 mg elemental calcium (calcium carbonate) plus 400 IU vitamin D3 daily for a mean of 7 years was associated with 1.06% higher bone density at the hip, but no significant reduction in total, hip, or spinal fractures (16). However, when data excluded participants with low adherence to the study medication, hip fracture rates were reduced by a significant 29% with calcium and vitamin D supplementation. Of note, calcium supplementation was associated with an increased risk for kidney stones in this study.

- In a double-blind, placebo-controlled study, 240 postmenopausal women were randomly assigned to receive 1,000 mg elemental calcium as calcium carbonate plus 560 IU vitamin D3, or a placebo for 2 years. BMD of the lumbar spine increased significantly in calcium-supplemented subjects at 1 and 2 years. An insignificant trend of greater hip BMD was seen with calcium supplementation. There were no significant changes from baseline values noted in the BMD of the distal forearm in either group. The authors concluded: "A positive effect on BMD was demonstrated, even in a group of early postmenopausal women, with a fairly good initial calcium and vitamin D status" (17).

- In a placebo-controlled study, 60 older postmenopausal women were randomly assigned to receive one of three treatments for 2 years: (*a*) milk supplementation (4 cups, mean calcium intake = 1,028 mg/day); (*b*) 1,000 mg calcium carbonate divided into two doses (mean calcium intake = 1,633 mg/day); or (*c*) a placebo (mean dietary calcium intake = 683 mg/day). The placebo subjects had significant losses in their greater trochanteric (hip) BMD, whereas the calcium-supplemented group had no bone loss and showed a significant increase in spinal and femoral neck BMD. The dietary group sustained minimal losses from the greater trochanteric BMD, but this did not reach statistical significance. In all groups, serum 25-OH vitamin D levels decreased during the winter, and parathyroid hormone (PTH) levels increased. The authors concluded: "Calcium supplementation prevents bone loss in elderly women by suppressing bone turnover during the winter when serum 25-OH vitamin D decreases and serum PTH increases" (18).

- In a double-blind, placebo-controlled study, two groups of elderly women (older than 60 years), one with prevalent fractures (n = 94) and the other without (n = 103), were randomly assigned to receive 1,200 mg calcium as calcium carbonate or a placebo for a mean of 4 years. Annual lateral spine radiographs and semiannual forearm bone density were measured during 4.3 years. The subjects with fractures who took calcium supplements (15 of 53) had significantly fewer incident fractures than the subjects with fractures using the placebo (21 of 41). Calcium supplementation did not reduce the incidence rate of fractures in the subjects without fractures. In subjects with fractures, subjects who took calcium supplements had significantly greater forearm bone mass than did subjects in the placebo group. There were no statistical differences in subjects without fractures. The authors concluded that in elderly, postmenopausal women with spinal fractures and self-selected calcium intakes of less than 1,000 mg/day, a calcium supplement may reduce the incidence of spinal fractures and halt bone loss (19).

◆ In a placebo-controlled study, 389 subjects older than 65 years were randomly assigned to receive 500 mg calcium plus 700 IU vitamin D3/day or a placebo for 3 years. Compared with the placebo group, the subjects taking calcium plus vitamin D, there was a significantly greater BMD at the femoral neck and spine and total-body BMD after 1 year, which remained significant for total body BMD in the following 2 years after the intervention ended. Of the 37 subjects who experienced nonvertebral fractures during the study, significantly more were in the placebo group (n = 26) than the supplemented group (n = 11) (20).

◆ To determine whether BMD gains remained when calcium supplements were discontinued, subjects from the previous study (20) were followed up for 2 years. For the women, benefits in total body BMD or at any bone site did not last. After they stopped calcium supplementation, the men lost the supplement-induced increases in spinal and femoral neck BMD, but they did continue to show small benefits in total body BMD (21).

◆ In a double-blind, placebo-controlled trial, 84 elderly women (ages 54 to 74 years) more than 10 years after menopause were randomly assigned to receive 1,000 mg elemental calcium or a placebo daily for 4 years. BMD was assessed using dual-energy x-ray absorptiometry at 2 and 4 years. In the treatment group, 49 subjects did not continue after the first 2 years ("noncompliant"), and only 14 took the supplements for the entire duration of the study. The reasons for dropout were not clearly described. In the control group (mean calcium intake = 952 mg/day) BMD decreased significantly more than in the calcium-supplemented group (mean calcium = 1,988 mg/day) at all sites of the hip and ankle. After 2 years, BMD at the ankle decreased significantly more in the noncompliant group than in the supplement group. BMD in the spine was maintained in all groups during the 4 years (22).

◆ In a double-blind, placebo-controlled study of adolescent twins, one twin in each pair (42 female twin pairs, mean age 14 years) was randomly assigned to receive 1,000 mg calcium while the other twin received a placebo daily for 12 to 18 months. Compliance was similar in both groups (85% placebo, 83% calcium). At the end of the first 6 months, the twin taking the calcium had significantly greater BMD at the spine and hip., which stabilized throughout the remainder of the study. After 18 months, there was only a significant increase in BMD at the spine (23).

Calcium and Hypertension

◆ According to a meta-analysis of 22 randomized clinical trials testing the effect of calcium supplements (500 to 2,000 mg) on blood pressure in hypertensive and normotensive subjects (n = 1,231), pooled estimates showed a significant decrease in systolic blood pressure (−1.68 mm Hg) with calcium supplementation for subjects with hypertension. There was also a significant decrease in systolic blood pressure for the overall sample of normotensive and hypertensive subjects. There was no significant effect on diastolic blood pressure in either subgroup. The authors concluded: "The effect was too small to support the use of calcium supplementation for preventing or treating hypertension" (24).

◆ A study assessing the long-term effects of calcium on body weight and blood pressure (a substudy of an ongoing, double-blind, randomized, placebo-controlled trial of calcium supplementation in postmenopausal women) was conducted at a university medical center in New Zealand. The mean age of the 732 subjects was 74 years and the mean body weight was 67 kg. Baseline mean blood pressure was within normal limits. Subjects were randomly assigned to take either 1 g/day calcium (Citracal, Mission Pharmacal, San Antonio, TX) or placebo divided into two doses taken prior to meals. Results showed that calcium supplementation, but not dietary calcium, was associated with stable systolic blood pressure over 30 months whereas systolic blood pressure increased significantly in the placebo group over the same time period. Diastolic blood pressure, body weight, and percent body fat were not significantly different across groups at the end of 30 months of intervention. Regardless of baseline calcium intake, calcium supplementation did not results in a significant improvement in blood pressure at 30 months, although a trend toward improvement was shown among women with dietary calcium intake below 600 mg/day at baseline (25).

◆ A meta-analysis of 33 randomized, controlled trials (n = 2,412) that lasted at least 2 weeks tested the effect of calcium supplementation (800 to 2,000 mg) on blood pressure in normotensive and hypertensive subjects. The pooled analysis showed a significant reduction in systolic blood pressure and an insignificant reduction in diastolic blood pressure in subjects taking the calcium supplements (26).

◆ In a double-blind, placebo-controlled study, 193 men and women (ages 30 to 74 years) were randomly assigned to receive 1,000 to 2,000 mg/day of elemental calcium or placebo daily for 4 months (for cholesterol determinations) and 6 months (for blood pressure data). Serum total cholesterol, HDL cholesterol, and systolic and diastolic blood pressure were measured. There was no change in blood pressure until 6 months, when the mean systolic and diastolic blood pressure decreased by 0.5%, but this was not statistically significant. There was also a trend toward a 2% to 4% reduction in total cholesterol, but this was not statistically significant (27).

◆ While not a study of supplemental calcium, the DASH study (a randomized, multi-center trial) has shown dietary calcium intake to have clinical efficacy in terms of blood pressure control. In the DASH trial, 459 subjects with systolic blood pressure less than 160 mm Hg and diastolic blood pressure of 80 to 95 mm Hg were randomly assigned to one of three diets for 8 weeks: (*a*) control diet, low in fruits and vegetables and low-fat dairy products, and a fat content typical of the average diet in the United States (dietary fat = 37% of energy; mean dietary calcium intake = 443 mg); (*b*) diet rich in fruits and vegetables (dietary fat = 37% fat; mean calcium intake = 534 mg); or (*c*) combination diet rich in fruits and vegetables and low-fat dairy products and with reduced saturated fat and total fat (dietary fat = 25%; mean calcium intake = 1,265 mg). Subjects consumed lunch or dinner on-site on weekdays and picked up all other meals from the preparation site. Before the study, all subjects were fed control diets for 3 weeks. Sodium intake and body weight were maintained at constant levels. The combination diet resulted in a significant reduction in systolic (–5.0 mm Hg) and diastolic (–3.0 mm Hg) blood pressure compared with the control diet. The diet rich in fruits and vegetables resulted in a significant reduction of systolic (–2.8 mm Hg) and diastolic (–1.1 mm Hg) compared with the control diet. Among the 133 subjects with hypertension, the combination diet significantly reduced systolic and diastolic pressure by 11.4 and 5.5 mm Hg more, respectively, than did the control diet. Subjects without hypertension who consumed the combination diet also experienced significant reductions of systolic and diastolic blood pressure by 3.5 mm Hg and 2.1 mm Hg. The authors concluded that a diet rich in fruits, vegetables, and low-fat dairy foods and with reduced saturated and total fat can substantially reduce blood pressure (28). They found similar results when data were analyzed by subgroups (race, sex, age, BMI, years of education, income, physical activity, alcohol intake, and hypertension status) (29).

♦ One review of nine controlled studies and a meta-analysis of six controlled studies concluded that calcium supplementation during pregnancy seems to reduce the risk of pregnancy-induced hypertension, especially in women at high risk and in those with low dietary calcium intakes (6,30). There was no overall effect of calcium supplements on the risk of preterm delivery, although there was a significant reduction in risk in women classified as high risk for developing hypertension. Also, there was no evidence of any effect of calcium supplements on stillbirth or death before discharge from hospital (6).

Calcium and Colon Cancer

♦ In a pooled analysis of 10 cohort studies (total n = 534,536), 4,992 incident cases of colorectal cancer were diagnosed between 6 and 16 years of follow-up. Dietary calcium intake, milk intake, and total calcium intake (dietary plus supplemental) were all associated with a significantly reduced risk for developing colorectal cancer, regardless of age or gender. Daily consumption of 250 g milk reduced risk for colorectal cancer by 15%. Total calcium intake of more than 1,000 g/day (vs total intake less than 500 mg/day) was associated with a 24% reduction in risk of colorectal cancer. Assessment of dietary calcium intake was completed using validated instruments in all of these studies, but it is not clear that data on supplemental calcium intake were collected consistently across all studies or that validated instruments were always used. This study also showed that the risk reduction improved to a 22% reduced risk when dietary *and* supplemental sources of calcium were combined in the analysis to show a "synergistic" effect (31). The role of supplemental calcium alone was not analyzed, and thus it is not known whether dietary and supplemental calcium had similar protective effects in this study.

♦ A Cochrane systematic review assessed the effect of supplementary calcium on the development of colon cancer and adenomatous polyps in humans. Only two studies (total n = 1,346 subjects) were included. These studies were randomized, controlled trials providing 1,200 or 2,000 mg supplemental calcium daily for 3 to 4 years. The reviewers concluded that, although the data from these two trials suggested that calcium supplementation may contribute moderate protection against adenomatous polyps, these data do not constitute sufficient evidence to warrant the recommendation of calcium supplementation for the prevention of colorectal cancer (32).

♦ The effect of calcium supplementation (vs placebo) on adenoma recurrence in the colon was assessed in 803 of 930 subjects randomly assigned in a double-blind fashion. Mean age was 61 years and the majority (> 70%) of subjects were men. Calcium supplementation was provided in the form of 3.0 g calcium carbonate providing 1.2 g elemental calcium daily for a period of 4 years. If subjects had low vitamin D status, calcium supplementation was not associated with reduced risk of adenoma recurrence, but if subjects had normal vitamin D nutriture, calcium supplementation reduced risk of recurrence by 29% (33).

♦ Data from the large prospective Nurses' Health Study and the Health Professionals' Follow-up Study from Harvard University suggest that calcium intake more than 1,250 mg/day vs less than 500 mg/day was associated with a 35% reduction in risk of distal colon cancer. Sex-specific protection could not be determined because the total number of cases was not large enough to distinguish sex-specific significance. This analysis was based on reported intake of dietary calcium, and calcium supplement users were excluded from the analysis (34).

♦ In a double-blind, placebo-controlled study, 930 subjects (mean age 61 years) with a recent history of colorectal adenoma were randomly assigned to receive 1,200 mg elemental calcium as calcium carbonate or a placebo daily, with follow-up colonoscopies 1 and 4 years after study entry. Risk ratios for adenoma recurrence were adjusted for age, sex, lifetime number of adenomas before the study, clinical center, and length of surveillance period. Subjects in the calcium supplement arm of the study had a significantly reduced risk of recurrent adenomas compared with subjects in the placebo arm. The adjusted risk ratio of the mean number of adenomas in the calcium group compared with that in the placebo group was 0.76. The effect of calcium was independent of initial dietary fat and calcium intake (35).

♦ According to a review of five uncontrolled trials, nine small-scale trials, and three large-scale randomized trials, calcium supplementation does not seem to substantially reduce colorectal epithelial cell proliferation rates (biomarker for increased risk of colon cancer) in humans, but it may normalize the distribution of proliferating cells within colon crypts where new colon cells evolve. All of the uncontrolled trials indicated significant decreases in cancer cell proliferation rates, whereas the controlled studies reported conflicting results (36).

Calcium and Weight Control

♦ A review article described a possible mechanism for a protective role of dietary calcium in adiposity. The authors hypothesize that dietary calcium reduces levels of circulating calcitriol, which decreases the level of intracellular calcium in the fat cell, thus stimulating fat breakdown (lipolysis) (37).

◆ A randomized, placebo-controlled weight-loss intervention (500 kcal/day energy deficit) was conducted among 32 obese adults assigned to (*a*) energy deficit alone, (*b*) energy deficit plus 800 mg calcium supplementation, or (*c*) energy deficit and 1,200 to 1,300 mg dietary calcium plus placebo. All three groups lost weight: subjects in the diet-only group lost 6.4% of initial body weight, compared with 8.6% weight loss for the supplement group and 10.9% weight loss for the high–dietary dairy group (38). Reductions in body fat and truncal fat were also enhanced in the supplement group and even more so in the dietary calcium group as compared with energy restriction alone.

◆ In a double-blind, placebo-controlled study, 100 overweight or obese women were randomly assigned to receive either 1,000 mg elemental calcium or placebo daily. After 25 weeks of energy restriction, there were no significant differences in body weight or fat mass between groups. The placebo group lost a mean of 6.2 kg body weight whereas the calcium supplemented group lost 7.0 kg body weight, this difference was not statistically significant (39).

Calcium and PMS

◆ A case-control study within the prospective Nurses' Health Study II cohort assessed a subset of 2,966 women who reported that they had been given a physician diagnosis of PMS during the previous 10 years of the Nurses' Health Study and 2,570 who reported that they had not received such a diagnosis. These women were then mailed the Calendar of PMS Experiences, which includes 26 PMS symptoms, to more objectively identify subjects with PMS. From their responses, 1,057 subjects with PMS (35.6% of those who reported a diagnosis) were identified, as well as 1,968 control subjects (78.6% of those who had not reported a diagnosis. Analysis of the diet information from a food-frequency questionnaire showed that women in the highest quintile of total vitamin D intake (median: 706 IU/day) had a 41% lower risk for developing PMS diagnosis (95% CI = 0.40–0.86) compared with those in the lowest quintile (median: 112 IU/day) (P for trend = .01). Calcium intake from food was also inversely related to PMS: compared with women with a low intake (median: 529 mg/day), participants with the highest intake (median: 1,283 mg/day) had a relative risk of 0.70 (95% CI = 0.50–0.97); (P = .02 for trend). Nonfat or low-fat milk consumption was also associated with a lower risk of PMS (P < .001) (40).

◆ In a prospective, double-blind, placebo-controlled study, 466 premenopausal women (ages 18 to 45 years) were randomly assigned to receive 1,200 mg elemental calcium (as calcium carbonate) or a placebo daily for three menstrual cycles. Subjects recorded symptoms and adverse effects daily, and underwent routine blood and urine analysis. The primary outcome measure was a 17-parameter symptom complex score. There were no differences in age, weight, height, oral contraceptive use, or menstrual length between groups. There were also no differences in the initial screening symptom complex score of the luteal, menstrual, or intermenstrual phase between groups. During the luteal phase of the treatment cycle, mean symptom complex score was significantly less in the calcium group for the third menstrual cycles.

The authors concluded: "Calcium supplementation is a simple and effective treatment in premenstrual syndrome, resulting in a major reduction in overall luteal phase symptoms" (41).

◆ In a double-blind, placebo-controlled, crossover study, 33 women with a history of recurrent PMS symptoms received in random order 1,000 mg calcium carbonate (400 mg elemental calcium) or a placebo daily for 3 months each. Efficacy was determined prospectively by measuring changes in daily symptom scores throughout a 6-month period and retrospectively by an overall global assessment. There was a significant reduction in daily PMS scores during calcium treatment during the luteal and menstrual phases, but not during the intermenstrual phase. Premenstrual factors (negative affect, water retention, pain) and pain during menstruation were significantly improved for those taking calcium supplements. When subjects were asked to assess effectiveness retrospectively, 73% reported fewer symptoms with calcium, 15% reported fewer symptoms with the placebo, and 12% reported no differences between treatments (42).

References

1. Weaver CM, Heaney RP. Calcium. In: Shils ME, Olson JA, Shike M, Ross AC, eds. *Modern Nutrition in Health and Disease.* 9th ed. Baltimore, Md: Williams & Wilkins; 1999:141–155.
2. Food and Drug Administration. Food labeling: health claims; calcium and osteoporosis. *Federal Register.* 1993;58:2665–2681.
3. National Institutes of Health. Optimal calcium intake. *NIH Consens Statement.* 1994;12:1–31.
4. Institute of Medicine. *Dietary Reference Intakes: Calcium, Phosphorus, Magnesium, Vitamin D, and Fluoride.* Washington, DC: National Academy Press; 1997.
5. Curhan GC. Dietary calcium, dietary protein, and kidney stone formation. *Miner Electrolyte Metab.* 1997;23:261–264.
6. Atallah AN, Hofmeyr GJ, Duley L. Calcium supplementation during pregnancy for preventing hypertensive disorders and related problems. *Cochrane Database Syst Rev.* 2000;2:CD001059.
7. Harvey JA, Kenny P, Poindexter J, et al. Superior calcium absorption from calcium citrate than calcium carbonate using external forearm counting. *J Am Coll Nutr.* 1990;9:583–587.
8. Heaney RP. Calcium supplements: practical considerations. *Osteoporos Int.* 1991;1:65–71.
9. Cook JD, Dassenko SA, Whittaker P. Calcium supplementation: effect on iron absorption. *Am J Clin Nutr.* 1991;53:106–111.
10. Reid IR. The roles of calcium and vitamin D in the prevention of osteoporosis. *Endocrinol Metab Clin North Am.* 1998;27:389–398.
11. Chiu KM. Efficacy of calcium supplements on bone mass in postmenopausal women. *J Gerontol.* 1999;54:M275-M280.

12. Pennington JAT. *Bowes and Church's Food Values of Portions Commonly Used.* 17th ed. Philadelphia, Pa: Lippincott-Raven Publishers; 1998.

13. Whiting SK, Wood R, Kim K. Calcium supplementation. *J Am Acad Nurse Pract.* 1997;9:187–192.

14. Recker RR. Calcium absorption and achlorhydria. *N Engl J Med.* 1985;313:70–73.

15. Levenson DI, Bockman RS. A review of calcium preparations. *Nutr Rev.* 1994;52: 221–232.

16. Jackson RD, LaCroix AZ, Gass M, et al. Calcium plus vitamin D supplementation and risk of fractures. *New Engl J Med.* 2006;354:669–683.

17. Baeksgaard L, Andersen KP, Hyldstrup L. Calcium and vitamin D supplementation increases spinal BMD in healthy, postmenopausal women. *Osteoporos Int.* 1998;8: 255–260.

18. Storm D, Eslin R, Porter ES, et al. Calcium supplementation prevents seasonal bone loss and changes in biochemical markers of bone turnover in elderly New England women: a randomized placebo-controlled trial. *J Clin Endocrinol Metab.* 1998;83: 3817–3825.

19. Recker RR, Hinders S, Davies KM, et al. Correcting calcium nutritional deficiency prevents spine fractures in elderly women. *J Bone Miner Res.* 1996;11:1961–1966.

20. Dawson-Hughes B, Harris SS, Krall EA, et al. Effect of calcium and vitamin D supplementation on bone density in men and women 65 years of age or older. *N Engl J Med.* 1997;337:670–676.

21. Dawson-Hughes B, Harris SS, Krall EA, et al. Effect of withdrawal of calcium and vitamin D supplements on bone mass in elderly men and women. *Am J Clin Nutr.* 2000;72:745–750.

22. Devine A, Dick IM, Heal SJ, et al. A 4-year follow-up study of the effects of calcium supplementation on bone density in elderly postmenopausal women. *Osteoporos Int.* 1997;7:23–28.

23. Nowson CA, Green RM, Hopper JL, et al. A co-twin study of the effect of calcium supplementation on bone density during adolescence. *Osteoporos Int.* 1997;7:219–225.

24. Allender PS, Cutler JA, Follman D, et al. Dietary calcium and blood pressure: a meta-analysis of randomized clinical trials. *Ann Intern Med.* 1996;124:825–831.

25. Reid IR, Horne A, Mason B, et al. Effects of calcium supplementation on body weight and blood pressure in normal older women: a randomized controlled trial. *J Clin Endocrinol Metab.* 2005;90:3824–3829.

26. Bucher HC, Cook RJ, Guyatt GH, et al. Effects of dietary calcium supplementation on blood pressure. A meta-analysis of randomized controlled trials. *JAMA.* 1996;275:1016–1022.

27. Bostick RM, Fosdick L, Grandits GA, et al. Effect of calcium supplementation on serum cholesterol and blood pressure. A randomized, double-blind, placebo-controlled, clinical trial. *Arch Fam Med.* 2000;9:31–39.

28. Appel LJ, Moore TJ, Obarzanek E, et al. A clinical trial of the effects of dietary patterns on blood pressure. DASH Collaborative Research Group. *N Engl J Med.* 1997;336: 1117–1124.

29. Svetkey LP, Simons-Morton D, Vollmer VM, et al. Effects of dietary patterns on blood pressure: subgroup analysis of the Dietary Approaches to Stop Hypertension (DASH) randomized clinical trial. *Arch Intern Med.* 1999;159:285–293.
30. Villar J, Belizan JM. Same nutrient, different hypotheses: disparities in trials of calcium supplementation during pregnancy. *Am J Clin Nutr.* 2000;71(5 Suppl): 1375S–1379S.
31. Cho E, Smith-Warner SA, Spiegelman D, et al. Dairy foods, calcium, and colorectal cancer: A pooled analysis of 10 cohort studies. *J Natl Cancer Inst.* 2004;96:1015–1022.
32. Weingarten MA, Zalmanovici A, Yaphe J. Dietary calcium supplementation for preventing colorectal cancer and adenomatous polyps. *Cochrane Database Syst Rev.* 2004;1:CD003548.
33. Grau MV, Baron JA, Sandler RS, et al. Vitamin D, calcium supplementation, and colorectal adenomas: results of a randomized trial. *J Natl Cancer Inst.* 2003;95:1765–1771.
34. Wu K, Willett WC, Fuchs CS, et al. Calcium intake and risk of colon cancer in women and men. *J Natl Cancer Inst.* 2002;94:437–446.
35. Baron JA, Beach M, Mandel JS, et al. Calcium supplements for the prevention of colorectal adenomas. Calcium Polyp Prevention Study Group. *N Engl J Med.* 1999;340:101–107.
36. Bostick RM. Human studies of calcium supplementation and colorectal epithelial cell proliferation. *Cancer Epidemiol Biomarkers Prev.* 1997;6:971–980.
37. Zemel MB, Miller SL. Dietary calcium and dairy modulation of adiposity and obesity risk. *Nutr Rev.* 2004;62:125–131.
38. Zemel MB, Thompson W, Milstead A, et al. Calcium and dairy acceleration of weight and fat loss during energy restriction in obese adults. *Obes Res.* 2004;12:582–590.
39. Shapses SA, Heshka S, Heymsfield SB. Effect of calcium supplementation on weight and fat loss in women. *J Clin Endocrinol Metab.* 2004;89:632–637.
40. Bertone-Johnson ER, Hankinson SE, Bendich A, et al. Calcium and vitamin D intake and risk of incident premenstrual syndrome. *Arch Intern Med.* 2005;165:1246–1252.
41. Thys-Jacobs S, Starkey P, Bernstein D, et al. Calcium carbonate and the premenstrual syndrome: effects on premenstrual and menstrual symptoms. Premenstrual Syndrome Study Group. *Am J Obstet Gynecol.* 1998;179:444–452.
42. Thys-Jacobs S, Ceccarelli S, Bierman A, et al. Calcium supplementation in premenstrual syndrome: a randomized crossover trial. *J Gen Intern Med.* 1989;4:183–189.

Carnitine (L-Carnitine)

Synthesized in the body from lysine and methionine, L-carnitine is a short-chain carboxylic acid containing nitrogen. It plays a central role in fatty acid metabolism by transporting long-chain fatty acids into mitochondria for beta oxidation. L-carnitine also affects the metabolism of acetyl-coenzyme-A. Approximately 95% of the body's carnitine stores are located in skeletal and cardiac muscle.

Carnitine has not been considered essential because low dietary intakes are compensated for by increased synthesis and limited renal clearance. Although not essential in healthy individuals, carnitine becomes conditionally essential when carnitine function is impaired, as in congenital deficiency, defects in liver or kidney function, certain inborn errors of metabolism, or increased catabolism. The FDA has approved L-carnitine supplementation for treatment of deficiencies associated with end-stage renal disease and certain inborn errors of metabolism. Carnitine deficiency is associated with muscle weakness, cardiomyopathy, and fatty acid accumulation (1). Different molecules of carnitine have been studied. L- and propionyl-L-carnitine have been examined for their effects on the heart, and acetyl-L-carnitine has been investigated for its potential neurological effects.

Media and Marketing Claims	Efficacy
Improves heart health	↑?
Improves athletic perfromance	NR
Increases energy in people with chronic fatigue syndrome or cancer	NR
Improves mental function in Alzheimer's disease	NR
Improves thyroid function	NR
Reduces male infertility	↔
Improves immune function	NR
Assists weight reduction	NR

Safety

- No serious adverse effects have been reported with L-carnitine dosages ranging from 0.5 to 6 g/day. Larger dosages have been associated with nausea and diarrhea (2).
- In the cited studies, only L-carnitine, propionyl L-carnitine, and acetyl L-carnitine hydrochloride were used. The safety, bioavailability, and efficacy of other forms of L-carnitine available as dietary supplements may differ. The D- or DL-carnitine forms may be associated with impaired exercise performance (3), and the D-carnitine form competes with L-carnitine for absorption, possibly leading to L-carnitine deficiency.
- Avoid L-carnitine in hypothyroidism; L-carnitine may inhibit thyroid hormone activity.

Drug/Supplement Interactions

- Some drugs may deplete body stores of L-carnitine, including valproic acid (anticonvulsant), pivalic acid–containing drugs (antibiotic), doxorubicin (chemotherapeutic agent), zidovudine (AZT) for HIV infection, carbamazepene (Tegretol), phenobarbital, and phenytoin (Dilantin).

- Transport of L-carnitine may be competitively inhibited by D-carnitine; avoid use of D- or DL-carnitine.

- L-carnitine increases the effects of the anticoagulant acenocoumarol (Sintrom), which is similar to warfarin (Coumadin) but is shorter acting; there is insufficient evidence that the interaction also occurs with warfarin.

Key Points

- Excellent reviews of the current evidence regarding the kinetics, pharmacokinetics, and health benefits of L-carnitine are provided in the November 2004 issue of *Annals of the New York Academy of Sciences.*

- Additional research is needed to evaluate the role of L-carnitine supplementation on cardiovascular outcomes/disorders such as ischemia, myocardial infarction, peripheral vascular disease, congestive heart failure, and arrhythmias. Benefits for cardiomyopathy are promising.

- Athletes do not seem to have increased needs for carnitine and are not at risk for carnitine deficiency. The small studies that have been published have reported no improvements in exercise performance with L-carnitine supplementation.

- Supplemental carnitine provides "extra" energy only if a true clinical carnitine deficiency exists. Deficiency is associated with muscle weakness, cardiomyopathy, and dysfunctional fat metabolism. There is no evidence that L-carnitine supplementation in healthy individuals improves energy or enhances fat loss. However, in individuals with chronic fatigue syndrome (CFS), there is some evidence that reduced serum carnitine levels are related to symptoms, and one preliminary study suggested that carnitine supplementation may be beneficial for people with CFS. Additional research is needed to verify these findings. One small study evaluated carnitine supplementation for cancer-related fatigue and showed a significant improvement in self-reported symptoms of fatigue.

- Studies of L-carnitine for Alzheimer's disease are conflicting, with little indication of efficacy.

- L-carnitine supplementation seems to reduce the symptoms of hyperthyroidism, but more studies are needed.

- Sperm motility may be increased in infertile males during L-carnitine supplementation when combined with acetyl-L-carnitine supplementation and use of NSAIDs, but data are insufficient to date.

- Studies suggest that people with AIDS often present with carnitine deficiency. Preliminary trials suggest that L-carnitine may improve some parameters of immune function in individuals with AIDS. Several open trials (not discussed here) have reported patient improvements. At this time, no studies have tested the effects of carnitine supplements on the morbidity and/or mortality in these individuals.

- Studies testing L-carnitine for weight loss are limited and, to date, do not support this use.

Food Sources

Carnitine is found mainly in meat—specifically red meats—and dairy products. Very small amounts are found in fruits, vegetables, grains, and eggs. The average nonvegetarian diet provides approximately 100 mg to 300 mg carnitine/day.

Food	Carnitine, mg/Serving
Beef, ground, raw (4 oz)	106
Milk, whole (1 cup)	8
Codfish (3 oz)	4.7
Chicken breast, raw (½ breast)	3.3
Ice cream (½ cup)	2.5
Cheese, American (2 oz)	2.1
Asparagus (½ cup)	0.1
Bread, whole-wheat (1 slice)	0.1

Source: Data are calculated from reference 1.

Dosage Information/Bioavailability

Carnitine is sold in capsules or tablets in the form of L-carnitine or propionyl-L-carnitine. An esterified form, acetyl-L-carnitine, is also sold as a supplement. Carnitine is also available as a prescription drug for the treatment of carnitine deficiency resulting from clinically diagnosed metabolic disorders. Most studies used 2 to 4 g L-carnitine divided into two or three doses. Supplemental carnitine increases plasma levels but also increases renal clearance of carnitine (1). The bioavailability/absorption of a 2-g dose is approximately 16% of the oral dose and decreases as the dose increases (4). Muscle carnitine content is increased after long-term supplementation, but not with supplementation lasting less than 2 weeks (5). There is preliminary evidence that supplemental choline maintains carnitine status by reducing urinary carnitine excretion (6). In contrast, valproic acid (anticonvulsant) and drugs containing pivalic acid (antibiotic) negatively affect carnitine status in humans (1).

Relevant Research

Carnitine and Cardiovascular Disorders

◆ Animal studies and clinical trials have suggested that carnitine supplementation may have potential benefits in various cardiovascular disorders, including ischemia, myocardial infarction, peripheral vascular disease, congestive heart failure, arrhythmias, and cardiotoxicity associated with anthracyclin therapy. In subjects with systemic carnitine deficiency, carnitine administration has been shown to reverse cardiomyopathy (7,8).

♦ Eighty subjects with heart failure caused by dilated cardiomyopathy were randomly assigned to receive 2 g L-carnitine or a placebo daily for about 3 years. There were no statistical differences between groups at baseline examination or in hemodynamic parameters, exercise tests, peak oxygen intake, arterial and pulmonary blood pressure, or cardiac output. After a mean of 33.7 months, 70 subjects were in the study (33 in the placebo group, 37 in the carnitine group). At the time of analysis, 63 subjects were alive (six deaths occurred in the placebo group and one death in the carnitine group). Analysis showed that survival rate was significantly higher among subjects taking carnitine supplements (9).

♦ In a study of 94 subjects with newly diagnosed type 2 diabetes and hypercholesterolemia who were randomly assigned to either 1 g L-carnitine twice per day or placebo for 6 months, supplementation with carnitine significantly reduced plasma lipoprotein a Lp(a) levels as compared with baseline (at 3 or 6 months) and as compared with placebo at 6 months. However, no significant differences were demonstrated for other cardiovascular or anthropometric variables including body weight, BMI, fasting glucose, plasma insulin, triglycerides, A1C, total cholesterol, apo A-I, or apo B, suggesting that the significant difference seen with Lp(a) may have been related to statistical chance (10).

♦ In a double-blind, placebo-controlled study, 245 subjects with intermittent claudication were randomly assigned to receive 1 g propionyl-L-carnitine or a placebo for 6 months. Only 187 subjects completed the study (87 in the carnitine group and 102 in the placebo group) because of lack of compliance and other unspecified reasons. The study was preceded by a 2-week run-in period to assess maximal walking distance and allow for washout of medications used for claudication. Quality of life (physical, emotional, social) as measured by the McMaster Health Index Questionnaire revealed a small but statistically significant improvement with carnitine compared with placebo. In subjects with a maximal walking distance less than 250 meters at baseline, physical function was significantly improved, but not in subjects walking more than 250 meters at baseline (11). One review article criticized this study for failing to use intention-to-treat analysis and for the high dropout rate of subjects (12).

♦ In a double-blind, placebo-controlled study, 155 subjects with claudication were randomly assigned to receive 2 g propionyl-L-carnitine or a placebo daily for 6 months. Subjects were assessed at baseline and months 3 and 6 using a graded treadmill test and a questionnaire on functional status. Subjects taking carnitine significantly increased their maximal walking time by 54% as compared with a 25% increase for those taking the placebo. Subjects taking carnitine also significantly improved in walking distance and walking speed, and functional status was enhanced compared with the placebo (13).

♦ In a double-blind, placebo-controlled trial, 101 subjects with suspected myocardial infarction were randomly assigned to receive 2 g L-carnitine or a placebo daily for 28 days. When compared with the placebo group, subjects taking carnitine supplements had a significant reduction in mean infarct size, assessed by cardiac enzymes and electrocardiographic tests, serum aspartate transaminase and lipid peroxides, and lactate dehydrogenase (day 6 postinfarction). Angina pectoris, heart failure plus left ventricular enlargement, and total arrhythmias were significantly less in the carnitine group. The authors concluded: "It is possible that L-carnitine supplementation in patients with suspected acute myocardial infarction may be protective against cardiac necrosis and complications during the first 28 days" (14).

Carnitine and Exercise Performance

◆ Several theories may explain the potential for carnitine to improve physical performance. An increase in carnitine from dietary supplements may increase fatty acid oxidation, thus sparing glycogen and glucose. L-carnitine may affect the acetyl CoA:CoA ratio by enhancing conversion of pyruvate to acetyl CoA. This would decrease lactic acid production, thereby improving exercise performance (5).

◆ In a double-blind, placebo-controlled, crossover study, 14 healthy male subjects were randomly assigned to receive an acute dose of intravenous L- carnitine (185 µmol/kg) or a placebo 2 hours before starting three different bicycle ergometer protocols, separated by 1-month washout periods. Each exercise protocol was done twice in random order, once with the placebo and once with carnitine. Carnitine administration had no effect on muscle carnitine content, respiratory exchange ratio, muscle lactate accumulation, plasma lactate concentration, muscle glycogen utilization, or plasma ß-hydroxybutyrate concentration during exercise. The authors concluded that muscle carnitine is segregated from large shifts in the plasma carnitine pool, and that short-term administration of carnitine has no significant effect on fuel metabolism during exercise (15).

◆ In a randomized, double-blind, placebo-controlled, crossover study, 20 collegiate swimmers completed a control trial of swim sprints, followed by a week of daily supplementation with 4 g L-carnitine in a citrus drink or a placebo drink. After the week of supplementation, subjects completed a second sprint trial. The treatment group had elevated serum carnitine levels and free and short-chain serum carnitine fractions compared with the placebo but no differences in blood pH, lactate, or base excess were seen between the two groups. There were no differences between trials or between groups on sprint performance time. The authors concluded: "L-carnitine supplementation does not provide an ergogenic benefit during repeated bouts of high-intensity anaerobic exercise in highly-trained swimmers" (16).

Carnitine and Fatigue in Cancer or Chronic Fatigue Syndrome

◆ In an open-label Phase I study, the effects of various dosages of carnitine on plasma carnitine levels were assessed in 13 subjects with cancer and demonstrated carnitine deficiency. Subjects reported significant fatigue, depression, sleep disruption, and overall reduced functional status at baseline, and after taking supplemental L-carnitine daily for 1 week, their fatigue, depression, and sleep disruption scores all improved significantly over baseline measures. However, overall functional status did not change. Dose was variable across subjects. Currently the investigative group is following up with a randomized, double-blind, placebo-controlled trial that will have adequate number of subjects to statistically test this hypothesis (17).

♦ In an open-label study comparing acetylcarnitine, or propionylcarnitine, or combination (2 g/day for 24 weeks) among 90 subjects with chronic fatigue syndrome (CFS), acetylcarnitine supplementation resulted in a significant improvement in mental fatigue (Stroop attention concentration score) compared with baseline, whereas propionylcarnitine was associated with a significant improvement in general fatigue score (Multidimensional Fatigue Inventory). Subjects receiving the combination therapy less frequently reported improvements in symptoms. Fatigue scores were worse in all groups when measured 2 weeks after discontinuing supplementation. Pain scores were not modulated by carnitine supplementation (18). This study is among the largest completed to date; however, the open-label approach and lack of placebo group reduce the validity of the study.

♦ Decreased carnitine levels have previously been reported in subjects with CFS (19–21). However, more recent controlled trials have reported normal blood and urine carnitine levels in subjects with CFS (22–24).

♦ In a parallel-design, crossover (not blinded) study, 30 subjects clinically diagnosed with CFS were given, in random order, 3 g L-carnitine or 100 mg amantadine (a medication used to treat fatigue in multiple sclerosis) for 2 months each, with a 2-week washout period. Subjects were assessed before, during, and after treatment. All subjects underwent detailed clinical evaluation including the Fatigue Severity Scale (FSS), the Beck Depression Inventory (BDI), the Symptom Checklist 90-R consisting of multiple psychological test categories and general summary scales (SCL-90-R), and the CFS Impairment Index (CFS-II), which consists of physical and mental subsets. The degree of improvement in each of the psychometric parameter studies (total of 18) was calculated by subtracting the baseline results from the 8-week results. Amantadine was poorly tolerated (only 50% of the subjects completed all 8 weeks). In those who completed 8 weeks of amantadine treatment, there was no significant change in any of the clinical parameters measured. After 4 weeks of L-carnitine treatment, 5 of 18 outcome measures showed a significant improvement. After 8 weeks, L-carnitine treatment resulted in a significant clinical improvement in 12 of the 18 studied parameters. No statistical comparison between L-carnitine and amantadine was done (25).

Acetyl-L-Carnitine and Alzheimer's Disease

♦ In a double-blind, placebo-controlled study, 431 subjects older than 50 years with mild to moderate probable Alzheimer's disease (AD) were randomly assigned to receive 3 g acetyl-L-carnitine hydrochloride or a placebo divided into three doses daily for 1 year. Eighty-three percent of the subjects completed the trial. The Alzheimer's Disease Assessment Scale cognitive component and the Clinical Dementia Rating Scale were used to assess participants every 3 months. Overall, both treatments were associated with the same rate of decline on tests. However, subanalysis (comparing early-onset subjects [age 65 years or younger] to late-onset subjects [older than 66]) revealed an insignificant trend for early-onset subjects taking carnitine to decline more slowly than early-onset patients on placebo. Early-onset subjects as a whole tended to decline more rapidly than did older subjects in the placebo group. Conversely, late-onset/older subjects taking carnitine supplements tended to decline more rapidly than did early-onset subjects on carnitine. The authors concluded: "A subgroup of AD patients aged 65 or younger may benefit from treatment with acetyl-L-carnitine, whereas older individuals may do more poorly" (26).

- In a double-blind, placebo-controlled trial, 30 subjects with mild to moderate probable AD were randomly assigned to receive acetyl-L-carnitine hydrochloride (2.5 g/day for 3 months, followed by 3 g/day for 3 months) or a placebo. Subjects were given tests of memory, language, and visuospatial and constructional abilities, and the level of carnitine was measured in cerebrospinal fluid. After 6 months, there was significantly less deterioration in timed cancellation tasks and Digit Span (a test of the number of digits a person can recall and repeat in sequence) and an insignificant trend toward less deterioration in the timed verbal fluency task in subjects taking carnitine. No differences were found in any other neurological tests. A subgroup with the lowest baseline scores and who received carnitine had significantly less deterioration on the verbal memory test and a significant increase in cerebrospinal fluid levels of carnitine compared with the placebo group. The authors concluded: "Acetyl L-carnitine may retard the deterioration in some cognitive areas in patients with AD" (27).

- In a double-blind, placebo-controlled, multicenter study, 130 individuals diagnosed with AD were randomly assigned to receive 2 g acetyl-L-carnitine or a placebo divided into four doses or a placebo daily for 1 year. Fourteen outcome measures were used to assess functional and cognitive impairment. After 1 year, both groups worsened, but the group who took carnitine had a slower rate of deterioration in 13 of the 14 outcome measures, reaching statistical significance for the Blessed Dementia Scale, logical intelligence, ideomotor and buccofacial apraxia, and selective attention. After results were adjusted for initial scores, the subjects who took carnitine had better scores on all outcome measures compared with subjects in the placebo group, reaching statistical significance for the Blessed Dementia Scale, logical intelligence, verbal critical abilities, long-term verbal memory, and selective attention (28).

- In a double-blind, placebo-controlled study, 229 subjects, age 45 to 65 years, with a diagnosis of probable AD were randomly assigned to receive 3 g acetyl-L-carnitine or a placebo divided into three doses daily for 1 year. Primary outcome measures were the Alzheimer's Disease Assessment Scale and the Clinical Dementia Rating Scale. Overall, there were no significant differences between groups on the change from baseline to endpoint. There were no differences in incidence of adverse effects between groups (29).

L-Carnitine and Thyroid Function

- L-carnitine is a naturally occurring thyroid hormone antagonist. A double-blind, placebo-controlled crossover study was conducted among 50 women with hyperthyroid disease who were taking levothyroxine (4). Symptoms (palpitations, anxiety, nervousness, etc) and biochemical parameters of thyroid function worsened during periods of placebo and improved with on L-carnitine supplementation of 2 or 4 g/day. The authors concluded that L-carnitine supplementation at either dosage could prevent or reverse symptoms of hyperthyroidism (30). Additional well-designed trials are needed.

L-Carnitine and Male Infertility

◆ L-carnitine is concentrated in epididymis and spermatozoa and plays a key role in sperm respiration and motility. Sperm counts and motility correlate with carnitine nutriture (31).

◆ Male infertility has been related to select disorders in mitochondrial function. Whether carnitine supplementation can overcome this defect has not been explored. In a study of 30 subjects with male infertility (asthenozoospermia), individuals were given placebo for 3 months, followed by a 3-month intervention of 2 g L-carnitine per day. Sperm health measures were taken at baseline, after placebo, and after carnitine treatment. Results showed that only subjects with normal mitochondrial function were responsive to L-carnitine supplementation, showing a significant increase in sperm motility above baseline and placebo levels (32). The mixed efficacy results from other trials may be related to the inclusion of infertile men with mitochondrial dysfunction.

◆ A placebo-controlled, randomized study of L-carnitine combined with L-acetyl-carnitine among 60 men with either low sperm count, reduced sperm motility, or atypical sperm was conducted to determine if supplementation would reduce infertility measures. Fifty-six subjects completed the study that randomly assigned men to either 2 g L-carnitine plus 1 g L-acetyl-carnitine or placebo daily for 2 months. Sperm count, motility, and form significantly improved in men receiving the supplement, with the greatest difference shown in forward motility in those men with the lowest motility levels at baseline (33).

◆ Ninety-eight men with inflammation of the prostatovesicular anatomy and increased seminal white counts leading to infertility were randomly assigned to receive (*a*) 1 g carnitine for 4 months, (*b*) an NSAID for 4 months, (*c*) an NSAID for 2 months followed by carnitine for 2 months, or (*d*) combined therapy for 4 months. Carnitine alone had little effect on semen count, sperm motility, production of reactive oxygen species in sperm, or pregnancy outcomes, whereas the group who took NSAIDs for 2 months followed by carnitine for 2 months had the greatest improvement in fertility measures (34). Further research is warranted.

Carnitine and Immune Function/AIDS

◆ Reduced levels of serum carnitine have been reported in individuals with AIDS who are treated with zidovudine (AZT) (35).

◆ In a randomized, placebo-controlled study, 20 men with advanced AIDS and normal serum levels of carnitine were treated with 6 g L-carnitine or a placebo daily for

2 weeks. Serum and peripheral blood mononuclear cell (PBMC) carnitine levels, CD4 cell counts, serum triglycerides, and lymphocyte proliferation to mitogen stimulation were measured at baseline and at the end of the study. Concentrations of total carnitine in PBMC in subjects with AIDS were less than levels in healthy control subjects. Compared with baseline, cellular carnitine content increased significantly and lymphocyte proliferative responsiveness to mitogens improved in subjects who took carnitine supplements. There was also a significant reduction in serum triglycerides compared with baseline (36).

Carnitine and Weight Loss

- ◆ In a double-blind, placebo-controlled study, 36 moderately overweight premenopausal women were pair-matched for BMI and randomly assigned to receive 4 g L-carnitine (divided into two doses) or placebo daily for 8 weeks. All subjects walked for 30 minutes at 6% to 70% maximum heart rate 4 days per week. Body composition, resting energy expenditure (REE), and substrate utilization were estimated before and after treatment. There were no significant changes in mean total body mass, fat mass, and resting lipid utilization. REE increased significantly for all subjects, but no difference was observed between treatments. Five of the carnitine subjects experienced nausea and diarrhea and consequently dropped out of the study (37).

References

1. Rebouche CJ. Carnitine. In: Shils ME, Olson JA, Shike M, Ross AC, eds. *Modern Nutrition in Health and Disease.* 9th ed. Baltimore, Md: Williams & Wilkins; 1999: 505–512.
2. Wiseman LR, Brogden RN. Propionyl-L-carnitine. *Drugs Aging.* 1998;12:243–248.
3. Watanabe S, Ajisaka R, Masuoka T, et al. Effects of L- and DL-carnitine on patients with impaired exercise tolerance. *Jpn Heart J.* 1995;36:319–331.
4. Harper P, Elwin CE, Cederblad G. Pharmacokinetics of intravenous and oral bolus doses of L-carnitine in healthy subjects. *Eur J Clin Pharmacol.* 1988;35:555–562.
5. Kanter MM, Williams MH. Antioxidants, carnitine, and choline as putative ergogenic aids. *Int J Sport Nutr.* 1995;5(Suppl):S120-S131.
6. Dodson WL, Sachan DS. Choline supplementation reduces urinary carnitine excretion in humans. *Am J Clin Nutr.* 1996;63:904–910.
7. Atar D, Spiess M, Mandinova A, et al. Carnitine—from cellular mechanisms to potential clinical applications in heart disease. *Eur J Clin Invest.* 1997;27:973–976.
8. Pauly DF, Pepine CJ. The role of carnitine in myocardial dysfunction. *Am J Kidney Dis.* 2003;41(Suppl):S35-S43.
9. Rizos I. Three-year survival of patients with heart failure caused by dilated cardiomyopathy and L-carnitine administration. *Am Heart J.* 2000;139(2 Pt 3):S120-S123.
10. Derosa G, Cicero AF, Gaddi A, et al. The effect of L-carnitine on plasma lipoprotein(a) levels in hypercholesterolemic patients with type 2 diabetes mellitus. *Clin Ther.* 2003;25:1429–1439.

11. Brevetti G, Perna S, Sabba C, et al. Effect of propionyl-L-carnitine on quality of life in intermittent claudication. *Am J Cardiol.* 1997;79:777–780.
12. Deckert J. Propionyl-L-carnitine for intermittent claudication. *J Fam Pract.* 1997;44: 533–534.
13. Hiatt WR, Regensteiner JG, Creager MA, et al. Propionyl-L-carnitine improves exercise performance and functional status in patients with claudication. *Am J Med.* 2001;110:616–622.
14. Singh RB, Niaz MA, Agarwal P, et al. A randomized, double-blind, placebo-controlled trial of L-carnitine in suspected acute myocardial infarction. *Postgrad Med J.* 1996;72:45–50.
15. Brass EP, Hoppel CL, Hiatt WR. Effect of intravenous L-carnitine on carnitine homeostasis and fuel metabolism during exercise in humans. *Clin Pharmacol Ther.* 1994;55:681–692.
16. Trappe SW, Costill DL, Goodpaster B, et al. The effects of L-carnitine supplementation on performance during interval swimming. *Int J Sports Med.* 1994;15:181–185.
17. Cruciani RA, Dvokin E, Homel P, et al. L-carnitine supplementation for the treatment of fatigue and depressed mood in cancer patients with carnitine deficiency: a preliminary analysis. *Ann N Y Acad Sci.* 2004;1033:168–176.
18. Vermeulen RC, Scholte HR. Explanatory open label, randomized study of acetyl-and propionylcarnitine in chronic fatigue syndrome. *Psychosom Med.* 2004;66:276–282.
19. Kuratsune H, Yamaguti K, Lindh G, et al. Low levels of serum acylcarnitine in chronic fatigue syndrome and chronic hepatitis C, but not seen in other diseases. *Int J Mol Med.* 1998;2:51–56.
20. Kuratsune H, Yamaguti K, Takahashi M, et al. Acylcarnitine deficiency in chronic fatigue syndrome. *Clin Infect Dis.* 1994;18(Suppl 1):S62-S67.
21. Plioplys AV, Plioplys S. Serum levels of carnitine in chronic fatigue syndrome: clinical correlates. *Neuropsychobiology.* 1995;32:132–138.
22. Soetekouw PM, Wevers RA, Vreken P, et al. Normal carnitine levels in patients with chronic fatigue syndrome. *Neth J Med.* 2000;57:20–24.
23. Soetekouw PM, Wevers RA, Vreken P, et al. Normal carnitine levels in patients with chronic fatigue syndrome. *Neth J Med.* 2000;57:20–24.
24. Jones MG, Goodwin CS, Amjad S, et al. Plasma and urinary carnitine and acylcarnitines in chronic fatigue syndrome. *Clin Chim Acta.* 2005;360:173–177.
25. Plioplys AV, Plioplys S. Amantadine and L-carnitine treatment of chronic fatigue syndrome. *Neuropsychobiology.* 1997;35:16–23.
26. Thal LJ, Carta A, Clarke WR, et al. A one-year multicenter placebo-controlled study of acetyl-L-carnitine in patients with Alzheimer's disease. *Neurology.* 1996;47: 705–711.
27. Sano M, Bell K, Cote L, et al. Double-blind parallel design pilot study of acetyl levocarnitine in patients with Alzheimer's disease. *Arch Neurol.* 1992;49:1137–1141.
28. Spagnoli A, Lucca U, Menasce G, et al. Long-term acetyl-L-carnitine treatment in Alzheimer's disease. *Neurology.* 1991;41:1726–1732.
29. Thal LJ, Calvani M, Amato A, et al. A one year controlled trial of acetyl-L-carnitine in early onset Alzheimer's disease. *Neurology.* 2000;55:805–810.

30. Benvenga S, Ruggeri RM, Russo A, et al. Usefulness of L-carnitine, a naturally occurring peripheral antagonist of thyroid hormone action, in iatrogenic hyperthyroidism: a randomized, double-blind, placebo-controlled clinical trial. *J Clin Endocrinol Metab.* 2001;86:3579–3594.

31. Ng CM, Blackman MR, Wang C, et al. The role of carnitine in the male reproductive system. *Ann N Y Acad Sci.* 2004;1033:177–188.

32. Garolla A, Maiorino M, Roverato A, et al. Oral carnitine supplementation increases sperm motility in asthenozoospermic men with normal sperm phospholipid hydroperoxide glutathione peroxidase levels. *Fertil Steril.* 2005;83:355–361.

33. Lenzi A, Sgro P, Salacone P, et al. A placebo-controlled double-blind randomized trial of the use of combined l-carnitine and l-acetyl-carnitine treatment in men with asthenozoospermia. *Fertil Steril.* 2004;81:1578–1584.

34. Vicari E, La Vignera S, Calogero AE. Antioxidant treatment with carnitines is effective in infertile patients with prostatovesiculoepididymitis and elevated seminal leukocyte concentrations after treatment with nonsteroidal anti-inflammatory compounds. *Fertil Steril.* 2002;78:1203–1208.

35. Mintz M. Carnitine in human immunodeficiency virus type 1 infection/acquired immune deficiency syndrome. *J Child Neurol.* 1995;10(Suppl 2):S40-S44.

36. De Simone C, Famularo G, Tzantzoglou S, et al. Carnitine depletion in peripheral blood mononuclear cells from patients with AIDS: effect of oral L-carnitine. *AIDS.* 1994;8:655–660.

37. Villani RG, Gannon J, Self M, et al. L-carnitine supplementation combined with aerobic exercise does not promote weight loss in moderately obese women. *Int J Sport Nutr Exerc Metab.* 2000;10:199–207.

Cat's Claw *(Uncaria tomentosa)*

A high-climbing woody vine, cat's claw grows extensively in the Amazon regions of Peru, Columbia, and Ecuador. The useable parts of the vine are the bark and root. Thorns located on the base of the leaves allow the vine to climb and create a canopy, thus the name "cat's claw." Cat's claw has been used in the Amazon for hundreds of years to treat autoimmune disorders and gastrointestinal problems. There are more than 10 species of cat's claw; *Uncaria tomentosa* is the species that is most commonly imported to the United States.

Media and Marketing Claims	Efficacy
Reduces inflammation associated with rheumatoid arthritis or osteoarthritis	NR
Antioxidant properties	NR

Safety

- The *Uncaria tomentosa* species of cat's claw is generally considered safe, with only minor side effects of stomach upset or diarrhea.
- *Acacia greggi* is also sold as cat's claw, but it is not the same, and it is highly toxic.
- Cat's claw has been safely used for up to 6 months (1).
- Acute renal failure has been reported in an individual with systemic lupus erythematosus (2).

Drug/Supplement Interactions

- Because it may have an additive effect, cat's claw should not be taken with antihypertensive or anticoagulant medications.
- Although direct evidence is not available, cat's claw—especially that of the *Unicaria tomentosa* species with tetracyclic alkaloid content—may augment the effects of immunosuppressive drug therapies whereas the pentacyclic form may counteract the immunosuppressive effects.

Key Points

- Due to the increased interest in cat's claw in the past 25 years, the country of Peru has given it protective status to prevent overharvesting and protect the integrity of the plant species.
- Preliminary evidence from two human studies suggests that cat's claw may improve clinical measures of pain in subjects with osteoarthritis or rheumatoid arthritis (3,4). However, much more controlled research is needed before recommendations can be made.
- Animal and cell culture studies suggest that cat's claw has antioxidant properties. Human studies are lacking.

Food Sources

None

Dosage Information/Bioavailability

The optimal dosage is not known, but one study (3) found 100 mg/day orally to be effective in the treatment of osteoarthritis. For clinical trials, *Uncaria guianensis* (cat's claw bark) is more commonly used than *Unicaria tomentosa*. In South America, *Uncaria guianensis* and *Unicaria tomentosa* are considered interchangeable. However, *Unicaria tomentosa* has two separate subspecies: one comprised predominantly of pentacyclic alkaloids associated with immune stimulation and the other containing tetracyclic alkaloids, which affect central nervous system function and may counteract immune stimulatory effects. The pentacyclic form (containing at least 1.3% pentacyclic alkaloids) of *Unicaria tomentosa* should be recommended over other forms of cat's claw.

A common plant found in the United States, *Acacia greggi*, is sometimes marketed as cat's claw, but it is not and it may be toxic.

Relevant Research

Cat's Claw and Rheumatoid Arthritis or Osteoarthritis

- In a prospective, multicenter, randomized, placebo-controlled, double-blind study conducted among 45 subjects with symptomatic osteoarthritis of the knee (requiring anti-inflammatory medications for at least 3 months), subjects were randomly assigned in a 2:1 ratio to either 100 mg aqueous extraction of freeze-dried *Unicaria guianensis* (plus excipient) or placebo following a 7-day washout from all medications for osteoarthritis (3). Pain was assessed at rest, at night, and with physical activity, along with biological markers of disease severity. At the end of treatment, only the cat's claw group showed an improvement in pain associated with activity, and both physicians and subjects reported significant improvements in symptom scores for those receiving cat's claw compared with placebo. Pain at night and at rest and knee circumference did not change significantly above baseline in either group, nor did tumor necrosis factor α or prostaglandin E 2 production. Studies with larger sample sizes are warranted.

- In a double-blind, randomized, placebo-controlled trial, 40 subjects (older than 20 years) being treated with sulfasalazine or hydroxychloroquine for treatment of rheumatoid arthritis (as defined by the College of Rheumatology Criteria for rheumatoid arthritis to include those with Steinbrocher Functional Class II or III) were given cat's claw extract or placebo in the first phase (24 weeks) of the two-phase study. Dosage for this study was 20 mg acid-extracted dry extract of *Radix Uncaria tomentosa* three times daily. In the second phase, all subjects received the extract for a period of 28 weeks. No washout period was described between the two treatment phases. Subjects received no steroid injections for 4 weeks before or during the study. Two subjects, one from each group, dropped out of the study due to adverse events (not described). Although both groups showed clinical improvement over time, subjects receiving the cat's claw extract during the first phase reported significantly fewer painful joints as compared with those receiving the placebo (53% reduction vs 24%). During phase two, subjects had fewer painful and swollen joints as well as reductions in the Ritchie Index (4).

- The anti-inflammatory activity of cat's claw extracts was assessed using the carrageenan-induced paw edema model in mice, analysis of nuclear factor (NF)—κB activity, and cyclooxygenase activity. A spray-dried hydroalcoholic extract and an aqueous freeze-dried extract significantly and dose-dependently decreased carrageenan-induced paw edema compared with controls, with the hydroalcoholic extract being the more potent. The hydroalcoholic extract was also more effective in the inhibition of NF-κB. Both extracts had weak and nonsignificant inhibitory activity against cyclooxygenase 1 and 2 (5).

◆ Extracts of cat's claw were fed to male mice for 8 days before ozone exposure to determine whether this could reduce the inflammatory effects of ozone on lung tissue in mice. Compared with untreated control mice, mice pretreated with cat's claw extract had significantly less lung inflammation as shown by lower levels of protein in bronchoalveolar lavage fluid, less epithelial necrosis, and fewer polymorphonuclear cells in the bronchiolar lumen (6).

Cat's Claw As an Antioxidant

◆ Antioxidant properties of cat's claw have been characterized in cell culture models using radical scavenging assays that quantify antioxidant capacity. This study tested the inflammatory marker production using an in vivo model of gastric inflammation to which cat's claw was added. It was found that non-alkaloid High Performance Liquid Chromatography fractions from cat's claw decreased lipopolysaccharide (LPS)–induced TNFα and nitrite formation by a specific cell line called RAW 264.7. Likewise, pretreatment with oral cat's claw was protective against indomethacin-induced gastritis in vivo (7). Whether these same anti-inflammatory and antioxidant effects will be demonstrated in vivo and in human clinical trials remains to be shown.

References

1. Keplinger K, Laus G, Wurm M, et al. *Uncaria tomentosa* (Wild.) DC—ethnomedicinal use and new pharmacological, toxicological, and botanical results. *J Ethnopharmacol.* 1999;64:23–34.
2. Hilepo JN, Bellucci AG, Mossey RT. Acute renal failure caused by "cat's claw" herbal remedy in a patient with systemic lupus erythematosus. *Nephron.* 1997;77:361.
3. Piscoya J, Rodriguez Z, Bustamante SA, et al. Efficacy and safety of freeze-dried cat's claw in osteoarthritis of the knee: mechanisms of action of the species *Uncaria guianensis*. *Inflamm Res.* 2001;50:442–448.
4. Mur E, Hartig F, Eibl G, et al. Randomized double-blind trial of an extract from the pentacyclic alkaloid-chemotype of *Uncaria tomentosa* for the treatment of rheumatoid arthritis. *J Rheumatol.* 2002;29:678–681.
5. Aguilar JL, Rojas P, Marcelo A, et al. Anti-inflammatory activity of two different extracts of *Uncaria tomentosa* (Rubiaceae). *J Ethnopharmacol.* 2002;81:271–276.
6. Cisneros FJ, Jayo M, Niedziela L. An *Uncaria tomentosa* (cat's claw) extract protects mice against ozone-induced lung inflammation. *J Ethnopharmacol.* 2005;96:355–364.
7. Sandoval M. Anti-inflammatory and antioxidant activities of cat's claw (*Uncaria tomentosa* and *Uncaria guianensis*) are independent of their alkaloid content. *Phytomedicine.* 2002;9:325–337.

Chitosan

Chitosan is an amino polysaccharide that has a chemical structure similar to the dietary fiber cellulose. It differs from other fibers in that it contains an amino group. Chitosan is derived by the deacetylation of chitin that is naturally found in the exoskeleton of insects and crustaceans and in the cell walls of fungi. Chitosan cannot be hydrolyzed by human digestive enzymes. When solubilized in acid environments such as the gastrointestinal tract, chitosan has a positive charge and binds with negatively charged molecules such as fat and bile. Because of its ability to bind with lipids, chitosan has been promoted in the dietary supplement industry as a weight-loss aid and cholesterol-lowering agent. It has also been investigated as a food and feed additive, a cationic agent for waste or water treatment, and for use in biomedical and pharmaceutical materials (1–4).

Media and Marketing Claims	Efficacy
Promotes weight loss by reducing absorption of dietary fat	↓?
Reduces lipid levels for heart disease prevention	↔
Reduces plaque formation on teeth	NR

Safety

- There are no long-term controlled trials in humans testing the safety of chitosan supplements.

- Although chitosan is a fiber, it is plausible that a residual protein could remain in a chitosan product derived from shellfish. Therefore, it may be prudent for individuals with allergies to shellfish to avoid chitosan products.

- Chitosan binds with fat and may reduce the absorption of fat-soluble vitamins and minerals. In one study of rats fat a high-fat diet with large amounts of chitosan for 2 weeks, chitosan caused a decrease in mineral absorption and bone mineral content compared with rats fed high-fat diets containing cellulose or glucosamine. Chitosan also reduced serum vitamin E levels in this study (5).

- Individuals with malabsorption disorders should avoid using chitosan because it may aggravate symptoms and could potentially exacerbate nutrient deficiencies (6).

- In one study, 800 mg chitosan increased serum triglycerides in normocholesterolemic obese subjects (7).

- A possible adverse effect of long-term intake of chitosan is that it may negatively alter the normal intestinal flora, thus affecting lipid and bile acid metabolism and promoting the growth of intestinal pathogens (6).

- Chitosan may reduce serum cholesterol, urea, and creatinine, and increase hemoglobin in individuals on hemodialysis.

Drug/Supplement Interactions

- Chitosan decreases absorption of fat-soluble vitamins and minerals.
- Chitosan may interfere with absorption of medications that bind with dietary fibers.

Key Points

- Research regarding the role of chitosan in weight control, particularly via reduced absorption of dietary fat, is conflicting and generally does not suggest a clinically relevant effect. More efficacy and safety data from controlled trials lasting longer than 6 months are needed to determine the effect of chitosan on weight control.
- Preliminary data from animal and human studies are conflicting with regard to the potential cholesterol-lowering effect of chitosan. However, in one human study, chitosan reduced LDL cholesterol, had no effect on HDL cholesterol, and increased triglyceride levels. More information is needed to determine the exact effect that chitosan may have on lipid control and whether it is safe for long-term use.
- Chitosan interferes with the absorption of some vitamins and minerals. Therefore, the long-term consequences of supplemental chitosan on bone health, nutrient deficiencies, growth, and malabsorption syndromes need to be determined.
- More research is needed to determine the effect of a chitosan mouth rinse on reducing plaque formation and its role in improving overall dental health.

Food Sources

None in significant quantities. Chitosan is derived from exoskeleton of shellfish.

Dosage Information/Bioavailability

Chitosan is sold in capsules providing approximately 500 mg of chitosan, with manufacturers recommending a dosage of 1,500 mg/day. Labels suggest taking chitosan with meals, especially fatty foods.

Relevant Research

Chitosan and Weight Loss

- In a well-designed, randomized, controlled weight-loss study with 250 overweight adult subjects, chitosan supplementation of 3 g/day resulted in small but significant improvements in weight loss (8). All subjects received weight-loss counseling, half were randomly assigned to receive the daily chitosan supplement, and half received a placebo. The study was conducted for 24 weeks. Supplementation was associated with a mean reduction in body weight of 0.4 kg, whereas the placebo group gained 0.2 kg. An intention-to-treat analysis was used.

◆ In a meta-analysis, researchers summarized data from five randomized, double-blind, placebo-controlled trials examining chitosan supplementation for weight loss. None of the studies was cited in searchable databases; all were retrieved by contacting one manufacturer. All of the studies were done in Italy, had nearly identical designs, and were published in the same Italian peer-reviewed journal during a 2-year period. Each study administered chitosan or a placebo in addition to a hypocaloric diet for 28 days, and all reported significantly greater weight loss with chitosan. Content of chitosan tablets was not described; the study noted only that four tablets per day were supplemented. Pooled results from these trials suggest a significant and clinically relevant reduction of body weight in overweight individuals on a hypocaloric diet. In addition, in three of the trials, chitosan was associated with reductions in blood lipids. However, the authors of the meta-analysis raised some concerns about the study designs and potential bias in that all studies were supported by one manufacturer. The researchers concluded that the clinical effectiveness of chitosan for weight control needs to be confirmed by independent, rigorous trials (9).

◆ In a double-blind, placebo-controlled study, 34 overweight subjects (28 women, 6 men) were randomly assigned to receive four capsules of chitosan (1,000 mg total) or a placebo daily for 28 days. Subjects were told to maintain their normal diet and keep a detailed food diary. Measurements (weight, height, blood pressure, blood samples, and quality of life) were taken at baseline, day 14, and day 28 of the study. At the end of the study, there were no significant differences between groups on weight, BMI, blood pressure, total cholesterol, triglycerides, serum beta carotene, vitamin A, vitamin D3, or vitamin E. An analysis of the chitosan capsules was performed and revealed that they contained 42% chitosan, less than the 71% (250 mg) stated by the distributor (10).

◆ One proposed hypothesis, which has not been tested, is that chitosan may bind to dietary fat, thereby reducing absorption. In a study measuring fecal fat excretion among 12 adults consuming a standard diet followed by diet plus 2.5 g chitosan supplementation per day, fecal fat excretion increased by 1.8 g/day with supplementation. This level of increased fecal fat excretion is likely clinically insignificant and may account for the negative results of larger trials looking at modulation of body weight and/or lipid levels (11).

◆ In a randomized, open-label, two-period crossover study, the effects of chitosan and orlistat on fecal fat excretion were compared in 12 healthy adults. After an initial 1 week wash-out period, subjects were randomly assigned to 890 mg chitosan (Fat Binder, East Anglia Pharmaceuticals, UK) or 120 mg orlistat three times daily for 7 days and then switched over to a 7-day intervention with the alternate agent (chitosan or orlistat). All subjects followed a weight maintenance diet with 30% of energy from fat (83 g/day) and 300 mg cholesterol daily throughout the 21-day study (12). Orlistat resulted in a significant increase in fecal fat excretion. However, chitosan had no effect. No placebo group was included, and there was no washout between treatments. Thus, the validity of the study is limited.

Chitosan and Cholesterol

- Microcrystalline chitosan was used in a randomized controlled trial evaluating the effect of chitosan on lipid levels in healthy adults. One hundred thirty subjects with mild abnormalities in lipid levels were randomly assigned to receive a placebo for 1 month, followed by either 1.2 g/day of placebo or chitosan for 3 months, followed by a 3-month placebo washout period. Then both groups were given chitosan for 3 months. There were no significant changes or differences across study groups in plasma lipids over time (13).

- A randomized, double-blind, controlled clinical trial was conducted among 90 women (mean age 56.6 years) who demonstrated mild to moderate abnormalities in blood lipid levels. After 28 and 56 days of treatment (for the 84 women who completed the trial), 1.2 g chitosan divided into equal doses given after each of three meals daily was associated with a significant decrease in total cholesterol compared with baseline levels, but LDL cholesterol levels decreased only in women older than 60 (n = 20 receiving chitosan). No significant change over time was shown in the placebo group. Overall, the reduction in cholesterol was small and of limited clinical significance (14).

- In a double-blind, placebo-controlled study in Finland, 51 healthy obese women with normal cholesterol levels were randomly assigned to receive microcrystalline chitosan containing 800 mg chitosan or a placebo just before meals for 8 weeks. Weight, serum lipids, and safety laboratory parameters were measured before the trial and at weeks 4, 6, and 8 of treatment. Subjects were told to maintain their normal eating habits. One subject in the chitosan group and three subjects in the placebo group reported that they had changed their eating habits during the study. No reductions in weight were observed in any of the treatment groups. After 4 weeks (but not after 8 weeks), there was a significant decrease in LDL cholesterol in the chitosan group compared with the placebo group. There was no significant difference between groups in serum total or HDL cholesterol. However, serum triglycerides increased significantly in the chitosan group compared with the placebo group. The authors note that similar increases in triglycerides have been reported with bile acid–binding resin (cholesterolyamine). A subset of subjects with a BMI of 30 or more who had not changed their eating habits was analyzed separately. In this subset, serum LDL levels decreased significantly at weeks 4 and 8 in the chitosan group compared with the placebo group (7).

- Forty Chinese subjects with type 2 diabetes and hypercholesterolemia who were taking oral hypoglycemics were recruited for a two-part study. In part A, 19 subjects underwent a mixed meal test for 8 hours. Subjects received 450 mg chitosan three times per day or a placebo. Blood samples were drawn hourly to determine blood glucose and triglyceride concentrations. There were no differences in blood values between the two groups. In part B of the study, 33 of 40 subjects completed a randomized, double-blind, placebo-controlled, crossover study lasting 16 weeks. Subjects were randomly assigned to receive either 450 mg chitosan three times per day or a placebo daily and were switched to the other treatment after 8 weeks. Plasma total cholesterol and LDL cholesterol levels were significantly less in the chitosan recipients than those in the placebo group, with no other differences in triglycerides, HDL cholesterol, ratio of total:HDL cholesterol, A1C, or fasting glucose values between groups (15).

Chitosan and Dental Plaque Formation

♦ A randomized, blinded, placebo-controlled crossover study among 24 adults evaluated use of a 0.5% chitosan rinse for 14 days. Subjects rinsed twice daily with a 20 mL solution and then switched to the alternate treatment after a 14-day washout period. Compared with baseline levels, use of the chitosan rinse was associated with significant reductions in plaque formation and salivary streptococci counts (16). The biological mechanism by which chitosan may reduce dental plaque formation is not described. Further research in larger numbers of subjects is warranted.

References

1. Omrod DJ, Holmes CC, Miller TE. Dietary chitosan inhibits hypercholesterolemia and atherogenesis in the apolipoprotein E-deficient mouse model of atherosclerosis. *Atherosclerosis.* 1998;138:329–334.
2. Illum L. Chitosan and its use as a pharmaceutical excipient. *Pharm Res.* 1998;15: 1326–1321.
3. LeHoux JG, Grondin F. Some effects of chitosan on liver function in the rat. *Endocrinology.* 1993;132:1078–1084.
4. Hirano S. Chitin biotechnology applications. *Biotechnol Annu Rev.* 1996;2:237–258.
5. Deuchi K, Kanauchi O, Shizukuishi M, et al. Continuous and massive intake of chitosan affects mineral and fat-soluble vitamin status in rats fed on a high-fat diet. *Biosci Biotechnol Biochem.* 1995;59:1211–1216.
6. Koide SS. Chitin-chitosan: properties, benefits and risks. *Nutr Res.* 1998;18: 1091–1101.
7. Wuolijoki E, Hirvela T, Ylitalo P. Decrease in serum LDL cholesterol with microcrystalline chitosan. *Methods Find Exp Clin Pharmacol.* 1999;21:257–361.
8. Mhurchu CN, Poppitt SD, McGill AT, et al. The effect of dietary supplement chitosan on body weight: a randomized controlled trial in 250 overweight and obese adults. *Int J Obes Relat Metab Disord.* 2004;28:1149–1156.
9. Ernst E, Pittler MH. A meta-analysis of chitosan for body weight reduction. *Perfusion.* 1998;11:461–465.
10. Pittler HM, Abbot NC, Harkness EF, et al. Randomized, double-blind trial of chitosan for body weight reduction. *Eur J Clin Nutr.* 1999;53:379–381.
11. Gades MD, Stern JS. Chitosan supplementation and fat absorption in men and women. *J Am Diet Assoc.* 2005;105:72–77.
12. Guerciolini R, Radu-Radulescu L, Boldrin M, et al. Comparative evaluation of fecal fat excretion induced by orlistat and chitosan. *Obes Res.* 2001;9:364–367.
13. Metso S, Ylitalo R, Nikkila M, et al. The effect of long term microcrystalline chitosan therapy on plasma lipids and glucose concentrations in subjects with increased plasma

total cholesterol: a randomized placebo-controlled double-blind crossover trial in healthy men and women. *Eur J Clin Pharmacol.* 2003;59:741–746.

14. Bokura H, Kobayashi S. Chitosan decreases total cholesterol in women: a randomized, double-blind, placebo-controlled trial. *Eur J Clin Nutr.* 2003;27:721–725.
15. Tsai-Sung, T, Sheu WHH, Lee WJ, et al. Effect of chitosan on plasma lipoprotein concentrations in type 2 diabetic subjects with hypercholesterolemia [letter]. *Diabetes Care.* 2000;23:1703–1704.
16. Sano H, Shibasaki K, Matsukubo T, et al. Effect of chitosan rinsing on reduction of dental plaque formation. *Bull Tokyo Dent Coll.* 2003;44:9–16.

Choline. *See* Lecithin/Choline.

Chondroitin Sulfate

Chondroitin sulfate (CS) is the most abundant glycosaminoglycan in articular cartilage. (Glycosaminoglycans are the ground substance in which collagen fibers are embedded in cartilage.) CS is made endogenously and consists of repeating disaccharide units of glucuronic acid and galactosamine sulfate. Chondroitin seems to inhibit degradative enzymes that break down the cartilage matrix and synovial fluid. Normally secreted by the cells that form cartilage (chondrocytes), chondroitin provides elasticity to joints by pulling fluid into cartilage tissue. Because of these effects, CS supplements have been investigated for their potential in treating osteoarthritis (1–3).

Media and Marketing Claims	Efficacy
Relieves osteoarthritis pain	↑?
Protects joints and tendons from sports injury	NR

Safety

- No reported adverse events.
- Chondroitin has been used safely in studies from 2 months to 6 years in duration.
- CS may worsen symptoms of asthma; use with caution.
- Men with prostate cancer or an increased risk for prostate cancer should avoid CS. Preliminary research suggests chondroitin may cause the spread or recurrence of prostate cancer.
- CS may cause epigastric pain, nausea, diarrhea, constipation.

Drug/Supplement Interactions

- No reported adverse interactions.
- High dosages of CS (2,400 mg/day) combined with high dosages of glucosamine (3,000 mg/day) may enhance the effects of warfarin. No interactions have been reported at recommended dosages.

Caution

Actual contents of products containing chondroitin or chondroitin plus glucosamine vary by as much as 115% from what is stated on product labels.

Key Points

- Preliminary evidence suggests that CS reduces pain associated with osteoarthritis of the knee compared with placebo. However, the potential for confounding by concomitant use of NSAIDs make the studies difficult to interpret.
- Several meta-analyses have reviewed the efficacy of chondroitin in the treatment of osteoarthritis, and each supports clinical efficacy in reducing symptoms but also recommended improving study design (4–6).
- There are currently no clinical trials in humans specifically testing the role of CS supplements in protecting joints from sports injuries.
- *See also* Glucosamine.

Food Sources

None (CS is derived from bovine trachea).

Dosage Information/Bioavailability

CS is typically sold in 250- to 750-mg capsules, often combined with glucosamine (*see* Glucosamine) and mucopolysaccharides, which are also promoted for their potential role in joint protection. Most products suggest taking 1,200 mg CS per day in split doses. The CS in supplements is usually derived from bovine trachea or shark cartilage. Intestinal absorption of CS depends on chain length. Despite the high molecular mass and charge density, there is evidence that CS is effectively absorbed in the human intestine (1,7). In one study, the absolute bioavailability was 12% in humans, with peak levels reached in 1 to 4 hours (7). Iodine-labeled CS administered orally in humans was found to be distributed to the synovial fluid and cartilage (7). In contrast, another study reported that neither intact nor depolymerized CS administered orally increased serum glycosaminoglycans (8).

Relevant Research

Chondroitin Sulfate and Osteoarthritis

- To assess the long-term effects of chondroitin supplementation on symptoms of osteoarthritis of the knee, a randomized, double-blind, placebo-controlled, crossover study was conducted. Investigators randomly assigned 120 symptomatic subjects with osteoarthritis of the knee to receive 800 mg CS or placebo every day for 3 months, followed by a 6-month interval without treatment, and then 3 months on the alternate treatment. One hundred ten subjects completed the study. Subjects in the CS group showed a 36% improvement in knee pain and a significant stabilization of joint space width (which is associated with reduced pain) over time compared with the placebo group (9). Additional studies using intermittent supplementation are required before clinical recommendations can be made.

- In a double-blind, parallel multicenter study, 127 subjects older than 45 years with knee osteoarthritis were randomly assigned to receive one of three treatments for 3 months: (*a*) 1,200 mg CS gel in one dose; (*b*) 1,200 mg CS capsules divided into three doses; or (*c*) a placebo. Subjects were assessed at days 0, 14, 42, and 91. Subjects were permitted to take authorized NSAIDs if needed, and daily ingestion was recorded. In both CS groups, clinical symptoms decreased significantly according to the Lesquesne's Index (assessment of functional status and quality of life) and spontaneous joint pain measured by a visual analogue scale (VAS). In the placebo group, there was a significant reduction on the VAS, but not for the Lesquesne's Index. There were no differences in the efficacy of single vs multiple doses of CS on clinical parameters. CS was rated by physicians and subjects as significantly more effective than the placebo. There was an insignificant trend toward less NSAID use in the CS groups compared with the placebo group (10).

- In a double-blind, placebo-controlled study (at two centers), 85 subjects (ages 39 to 83 years) with knee osteoarthritis were randomly assigned to receive a placebo or 800 mg CS per day (divided into two doses) for 6 months. Five subjects dropped out of the study for reasons unrelated to treatment. Subjects were assessed at months 0, 1, 3, and 6. Subjects were permitted to take paracetamol (an analgesic, also known as acetaminophen) as needed. Consumption was recorded as total number of tablets taken during the study. In the CS group, the Lesquesne's Index and spontaneous joint pain significantly decreased. In the CS group, walking time for a 20-meter walk was significantly reduced at 6 months. Global assessment of efficacy by physicians and subjects was significantly in favor of CS compared with the placebo. There was an insignificant trend for subjects in the CS group to consume less paracetamol for pain than subjects in the placebo group (11).

- In a double-blind, placebo-controlled study, 60 subjects (age 35 to 78 years) with knee osteoarthritis were randomly assigned to receive 800 mg CS daily (divided into two doses) or a placebo for 1 year. Eighteen subjects (nine in each group) did not complete the study. Subjects were assessed at months 0, 3, 6, and 12 and were given free access to paracetamol as a rescue medication, but use was not recorded. There were no significant differences in knee pain between groups at baseline. At month 12, joint pain and overall mobility were significantly improved in the CS group. In the CS group, the metabolism of bone and joints (assessed by various biochemical markers in serum) was normalized, whereas it remained abnormal in subjects taking the placebo. The authors hypothesized that CS may have an effect on the subchondral bone by inhibiting the degradation of collagen. They concluded: "Further trials, including more patients and over longer periods of time, are definitely necessary to confirm the possible structure-modifying properties of CS" (12).

◆ In a double-blind, parallel-group study, 146 subjects (ages 40 to 75 years) with knee osteoarthritis were randomly assigned to receive either diclofenac sodium (an NSAID) or 400 mg CS three times a day for 1 month. In months 2 and 3, the diclofenac group was given only a placebo, whereas the chondroitin group continued taking CS. During months 4 through 6, both groups received a placebo. Subjects taking diclofenac showed immediate reduction of symptoms, which reappeared at the end of treatment. Subjects taking chondroitin had a delay in therapeutic improvement, but it lasted for up to 3 months after the end of treatment. At the end of the 4- to 6-month period, the Lesquesne's Index score was 64.4% less than baseline levels in the chondroitin group, whereas in the diclofenac group this value was 29.7% less than the baseline. The difference between groups was significant. At days 10 and 20, reduction of paracetamol consumption was more evident in the diclofenac group than in the chondroitin group (significant). At day 30, the reduction in paracetamol consumption was not different between groups. At the end of treatment with CS (day 90), there was an 88% reduction in paracetamol use compared with baseline values, whereas the reduction with diclofenac was 37.8%. The difference between groups was significant, with CS showing greater efficacy (13).

References

1. Conte A, Volpi N, Palmieri L, et al. Biochemical and pharmacokinetic aspects of oral treatment with chondroitin sulfate. *Arzneimittelforschung*. 1995;45:918–925.
2. Paroli E, Antonilli L, Biffoni M. A pharmacological approach to glycosaminoglycans. *Drugs Exp Clin Res*. 1991;17:9–20.
3. Hardingham T. Chondroitin sulfate and joint disease. *Osteoarthritis Cartilage*. 1998;6 (Suppl A):3–5.
4. Leeb BF, Schweitzer H, Montag K, et al. A meta-analysis of chondroitin sulfate in the treatment of osteoarthritis. *J Rheumatol*. 2000;27:205–211.
5. McAlindon TE, LaValley MP, Gulin JP, et al. Glucosamine and chondroitin for treatment of osteoarthritis: a systematic quality assessment and meta-analysis. *JAMA*. 2000;283:1469–1475.
6. Richy F, Bruyere O, Ethgen O, et al. Structural and symptomatic efficacy of glucosamine and chondroitin in knee osteoarthritis: a comprehensive meta-analysis. *Arch Intern Med*. 2003;163:1514–1522.

7. Ronca F, Palmieri L, Panicucci P, et al. Anti-inflammatory activity of chondroitin sulfate. *Osteoarthritis Cartilage*. 1998;6(Suppl A):14–21.
8. Baici A, Horler D, Moser B, et al. Analysis of glycosaminoglycans in human serum after oral administration of chondroitin sulfate. *Rheumatol Int*. 1992;12:81–88.
9. Uebelhart D, Malaise M, Marcolongo R, et al. Intermittent treatment of knee osteoarthritis with oral chondroitin sulfate: a one-year, randomize, double-blind, multicenter study versus placebo. *Osteoarthritis Cartilage*. 2004;12:269–276.
10. Bourgeois P, Chales G, Dehais J, et al. Efficacy and tolerability of chondroitin sulfate 1,200 mg/day vs chondroitin sulfate 3 × 400 mg/day vs placebo. *Osteoarthritis Cartilage*. 1998;6(Suppl A):25–30.
11. Bucsi L, Poor G. Efficacy and tolerability of oral chondroitin sulfate as a symptomatic slow-acting drug for osteoarthritis (SYSADOA) in the treatment of knee osteoarthritis. *Osteoarthritis Cartilage*. 1998;6(Suppl A):31–36.
12. Uebelhart D, Thonar EJ, Delmas PD, et al. Effects of oral chondroitin sulfate on the progression of knee osteoarthritis: a pilot study. *Osteoarthritis Cartilage*. 1998;6(Suppl A):39–46.
13. Morreale P, Manopulo R, Galati M, et al. Comparison of the anti-inflammatory efficacy of chondroitin sulfate and diclofenac sodium in subjects with knee osteoarthritis. *J Rheumatol*. 1996;23:1385–1391.

Chondroitin Sulfate and Glucosamine Combinations and Osteoarthritis. *See* Glucosamine.

Chromium

Chromium is an essential trace mineral that, in the form of a low–molecular weight chromium binding substance, potentiates insulin, which influences carbohydrate, lipid, and protein metabolism (1). Chromium in its biologically active form may stimulate insulin receptor protein tyrosine kinase activity after the receptor is activated by insulin. Because of its potential effect on metabolism by potentiating insulin, chromium has been promoted as a weight-loss aid and muscle builder.

Media and Marketing Claims	Efficacy
Helps with blood glucose control in individuals with diabetes	↔
Reduces serum cholesterol, prevents heart disease	↓?
Promotes weight loss	↓?
Promotes increased muscle mass and decreases body fat	↓

Safety

- The long-term effects of increased cellular concentrations of chromium in the body are not known. It has been hypothesized that 5 years of consuming 600 μg of chromium picolinate (300 μg elemental chromium) could possibly lead to an accumulation in some tissues, similar to levels that caused DNA damage observed in animals and in vitro studies (2,3).

- Researchers investigating the safety of chromium supplements (picolinate or chloride) found that supplementing rats with several thousand times the equivalent of the upper limit of the Estimated Safe and Adequate Dietary Intake (ESSADI) for humans resulted in no toxicity (4).

- A Tolerable Upper Intake Level (UL) has not been established.

- Long-term effects of high doses are not known.

- There have been reports of headaches, sleep disturbances, and mood swings with chromium supplements (5).

- Chromium exists in two forms: trivalent (occurs mainly in nature) and hexavalent (occurs mainly in industrial settings). The hexavalent form is a synthetic compound that is very toxic and carcinogenic (2).

- One review cautioned that chromium may compete with iron for serum protein binding sites and questioned the safety of picolinate (6).

- A dosage of 1,200 to 2,400 μg chromium picolinate daily for 5 months resulted in liver dysfunction and renal failure in one 33-year-old woman taking the supplement for weight loss (7).

- Avoid use of chromium polynicotinate with existing liver disease.

- Avoid chromium supplements with existing renal dysfunction.

- Dosages of chromium picolinate as low as 200 to 400 μg/day may cause cognitive, perceptual, and motor dysfunction in some individuals.

- Chromium may cause allergic reactions in individuals with chromate or leather contact allergies.

Drug/Supplement Interactions

- Vitamin C and NSAIDs, including aspirin, ibuprofen, indomethacin, and naproxen, may increase chromium absorption.

- Antacids, zinc, H2-blockers (cimetidine, ranitidine, nizatidine, famotidine), and proton pump inhibitors (PPIs—omepraxole, lansoprazole, arbeprazole, pantoprazole, esomeprazole) may decrease chromium absorption.

- In theory, chromium could enhance the blood glucose–lowering effects of diabetes medications and injected insulin.

- Herbs containing chromium (horsetail and caccara) may increase the risk of chromium toxicity if used chronically or with chromium supplementation.

◆ Corticosteroids can increase chromium excretion and cause chromium deficiency or hyperglycemia.

Key Points

◆ According to national consumption surveys, the average American diet meets the AI for chromium. A varied diet consisting of foods rich in chromium is recommended to meet the AI; chromium status may be maximized by choosing a diet low in simple sugars and rich in whole, unprocessed foods.

◆ According to one study, high-dose chromium supplements (1,000 μg/day) may benefit individuals with type 1 or type 2 diabetes with low chromium status by improving A1C, glucose, insulin, and cholesterol levels. Long-term research is needed to determine the safety and efficacy of high-dose supplements and whether chromium supplements have a beneficial effect on retinopathy, nephropathy, and mortality associated with diabetes.

◆ A recent FDA review concludes that a "relationship between chromium piccolinate and insulin resistance is inconclusive."

◆ Preliminary evidence suggests that chromium positively affects blood lipids, specifically HDL cholesterol and triglycerides. However, results are inconsistent regarding which blood lipids were affected. There are currently no studies investigating the effects of chromium supplements on morbidity or mortality associated with cardiovascular disease.

◆ It is likely that the positive effects of chromium on blood glucose, lipid metabolism, and even cardiovascular risk factors are only demonstrated in people with depleted chromium stores, such as is seen in individuals with long-term type 2 diabetes (8).

◆ There is little evidence from well-designed studies that chromium increases lean body mass or decreases body fat.

◆ Although it has been hypothesized that athletes may require additional chromium in their diets due to increased chromium losses from exercise, there is currently no evidence that supplements are anabolic or have other benefits for healthy athletes.

Food Sources

Brewer's yeast, black pepper, cheese, broccoli, and beans, seeds, wine, and beer are good sources of chromium. The process of refining wheat removes chromium in the germ and bran. It is estimated that the average American diet provides 15 μg per 1,000 kcal (2,9). The chromium content of foods varies widely, and a significant portion of chromium present in foods may be introduced externally during growing, processing, preparation, fortification, and handling (10).

Food	Chromium, µg/serving
Cheese (2 oz)	56
Liver (2 oz)	55
Wine (3 oz)	45
Broccoli (1 cup)	22
Ham (3 oz)	3.6
Potatoes, mashed (1 cup)	2.7
Beans, green (1 cup)	2.2
Turkey breast (3 oz)	1.7
Apple (1 medium)	1.4
Rice, white (1 cup)	1.2
Banana (1 medium)	1.0
Bread, whole-wheat (1 slice)	0.98

Dosage Information/Bioavailability

Chromium in the form of chromium picolinate, nicotinic acid, or chloride is sold in doses ranging from 50 to 600 µg. Chromium is also found in smaller amounts in multivitamin/mineral supplements. Chromium picolinate (tripicolinate) and nicotinic acid and chromium from brewer's yeast (organic complexes) apparently are absorbed and retained better than the chromium chloride form (inorganic complex) (11). Chromium absorption seems to vary with dosage. A dietary intake of 10 µg chromium had a 2% absorption rate, whereas a dietary intake of 40 µg had an absorption rate of 0.5% (12). Vitamin C and aspirin may enhance absorption, whereas antacids may decrease absorption of chromium (2,13).

The Food and Nutrition Board has set AIs for chromium, but the board did not set an RDA due to insufficient evidence (14). The new AI is 35 µg/day for men age 19 to 50 years; for women in this age range, the AI is 25 µg/day. For adults older than 50, the AI is 30 µg/day for men and 20 µg/day for women. These values differ from the previous ESADDI of 50 to 200 µg for individuals age 7 and older (15). However, the newer research suggests that the actual chromium requirements for healthy adults is substantially less than originally thought, which was based on dietary intake data from the early 1980s when methods of chromium analysis in foods were less accurate (9,16). The World Health Organization recommended a basal chromium intake of 25 µg/day to prevent pathological symptoms of deficiency, and a daily intake of 33 µg to maintain desirable tissue storage concentrations (9,16).

Diets high in simple sugars (35% simple sugars, 15% complex carbohydrates) increase urinary chromium excretion compared with diets low in sugar (15% simple sugars, 35% complex carbohydrates). This may be a result of increased chromium use in response to the increase in glucose metabolism (17–19). A study of acute glucose response to meals with or without chromium supplementation (400 or 800 mg) suggests that chromium may blunt postprandial glucose response, but large individual variability exists and studies in larger numbers of subjects are needed (20).

Strenuous exercise and physical trauma may also increase urinary excretion of chromium (21–23). However, urinary chromium losses with exercise have been associated with accompanying increases in chromium absorption (24).

Relevant Research

Chromium and Diabetes

+ A meta-analysis of 618 subjects enrolled in 15 studies indicated that in individuals without diabetes chromium had no association with blood glucose, insulin, or A1C. In subjects from China with diabetes (n = 155), chromium was associated with improved glucose response, but combined data from other studies were negative. Chromium deficiency may be more prevalent in China, and therefore supplementation is more likely to be efficacious than in the United States (25).

+ In a study of chromium piccolinalte supplementation (200 µg twice daily for 3 weeks) among 39 elderly subjects with diabetes and 39 control group elderly subjects, the subjects with diabetes had a significant reduction in A1C (8.5% to 7.6%) and fasting blood glucose (190 mg/dL to 150 mg/dL) as well as total serum cholesterol (235 mg/dL to 213 mg/dL). However, subjects were also placed on a 1,500-kcal diet and weight change was not reported; energy restriction likely also contributed to the metabolic improvements (26).

+ In a study of subjects with impaired glucose tolerance but not diagnosed diabetes, chromium supplementation did not improve glucose levels, insulin sensitivity, or lipid profiles (27).

+ In a double-blind, placebo-controlled study, 180 subjects with type 2 diabetes were randomly assigned among three groups to take (*a*) a placebo; (*b*) 200 µg chromium picolinate (100 µg elemental chromium) divided into two doses; or (*c*) 1,000 µg chromium picolinate (500 µg elemental chromium) divided into two doses. Subjects maintained their usual diet and medication throughout the 4-month study. A1C values significantly improved after 2 months in the high-dose chromium group and were less in both chromium groups after 4 months compared with placebo. Fasting and 2-hour insulin values were significantly less in both chromium groups at 2 and 4 months. However, only the subjects taking high-dose chromium had significantly lower 2-hour glucose values and lower plasma total cholesterol (28).

+ In a double-blind, placebo-controlled crossover study, 78 individuals with type 2 diabetes in Saudi Arabia received in random order brewer's yeast (23 µg chromium) and 200 µg chromium from chromium chloride for 4 weeks each. In all subjects, there were four 8-week phases in the study. Each phase of chromium supplementation was followed by placebo administration for 8 weeks. At the beginning and end of each phase, weight, diet, drug use, and blood and urine glucose and lipids were recorded. Both forms of chromium resulted in a significant decrease in levels of mean glucose (fasting and 2-hour postprandial), fructosamine, and triglycerides. Mean HDL cholesterol and serum and urinary chromium levels all increased during chromium intake. After either chromium phase, mean drug dosage tended to decrease, but was not significant, except with the drug glibenclamide. There were no changes in dietary intakes or BMI. Overall, brewer's yeast was associated with chromium retention and more positive effects than the chromium chloride form (29).

♦ In a prospective, double-blind, placebo-controlled crossover study, 28 subjects with type 2 diabetes received in random order 200 μg chromium picolinate or a placebo for 2 months each, with a 2-month washout period. There was no change in fasting glucose control or plasma HDL or LDL cholesterol concentrations. However, during chromium supplementation, mean triglyceride concentrations decreased significantly (by 17.4%). The authors acknowledged that long-term studies are needed to determine whether the short-term change in triglycerides can be sustained (30).

♦ In a review, researchers examined 15 studies on chromium supplementation (picolinate and chloride forms) and concluded (*a*) overt chromium deficiency results in insulin resistance; (*b*) insulin resistance due to chromium deficiency can be improved with chromium supplementation; and (*c*) chromium deficiency, although rare, may be a cause of insulin resistance in deficient populations (31).

♦ According to another review, consumption of low-chromium diets (< 20 μg) by healthy control subjects does not seem to affect blood glucose or insulin variables. In addition, control subjects with good glucose tolerance (glucose = 5.6 mmol/L 90 minutes after a glucose challenge) on low-chromium diets do not show signs of deficiency, and supplementation of 200 μg elemental chromium daily for 5 weeks is without effect on glucose or insulin variables (16).

♦ An evidenced-based review found that the evidence that chromium picolinate reduces insulin resistance is uncertain or inconclusive (32).

Chromium and Cardiovascular Disease

♦ In a double-blind, placebo-controlled study, 72 male subjects using beta blockers were randomly assigned to receive 600 μg chromium picolinate (300 μg elemental chromium) divided into three doses or a placebo daily for 8 weeks. Fasting lipids were measured before and after treatment, and 8 weeks after the completion of the study. There was a significant increase in mean HDL cholesterol concentrations in the group taking chromium supplements after adjusting for baseline HDL and total cholesterol concentrations, age, and weight change. There were no differences in total cholesterol, triglycerides, or body weight between groups (33).

♦ In a placebo-controlled (not blinded) study, 76 subjects with atherosclerosis (25 of whom had stable type 2 diabetes) were randomly assigned to receive 250 μg chromium as chromium chloride or a placebo daily for 7 to 16 months. Blood samples were taken at the beginning, at 3 months, and at the end of the study. There was a significant increase in serum chromium and decrease in triglyceride concentrations at 3 and 6 months in the chromium group compared with placebo group. At 6 months only, there was a significant increase in serum HDL cholesterol concentrations in the chromium group compared with the placebo group. Chromium supplements had no effect on blood glucose or total cholesterol levels (34). The results of this study would be strengthened if the study were done with a double-blind design.

◆ In a double-blind, placebo-controlled crossover study, 28 healthy subjects received, in random order, 200 μg elemental chromium as chromium picolinate or a placebo daily for 42 days. Chromium supplements resulted in a significant decrease in total cholesterol and LDL cholesterol. Apolipoprotein A-I (the principal protein in HDL) increased during the chromium supplementation phase, although the HDL level did not increase significantly (35).

Chromium and Obesity

◆ A meta-analysis of chromium supplementation for weight loss that included only randomized, double-blind study designs showed a significant improvement in weight loss (mean = 1.1 kg) among 489 subjects receiving chromium picolinate supplementation. Clinical significance of such a small difference may not support chromium supplementation for weight loss (36).

◆ In double-blind, placebo-controlled study, 43 obese female subjects were randomly assigned to one of four groups for 9 weeks: (*a*) chromium picolinate (400 μg elemental chromium per day) with no exercise; (*b*) chromium with exercise; (*c*) placebo with exercise; or (*d*) chromium nicotinate supplementation (400 μg elemental chromium per day) with exercise. Chromium picolinate supplementation without exercise resulted in a statistically significant weight gain but no statistical change in body fat, fat-free mass, or fat mass as assessed by hydrostatic weighing. The chromium nicotinate group experienced significant weight loss and a reduced insulin response to an oral glucose loading test. The authors speculated that the high dose of chromium picolinate used (double the amount in most of the earlier studies) may have caused the weight gain, although they did not attempt to explain the possible mechanism of action. Although their sample size was small, the authors concluded that chromium picolinate may be contraindicated in nonexercising, young, obese women (37).

◆ In a double-blind, placebo-controlled study, 95 overweight Navy personnel subjects were randomly assigned to receive 400 μg chromium picolinate (200 μg elemental chromium) or a placebo daily for 16 weeks. Subjects completed 30 minutes of exercise training (unsupervised) at least three times per week during the study. Chromium had no effect on the percentage of body fat (computed from body circumference and height), body weight, or lean body mass compared with placebo. The authors concluded: "Chromium picolinate was ineffective in enhancing body fat reductions in this group and could not be recommended as an adjuvant to Navy weight-loss programs in general" (38).

Chromium for Strength Training and Body Mass

◆ In a double-blind, randomized, placebo-controlled study of chromium supplementation in 44 obese women involved in weight-training and participating in a 12-week walking program, chromium supplementation of 400 μg/day was not associated with significant differences in body composition, resting energy expenditure, glucose, lipids, or C-peptide. However, improvements in total cholesterol were demonstrated in both the group taking chromium and the control group (39).

- In a double-blind, placebo-controlled study, 36 male weight-trained subjects were randomly assigned to receive 170 to 180 µg chromium (as chromium picolinate or chromium chloride), or a placebo daily during an 8-week resistance training program. Both chromium supplements increased serum and urinary chromium concentrations. However, chromium had no effect on strength, mesomorphy, or body composition (x-ray absorptiometry, skinfolds) compared with the placebo (40).

- In a double-blind, placebo-controlled study, 59 college students were enrolled in a 12-week weightlifting program and were randomly assigned to receive 200 µg chromium (as chromium picolinate) or a placebo. No treatment effects of chromium were seen on strength (one-repetition maximum for the squat and bench press), skinfold, and circumference measures. However, in the group taking chromium picolinate body weight increased significantly in female weightlifters but did not change in the male weightlifters. It was not clear whether the weight gain was fat or lean body mass, although the authors hypothesized the gain was muscle mass because of a insignificant decrease in skinfold measures (41).

- In a double-blind, placebo-controlled study, 38 football players were randomly assigned to receive 200 µg chromium as chromium picolinate or a placebo daily for 9 weeks. Subjects were assessed for strength and body composition, measured by hydrostatic weighing pre-, mid-, and posttreatment. There was no change in body composition or strength (maximal isometric actions for each muscle group) during intensive weight-training compared with the placebo group. Among those taking chromium supplement, urinary chromium excretion increased 5-fold compared with the placebo group (42).

- A review article concluded: (*a*) Athletes may be at risk for negative chromium balance and may have increased chromium requirements because of increased urinary and sweat losses, and (*b*) anabolic steroid–like muscle mass increases after chromium supplementation are very unlikely (6).

References

1. Davis CM, Vincent JB. Chromium oligopeptides activates insulin receptor tyrosine kinase activity. *Biochemistry.* 1997;36:4382–4385.
2. Nielsen FH. Controversial chromium. *Nutr Today.* 1996;31:226–233.
3. Stearns DM, Belbruno JJ, Wetterhahn KE. A prediction of chromium (III) accumulation in humans from chromium dietary supplements. *FASEB J.* 1995;9:1650–1657.
4. Anderson RA, Bryden NA, Polansky MM. Lack of toxicity of chromium chloride and chromium picolinate in rats. *J Am Coll Nutr.* 1997;16:273–279.
5. Schrauzer GN, Shrestha KP, Arce MF. Somatopsychological effects of chromium supplementation. *J Nutr Med.* 1992;3:42–48.
6. Lefavi RG, Anderson RA, Keith RE, et al. Efficacy of chromium supplementation in athletes: emphasis on anabolism. *Int J Sport Nutr.* 1992;2:111–122.

7. Cerulli J, Grabe DW, Gauthier I, et al. Chromium picolinate toxicity. *Ann Pharmacother.* 1998;32:428–431.

8. Cefalu WT, Hu FB. Role of chromium in human health and in diabetes. *Diabetes Care.* 2004;27:2741–2751.

9. Stoecker BJ. Chromium. In: Shils ME, Olson JA, Shike M, Ross AC, eds. *Modern Nutrition in Health and Disease.* 9th ed. Baltimore, Md: Williams & Wilkins; 1999: 277–282.

10. Anderson RA, Bryden NA, Polansky MM. Dietary chromium intake: freely chosen diets, institutional diets, and individual foods. *Biol Trace Elem Res.* 1992;32:117–121.

11. Olin KL, Stearns D, Armstrong W, et al. Comparative retention/absorption of [51]chromium (^{51}Cr) from ^{51}Cr chloride, ^{51}Cr nicotinate, and ^{51}Cr picolinate in a rat model. *J Trace Electrolytes Health Dis.* 1994;11:182–186.

12. Anderson RA, Kozlovsky AS. Chromium intake, absorption, and excretion of subjects consuming self-selected diets. *Am J Clin Nutr.* 1985;41:1177–1183.

13. Seaborn CD, Stoecker BJ. Effects of antacid or ascorbic acid on tissue accumulation and urinary excretion of [51]chromium. *Nutr Res.* 1990;10:1401–1407.

14. Institute of Medicine. *Dietary Reference Intakes for Vitamin A, Vitamin K, Arsenic, Boron, Chromium, Copper, Iodine, Iron, Manganese, Molybdenum, Nickel, Silicon, Vanadium, and Zinc.* Washington, DC: National Academy Press; 2001.

15. Institute of Medicine. *Recommended Dietary Allowances.* 10th ed. Washington, DC: National Academy Press; 1989.

16. Anderson RA. Nutritional factors influencing the glucose/insulin system: chromium. *J Am Coll Nutr.* 1997;16:404–410.

17. Kozlovsky AS, Moser PB, Reiser S, et al. Effects of diets high in simple sugars on urinary chromium losses. *Metabolism.* 1986;35:515–518.

18. Anderson RA, Bryden NA, Polansky MM, et al. Urinary chromium excretion and insulinogenic properties of carbohydrates. *Am J Clin Nutr.* 1990;51:864–868.

19. Anderson RA, Polansky MM, Bryden NA, et al. Urinary chromium excretion of human subjects: effects of chromium supplementation and glucose loading. *Am J Clin Nutr.* 1982;36:1184–1193.

20. Frauchiger MT, Wenk C, Colombani PC. Effects of acute chromium supplementation on postprandial metabolism in healthy young men. *J Am Coll Nutr.* 2004;23:351–357.

21. Anderson RA, Bryden NA, Polansky MM, et al. Exercise effects on chromium excretion of trained and untrained men consuming a constant diet. *J Appl Physiol.* 1988;64: 249–252.

22. Campbell WW, Anderson RA. Effects of aerobic exercise and training on the trace minerals chromium, zinc, and copper. *Sports Med.* 1987;4:9–18.

23. Borel JS, Majerus TC, Polansky MM, et al. Chromium intake and urinary chromium excretion of trauma patients. *Biol Trace Elem Res.* 1984;6:317–326.

24. Rubin MA, Miller JP, Ryan AS, et al. Acute and chronic resistive exercise increase urinary chromium excretion in men as measured with an enriched chromium stable isotope. *J Nutr.* 1998;128:73–78.

25. Althius MD, Jordon NE, Ludington EA, et al. Glucose and insulin responses to dietary chromium supplements: a meta-analysis. *Am J Clin Nutr.* 2002;76:148–155.

26. Rabinovitz H, Friedensohn A, Leibovitz A, et al. Effect of chromium supplementation on blood glucose and lipid levels in type 2 diabetes mellitus elderly patients. *Int J Vitam Nutr Res.* 2004;74:178–182.

27. Gunton JE, Cheung NW, Hitchman R, et al. Chromium supplementation does not improve glucose tolerance, insulin sensitivity, or lipid profile: a randomized, placebo-controlled, double-blind trial of supplementation in subjects with impaired glucose tolerance. *Diabetes Care.* 2005;28:712–713.

28. Anderson RA, Cheng N, Bryden NA, et al. Elevated intakes of supplemental chromium improve glucose and insulin variables in individuals with type 2 diabetes. *Diabetes.* 1997;46:1786–1791.

29. Bahijiri SM, Mira SA, Mufti AM, et al. The effects of inorganic chromium and brewer's yeast supplementation on glucose tolerance, serum lipids, and drug dosage in individuals with type 2 diabetes. *Saudi Med J.* 2000;21:831–837.

30. Lee NA, Reasner CA. Beneficial effect of chromium supplementation on serum triglyceride levels in NIDDM. *Diabetes Care.* 1994;17:1449–1452.

31. Mertz W. Chromium in human nutrition: a review. *J Nutr.* 1993;123:626–633.

32. Trumbo PR, Ellwood KC. Chromium picolinate intake and risk of type 2 diabetes: an evidence-based review by the United States Food and Drug Administration. *Nutr Rev.* 2006;64:357–363.

33. Roeback JR, Hla KM, Chambless LE, et al. Effects of chromium supplementation on serum high-density-lipoprotein cholesterol levels in men taking ß-blockers. A randomized, controlled trial. *Ann Intern Med.* 1991;115:917–924.

34. Abraham AS, Brooks BA, Eylath U. The effect of chromium supplementation on serum glucose and lipids in patients with and without non-insulin-dependent diabetes. *Metabolism.* 1992;41:768–771.

35. Press RI, Geller J, Evans GW. The effect of chromium picolinate on serum cholesterol and apolipoprotein fractions in human subjects. *West J Med.* 1990;152:41–45.

36. Pittler MH, Stevinson C, Ernst E. Chromium picolinate for reducing body weight: meta-analysis of randomized trials. *Int J Obes Relat Metab Disord.* 2003;27:522–529.

37. Grant KE, Chandler RM, Castle AL, et al. Chromium and exercise training: effect on obese women. *Med Sci Sports Exerc.* 1997;29:992–998.

38. Trent LK, Thieding-Cancel D. Effects of chromium picolinate on body composition. *J Sports Med Phys Fitness.* 1995;35:273–280.

39. Volpe SL, Huang HW, Larpadisorn K, Lesser II. Effect of chromium supplementation and exercise on body composition, resting metabolic rate and selected biochemical parameters in moderately obese women following an exercise program. *J Am Coll Nutr.* 2001;20:293–306.

40. Lukaski HC, Bolonchuk WW, Siders WA, et al. Chromium supplementation and resistance training: effects on body composition, strength, and trace element status of men. *Am J Clin Nutr.* 1996;63:954–965.

41. Hasten DL, Rome EP, Franks BD, et al. Effects of chromium picolinate on beginning weight training students. *Int J Sport Nutr.* 1992;2:343–350.

42. Clancy SP, Clarkson PM, DeCheke ME, et al. Effects of chromium picolinate supplementation on body composition, strength, and urinary chromium loss in football players. *Int J Sport Nutr.* 1994;4:142–153.

Cobalamin. *See* Vitamin B-12 (Cobalamin).

Coenzyme Q$_{10}$

Coenzyme Q$_{10}$ (CoQ$_{10}$), or ubiquinone, is an electron and proton carrier supporting ATP synthesis in the lipid phase of the mitochondria membrane. It is synthesized endogenously within the intracellular environment throughout the body, specifically in the heart, liver, kidney, and pancreas. The CoQ$_{10}$ content of human tissue seems to be related to age, peaking at age 20, and subsequently decreasing (1). CoQ$_{10}$ has demonstrated antioxidant activity in experimental studies (2–4). Because of its potential antioxidant role and involvement in mitochondrial function, CoQ$_{10}$ has been investigated in cardiovascular disease, exercise performance, cancer, HIV/AIDS, and neurodegenerative diseases.

Media and Marketing Claims	Efficacy
Improves health of people with heart disease and hypertension	↑
Improves exercise performance	↓
Reduces cancer risk	NR
Improves immune function in individuals with HIV	NR
Helps with neurological disorders	NR
Prevents migraine headache	NR

Safety

◆ High doses of CoQ$_{10}$ (1,200, 1,800, 2,400, or 3,000 mg/day) with 1,200 IU of vitamin E were given to 17 patients with Parkinson's disease for 2 weeks. Plasma levels were maximized at 2,400 mg/day. No serious adverse events were associated with short term supplementation. Mild dyspepsia was reported in some subjects (5).

◆ In a small study of individuals with Parkinson's disease (n = 15), patients were randomly assigned to 200, 400 or 800 mg CoQ$_{10}$ per day plus 400 IU vitamin E for 1 month. Supplementation with CoQ$_{10}$ plus vitamin E at the 200 and 400 mg/day doses resulted in a nonsignificant increase in complex I: citratesynthetase ratio, an effect that has been shown to be associated with reduced Parkinsonian symptoms. The authors suggested that if CoQ$_{10}$ is supplemented at doses more than 600 mg/day, it would be prudent to periodically monitor renal function (6).

◆ No serious adverse effects have been reported for 200 mg CoQ$_{10}$ daily for 1 year and 100 mg daily for up to 6 years (7).

♦ Potential side effects may include mild gastrointestinal distress, including nausea, vomiting, diarrhea, appetite suppression, and heartburn.

Drug/Supplement Interactions

♦ HMG-CoA reductase inhibitor drugs (statins) used for cholesterol reduction may deplete blood coenzyme Q_{10} levels.

♦ Smoking depletes body stores of coenzyme $Q_{10.}$

♦ Endogenous synthesis of coenzyme Q_{10} is dependent on adequate vitamin B-6 status.

♦ CoQ_{10} may reduce blood pressure and have an additive effect with antihypertensive drugs.

♦ CoQ_{10} may reduce effectiveness of chemotherapeutic drugs that induce oxidative stress (cyclophosphamide, cytoxan).

♦ CoQ_{10} may reduce effectiveness of warfarin (Coumadin) as an anticoagulation agent; patients on warfarin should not use CoQ_{10} supplements.

Key Points

♦ Some evidence from controlled human studies suggests that CoQ_{10} supplementation may improve the symptoms and outcome of cardiac surgery, myocardial infarction, and congestive heart failure. However, not all research report benefits from CoQ_{10} supplementation. More studies are needed to determine the dosage, timing, and safety of supplementation in this population.

♦ Controlled trials do not support CoQ_{10} supplementation for athletes because it does not seem to enhance exercise performance or reduce oxidative stress induced by exercise.

♦ Although blood CoQ_{10} concentrations seem to be decreased in individuals with breast cancer, controlled trials are lacking to support the claim that CoQ_{10} prevents or treats cancer. Some people with cancer do show reduced levels of CoQ_{10}. Current studies are poorly designed to answer the question. There is some suggestion that CoQ_{10} may reduce the cardiac toxicity of select chemotherapeutic drugs.

♦ Likewise, controlled research is lacking and is needed to determine the potential role of CoQ_{10} supplements in immune function in AIDS. Case studies and uncontrolled trials suggesting a beneficial effect of CoQ_{10} supplements in people with AIDS and healthy subjects do not provide adequate information to make recommendations for this population.

♦ Controlled clinical trials are lacking and are necessary to determine the potential role of CoQ_{10} supplements in neurodegenerative diseases.

♦ Although blood CoQ_{10} concentrations seem to decrease with age, there is currently no evidence suggesting that supplements slow the human aging process.

◆ Although preliminary evidence suggests CoQ-10 supplementation may reduce the frequency of migraines in chronic sufferers, more research is needed.

Food Sources

An analysis of the CoQ_{10} content of the Danish diet (US data are not available) revealed a mean intake of 3 to 5 mg/day, mainly from meat and poultry. Frying foods destroys 14% to 34% of the CoQ_{10} content, whereas boiling causes no detectable destruction (8).

Food	CoQ_{10}, mg/serving
Beef (3 oz)	2.6
Chicken (3 oz)	1.4
Pork chop (3 oz)	1.2
Trout (3 oz)	0.9
Salmon (3 oz)	0.4
Orange (1 medium)	0.4
Broccoli (½ cup)	0.2

Source: Data are from reference 8.

Dosage Information/Bioavailability

Because CoQ_{10} is not an essential nutrient, no RDA has been set. CoQ_{10} is sold in capsules and tablets in doses ranging from 10 to 130 mg per capsule. One study found that CoQ_{10} in both food and dietary supplement sources significantly increased serum concentrations (9). Another study found a new soluble form of CoQ_{10} was absorbed more efficiently than were other commercially available forms, and therefore lower doses of that form could be used to raise increase levels (10).

Relevant Research

Tissue and Blood Concentrations of CoQ₁₀ in Cardiovascular Disease

◆ A review article cited several studies suggesting that CoQ_{10} concentrations are reduced in heart tissue measured from biopsies obtained during catheterization in individuals with cardiovascular disease. The lowest tissue levels were observed in subjects with advanced heart failure (11).

◆ In a cross-sectional study of 94 hospital patients, subjects with very low serum CoQ_{10} levels had a significant increased risk of dying or having congestive heart failure and/or myalgia (12).

◆ Several studies have reported decreased blood concentrations of CoQ_{10} in subjects treated with HMG-CoA reductase inhibitors (cholesterol-lowering medications such as pravastatin) (13–15), although not all studies have been consistent (16).

CoQ_{10} Supplements and Cardiovascular Disease

◆ A randomized, double-blind, controlled study of 144 subjects with a history of myocardial infarct compared the efficacy of CoQ_{10} supplementation with B-complex vitamin supplementation (control) in the prevention of recurrent cardiac events. In this study, 120 mg/day of CoQ_{10} was associated with a significant reduction in total and nonfatal cardiac events as well as lower rates of reported fatigue as compared with the control group. CoQ_{10} was also associated with significant increase in plasma vitamin E and HDL cholesterol and a reduction of lipid peroxidation as measured by thiobarbituric acid reactions substances (TBARS) and malondialdehyde (MDA) (17).

◆ In a double-blind study, 32 individuals awaiting heart transplantation were randomly assigned to receive 60 mg CoQ_{10} or placebo for 3 months along with their usual medication therapies. Of the 27 subjects who completed the study, those receiving CoQ_{10} demonstrated a significant improvement in a 6-minute walk test, fatigue, and the Minnesota Living with Heart Failure Questionnaire, but no significant changes in electrocardiogram were shown. Small sample size and brief duration of intervention limit study interpretation, but supplementation may prove beneficial for the increasing number of people awaiting cardiac transplantation (18).

◆ In a double-blind, placebo-controlled, crossover study, 30 individuals with ischemic or idiopathic dilated cardiomyopathy and chronic left ventricular dysfunction were randomly assigned to receive CoQ_{10} or a placebo for 3 months each. Right heart pressures, cardiac output, echocardiographic left ventricular volumes, and quality of life (measured using the Minnesota Living with Heart Failure Questionnaire) were assessed at baseline and after each treatment. Plasma levels of CoQ_{10} increased to more than twice basal values. There were no significant differences between treatments in left ventricular ejection fraction, cardiac volumes, hemodynamic indexes, or quality of life measures (19).

◆ In a double-blind, placebo-controlled trial, 144 subjects with acute myocardial infarction were randomly assigned to receive 120 mg CoQ_{10} or a placebo daily for 28 days, starting within 3 days after infarction. The extent of cardiac disease, increase in cardiac enzymes, and oxidative stress were similar between groups at baseline. After treatment, angina pectoris, total arrhythmias, and poor left ventricular function were significantly improved in the CoQ_{10} group compared with the placebo group. Total cardiac events, including cardiac deaths and nonfatal infarction, were also significantly reduced in the CoQ_{10} group compared with the placebo group (15.0% vs 30.9%). The authors concluded that further studies with a larger number of subjects and long-term follow-up are needed to confirm their results (20).

◆ A meta-analysis of eight clinical trials of CoQ_{10} in individuals with congestive heart failure (CHF) found that supplemental CoQ_{10} was associated with a significant improvement in stroke volume, ejection fraction, cardiac output, cardiac index, and diastolic volume index (21).

◆ In a double-blind, placebo-controlled study, 322 subjects with chronic CHF were randomly assigned to receive 2 mg CoQ_{10}/kg/day or a placebo for 1 year. The number of episodes of pulmonary edema or cardiac asthma were significantly less in the CoQ$_{10}$ group than in the placebo group. In addition, subjects taking CoQ$_{10}$ supplements had significantly fewer hospitalizations (22).

◆ In a double-blind, placebo-controlled study, 55 individuals with CHF were randomly assigned to receive 200 mg CoQ$_{10}$ or a placebo daily for 6 months. Cardiac performance (ventricular ejection fraction), peak oxygen consumption, and exercise duration were measured at baseline and at study's end. Subjects receiving CoQ$_{10}$ supplements had higher serum concentrations of CoQ$_{10}$, but there were no differences in any of the parameters measured when compared with the placebo (23).

◆ In a 12-week, randomized, double-blind, placebo-controlled, 2 × 2 factorial design trial, CoQ$_{10}$ was compared with fenofibrate or a combination to assess changes in blood glucose and blood pressure in patients with type 2 diabetes and dyslipidemia. This was a secondary analysis conducted in the context of an on-going study to determine the effects of these agents on cardiac function. CoQ$_{10}$ was administered at a dose of 100 mg twice daily and fenofibrate at a dose of 200 mg daily. Despite significant increases in plasma CoQ-10 levels, A1C was not clinically significantly changed with any supplement. Blood pressure was significantly reduced with CoQ$_{10}$ (−6.1 mmHg reduction in systolic blood pressure and −2.9 mmHg in diastolic blood pressure). These findings support the need for more research on the effects of CoQ$_{10}$ on blood (24).

CoQ$_{10}$ and Exercise Performance

◆ In a placebo-controlled study, 18 male endurance cyclists and triathletes were given 1 mg CoQ$_{10}$/kg/day or a placebo for 28 days. Subjects were evaluated during and following graded cycling to exhaustion, which was completed before and after the trial. Although CoQ$_{10}$ supplements significantly increased plasma concentrations of CoQ$_{10}$, there was no effect on submaximal or maximal performance measures (oxygen uptake, anaerobic and respiratory compensation thresholds, blood lactate, glucose and triglyceride levels, heart rate, and blood pressure). The authors noted that these results do not preclude the possibility that supplemental CoQ$_{10}$ may benefit athletes with a preexisting cellular CoQ$_{10}$ deficiency (25).

◆ In a double-blind, placebo-controlled study, 18 subjects were given 120 mg CoQ$_{10}$/day or a placebo for 22 days. The first week included normal physical activity, followed by 4 days of high-intensity anaerobic training, with a 7-day recovery period. There was a significantly greater increase in anaerobic performance in the placebo group compared with the CoQ$_{10}$ group. There were no significant differences between groups in VO$_{2max}$, submaximal and peak VO$_2$, perceived exertion, respiratory quotient, blood lactate, or heart rate (26).

◆ In a double-blind, placebo-controlled study, 37 moderately trained male marathon runners were randomly assigned to receive 90 mg CoQ$_{10}$ plus 13.5 mg α-tocopherol or a placebo daily for 3 weeks before a marathon. Just before the run, there was a significant 282% increase in plasma CoQ$_{10}$ and a 16% increase in plasma vitamin E in subjects in the supplement group compared with the placebo group. Also, the proportion of plasma ubiquinol of total CoQ_{10}, an indication of plasma redox status in vivo, was significantly higher in subjects in the supplement group. Additionally, the susceptibility of the VLDL plus LDL fraction, to ex vivo copper-induced oxidation, was significantly reduced after CoQ_{10} and vitamin E supplementation compared with placebo. The marathon race increased lipid peroxidation in both groups. However, supplementation of CoQ_{10} plus vitamin E had no effect on lipid peroxidation or on the muscular damage (increase in serum creatine kinase activity or in plasma lactate levels) induced by the marathon race (27).

CoQ_{10} and Cancer

- Observational studies of women diagnosed with breast cancer have reported reduced blood CoQ_{10} concentrations (28). In one study, 200 women age 18 to 65 years hospitalized for the biopsy and/or ablation of a breast tumor had significantly reduced plasma CoQ_{10} levels compared with blood samples from 253 healthy control subjects age 18 to 65 years. There was no difference in plasma CoQ_{10} reduction between patients with malignant tumors (n = 80) and nonmalignant lesions (n = 120). There was also no correlation between age and CoQ_{10} levels (28).

- In an uncontrolled study, 32 subjects with metastasized breast cancer took a combination of antioxidants (vitamin C, selenium, beta carotene, and essential fatty acids) that included 90 mg CoQ_{10}. After 18 months, the authors reported partial remission in six subjects (29). An article by the same researchers reported regression of metastases in 10 women with breast cancer who took 390 mg CoQ_{10} daily for 3 to 5 years (30). However, these results should be viewed with caution because it is impossible to evaluate the efficacy of CoQ_{10} from case studies and uncontrolled trials. They are included here because they are often cited to support marketing claims.

CoQ_{10} and Immunity and HIV/AIDS

- One study reported that individuals with AIDS had reduced CoQ_{10} blood concentrations compared with control subjects (31).

- Three uncontrolled trials of supplemental CoQ_{10} in small numbers of healthy subjects and individuals with cancer showed improvement in immune parameters (31–34). These studies are included, despite their methodological flaws, because they are often cited to support marketing claims.

CoQ_{10} and Neurodegenerative Disease

- Eighty subjects with early Parkinson's disease (PD) were randomly assigned to either placebo or increasing dosages of CoQ_{10} at 300, 600, or 1,200 mg/day for up to 16 months. Based on the Unified Parkinson's Disease Rating Scale, CoQ_{10} supplementation at 1,200 mg/day was associated with a significant improvement in function. There was a trend for significance at lower dosages, which did not reach statistical significance. The clinical relevance or long-term efficacy of supplementation was not evaluated or discussed (35).

♦ In an uncontrolled pilot study, 15 subjects with PD (age 54 to 70 years) took one of three dosages of CoQ$_{10}$ plus 400 IU vitamin E. Subjects 1 through 5 were given 400 mg CoQ$_{10}$ per day, subjects 6 through 10 were given 600 mg CoQ$_{10}$ per day, and subjects 11 through 15 were given 800 mg CoQ$_{10}$ per day for 1 month. Plasma CoQ$_{10}$ levels increased with all dosages. CoQ$_{10}$ plus vitamin E did not change the mean score on the motor portion of the Unified Parkinson's Disease Rating Scale. There was a trend toward an increase in complex I activity of the mitochondrial electron-transport chain (reduced in the platelets and substatia niagra of patients with PD). The authors noted that any symptomatic effect caused by CoQ$_{10}$ would likely have been overshadowed by the effect of medication that the subject continued to take during the study (6).

CoQ$_{10}$ and Migraines

♦ In a double-blind study, 42 individuals with chronic migraines were randomly assigned to receive 100 mg CoQ$_{10}$ three times daily or a placebo for 3 months. Migraine frequency rates were reduced 14.4% in the placebo group and 47.6% in the CoQ$_{10}$ group, offering preliminary evidence of a protective effect of CoQ$_{10}$ on migraines (36).

♦ In an uncontrolled study of 32 individuals with episodic migraines, 150 mg CoQ$_{10}$ daily was associated with a 50% reduction in number of days with migraine in 61.3% of subjects (total days with migraine decreased from 7.34 during the initial 3 month observational period to 2.95 during the 3-month intervention period). This study was small and was not placebo-controlled. Further research in this area is warranted (37).

References

1. Kalen A, Appelkvist EL, Dallner G. Age-related changes in the lipid composition of rat and human tissue. *Lipids.* 1989;24:579–584.
2. Mordente A, Martorana GE, Santini SA, et al. Antioxidant effect of coenzyme Q on hydrogen peroxide-activated myoglobin. *Clin Investig.* 1993;71(8 Suppl):S92-S96.
3. Ernster L, Forsmark-Andree P. Ubiquinol: an endogenous antioxidant in aerobic organisms. *Clin Investig.* 1993;71(8 Suppl):S60-S65.
4. Weber C, Sejersgard Jakobsen T, Mortensen SA, et al. Antioxidative effect of dietary coenzyme Q$_{10}$ in human blood plasma. *Int J Vitam Nutr Res.* 1994;64:311–315.
5. Shults CW, Flint Beal M, Song D, et al. Pilot trial of high dosages of coenzyme Q$_{10}$ in patients with Parkinson's disease. *Exp Neurol.* 2004;188:491–494.
6. Shults CW, Beal MF, Fontaine D, et al. Absorption, tolerability, and effects on mitochondrial activity of oral coenzyme Q$_{10}$ in parkinsonian patients. *Neurology.* 1998;50:793–795.
7. Overvad K, Diamant B, Holm L, et al. Coenzyme Q$_{10}$ in health and disease. *Eur J Clin Nutr.* 1999;53:764–770.
8. Weber C, Bysted A, Holmer G. The coenzyme Q$_{10}$ content of the average Danish diet. *Int J Vitam Nutr Res.* 1997;67:123–129.

9. Weber C, Bysted A, Holmer G. Coenzyme Q_{10} in the diet—daily intake and relative bioavailability. *Mol Aspects Med.* 1997;18(Suppl):S251-S254.

10. Chopra RK, Goldman R, Sinatra ST, et al. Relative bioavailability of coenzyme Q_{10} formulations in human subjects. *Int J Vitam Nutr Res.* 1998;68:109–113.

11. Mortensen SA. Perspectives on therapy of cardiovascular diseases with coenzyme Q_{10} (ubiquinone). *Clin Investig.* 1993:71(8 Suppl):S116-S123.

12. Jameson S. Statistical data support prediction of death within 6 months on low levels of coenzyme Q_{10} and other entities. *Clin Investig.* 1993;71(8 Suppl):S137-S139.

13. Appelkvist EL, Edlund C, Low P, et al. Effects of inhibitors of hydroxymethylglutaryl coenzyme A reductase on coenzyme Q and dolichol biosynthesis. *Clin Investig.* 1993;71(8 Suppl):S97-S102.

14. De Pinieux G, Chariot P, Ammi-Said M, et al. Lipid-lowering drugs and mitochondrial function: effects of HMG-CoA reductase inhibitors on serum ubiquinone and blood lactate/pyruvate ratio. *Br J Clin Pharmacol.* 1996;42:333–337.

15. Bargossi AM, Battino M, Gaddi A, et al. Exogenous CoQ_{10} preserves plasma ubiquinone levels in patients treated with 3-hydroxy-3methylglutaryl coenzyme A reductase inhibitors. *Int J Clin Lab Res.* 1994;24:171–176.

16. Laaksonen R, Jokelainen K, Sahi T, et al. Decreases in serum ubiquinone concentrations do not result in reduced levels in muscle tissue during short-term simvastatin treatment in humans. *Clin Pharmacol Ther.* 1995;57:62–66.

17. Singh RB, Neki NS, Kartikey K, et al. Effect of coenzyme Q10 on risk of atherosclerosis in patients with recent myocardial infarction. *Mol Cell Biochem.* 2003;246:75–82.

18. Berman M, Erman A, Ben-Gal T, et al. Coenzyme Q_{10} in patients with end-stage heart failure awaiting cardiac transplantation: a randomized, placebo-controlled study. *Clin Cardiol.* 2004;27:295–299.

19. Watson PS, Scalia GM, Galbraith A, et al. Lack of effect of coenzyme Q on left ventricular function in patients with congestive heart failure. *J Am Coll Cardiol.* 1999;33:1549–1552.

20. Singh RB, Wander GS, Rastogi A, et al. Randomized, double-blind, placebo-controlled trial of coenzyme Q_{10} in patients with acute myocardial infarction. *Cardiovasc Drugs Ther.* 1998;12:347–353.

21. Soja AM, Mortensen SA. Treatment of congestive heart failure with coenzyme Q_{10} illuminated by meta-analyses of clinical trials. *Mol Aspects Med.* 1997;18(Suppl):S159–S168.

22. Morisco C, Trimarco B, Condorelli M. Effect of coenzyme Q_{10} therapy in patients with congestive heart failure: a long-term multicenter randomized study. *Clin Investig.* 1993;71(8 Suppl):S134-S136.

23. Khatta M, Alexander BS, Krichten CM, et al. The effect of coenzyme Q_{10} with congestive heart failure. *Ann Intern Med.* 2000;132:636–640.

24. Hodgson JM, Watts GF, Playford DA, et al. Coenzyme Q_{10} improves blood pressure and glycaemic control: a controlled trial in subjects with type 2 diabetes. *Eur J Clin Nutr.* 2002;56:1137–1142.

25. Weston SB, Zhou S, Weatherby RP, et al. Does exogenous coenzyme Q_{10} affect aerobic capacity in endurance athletes? *Int J Sport Nutr.* 1997;7:197–206.

26. Malm C, Svensson M, Ekblom B, et al. Effects of ubiquinone-10 supplementation and high intensity training on physical performance in humans. *Acta Physiol Scand.* 1997;161:379–384.
27. Kaikkonen J, Kosonen L, Nyyssonen K, et al. Effect of combined coenzyme Q_{10} and d-alpha-tocopherol acetate supplementation on exercise-induced lipid peroxidation and muscular damage: a placebo-controlled, double-blind study in marathon runners. *Free Radic Res.* 1998;29:85–92.
28. Jolliet P, Simon N, Barre J, et al. Plasma coenzyme Q_{10} concentrations in breast cancer: prognosis and therapeutic consequences. *Int J Clin Pharmacol Ther.* 1998;36:506–509.
29. Lockwood K, Moesgaard S, Hanioka T, et al. Apparent partial remission of breast cancer in 'high risk' patients supplemented with nutritional antioxidants, essential fatty acids and coenzyme Q_{10}. *Mol Aspects Med.* 1994;15(Suppl):S231-S240.
30. Lockwood K, Moesgaard S, Yamamoto T, et al. Progress on therapy of breast cancer with vitamin Q_{10} and the regression of metastases. *Biochem Biophys Res Commun.* 1995;212:172–177.
31. Folkers K, Langsjoen P, Nara Y, et al. Biochemical deficiencies of coenzyme Q_{10} in HIV-infection and exploratory treatment. *Biochem Biophys Res Commun.* 1988;153:888–896.
32. Folkers K, Hanioka T, Xia LJ, et al. Coenzyme Q_{10} increases T4/T8 ratios of lymphocytes in ordinary subjects and relevance to patients having the AIDS related complex. *Biochem Biophys Res Commun.* 1991;176:786–791.
33. Folkers K, Morita M, McRee J. The activities of coenzyme Q_{10} and vitamin B_6 for immune responses. *Biochem Biophys Res Commun.* 1993;193:88–92.
34. Folkers K, Brown R, Judy WV, et al. Survival of cancer patients on therapy with coenzyme Q_{10}. *Biochem Biophys Res Commun.* 1993;192:241–245.
35. Shults CW, Oakes D, Kieburtz K, et al. Effects of coenzyme Q_{10} in early Parkinson disease: evidence of slowing of the functional decline. *Arch Neurol.* 2002;59:1541–1550.
36. Sandor PS, Di Clemente L, Coppola G, et al. Efficacy of coenzyme Q_{10} in migraine prophylaxis: a randomized controlled trial. *Neurology.* 2005;64:713–715.
37. Rozen TD, Oshinsky ML, Gebeline CA, et al. Open label trial of coenzyme Q_{10} as a migraine preventive. *Cephalagia.* 2002;22:137–141.

Colostrum/Bovine Colostrum

Colostrum is the premilk fluid secreted from the mammary glands during the first few days after birth. In addition to supplying both macro- and micronutrients to the newborn, colostrum is a source of several growth and immune factors that contribute to the neonate's development and immune defense. Both bovine and human colostrum contain a variety of peptide growth factors, including insulin-like growth factors (IGF-1, IGF-2), insulin, transforming growth factor (TGF)-α and -β, and epidermal growth factor (EGF) (1–3). Colostrum also contains several antimicrobial compounds, including immunoglobulins, lactoferrin, lysozyme, and lactoperoxidase. Immunoglobulins are largely responsible for the antimicrobial activity of bovine colostrum. Immunoglobulin (Ig) G1 is the most abundant type of immunoglobulin in colostrum, whereas IgG2, IgM, and IgA are found at much lower levels. Immunoglobulins from colostrum play an important role in protecting newborn calves from infectious enteric and respiratory diseases. Lactoferrin, an iron-binding glycoprotein, is another antimicrobial compound found in colostrum (1–3).

Researchers have discovered that hyperimmunizing cows with repeated injections of vaccines can increase the immunoglobulin content of the milk (1). The resulting product is referred to as "hyperimmune colostrum" but this product differs from commercially available colostrum and it is not sold as a dietary supplement in the United States. Bovine colostrum has been marketed as a dietary supplement for digestive health, immunity, weight loss, skin health, and other conditions (2,3).

Media and Marketing Claims	Efficacy
Improves digestive health	↑(hyperimmune colostrum) NR (nonimmune colostrum)
Supports immune function in people with HIV	NR
Improves athletic performance	↔

Safety

- No serious adverse effects have been reported with hyperimmune or nonimmune colostrum products.

- Products need to be properly processed by pasteurization or microfiltration. Colostrum suppliers need to certify that products are free of bovine spongiform encephalopathy (BSE, ie, mad cow disease) and other bovine diseases. Additionally, products should be screened for the presence of heavy metals, pesticides, herbicides, and pathogens, and also tested to verify that the final product is biologically active.

- Colostrum could cause mild gastrointestinal discomfort in individuals with lactose-intolerance, because the products do contain a small amount of lactose.

- There is a potential risk that supplements derived from cows could be contaminated with BSE. However, there is no research showing that colostrum can be contaminated with BSE, and disease transmission to humans by this route has not been reported. Avoid products produced in countries where BSE has been found.

- Individuals with cow's milk allergy should avoid colostrum.

Drug/Supplement Interactions

- No adverse interactions have been reported.
- Colostrum taken may have a beneficial effect on the gut when taken with NSAIDs.

◆ Antibody activity of hyperimmune bovine colostrum (produced by cows immunized against specific pathogens) may be decreased if taken with food due to increase in stomach acid and digestive enzyme activity.

Key Points

◆ Large-scale, controlled clinical trials of nonimmune colostrum are needed to determine its efficacy for use with intestinal diseases.

◆ Although several uncontrolled trials have suggested that bovine colostrum may be helpful for patients with AIDS-related diarrhea, controlled trials are needed to determine efficacy for this population. No recent studies have been published in this area.

◆ Small intervention trials are conflicting, but have shown some positive effects on exercise performance.

Food Sources

Colostrum is not a constituent of food (except for human breastmilk). Regular cow's milk contains negligible amounts of the immune and growth factors found in bovine colostrum.

Dosage Information/Bioavailability

Colostrum sold in supplements is typically collected during the first 72 hours after a cow gives birth. Supplements may either be pasteurized at minimum heat after filtration and homogenization or sterilized through microfiltration and vacuum packaging (4). Ideally, colostrum products should be taken from several pasture-fed cows to insure a wide spectrum of antibodies and growth factors. Colostrum is available in capsules, chewable tablets, powders, liquid, energy bars and protein powders, and in topical skin creams and lotions. Manufacturers suggest taking 2,000 to 5,000 mg of colostrum (approximately 8 to 10 capsules) daily, although some studies have used 20-g doses.

A unique study was conducted to determine if exposure to rotavirus antibodies in the form of milk from immunized cattle would result in the positive presence of these antibodies in the feces, which could suggest a reduction in risk for this infection. In the study, 105 preschoolers were supplemented with hyperimmune colostrum (100 mL milk consumed three times daily for 6 days) from cows immunized against rotavirus (rotavirus causes infectious diarrhea). Colostral antibodies were shown to survive passage through the gut and remained active according to ELISA measures of rotaviral activity (5).

Relevant Research

Colostrum and Intestinal Disorders

◆ In a double-blind, placebo-controlled study, 27 subjects (age 1 month to 18 years) with *E. coli*–associated diarrhea were randomly assigned to receive 7,000 mg bovine colostrum (from nonimmunized cows) or placebo daily for 2 weeks. Stool frequency and fecal excretion of the infecting strains were assessed. At the end of therapy, stool frequency decreased significantly in subjects treated with colostrum (from three stools to one). Subjects in the placebo group had no change in stool frequency. However, colostrum had no effect on the carriage of pathogens in feces (6).

◆ Other controlled clinical trials using colostrum from hyperimmunized cows have reported improvements in diarrhea in children infected with rotavirus (7,8) and in healthy adults with *Cryptosporidium parvum* infection (9).

Colostrum and NSAID-Induced Gut Injury

◆ In a placebo-controlled, crossover trial, seven healthy male subjects received in random order 375 mL bovine colostrum (nonimmune) or isocaloric placebo daily for 7 days each. There was a 2-week washout period between treatments. For the last 5 days of each study arm, subjects also took indomethacin (50 mg × 3). At the beginning and end of each test period, intestinal permeability was measured by quantifying lactulose, rhamnose, and mannitol sugar absorption. Gut permeability is a method of testing small intestinal injury. There were no significant differences in baseline permeability values. However, permeability significantly increased about three times in response to indomethacin in the placebo subjects, but not the colostrum-treated subjects. This pilot study was not blinded, and therefore the results should be viewed with caution (10).

◆ A second study was performed by the same researchers in 15 subjects who had regularly been taking a stable, substantive dose of a nonselective NSAID for at least 1 year. Subjects in a double-blind, crossover design were randomly assigned to receive 375 mL bovine colostrum or placebo daily for 7 days each, with a 2-week washout period. All subjects continued their NSAID therapies. Intestinal permeability was assessed at baseline and at the end of the study. At the study's end, colostrum had no significant effect on gut permeability (11).

Colostrum and AIDS-Related Diarrhea

◆ There is some evidence from small, uncontrolled trials that hyperimmune and/or nonimmune colostrum may benefit people with AIDS who are infected with the parasite *Cryptosporidium parvum*. In one in vitro study, hyperimmune colostrum inhibited *C. parvum* infection in human intestinal cells, whereas nonimmune colostrum did not (12).

◆ In an open study of 24 individuals with AIDS who had severe diarrhea, 21 days of hyperimmune colostrum treatment reduced stool weight (from 1,158 to 595 g/day at study's end) and stool frequency (from 6.6 to 5.4 bowel movements/day at study's end) (13). Because this study was not controlled, the results should be viewed with caution.

◆ There are also case reports of clinical improvement with hyperimmune colostrum in two patients with AIDS and diarrhea secondary to *C. parvum* (14,15).

Colostrum and Body Composition in Athletes

♦ In a double-blind, placebo-controlled study, 22 resistance- and aerobically trained subjects were randomly assigned to receive 20 g colostrum in powder form or placebo (whey protein) daily for 8 weeks. Subjects were instructed to maintain their current diet and exercise level. Body composition was assessed by dual x-ray absorptiometry. Also assessed were: treadmill time to exhaustion, one-repetition maximum strength during bench press, and the total number of repetitions done during one set to exhaustion at a submaximal load for bench. There were no significant differences between groups in baseline measures of age, height, weight, body composition, performance measures, or exercise training. The whey protein group experienced a significant increase in body weight, but no change in lean body mass (LBM), whereas the colostrum group had a significant increase in LBM (mean gain of 1.5 kg), but no significant change in body weight. There were no other differences in any other parameter measured (16).

Colostrum and Athletic Performance

♦ Thirty-four trained and untrained athletes took 60 g bovine colostrum or whey protein during an 8-week resistance training program. Trained athletes receiving bovine colostrum demonstrated a significant increase in arm circumference associated with an increase in subcutaneous fat whereas all athletes (both trained and untrained) showed an increase in voluntary isometric torque, regardless of supplement group (17). This study was neither blinded nor randomized, limiting the validity of the results.

♦ In a randomized, placebo-controlled, double-blind study, 51 males were given either bovine colostrum or whey protein for 8 weeks during resistance and plyometric training. At the end of the study, peak vertical jump and peak cycle power were significantly greater in the bovine colostrum group as compared with the placebo; however, the differences between the two groups had not been significant at 4 weeks. Plasma IGF-1 levels were not different across groups or over time. Anaerobic work capacity also did not change over time (18).

♦ In a small study of 35 male and female elite hockey players, 8 weeks of 60 g/day bovine colostrum supplementation vs placebo resulted in significant improvement in sprint test performance ($P = .02$) but no difference in vertical jump, body composition or endurance tests across groups (19).

♦ A randomized, double-blind, controlled study of bovine colostrum(60 g/day) vs whey protein among 30 physically-fit males showed minimal or no change in several performance factors and did not support the use of bovine colostrum supplementation for improved athletic performance (20).

References

1. Pakkanen R, Aalto J. Growth factors and antimicrobial factors of bovine colostrum. *Int Dairy J.* 1997;7:285–297.

2. Playford RJ, Macdonald CE, Johnson WS. Colostrum and milk-derived peptide growth factors for the treatment of gastrointestinal disorders. *Am J Clin Nutr.* 2000;72:5–14.
3. Lilius EM, Marnila P. The role of colostral antibodies in prevention of microbial infections. *Curr Opin Infect Dis.* 2001;14:295–300.
4. Maher TJ. *Bovine Colostrum Continuing Education Module.* Boulder, Colo: New Hope Institute of Retailing; 2000.
5. Pacyna J, Siwek K, Terry SJ, et al. Survival of rotavirus antibody activity derived from bovine colostrum after passage through the human gastrointestinal tract. *J Pediatr Gastroenterol Nutr.* 2001;32:162–167.
6. Huppertz HI, Rutkowski S, Busch DH, et al. Bovine colostrum ameliorates diarrhea in infection with diarrheagenic *Escherichia coli*, shiga toxin-producing *E. coli*, and *E. coli* expressing intimin and hemolysin. *J Pediatr Gastroenterol Nutr.* 1999;29:452–456.
7. Sarker SA, Casswall TH, Mahalanabis D, et al. Successful treatment of rotavirus diarrhea in children with immunoglobulin from immunized bovine colostrum. *Pediatr Infect Dis J.* 1998;17:149–154.
8. Mitra AK, Mahalanabis D, Ashraf H, et al. Hyperimmune cow colostrum reduces diarrhea due to rotavirus: a double-blind, controlled clinical trial. *Acta Paediatr.* 1995;84:996–1001.
9. Okhuysen PC, Chappell CL, Crabb J, et al. Prophylactic effect of bovine anti-*Cryptosporidium* hyperimmune colostrum immunoglobulin in healthy volunteers challenged with *Cryptosporidium*. *Clin Infect Dis.* 1998;26:1324–1329.
10. Playford, RJ, MacDonald CE, Calnan DP, et al. Co-administration of the health food supplement, bovine colostrums, reduces the acute non-steroidal anti-inflammatory drug induced increase in intestinal permeability. *Clin Sci (Lond).* 2001;100:627–638.
11. Playford RJ, MacDonald CE, Calnan DP, et al. Co-administration of the health food supplement, bovine colostrum, reduces the acute non-steroidal anti-inflammatory drug-induced increase in intestinal permeability. *Clin Sci (Lond).* 2001;100:627–633.
12. Flanigan T, Marshall R, Redman D, et al. In vitro screening of therapeutic agents against Crytosporidium: hyperimmune cow colostrum is highly inhibitory. *J Protozool.* 1991;38(suppl):S225-S227.
13. Greenberg PD, Cello JP. Treatment of severe diarrhea caused by *Cryptosporidium parvum* with oral bovine immunoglobulin concentrate in patients with AIDS. *J Acquir Immune Defic Syndr Hum Retrovirol.* 1996;13:348–354.
14. Shield J, Melville C, Novelli V, et al. Bovine colostrum immunoglobulin concentrate for cryptosporidiosis in AIDS. *Arch Dis Child.* 1993;69:451–453.
15. Ungar BL, Ward DJ, Fayer R, et al. Cessation of Cryptosporidium-associated diarrhea in an acquired immunodeficiency syndrome patient after treatment with hyperimmune bovine colostrum. *Gastroenterology.* 1990;98:486–489.
16. Antonio J, Sanders MS, Van Gammeren D. The effect of bovine colostrum supplementation on body composition and exercise performance in active men and women. *Nutrition.* 2001;17:243–247.
17. Brinkworth GD, Buckley JD, Slavotinek JP, et al. Effect of bovine colostrum supplementation on the composition of resistance of resistance trained and untrained limbs in healthy young men. *Eur J Appl Physiol.* 2004;91:53–60.

18. Buckley JD, Brinkworth GD, Abbott MJ. Effect of bovine colostrum on anaerobic exercise performance and plasma insulin-like growth factor I. *J Sports Sci.* 2003;21: 577–588.
19. Hofman Z, Smeets R, Verlaan G, et al. The effect of bovine colostrums supplementation on exercise performance in elite field hockey players. *Int J Sports Nutr Exerc Metab.* 2002;12:431–469.
20. Buckley JD, Abbott MJ, Brinkworth GD, et al. Bovine colostrum supplementation during endurance running training improves recovery, but not performance. *J Sci Med Sport.* 2002;5:65–79.

Conjugated Linoleic Acid

Conjugated linoleic acid (CLA) is a term used to describe a group of linoleic acid isomers in which the double bonds are conjugated at carbons 10 and 12 or 9 and 11 in the *cis* and *trans* configurations. CLA is a class of fatty acids produced naturally by microorganisms associated with digestion, particularly certain microorganisms in the rumen of cattle. It is found in low concentrations in human blood and tissues. Nine different isomers of CLA have been identified. Biological activity and effects on health vary by isoform. Researchers have not determined the mechanism for the potential anticarcinogenic activity of CLA. CLA has also been investigated for its effect on body composition. A specific CLA isomer (*trans*-10, *cis*-12) may be responsible for this by inhibiting several biochemical factors associated with lipid uptake. Some theorize that CLA inhibits heparin-releasable lipoprotein lipase, which cleaves triglycerides so that free fatty acids are absorbed into cells (1,2).

Media and Marketing Claims	Efficacy
Helps control weight, reduce body fat	↔
Stimulates immune function	↓
Prevents cancer	NR
Reduces risk for heart disease	↓
Improves glucose tolerance	↓

Safety

♦ Safety of CLA supplements for long term use has not been tested. CLA (3.9 g/day) had no adverse effects in a study lasting 93 days.

♦ The most common side effect of CLA is gastrointestinal upset, including diarrhea, nausea, loose stools, and dyspepsia; fatigue is also possible.

♦ The *trans*-10, *cis*-12 isomer of CLA increases insulin resistance in individuals with abdominal obesity or diabetes.

♦ A dosage of 4.2 g CLA daily for 1 month caused lipid peroxidation in obese men (3).

Drug/Supplement Interactions

CLA may increase storage of vitamin A (retinol) in liver and breast tissue.

Key Points

- An extensive review of the potential health benefits of CLA was published in the June 2004 supplement to the *American Journal of Clinical Nutrition*. In general, the biological mechanism for a role of CLA in weight control, cancer prevention, immunity, or glucose control have not been fully elucidated. Extensive human research is needed before clinical recommendations for supplementation can be made (4).

- Studies in animals suggest that CLA supplementation reduces body fat and increases lean body mass. Preliminary human research suggests that CLA does not seem to have the same favorable effects on body composition. One study completed in a metabolic unit showed no positive effect of CLA supplementation on weight loss, lean body mass, or appetite. More research in larger groups of subjects is needed before CLA can be recommended as adjunctive therapy for weight management.

- Although CLA seems to enhance immune function in animal models, one study reported no immune enhancement in healthy women and another suggested that CLA had a negative effect on immune parameters. Clearly, more human research is needed.

- Preliminary animal and in vitro studies suggest CLA may have anticarcinogenic properties. One epidemiological study found an association between increased dietary CLA and decreased risk for estrogen-related-negative breast cancer in premenopausal women. Well-controlled, clinical trials are needed to determine the effect of CLA supplements on cancer in humans.

- CLA had no effect on blood cholesterol (total, LDL, HDL), triglyceride levels, platelet function, or blood coagulation in healthy women with normal cholesterol levels. CLA had no effect on blood lipids in obese men. In one study, the *trans*-10, *cis*-12 form of CLA actually increased triglycerides and LDL:HDL ratios.

- There is preliminary research that CLA may benefit prediabetic obese rats. However, limited evidence from human trials (published in peer-reviewed journals) suggest that CLA does not significantly affect glucose or insulin levels in healthy or obese subjects. In fact, CLA may increase insulin resistance in individuals with diabetes. More research is needed to determine the effects of CLA on diabetes control.

Food Sources

CLA is primarily found in the milk and meat of ruminant animals. The CLA content of dairy products ranges from 2.3 to 11.3 mg per gram of fat, of which the majority is in the *cis*-9, *trans*-11 isomer form. Beef fat contains 3.1 to 8.5 mg CLA per gram of fat with the *cis*-9, *trans*-11 isomer predominating. Cooking has been shown to increase the CLA content of meat. Food products from nonruminant animals and plant oils have a CLA content of 0.6 to 0.9 mg per gram of fat. The CLA content of the US diet has been estimated at approximately 1 g/day (1), although another study suggested a much lower daily intake of approximately 150 to 200 mg CLA in the US diet (2).

Food	CLA, mg/serving
Lamb, uncooked (4 oz)	137
Beef, ground, uncooked (4 oz)	130
Butter (1 Tbsp)	54
Yogurt, low-fat (1 cup)	16.7
Yogurt, nonfat (1 cup)	11.2
Peanut butter (2 Tbsp)	3.3
Chicken, uncooked (½ chicken)	3.2
Oil, olive (1 Tbsp)	2.7
Shrimp, uncooked (3 oz)	0.9

Source: Data are calculated from values from reference 5.

Dosage Information/Bioavailability

CLA produced synthetically from sunflower oil is sold in capsules that provide approximately 60% to 80% CLA. Manufacturers typically recommend 1 to 4 g CLA/day. Many products contain the patented CLA formula Tonalin or Clarinol used in some research studies. These products contain the biologically active CLA isomers (*cis*-9, *trans*-11 and *trans*-10, *cis*-12). The amount of CLA in human adipose tissue and serum is significantly related to dietary milk fat intake (6,7).

Relevant Research

CLA and Body Composition/Obesity

◆ A 2003 review by Larsen et al emphasized that although animal studies continue to show efficacy for CLA supplementation in weight control, no human studies to date have provided sufficient support for this hypothesis (8). A few small studies have since been completed and are described below.

◆ In a double-blind, placebo-controlled study, 54 overweight adults experiencing weight cycling followed a very-low-calorie diet for 3 weeks followed by 13 weeks with either supplemental CLA (1.8 or 3.6 g/day) or placebo. The very-low-calorie diet resulted in significant weight reduction (mean loss of 7% body weight) at 3 weeks. Weight regain occurred after the diet in all subjects and was not associated with CLA supplementation. However, in those receiving CLA, weight regain was associated with a slightly higher increase in fat-free mass (FFM) during regain, which correlated with an increase in resting energy expenditure. The clinical relevance is minimal and does not support the use of CLA for weight control (9).

- Negative results were also shown in a double-blind, placebo-controlled study using two different isomers of CLA at two different levels of intake. Ninety overweight adults were randomly assigned to one of five beverages that contained: (*a*) 1.5 g *cis*-9, *trans*-11; (*b*) 3 g *cis*-9, *trans*-11; (*c*) 1.5 g *cis*-10, *trans*-12; (*d*) 3 g *cis*-10, *trans*-12; or (*e*) 3 g oleic sunflower oil Eighty-two subjects completed the trial. No significant changes over time or across treatment groups were seen for plasma insulin, blood glucose, weight, BMI, waist-to-hip ratio, or body fat during the 18-week intervention (10).

- A double-blind, placebo-controlled study of 180 overweight adults showed an inverse association between CLA supplements and body fat. Subjects were randomly assigned to receive CLA-free fatty acid (4.5 g with 3.6 g active CLA), CLA-triacyl-glycerol (4.5 g with 3.6 g active CLA), or placebo (4.5 g olive oil) for 1 year. Diet was not controlled. Whereas all groups had similar body composition at study onset, mean body fat mass was lower in those taking CLA than in the placebo group at 1 year. CLA-FFA supplementation was also associated with a significant increase in lean body mass. Lipoprotein(a) (Lp[a]) levels increased with CLA supplementation, and HDL decreased significantly in the CLA-triacylglycerol group (11). This study suggests that CLA may have favorable effects on body composition, but unfavorable changes in lipid levels may preclude use.

- In a double-blind, placebo-controlled study, 60 overweight or obese subjects were randomly assigned into five groups, receiving either a placebo (9 g olive oil) or 1.7, 3.4, 5.1, or 6.8 g CLA/day for 12 weeks. Dual-energy x-ray absorptiometry measured body composition at baseline, and at weeks 6 and 12. Forty-seven subjects completed the study. Body fat mass decreased in the CLA groups compared with the placebo group, with significant reductions observed in the 3.4-g and 6.8-g CLA groups. However, there were no differences among groups in lean body mass, BMI, blood safety variables, or blood lipids. There were no differences among groups regarding adverse events (12).

- In a randomized, controlled study, the effect of CLA (3 g/day for 64 days) vs a placebo (sunflower oil) was investigated in 17 healthy women confined to a metabolic suite for 94 days. Diet and activity were controlled and held constant. Subjects stayed in a metabolic suite for a control period lasting 30 days just before treatment. CLA supplementation had no effect on fat-free mass, fat mass, and percentage body fat compared with the placebo. In addition, CLA did not change the rate of appearance of glycerol, which indicates lipolytic rates, at rest or during exercise after 4 weeks of supplementation; nor did it affect 4-week or 8-week measures of energy expenditure (kcal/min), fat oxidation, and respiratory exchange ratios (13).

- In another report of the same subjects, the effects of CLA on circulating leptin levels, appetite, insulin, glucose, and lactate concentrations were examined. CLA supplementation was associated with a transient decrease in mean circulating leptin levels for 7 weeks, but then returned to baseline during the last 2 weeks of the study. Appetite parameters measured during the time when the greatest decreases in leptin levels were observed showed no significant effect of CLA compared with the placebo. No effects were seen on plasma glucose or lactate levels (14).

CLA and Immunity

♦ The effects on immunity of 3 g of *cis*-9 *trans*-11 CLA at increasing doses of 0.59, 1.19, and 2.38 g/day vs similar doses of *trans*-10, *cis*-12 CLA for 8 weeks were studied in healthy adults using a crossover design, with a 6-week washout. Both CLA supplements were associated with a significant, unwanted *decrease* in mitogen-induced T cell activation, which was dose-dependent. CLA was not able to modulate C-reactive protein, cytokines, or blood leukocyte counts (15).

♦ In a 93-day double-blind, placebo-controlled study, 17 women (ages 20 to 41 years) stayed in a metabolic research unit where exercise and diet were strictly controlled. Seven subjects were fed the basal diet (19%, 20%, and 51% energy from protein, fat, and carbohydrate, respectively). The remaining subjects were fed the basal diet for the first 30 days, followed by 3.9 g CLA daily for the next 63 days. Indexes of immune response (number of circulating white blood cells, granulocytes, monocytes, lymphocytes, and their subsets) were tested at weekly intervals, and delayed type hypersensitivity to a panel of six antigens was tested on days 30 and 90. All subjects were immunized with an influenza vaccine on day 65, with antibody titers collected on day 65 and day 92. CLA feeding had no effect on any of the parameters of immune status tested (16).

CLA and Cancer

♦ According to a review article that summarized animal model and cell culture studies of CLA and cancer, CLA inhibited proliferation in all cell lines, such as human malignant melanoma, and colorectal, breast, and lung cancer (17).

♦ No intervention data are available for CLA and cancer. One case-control study from the Western New York Breast Cancer Cohort suggested that at the highest dietary CLA intake levels there is a borderline significant decrease in risk for estrogen-receptor negative breast cancer (odds ratio [OR] = 0.4; 95% CI = 0.16–1.01) in premenopausal women that may warrant further study (18).

♦ In a population case-control study among Finnish women, dietary and serum CLA levels were significantly less in postmenopausal women diagnosed with breast cancer (n = 127) compared with control subjects who had no current or previous cancer (n = 133), as were serum myristic and *trans*-vaccenic acids (OR = 0.4; 95% CI = 0.2–0.9). No significant associations were demonstrated among premenopausal women (19).

CLA and Cardiovascular Disease

♦ A randomized, double-blind, placebo-controlled study of 25 obese men receiving 3 g *cis*-9 *trans*-11 CLA supplementation vs placebo for a period of 3 months showed adverse results. Men on the CLA supplement showed significant increases in lipid peroxidation biomarkers and decreased insulin resistance with supplementation. This would suggest that currently available supplements may actually increase risk for cardiovascular disease. Further research using well-defined supplements is warranted (20).

♦ In a separate study of healthy males, *cis*-9 *trans*-11 supplementation for 8 weeks at variable doses (0.6 to 2.4 g/day) or *trans*-10,*cis*-12 (0.6 to 2.5 g/day) showed variable effects that were dependent on the isoform of CLA. *Trans*-10, *cis*-12 supplementation had the detrimental effect of increasing serum triglyceride levels and LDL:HDL ratios, whereas *cis*-9,*trans*-11 decreased these cardiovascular outcomes. No change in body composition was shown (15).

♦ In a controlled study, 17 healthy women with normal lipids were randomly assigned to receive 3.9 g CLA or a placebo (equivalent amount of sunflower oil) for 63 days, following a 30-day stabilization period of no treatment. Subjects stayed in a metabolic research unit for the duration of the study. Subjects consumed a low-fat diet (30% of energy from fat). CLA had no significant effects on plasma cholesterol (total, LDL, and HDL) or triglyceride levels (21). Another article on the same subjects also reported that CLA had no effect on platelet aggregation or blood clotting parameters (22).

♦ In a double-blind, placebo-controlled study, 25 men with abdominal obesity (ages 39 to 64 years) were randomly assigned receive 4.2 g CLA/day or a placebo for 4 weeks. The main endpoints were differences between the two groups in sagittal abdominal diameter (SAD), serum cholesterol, LDL, HDL, triglycerides, free fatty acids, glucose, and insulin. At baseline, there were no significant differences between groups in anthropometric or metabolic variables. At the study's end, there was a significant decrease in SAD in the CLA group compared with the placebo group. However, there were no other differences in anthropometric measurements or biochemical parameters (23).

CLA and Diabetes

♦ A randomized, double-blind, placebo-controlled study of CLA supplementation in 32 subjects with type 2 diabetes showed that 3 g/day of 50% *cis*-9,*trans*-11 and 50% *trans*-10,*cis*-12 for 8 weeks resulted in a significant increase in fasting blood glucose concentration and reduced insulin sensitivity. HDL(2) cholesterol levels increased by 8% with CLA supplementation, and CLA reduced fibrinogen concentrations while showing no effect on C-reactive protein or interleukin-6 proinflammatory markers (24). This is among the first well-designed human studies in this area, and it raises substantial concern regarding the potential adverse effects of CLA supplements with regard to diabetes and chronic disease risk.

♦ In studies of subjects without diabetes, CLA had no significant effect on insulin or glucose levels (14,23).

References

1. Decker EA. The role of phenolics, conjugated linoleic acid, carnosine, and pyrroloquinoline quinone as nonessential dietary antioxidants. *Nutr Rev*. 1995;53:49–58.

2. Terpstra AH. Differences between humans and mice in efficacy of the body fat lowering effect of conjugated linoleic acid: role of metabolic rate. *J Nutr.* 2001;131: 2067–2068.

3. Basu S, Riserus U, Turpeinen A, et al. Conjugated linoleic acid induces lipid peroxidation in men with abdominal obesity. *Clin Sci (Colch).* 2000;99:511–516.

4. Pariza MW. Perspective on the safety and effectiveness of conjugated linoleic acid. *Am J Clin Nutr.* 2004;79(6 Suppl):S1132-S1136.

5. Rizenthaler KL, McGuire MK, Falen R, et al. Estimation of conjugated linoleic acid intake by written dietary assessment methodologies underestimates actual intake evaluated by food duplicate methodology. *J Nutr.* 2001;131:1548–1554.

6. Chin SF, Liu W, Storkson JM, et al. Dietary sources of conjugated dienoic isomers of linoleic acid, a newly recognized class of anticarcinogens. *J Food Comp Anal.* 1992;5:185–197.

7. Jiang J, Wolk A, Vessby B. Relation between the intake of milk fat and the occurrence of conjugated linoleic acid in human adipose tissue. *Am J Clin Nutr.* 2000;70:21–27.

8. Larsen TM, Toubro S, Astrup A. Efficacy and safety of dietary supplements containing CLA for the treatment of obesity: evidence from animal and human studies. *J Lipid Res.* 2003;44:2234–2241.

9. Kamphuis MM, Lejeune MP, Saris WH, et al. The effect of conjugated linoleic acid supplementation after weight loss on body weight regain, body composition, and resting metabolic rate in overweight subjects. *Int J Obes Relat Metab Disord.* 2003;27:840–847.

10. Malpuech-Brugere C, Verboeket-van de Venne WP, Mensick RP, et al. Effects of two conjugated linoleic acid isomers on body fat mass in overweight humans. *Obes Res.* 2004;12:591–598.

11. Gaullier JM, Halse J, Hoye K, et al. Conjugated linoleic acid supplementation for 1 y reduces body fat mass in healthy overweight humans. *Am J Clin Nutr.* 2004;79:1118–1125.

12. Blankson H, Stakkestad JA, Fagertun E, et al. Conjugated linoleic acid reduces body fat mass in overweight and obese humans. *J Nutr.* 2000;130:2943–2948.

13. Zambell KL, Keim NL, Van Loan MD, et al. Conjugated linoleic acid supplementation in humans: effects on body composition and energy expenditure. *Lipids.* 2000;35:777–782.

14. Medina EA, Horn WF, Keim NL, et al. Conjugated linoleic acid supplementation in humans: effects on circulating leptin concentrations and appetite. *Lipids.* 2000;35: 783–788.

15. Tricon S, Burdge GC, Kew S, et al. Effects of *cis*-9 *trans*-11 and *trans*-10, *cis*-12 conjugated linoleic acid on immune cell function in healthy humans. *Am J Clin Nutr.* 2004;80:1626–1633.

16. Park Y, Albright KJ, Storkson JM, et al. Changes in body composition in mice during feeding and withdrawal of conjugated linoleic acid. *Lipids.* 1999;34:243–248.

17. Parodi PW. Cow's milk fat components as potential anticarcinogenic agents. *J Nutr.* 1997;127:1055–1060.

18. McCann SE, Ip C, Ip MM, et al. Dietary intake of conjugated linoleic acids and risk of premenopausal and postmenopausal breast cancer, Western New York Exposures and Breast Cancer Study (WEB Study). *Cancer Epidemiol Biomarkers Prev.* 2004;13: 1480–1484.

19. Aro A, Mannisto S, Salminen I, et al. Inverse association between dietary and serum conjugated linoleic acid and risk of breast cancer in postmenopausal women. *Nutr Cancer.* 2000;38:151–157.

20. Riserus U, Vessby B, Arnlov J, et al. Effects of *cis*-9, *trans*-11 conjugated linoleic acid supplementation on insulin sensitivity, lipid peroxidation, and proinflammatory markers in obese men. *Am J Clin Nutr.* 2004;80:279–283.
21. Benito P, Nelson GJ, Kelley DS, et al. The effect of conjugated linoleic acid on plasma lipoproteins and tissue fatty acid composition in humans. *Lipids.* 2001;36:229–236.
22. Benito P, Nelson GJ, Kelley DS, et al. The effect of conjugated linoleic acid on platelet function, platelet fatty acid compostion, and blood coagulation in humans. *Lipids.* 2000;36:221–227.
23. Riserus U, Berglund L, Vessby B. Conjugated linoleic acid (CLA) reduced abdominal adipose tissue in obese middle-aged men with signs of the metabolic syndrome: a randomised controlled trial. *Int J Obes Relat Metab Disord.* 2001;25:1129–1135.
24. Moloney F, Yeow TP, Mullen A, et al. Conjugated linoleic acid supplementation, insulin sensitivity, and lipoprotein metabolism in patients with type 2 diabetes mellitus. *Am J Clin Nutr.* 2004;80:887–895.

Cranberry Extract

The cranberry *(Vaccinium macrocarpon)* is one of the few fruits native to North America. Cranberries get their name from Dutch and German settlers who called them "crane berries" because the vines and flowers resemble the head of a crane. Later, the name was shortened to cranberry. Native Americans used cranberries to help preserve food, as a dye, and in poultices to draw poison from arrow wounds. In the 20th century, cranberry juice was a folk remedy used to prevent urinary tract infections (UTIs). Early research from the 1920s through the 1970s proposed that cranberry helped UTIs by acidifying urine. Cranberry juice contains quinic acid, which was thought to cause excretion of hippuric acid in the urine, with the hippuric acid acting as an antibacterial agent. However, this theory has since been disproved. Cranberry juice also contains proanthocyanidins (tannins) that seem to prevent *Escherichia coli* bacteria from attaching to the bladder or kidney walls. Proanthocyanidins in blueberries also seem to have this effect. In addition, several compounds in cranberries, including fructose, interfere with *E. coli* adhesion to the urinary tract wall. Because of the potential positive effects of cranberry juice on the urinary tract, supplements containing cranberry juice extract have been marketed for urinary tract health (1–5).

Media and Marketing Claims	Efficacy
Prevents urinary tract infections (UTIs)	↑? (cranberry juice) NR (supplements)
Treats UTIs	↓?
Prevents UTIs in people with neurogenic bladder, such as individuals with spinal cord injury	NR (supplements)

Safety

- Cranberry juice or supplements are not a substitute for treatment with antibiotics during acute UTIs.
- Very large doses (3 to 4 liters of cranberry juice per day) can cause gastrointestinal upset and diarrhea.
- Long-term consumption of 1 liter of cranberry juice per day may increase risk of kidney stone formation because of the high oxalate content in cranberries (6). Data are conflicting (7).
- Individuals with aspirin allergy or asthma may have a theoretical risk of allergic reaction to salicylate in cranberry.

Drug/Supplement Interactions

- No reported adverse interactions.
- Preliminary evidence suggests that flavonoids in cranberry may inhibit cytochrome P450 2C9 (CYP2C9) enzymes, which could lead to decreased metabolism of CYP2C9 substrates such as amitriptyline, diazepam, zileuton, warfarin, and others (8).
- Theoretically, chronic consumption of large amounts of cranberry could have an additive effect on the anticoagulant activity of warfarin because of increased salicylate levels.

Key Points

- There is some evidence that drinking cranberry juice (approximately 10 ounces per day) may reduce the incidence of UTIs. However, many of the studies on cranberries have been criticized for poor design, high dropout rates, and small sample sizes.
- There is currently limited evidence that cranberry juice or pills may provide effective treatment for an *existing* UTI. To avoid serious kidney infection, individuals who think they may have a UTI should consult their health care provider for treatment.
- Although data are limited, patients with neurogenic bladder (spinal cord injury, etc) do not seem to benefit from cranberry juice prophylaxis.

Food Sources

Fresh or frozen cranberries, cranberry juice, dried cranberries. Approximately 4,400 cranberries make 1 gallon of juice (687 cranberries make 10 ounces of juice) (1).

Dosage Information/Bioavailability

Cranberry extract is available in pills and capsules. Manufacturers recommend dosages ranging from 400 to 2,400 mg daily (approximately 3 to 6 capsules/day). Many products are standardized to 5% proanthocyanidins, although the amount needed to have an antibacterial effect in the urinary tract is unknown. Some products are prepared from spray-dried cranberry juice, and these most closely resemble the juice product. The bio-availability of the proposed active components of cranberry (proanthocyanidins/tannins) is currently being tested in humans.

Relevant Research

Cranberry and UTIs

- In a the Cochrane Database Review System review of the evidence for cranberry juice and UTI prevention and treatment, seven trials were selected as scientifically sound. Two randomized controlled studies showed a 39% reduction in risk for developing a urinary tract infection for women after 12 months of supplementation at a dose of 50 mL concentrate daily in one study and a dose of 250 mL juice or tablet daily in the second study (9).

- A systematic review of controlled trials using cranberry in the prevention of UTIs in susceptible populations summarized the results of five trials that met inclusion criteria (total subjects = 304). Four of the studies compared cranberry juice to placebo juice or water, and one used cranberry capsules vs a placebo. Data from two of the five trials indicated that cranberries were effective for symptomatic or asymptomatic UTIs, but this result was not obtained in an intention-to-treat analysis. The overall quality of the trials was considered to be poor, the sample sizes small, and number of dropouts high. The authors noted that the large number of dropouts (20% to 55%) may indicate that juice may not be acceptable for long-term use. They concluded that further properly designed trials are needed to determine whether cranberry juice can prevent UTIs. Additionally, the dose, formulation, and duration need to be clarified (10).

- In an intervention trial among women (N = 150) who completed treatment for *E. coli* UTI, women were randomly assigned to receive (*a*) 50 mL cranberry-loganberry concentrate for 6 months, (*b*) 100 mL lactobacillus milk drink 5 days/week for 1 year, or (*c*) no intervention. Subjects receiving the cranberry-loganberry concentrate had significantly lower rates of recurrent infection than the other two groups (16% vs 36% to 39%) (11).

- In a double-blind, placebo-controlled, multicenter study, 192 elderly women were randomly assigned to receive 300 mL cranberry juice cocktail (sweetened with saccharin) or a placebo beverage (identical in taste, appearance, and vitamin C content) daily for 6 months. Baseline and monthly urine samples were analyzed for bacteriuria and the presence of white blood cells. One hundred twenty subjects completed the trial. Subjects in the cranberry group had odds of bacteriuria with pyuria that were 42% of the odds in the placebo group, and this difference was statistically significant. Furthermore, in subjects treated with cranberry, the odds of remaining bacteriuric-pyuric were 27% of the odds in the placebo group. There was no evidence that cranberry reduced the pH of the urine, indicating that urinary acidification was not responsible for the antibacterial effect (5).

◆ An in vitro study assessed whether cranberry juice inhibits encrustation and blockage of urethral catheters. Researchers assigned 24 healthy volunteers to drink cranberry juice (2 × 500 mL during 8 hours) or the equivalent amount of water (placebo). Urine was collected, then incubated for 24 or 48 hours in laboratory models of the catheterized bladder that were inoculated with *Proteus mirabilis* (a typical pathogen that causes encrustation and blockage in catheters). The amount of calcium and magnesium recovered from catheters did not differ between the two groups. However, there was significantly less encrustation on catheters in subjects who drank the water compared with juice drinkers. The authors concluded that drinking large volumes of cranberry juice did not result in the excretion of factors into urine that inhibit encrustation (12).

◆ In a prospective, randomized, double-blind, placebo-controlled crossover design study of the efficacy of a supplement of 400 mg cranberry extract (400 mg three times daily for 4 weeks) in reducing UTIs in individuals with neurogenic bladders secondary to spinal cord injury (n = 21), there was clinical improvement with cranberry use. Although the sample size was small, this study may suggest that there is a biological difference in response depending on the underlying physical condition contributing to risk of a UTI (13).

References

1. Ocean Spray Cranberries. About cranberries. Available at: http://www.oceanspray.com. Accessed July 3, 2002.
2. Howell AB, Vorsa N, Der Marderosian A, et al. Inhibition of the adherence of P-fimbriated *Escherichia coli* to uroepithelial-cell surfaces by proanthocyanidin extracts from cranberries. *N Engl J Med.* 1998;339:1085–1086.
3. Foo LY, Lu Y, Howell AB, et al. A-type proanthocyanidin trimers from cranberry that inhibit adherence of uropathogenic P-fimbriated *Escherichia coli*. *J Nat Prod.* 2000;63:1225–1228.
4. Kerr KG. Cranberry juice and prevention of recurrent urinary tract infection. *Lancet.* 1999;353:673.
5. Avorn J, Monane M, Gurwitz JH, et al. Reduction of bacteriuria and pyuria after ingestion of cranberry juice. *JAMA.* 1994;271:751–754.
6. Rogers J. Clinical: Pass the cranberry juice. *Nurs Times.* 1991;27:36–37.
7. Massey L, Roman-Smith H, Sutton RAL. Effect of dietary oxalate and calcium on urinary oxalate and risk of formation of calcium oxalate kidney stones. *J Am Diet Assoc.* 1993;93:901–906.
8. Grant P. Warfarin and cranberry juice: an interaction? *J Heart Valve Dis.* 2004;13:25–26.
9. Jepson RG, Mihaljevic L, Craig J. Cranberries for treating urinary tract infections. *Cochrane Database Syst Rev.* 2004;2:CD001322.
10. Jepson RG, Mihaljevic L, Craig L. Cranberries for preventing urinary tract infections. *Cochrane Database Syst Rev.* 2001;3:CD001321.

11. Kontiokari T, Sundqvist K, Nuutinen M, et al. Randomised trial of cranberry-lingonberry juice and Lactobacillus GG drink for the prevention of urinary tract infections in women. *BMJ.* 2001;322:1571.
12. Morris NS, Stickler DJ. Does drinking cranberry juice produce urine inhibitory to the development of crystalline, catheter-blocking *Proteus mirabilis* biofims? *BJU Int.* 2001;88: 192–197.
13. Linsenmeyer TA, Harrison B, Oakley A, et al. Evaluation of cranberry supplement for reduction of urinary tract infections in individuals with neurogenic bladders secondary to spinal cord injury. A prospective, double-blinded, placebo-controlled, crossover study. *J Spinal Cord Med.* 2004;27:29–34.

Creatine

Creatine is synthesized from amino acids (glycine, arginine, methionine) in the liver, pancreas, and kidneys at a rate of approximately 1 g/day. Skeletal muscle holds 95% of the 120 to 140 g of creatine found in the body. In the muscle, creatine is converted into phosphocreatine, which is needed for ATP production. Studies suggest that consuming 20 to 25 g creatine per day (for 2 to 6 days) increases muscle creatine by 20% to 30%. The availability of phosphocreatine is believed to become a limiting factor during short bouts of high-intensity exercise. (Phosphocreatine is the major source of muscle energy during exercise lasting 2 to 30 seconds.) Therefore, it is thought if more phosphocreatine is available via creatine supplementation, there will be a faster recovery of ATP, which would improve high-power activity that is dependent on the ATP-phosphocreatine energy system. Numerous studies have tested the effects of supplemental creatine on exercise performance (1–6).

Media and Marketing Claims	Efficacy
Increases muscle strength and mass	↑?
Delays fatigue in athletes	NR
Increases strength in elderly	NR
Increases strength in muscular disease	NR
Increases strength in heart disease (congestive heart failure)	NR

Safety

- Creatine has been used safely for up to 5 years by healthy adults.
- It is not known whether supplementation suppresses endogenous creatine synthesis in humans (1).

- ◆ Very high doses may have adverse effects on renal, hepatic, or cardiac function, or lead to hypertension. More research is needed.

- ◆ Individuals should not exceed maintenance dosage (2 to 5 g/day).

- ◆ Creatine may cause weight gain/water retention, gastrointestinal pain, nausea, or diarrhea.

- ◆ The FDA has advised consumers to consult a physician before they use creatine because of reports of deaths caused by dehydration in wrestlers who were purportedly using creatine. However, further investigation by the CDC revealed that creatine was not the cause of the deaths. Nevertheless, there is a concern that athletes in sports in which competition assignment is based on weight classification, may resort to extreme weight-loss methods to decrease the extra water gain that occurs with creatine ingestion (2,7,8).

- ◆ Athletes tend to consume higher dosages of creatine than manufacturers recommend. In a survey of 52 collegiate athletes, 39 exceeded the maintenance dosage of 2 to 5 g/day, 16 reported diarrhea, 13 reported muscle cramping, and 7 reported dehydration. Individuals choosing to supplement with creatine must not exceed recommended dosages because of potential adverse effects (9). Health professionals should assess athletes for dietary supplement use (including creatine) and discourage the practice of exceeding recommended dosages.

- ◆ Theoretically, increased intramuscular water content could dilute electrolytes causing cramping and intracellular swelling, which could result in muscle tightness (2,7).

- ◆ No serious adverse effects have been reported; however, there are no controlled studies testing the safety of creatine supplementation for longer than 8 weeks (2).

- ◆ A patient with nephrotic syndrome who had been supplementing with creatine experienced a deterioration in renal function. Based on this, creatine supplementation should be avoided, especially by patients with renal disease/insufficiency (10). A case report of nephritis has also been published (11).

Drug/Supplement Interactions

- ◆ Creatine may interact negatively with ma huang (ephedra, a supplement that is banned in the United States).

- ◆ Creatine should not be used long-term with nephrotoxic drugs (NSAIDs, cyclosporine, ACE inhibitors).

Note

Creatine is permitted by the International Olympic Committee National Collegiate Athletic Association (NCAA), and professional sports. However, many creatine products may also contain banned substances, which could place the athlete at risk for disqualification.

Key Points

- There was some initial evidence that creatine supplementation may increase muscular strength/power during short bouts of exercise, but no recent peer-reviewed studies have been published. "Creatine supplementation has not been consistently shown to enhance performance in exercise tasks dependent on anaerobic glycolysis, but additional laboratory and field research is merited" (2).

- Creatine supplementation may be more effective in athletes with creatine deficiency, although more evidence of this is needed.

- The increase in muscle mass that has been noted is thought to be associated with increases in intermuscular water that dissipates approximately 28 days after supplementation.

- Additional research is needed to determine whether chronic creatine supplementation during training enhances overall competitive performance in actual sport activities.

- There is no evidence that creatine increases fat metabolism, although in some studies creatine in conjunction with resistance exercise has been associated with an increase in lean body mass in males. Several studies did not determine the composition of weight gain (ie, whether it was because of water retention or actual muscle mass). Additional research is needed to confirm the effect of creatine on body composition and field performance.

- A preliminary study in the elderly reported no benefit with creatine supplementation. Controlled, clinical trials of sufficient sample sizes are needed to verify claims that creatine increases strength in this population. Elderly patients choosing to supplement with creatine should be assessed for renal function because of potential adverse effects.

- There is preliminary and conflicting evidence that creatine may improve strength in patients with neuromuscular diseases. More controlled research is needed in this population.

- Preliminary evidence from one study suggest that creatine supplementation may improve strength in patients with congestive heart failure. Again, more controlled research is needed.

Food Sources

A mixed diet provides approximately 1 g creatine per day (1). Most dietary creatine comes from animal products; only trace amounts are found in plant foods.

Food	Creatine, mg/serving
Herring, raw (3 oz)	553–850
Pork, raw (3 oz)	425
Salmon, raw (3 oz)	383
Beef, raw (3 oz)	383

Food	Creatine, mg/serving
Cod, raw (3 oz)	255
Milk (1 cup)	24

Source: Data are calculated from values from reference 1.

Dosage Information/Bioavailability

Creatine is produced endogenously, so there are no set dietary requirements. Creatine is available as creatine monohydrate in pills, powders, and beverages, often with other supplements such as HMB (beta-hydroxy beta-methylbutyrate), amino acids, and carnitine. Studies have reported that the maximal muscle storage of creatine is achieved by supplementing 5 g creatine monohydrate four times per day for 5 to 6 days, followed by a maintenance phase of 2 g/day to replace daily turnover (2,4,12). In one study, consuming carbohydrates along with creatine supplements further enhanced intramuscular creatine uptake and glycogen deposition (13). Caffeine seems to inhibit phosphocreatine resynthesis during recovery from exercise; therefore, caffeine may interfere with any ergogenic effect of creatine (14). Vegetarians have lower muscle stores of creatine and absorb more from supplements than nonvegetarians with higher stores (15).

Relevant Research

Creatine and High-Intensity Exercise (Phosphocreatine-ATP System) in Laboratory Settings

- In a double-blind, randomized study, two groups of 25 collegiate football players (NCAA division IA) were pair-matched by total body weight and assigned to supplement their diet during off-season weight training for 28 days with a placebo (glucose-taurine-electrolyte mixture) or 15.75 g creatine monohydrate (plus glucose-taurine-electrolyte mixture) per day. Before and after the study, subjects performed a maximal repetition test on the isotonic bench press, squat, and power clean (Olympic weight-lifting exercise), and performed a sprint test on the cycle ergometer (12 × 6 sprints with 30-second rest recovery). Body weight, body water and composition by x-ray absorptiometry were also determined. Bench press lifting volume; the sum of weight lifted during the bench press, squat, and power clean exercises; and total work performed during the first five 6-second sprints increased significantly in the group taking creatine compared with placebo. Subjects in the creatine group also gained significantly more total body weight and fat-/bone-free mass compared with the placebo group, whereas no differences were observed in total body water (16).

- In a placebo-controlled study, two matched groups of 19 competitive rowers each were given a placebo or creatine (0.25 g creatine per kilogram body weight) for 5 days before completing a 1,000-meter simulated race. The control group showed no change in rowing performance, whereas 16 of 19 subjects taking the creatine supplement improved performance times, although these improvements did not reach statistical significance (17).

♦ Several other studies have shown significant improvement in short bouts of activities that require high levels of strength and power (knee extensions, bench press, running, and cycling sprints) (2,18–23). However, other studies did not show any benefit (2,24–26). The studies of endurance have generally not reported an ergogenic benefit (1,2,27).

Creatine and High-Intensity Exercise in Field Studies

♦ In a double-blind, placebo-controlled study, 18 highly trained subjects (male soccer players and female field hockey players) completed two testing sessions of three 60-meter distance running trials (control and postsupplement) 1 week apart. Subjects were pair-matched by gender and running speed. Run sessions were videotaped with high-speed cameras. Speed velocities were determined at 10 to 30 meters, 40 to 50 meters, and 50 to 60 meters. After the control session, subjects were randomly assigned to receive 20 g creatine plus 5 g glucose or a placebo (5 g glucose only) divided into five doses daily for 7 days, followed by the second 60-meter sprint. There were no statistically significant main or interaction effects on velocity between groups (28).

♦ In a double-blind, placebo-controlled study, 32 elite swimmers were tested on two occasions separated by 1 week (50-meter and 100-meter maximal-effort sprints with 10 minutes active recovery and a 10-second maximal leg ergometry test). Swimmers were divided into two groups matched for gender, stroke, and sprint time, and randomly assigned to 20 g creatine monohydrate (divided into four doses) or a placebo daily for 5 days prior to the second exercise trial. There were no significant differences between the group means for sprint times or between maximal leg ergometry power and work. The authors concluded: "This study does not support the hypothesis that creatine supplementation enhances single-effort sprint ability of elite swimmers" (29).

♦ In a double-blind, placebo-controlled study, 20 highly trained male and female swimmers were tested for blood ammonia and lactate concentrations after 25-, 50-, and 100-meter performance in their best stroke on two occasions 7 days apart. After the first trial, subjects were randomly assigned to receive 20 g creatine divided into four doses or a placebo (20 g lactose) for 5 days. There were no significant differences in performance times between trials. There was no effect on postexercise blood lactate levels. Postexercise blood ammonia decreased in the 50- and 100-meter trials in the creatine group, and in the 50-meter trial in the placebo group. The authors concluded: "Creatine supplementation cannot be considered as an ergogenic aid for sprint performance in highly trained swimmers after 5 days of creatine ingestion" (30).

Creatine and Body Composition

♦ Several studies in male subjects reported an increase in body mass averaging 0.7 to 2.0 kg following short-term creatine intake (20 to 25 g creatine per day for 5 to 14 days) (2,12,16,20,21,23,25). It is controversial whether the weight gain is because of water retention or actual muscle mass because most studies did not measure lean body mass (1,2). Some new research indicates that the increase in body mass is fat-free mass (31,32).

Creatine and Muscle Strength

◆ In a review of 22 studies assessing the association between creatine supplementation plus resistance training (or placebo) and muscle strength after resistance training, the author estimated a mean of 8% greater improvement in muscle strength with creatine vs placebo (33).Weight-lifting performance increased 26% on average in the creatine group vs 12% in the placebo group. However, individual response was highly variable and thus significance would only be reached in studies of large sample size, which to date have not been done.

Creatine and the Elderly

◆ In a double-blind, placebo-controlled study, 32 older men and women (ages 67 to 80 years) were randomly assigned to one of four groups for 8 weeks: (*a*) no exercise plus creatine, (*b*) no exercise plus placebo, (*c*) strength-training program plus creatine, and (*d*) strength-training program plus placebo. The strength program was performed 3 days per week for 8 weeks. The supplementation regimen consisted of 20 g creatine monohydrate plus 8 g glucose for 5 days, followed by 3 g of creatine plus 2 g glucose for the remainder of the study. Body mass, body fat, lower-limb muscular volume, 1- and 12-repetition maximums, and isometric intermittent endurance tests for leg press, leg extension, and chest press were measured before and after the study. No statistically significant changes in anthropometric measurements were found in any of the groups. The strength-trained subjects (both creatine and placebo groups) experienced significant increases in repetition maximums compared with control subjects (34).

Creatine and Muscular Disease

◆ Twenty individuals with myotonic dystrophy type 2 received either placebo or creatine supplementation for 3 months. No significant increase in muscle strength as assessed by hand grip dynamometry or Neuromuscular Symptom Score was shown with creatine supplementation; two patients with chronic myalgia showed minor improvements. More research in larger populations is needed because this pilot study suggests that any possible clinical benefit may be small (35).

◆ In a pilot study, 81 subjects with neuromuscular diseases were given 10 g creatine monohydrate for 5 days and 5 g/day for another 5 days. After finding improvements in strength, the authors then did a second study in which 21 subjects from the open trial were entered into a single-blinded, placebo-controlled trial of creatine (same dosage). The authors did not specify the reason for not using a double-blind design. Body weight, handgrip strength, dorsiflexion, and knee extensor strength were measured before and after treatment. Creatine resulted in a significant increase in all measurements in both pilot studies (36).

Creatine and Congestive Heart Failure

- In a double-blind, placebo-controlled study, 20 men (mean age 63 years) with congestive heart failure were assigned to receive 20 g creatine divided into four doses or a placebo for 5 days. Before and after supplementation, subjects performed handgrip exercises, 5-second contraction followed by 5-second rest for 5 minutes at 25%, 50%, and 75% of maximum voluntary contraction or until exhaustion. Blood was taken at rest and at 0 and 2 minutes after exercise to measure lactate and ammonia. After 30 minutes the procedure was repeated with fixed workloads. There was a significant increase in contractions until exhaustion at 75% maximum voluntary contraction after creatine treatment, but no effect in the placebo group. There was a significant decrease in ammonia levels per contraction at 75% maximum voluntary contraction compared with placebo, but no significant effect on lactate concentrations. The authors concluded: "Creatine supplementation in chronic heart failure augments skeletal muscle endurance and attenuates the abnormal skeletal muscle metabolic response to exercise" (37).

References

1. Balsom PD, Soderlund K, Ekblom B. Creatine in humans with special reference to creatine supplementation. *Sports Med.* 1994;18:268–280.
2. Williams MH, Branch JD. Creatine supplementation and exercise performance: an update. *J Am Coll Nutr.* 1998;17:216–234.
3. Greenhaff PL, Bodin K, Soderlund K, et al. Effect of oral creatine supplementation on skeletal muscle phosphocreatine resynthesis. *Am J Physiol.* 1994;266(pt 1):E725-E730.
4. Harris RC, Soderlund K, Hultman E. Elevation of creatine in resting and exercised muscle of normal subjects by creatine supplementation. *Clin Sci (Colch).* 1992;83: 367–374.
5. Volek JS Rawson ES. Scientific basis and practical aspects of creatine supplementation for athletes. *Nutrition.* 2004;20:609–614.
6. Kreider RB. Effects of creatine supplementation on performance and training adaptations. *Mol Cell Biochem.* 2003;244:89–94.
7. Feldman EB. Creatine: a dietary supplement and ergogenic aid. *Nutr Rev.* 1999;57:45–50.
8. Andres LPA, Sacheck J, Tapia S. A review of creatine supplementation: side effects and improvements in athletic performance. *Nutr Clin Care.* 1999;2:73–81.
9. Juhn MS, O'Kane JW, Vinci DM. Oral creatine supplementation in male collegiate athletes: a survey of dosing habits and side effects. *J Am Diet Assoc.* 1999;99:593–595.
10. Pritchard NR, Kalra PA. Renal dysfunction accompanying oral creatine supplements. *Lancet.* 1998;351:1252–1253.
11. Koshy KM, Griswold E, Schneeberger EE. Interstitial nephritis in patient taking creatine. *N Engl J Med.* 1999;340:814–815.
12. Greenhaff PL. Creatine and its application as an ergogenic aid. *Int J Sport Nutr.* 1995;5(Suppl):S100-S110.
13. Green AL, Sewell DA, Simpson L, et al. Creatine ingestion augments muscle creatine uptake and glycogen synthesis during carbohydrate feeding in man. *J Physiol.* 1996;491:63.

14. Vandenberghe K, Gillis N, Van Leemputte M, et al. Caffeine counteracts the ergogenic action of muscle creatine loading. *J Appl Physiol.* 1996;80:452–457.
15. Delanghe J, De Slypere JP, De Buyzere J, et al. Normal reference values for creatine, creatinine, and carnitine are lower in vegetarians. *Clin Chem.* 1989;35:1802–1803.
16. Kreider RB, Ferreira M, Wilson M, et al. Effects of creatine supplementation on body composition, strength, and sprint performance. *Med Sci Sports Exerc.* 1998;30:73–82.
17. Rossiter HB, Cannell ER, Jakeman PM. The effect of oral creatine supplementation on the 1,000-m performance of competitive rowers. *J Sports Sci.* 1996;14:175–179.
18. Greenhaff PL, Casey A, Short AH, et al. Influence of oral creatine supplementation on muscle torque during repeated bouts of maximal voluntary exercise in man. *Clin Sci (Colch).* 1993;84:565–571.
19. Harris RC, Viru M, Greenhaff PL, et al. The effect of oral creatine supplementation on running performance during maximal short-term exercise in man. *J Physiol.* 1993;467:74P.
20. Balsom PD, Ekblom B, Soderlund K, et al. Creatine supplementation and dynamic high-intensity intermittent exercise. *Scand J Med Sci Sports.* 1993;3:143–149.
21. Soderlund K, Balsom PD, Ekblom B. Creatine supplementation and high-intensity exercise: influence on performance and muscle metabolism. *Clin Sci.* 1994;87(suppl): S120–S121.
22. Birch R, Noble D, Greenhaff PL. The influence of dietary creatine supplementation on performance during repeated bouts of maximal isokinetic cycling in man. *Eur J Appl Physiol.* 1994;69:268–270.
23. Earnest CP, Snell PG, Rodriguez R, et al. The effect of creatine monohydrate ingestion on anaerobic power indices, muscular strength and body composition. *Acta Physiol Scand.* 1995;153:207–209.
24. Cooke WH, Grandjean PW, Barnes WS. Effect of oral creatine supplementation on power output and fatigue during bicycle ergometry. *J Appl Physiol.* 1995;78:670–673.
25. Earnest C, Rash J, Snell P, et al. Effect of creatine monohydrate ingestion on interme-diate length anaerobic treadmill running to exhaustion (Abstract). *Med Sci Sports Exerc.* 1995;27(suppl):S14.
26. Mujika I, Chatard JC, Lacoste L, et al. Creatine supplementation does not improve sprint performance in competitive swimmers. *Med Sci Sports Exerc.* 1996;28:1435–1441.
27. Balsom PD, Harridge SD, Soderlund K, et al. Creatine supplementation per se does not enhance endurance exercise performance. *Acta Physiol Scand.* 1993;149:521–523.
28. Redondo DR, Dowling EA, Graham BL, et al. The effect of oral creatine monohydrate supplementation on running velocity. *Int J Sport Nutr.* 1996;6:213–221.
29. Burke LM, Pyne DB, Telford RD. Effect of oral creatine supplementation on single-effort sprint performance in elite swimmers. *Int J Sport Nutr.* 1996;6:222–233.
30. Mujika I, Chatard JC, Lacoste L, et al. Creatine supplementation does not improve sprint performance in competitive swimmers. *Med Sci Sports Exerc.* 1996;28:1435–1441.
31. Becque MD, Lochmann JD, Melrose DR. Effects of oral creatine supplementation on muscular strength and body composition. *Med Sci Sports Exerc.* 2000;32:654–658.
32. Mihic S, MacDonald JR, McKenzie S, et al. Acute creatine loading increases fat-free mass, but does not affect blood pressure, plasma creatinine, or CK activity in men and women. *Med Sci Sports Exerc.* 2000;32:291–296.

33. Rawson ES, Volek JS. Effects of creatine supplementation and resistance training on muscle strength and weightlifting performance. *J Strength Cond Res.* 2003;17:822–831.
34. Bermon S, Venembre P, Sachet C, et al. Effects of creatine monohydrate ingestion in sedentary and weight-trained older adults. *Acta Physiol Scand.* 1998;164:147–155.
35. Schneider-Gold C, Beck M, Wessig C, et al. Creatine monohydrate in DM2/PROMM: a double-blind placebo-controlled clinical study. Proximal myotonic myopathy. *Neurology.* 2003;60:500–502.
36. Tarnopolsky M, Martin J. Creatine monohydrate increases strength in patients with neuromuscular disease. *Neurology.* 1999;52:854–857.
37. Andrews R, Greenhaff P, Curtis S, et al. The effect of dietary creatine supplementation on skeletal muscle metabolism in congestive heart failure. *Eur Heart J.* 1998;19:617–622.

Curcumin. *See* Turmeric *(Curcuma longa).*

Decosahexaenoic Acid (DHA). *See* Fish Oil.

Dehydroepiandrosterone (DHEA)

Dehydroepiandrosterone (DHEA) is the most abundant hormone secreted by the adrenal glands. Dehydroepiandrosterone-3-sulfate (DHEAS) is the metabolic precursor to DHEA, and they are interconvertible (1). In the peripheral tissues, both DHEA and DHEAS can be converted into active androgens and estrogens (2). Despite numerous studies investigating the potential role of DHEA in health and disease, little is known about the function of this hormone. Serum DHEA levels peak by 20 to 30 years of age, and decrease thereafter with age (3).

Media and Marketing Claims	Efficacy
Slows aging; improves age-related memory loss	NR
Improves immune function	↓
Improves heart health	↔
Helps prevent cancer	NR
Reduces symptoms of lupus	↑?
Improves health of individuals with AIDS	NR
Assists weight reduction	NR
Reduces menopausal symptoms	NR

Safety

♦ The safety of long-term administration of DHEA is unknown.

♦ Chronic supplementation with DHEA can alter levels of other hormones, which may have unknown adverse effects.

♦ Excess DHEA seems to increase levels of testosterone. In women, this promotes masculinization (increased facial hair, stimulated acne, increased hair loss, deepening of the voice, menstrual irregularities). In men, it may increase the risk of prostate cancer (4).

♦ DHEA also has estrogenic activity and may increase the risk of hormone-stimulated cancers such as breast and endometrial cancers (5). Individuals with estrogen receptor–positive cancers (breast, uterine, ovarian) and hormone-sensitive conditions (endometriosis, uterine fibroids, polycystic ovary syndrome) should avoid using DHEA.

♦ DHEA may decrease serum HDL cholesterol levels (6). Preliminary evidence suggests that DHEA may increase macrophage foam cell formation. Both of these can contribute to cardiac disease risk.

♦ DHEA may increase risk of adverse psychiatric events in individuals with a history of depression or bipolar disorder.

♦ DHEA may adversely increase liver function tests.

Drug/Supplement Interactions

♦ DHEA can overcome the estrogen receptor–antagonist activity of drugs such as fulvestrant and tamoxifen in estrogen receptor–positive cancer cells.

♦ DHEA may increase blood levels of triazolam (Halcion), a benzodiazepine used for insomnia, anxiety, and seizures.

♦ DHEA may inhibit cytochrome P450 3A4 (CYP3A4) enzymes, leading to decreased metabolism of substrates such as alfentanil, alprazolam, amitriptyline, amiodarone, buspirone, cerivastatin, citalopram, felodipine, fexofenadine, itraconazole, ketoconazole, lansoprazole, losartan, lovastatin, midazolam, ondansetron, prednisone, sertraline, sibutramine, sildenafil, simvastatin, verapamil, and many others.

♦ DHEA may interfere with anti-estrogen effects of aromatase inhibitors such as anastrozole, exemestane, and letrozole.

♦ Insulin use may decrease the effectiveness of DHEA supplements.

Note

DHEA is banned by the National Collegiate Athletic Association and the International Olympic Committee.

Key Points

- DHEA levels decrease with age; however, there is no evidence DHEA supplementation prevents aging or lengthens life span in humans.

- The role of serum DHEA levels in cognitive function in elderly subjects is unclear, although at this time epidemiological studies have not found a correlation between decreased DHEA levels and cognitive function. Although one controlled study showed an improvement in mood, other studies showed no effect on mood or memory. There is not enough evidence to substantiate claims that DHEA improves mood or memory.

- The impact of DHEA on immune function is conflicting, and even in the reports showing improved immune response, the magnitude of the effects in humans is modest (3).

- Epidemiological studies have provided conflicting reports on the association between DHEA levels and cardiovascular disease (CVD).

- There is no clear evidence about the role of DHEA in cancer risk or prevention.

- Some, but not all preliminary trials of DHEA supplement use by patients with lupus have shown some reduction in disease activity. More controlled research is needed in this population.

- Although DHEA levels may decrease with HIV infection, one uncontrolled trial of DHEA supplements in subjects with HIV showed no benefit. More research is needed before recommendations can be made for this population.

- DHEA supplements do not seem to have a beneficial effect on body composition or energy expenditure at either pharmacological or physiological replacement dosages for 1 to 3 months.

- DHEA has not been shown to alter body fat levels or insulin sensitivity (7).

- Studies of DHEA in menopausal women are conflicting. More research is needed to determine the effect of DHEA supplementation on symptoms of menopause.

- Overall, most of the effects of DHEA replacement have been extrapolated from epidemiological or animal model studies, and need to be investigated in human clinical trials (8). The long-term consequences of supplementing with DHEA are unknown, and the potential adverse effects may outweigh the possible benefits. Until more research is available about the safety, efficacy, and dosage of DHEA, supplementation with this hormone is not recommended unless a physician is supervising use.

Food Sources

None

Dosage Information/Bioavailability

DHEA supplements are available in capsules or tablets ranging in doses from 25 to 50 mg. Some products also contain pregnenolone, a direct precursor to DHEA. Numerous studies have used dosages ranging from 0.1 to 1,000 mg/kg body weight.

In a study of 45 DHEA products, 53% contained DHEA at 85% to 95% of the declared amounts; only one had no trace of DHEA; and four exceeded 100% of the amount stated on the label (9).

An oral dose of DHEA (400 mg) reached maximal serum androgen levels within 180 minutes to 240 minutes in postmenopausal women. This dose also was reported to increase serum DHEA by 6-fold, testosterone by 2.5-fold, dihydrotestosterone by 15-fold, and androstenedione by 12-fold compared with the baseline. After 4 weeks of supplementation in the same subjects, estrone and estradiol levels increased 2-fold compared with baseline (10). High-dose supplementation in women can cause acne, body hair growth, and deepening of the voice. A 50-mg dose has not been shown to increase estrone or estradiol or cause androgenic side effects (11). In another study, a single 200-mg dose increased DHEA concentrations by 5- to 6-fold in healthy subjects age 65 to 79 years. It also increased DHEAS by 5-fold in men and by 21-fold in women (12).

Relevant Research

Serum DHEA Levels and Age

- In a prospective study of 614 free-living men and women, DHEA concentrations were assessed every 5 years for 15 years. Overall, the mean decrease in DHEA was 5.6% per year, and the rate of decrease was directly related to age, but not gender, adiposity, or serum glucose. However, when analyzed by gender, DHEA levels were higher and decreased more rapidly in men age 20 to 49 years than in women in the same age group. After age 50 years, DHEA concentrations and rates of decrease were similar in men and women. The mean decrease in DHEAS after age 50 years was 2% per year and was not related to age, gender, adiposity, or glucose (13).

DHEA and Aging, Memory, Libido, and Mood

- In a prospective cohort study (Rancho Bernardo Study), DHEAS was assessed from plasma of 437 subjects (men older than 50 years and women older than 55 years) from an upper-middle-class community in 1972 to 1974. Subjects were screened for dementia in 1988 to 1991. (Mini-Mental Status Examination, Buschke selective reminding test, Trails B, category fluency, and Heaton Visual Reproduction Test were used.) DHEAS levels were higher in men than women, and decreased with age in both sexes. There were no significant differences in age-adjusted DHEAS levels in subjects having impaired performance on any cognitive test. Low baseline DHEAS levels were not associated with any record of dementia on death certificates (14).

- In a case-control study, 45 patients with Alzheimer's disease and cerebrovascular dementia had similar serum DHEA levels compared with healthy controls. However, DHEAS and DHEAS:DHEA ratio were reduced compared with control subjects. The authors concluded that the role of DHEA in dementia is unclear (15).

- In a study of sexual function and arousal in 12 premenopausal women, acute supplementation with 300 mg DHEA did not increase vaginal amplitude responses or subjective tests of libido (16). A similarly designed study in postmenopausal women did show efficacy for a 300 mg acute dose of DHEA to improve libido (n = 16) suggesting the benefit may be age-related in that postmenopausal women are more likely to demonstrate reduced DHEA levels that are responsive to supplementation (17).

♦ In a double-blind, placebo-controlled, crossover study, 30 healthy subjects ages 40 to 70 years were randomly assigned to receive, in random order, 50 mg DHEA or a placebo daily for 3 months each. At baseline, 3 months, and 6 months, fasting blood samples were taken. A subgroup of 13 subjects had several blood samples taken over a 24-hour period. Another subgroup of five subjects underwent a hyperinsulinemic euglycemic clamp. Subjects were instructed by a nutritionist to continue their current exercise and dietary regimens. DHEA had no effect on insulin sensitivity or body fat. There was a significant increase in serum insulin-like-growth-factor-I levels (IGF-I), a metabolic growth factor regulated by growth hormone. During DHEA supplementation, there was a significant increase in perceived physical and psychological well-being, but no effect on libido (11).

♦ In a double-blind, placebo-controlled study, 280 healthy men and women (age 60 to 79 years) were randomly assigned to receive 50 mg DHEA or a placebo daily for 1 year. Subjects were tested at baseline and at 1 year for bone turnover (assessed by dual energy x-ray absorptiometry). Libido, quality of life, and psycho-affective state were assessed by the General Well Being Scale of Dupuy. Muscular strength was measured by handgrip, and skin status was assessed by hydration, epidermal thickness, sebum production, and pigmentation. DHEA increased DHEAS levels to normal young adult levels after month 6 and 12 in men, and after month 12 in women (for month 6 in women, DHEAS levels exceeded those of normal young women). DHEA supplementation significantly increased bone turnover and decreased osteoclastic activity only in women older than 70 years compared with the placebo (18).

DHEA and Immunity

♦ In a double-blind, placebo-controlled study, 78 healthy, elderly subjects were randomly assigned to receive DHEAS injection (7.5 mg) or a placebo coadministered with the influenza vaccine (consisting of three antigens: H1N1, H3N2, and B). Immune responses to vaccine after weeks 0, 2, and 4 of DHEA supplementation were measured. No significant differences were found for antibody responses to the H1N1 and B antigens or vaccine-antigen induced lymphoproliferation (19).

♦ In a prospective, double-blind study, 71 healthy, elderly subjects (ages 61 to 89 years) were randomly assigned to receive 50 mg DHEA or a placebo for 4 days (starting 2 days before receiving three strains of influenza vaccine). Antibody response against the strains of vaccine was measured before and 28 days after vaccination, and compared between previously vaccinated and nonvaccinated subjects. As expected, DHEA levels increased 5- to 10-fold in the treatment group but were not affected in the placebo group. DHEA did not enhance established immunity as measured by antibody levels (20).

DHEA and Cardiovascular Disease

♦ A review of research regarding DHEA and CVD risk found contradictory results. Increased DHEA seems to be related to reduced obesity in males and females, but DHEA levels are not a prognostic indicator of CVD endpoints. The authors suggest that early studies supporting a protective effect were poorly designed and have not been successfully replicated, supporting the notion that DHEA effects in CVD risk reduction are mild to moderate at best (21).

♦ In a prospective cohort study, 1,971 subjects age 30 to 88 years were followed up for 19 years. After the first 12 years, high levels of plasma DHEAS were associated with a reduced risk of fatal CVD in men but an increased risk in women. After 19 years, DHEAS levels were not associated with CVD or ischemic heart disease (IHD) deaths when compared with control subjects without CVD or IHD. However, when compared with survivors of CVD, there was a significant, modestly reduced risk of fatal CVD in men with increased DHEAS and an insignificant increased risk of fatal CVD in women (22). In a follow-up analysis, after adjusting for age, cholesterol, blood pressure, smoking, estrogen replacement, obesity, blood glucose, and family history of heart disease, higher DHEAS levels were unrelated to the risk of fatal CVD in women (23).

♦ One review article reported on placebo-controlled human studies in which DHEA supplementation was associated with (*a*) inhibition of platelet aggregation (DHEA = 900 mg/day), and (*b*) reduced plasminogen activator inhibitor type 1 (DHEA = 150 mg/day). DHEA administration also reduced atherosclerosis in cholesterol-fed rabbits and reduced serum cholesterol in monkeys and dogs (3).

DHEA and Cancer

♦ In a prospective cohort study of 534 women age 50 to 79 years, DHEAS levels were obtained from 1972 to 1974, and subjects were followed up for 15 years. At the end of the study, there were 21 cases of incident breast cancer, 20 cases with earlier diagnosis, and 10 cases with unknown date of onset who were identified from death certificates only. After controlling for age, BMI, estrogen use, and smoking, DHEAS levels were not associated with risk for breast cancer (24).

♦ In a prospective, nested case-control study, 71 healthy postmenopausal subjects not on estrogen therapy when they donated blood and who were diagnosed with breast cancer up to 10 years later, were compared with matched controls. Increased serum DHEA and the metabolite 5-androstene-3 beta, 17 beta-diol (ADIOL) levels were associated with a significant increase in incidence of breast cancer. Women whose serum DHEAS was in the highest quartile also had a significantly increased risk of breast cancer. The authors concluded that the adrenal androgens, DHEA, and DHEAS may play a role in the etiology of breast cancer (5).

DHEA and Lupus

◆ A double-blind, randomized trial among 191 women with systemic lupus erythematosus (SLE) assessed whether DHEA supplementation would support a reduction in daily corticosteroid use for symptom control. Subjects were prescribed between 10 and 30 mg prednisone per day at study onset. They were randomly assigned to receive 100 or 200 mg of DHEA per day or placebo for 7 to 9 months. Prednisone therapy was reduced using the SLE Disease Activity Index Score on a monthly basis. Responders were able to reduce prednisone therapy to 7.5 mg/day or less over the treatment period. The percentage of responders was equivalent across groups; however, analysis of women who were in active disease at baseline, the 200-mg DHEA dose was associated with a significantly greater percentage of responders as compared with placebo (25). The results are promising but warrant further investigation.

◆ A similar therapeutic response was found in a multicenter study of 381 women with SLE. Subjects with active disease were randomly assigned to a 12-month intervention with standard medications plus 200 mg DHEA or placebo daily. Of the women receiving DHEA, 58.5% reported improvements in symptoms, whereas 44.5% of those on placebo showed improvement, a difference that was statistically significant ($P = .017$) (26).

◆ In a double-blind, placebo-controlled trial, 28 women with mild to moderate SLE were randomly assigned to receive 200 mg DHEA or a placebo daily for 3 months. There was an insignificant trend for subjects treated with DHEA to have greater improvement in SLE Disease Activity Index scores, physician overall assessment of disease activity, and a reduction in the dosage of prednisone when compared with the placebo group. The difference between the subjects' assessment of disease activity between groups was significant. Mild acne was a frequent side effect during DHEA supplementation (27).

◆ In an open label study, 50 women with mild to moderate SLE were treated with 50 to 200 mg DHEA daily for 6 to 12 months. DHEA increased the serum levels of DHEA, DHEAS, and testosterone. Compared with baseline, DHEA therapy was associated with a significant decrease in disease activity (SLE Disease Activity Index score) and significant improvement in subject and physician global assessment. Concurrent prednisone dosages were reduced significantly. Mild acne occurred in 54% of the subjects (28).

DHEA and HIV Infection

◆ Serum DHEA concentrations in individuals with HIV seem to progressively decrease as HIV disease advances (29).

◆ In an open, uncontrolled trial, 31 subjects with HIV disease were given 750 to 2,250 mg DHEA, divided into three doses daily for 16 weeks. There were no sustained improvements in CD4 counts or decreases in serum p24 antigen or beta-2 microglobulin levels. Serum neopterin levels decreased transiently by 23% to 40% at week

8 compared with baseline in all dosing groups. The authors concluded that DHEA was well tolerated by individuals with mild symptomatic HIV disease, but that randomized, controlled trials are needed to determine the efficacy of DHEA in HIV-related diseases (30).

DHEA and Body Composition

♦ In a randomized, double-blind, placebo-controlled trial, 56 elderly men and women (age 65 to 78 years) with age-related decreases in DHEA levels were assigned to receive daily dosages of 50 mg of DHEA or a placebo for 6 months. Fifty-two participants completed the study, with 97% compliance. Based on intention-to-treat analyses, DHEA vs placebo induced significant decreases in visceral fat area. The insulin area under the curve (AUC) during an oral glucose tolerance test was significantly reduced after 6 months of DHEA therapy compared with placebo. The AUC was unchanged despite lower insulin levels, resulting in a significant increase in insulin sensitivity in those who received DHEA compared with placebo. Researchers concluded that DHEA could play a role in preventing and treating metabolic syndrome associated with abdominal fat (31).

DHEA and Menopausal Symptoms

♦ In a double-blind, placebo-controlled study, 60 perimenopausal women with complaints of altered mood and well-being were randomly assigned to receive 50 mg DHEA per day or a placebo for 3 months. Changes in serum DHEA, DHEAS, and testosterone were significantly greater in the DHEA group than the placebo group. There were no differences between groups in the severity of perimenopausal symptoms, mood, dysphoria, libido, cognition, memory, or well-being (32).

References

1. Longcope C. Dehydroepiandrosterone metabolism. *J Endocrinol.* 1996;150(Suppl): S125–S127.
2. Labrie F, Belanger A, Simard J, et al. DHEA and peripheral androgen and estrogen formation: intracrinology. *Ann N Y Acad Sci.* 1995;774:16–28.
3. Svec F, Porter JR. The actions of exogenous dehydroepiandrosterone in experimental animals and humans. *Proc Soc Exp Biol Med.* 1998;218:174–191.
4. Dehydroepiandrosterone (DHEA). *Med Lett Drugs Ther.* 1996;38:91–92.
5. Dorgan JF, Stanczyk FZ, Longcope C, et al. Relationship of serum dehydroepiandrosterone (DHEA), DHEA sulfate, and 5-androstene-3 beta, 17 beta-diol to risk of breast cancer in postmenopausal women. *Cancer Epidemiol Biomarkers Prev.* 1997;6: 177–181.
6. Mortola JF, Yen SS. The effects of oral dehydroepiandrosterone on endocrine-metabolic parameters in postmenopausal women. *J Clin Endocrinol Metab.* 1990;71:696–704.
7. Clore JN. Dehydroepiandrosterone and body fat. *Obes Res.* 1995;3(Suppl 4): 613S–616S.

8. Watson RR, Huls A, Araghinikuam M, et al. Dehydroepiandrosterone and diseases of aging. *Drugs Aging.* 1996;9:274–291.

9. Thompson RD, Carlson M. Liquid chromatographic determination of dehydroepiandrosterone (DHEA) in dietary supplement products. *J AOAC Int.* 2000;83: 847–857.

10. Mortola JF, Yen SS. The effects of oral dehydroepiandrosterone on endocrine metabolic parameters in postmenopausal women [erratum in *J Clin Endocrinol Metab.* 1995;80:2799]. *J Clin Endocrinol Metab.* 1990;71:696–704.

11. Morales AJ, Nolan JJ, Nelson JC, et al. Effects of replacement dose of dehydroepiandrosterone in men and women of advancing age. *J Clin Endocrinol Metab.* 1994;78:1360–1367.

12. Frye RF, Kroboth PD, Kroboth FJ, et al. Sex differences in the pharmacokinetics of dehydroepiandrosterone (DHEA) after single- and multiple dose administration in healthy older adults. *J Clin Pharmacol.* 2000;40:596–605.

13. Nafziger AN, Bowlin SJ, Jenkins PL, et al. Longitudinal changes in dehydroepiandrosterone concentrations in men and women. *J Lab Clin Med.* 1998;131:316–323.

14. Barrett-Connor E, Edelstein SL. A prospective study of dehydroepiandrosterone sulfate and cognitive function in an older population: the Rancho Bernardo Study. *J Am Geriatr Soc.* 1994;42:420–423.

15. Yanase T, Fukahori M, Taniguchi S, et al. Serum dehydroepiandrosterone (DHEA) and DHEA-sulfate (DHEA-S) in Alzheimer's disease and in cerebrovascular dementia. *Endocr J.* 1996;43:119–123.

16. Meston CM, Heiman JR. Acute dehydroepiandrosterone effects on sexual arousal in premenopausal women. *J Sex Marital Ther.* 2002;28:53–60.

17. Hackbert L, Heiman JR. Acute dehydroepiandrosterone (DHEA) effects on sexual arousal in postmenopausal women. *J Womens Health Gend Based Med.* 2002;11:155–162.

18. Baulieu EE, Thomas G, Legrain S, et al. Dehydroepiandrosterone (DHEA), DHEA sulfate, and aging: contribution of the DHEAge Study to a sociobiomedical issue. *Proc Natl Acad Sci USA.* 2000;97:4279–4284.

19. Degelau J, Guay D, Hallgren H. The effect of DHEAS on influenza vaccination in aging adults. *J Am Geriatr Soc.* 1997;45:747–751.

20. Ben-Yehuda A, Danenberg HD, Zakay-Rones Z, et al. The influence of sequential annual vaccination and of DHEA administration on the efficacy of the immune response to influenza vaccine in the elderly. *Mech Ageing Dev.* 1998;102:299–306.

21. Tchernof A, Labrie F. Dehydroepiandrosterone, obesity and cardiovascular disease risk: a review of human studies. *Eur J Endocrinol.* 2004;151:1–14.

22 Barrett-Connor E, Goodman-Gruen D. The epidemiology of DHEAS and cardiovascular disease. *Ann N Y Acad Sci.* 1995;774:259–270.

23. Barrett-Connor E, Goodman-Gruen D. Dehydroepiandrosterone sulfate does not predict cardiovascular death in postmenopausal women. The Rancho Bernardo Study. *Circulation.* 1995;91:1757–1760.

24. Barrett-Connor E, Friedlander NJ, Khaw KT. Dehydroepiandrosterone sulfate and breast cancer risk. *Cancer Res.* 1990;50:6571–6574.

25. Petri MA, Lahita RG, Van Vollenhoven RF, et al. Effects of prasterone on corticosteroid requirements of women with systemic lupus erythematosus: a double-blind, randomized, placebo-controlled trial. *Arthritis Rheum.* 2002;46:1820–1829.
26. Petri MA, Mease PJ, Merrill JT, et al. Effects of prasterone on disease activity and symptoms in women with active systemic lupus erythematosus. *Arthritis Rheum.* 2002;50:2858–2868.
27. van Vollenhoven RF, Engleman EG, McGuire JL. Dehydroepiandrosterone in systemic lupus erythematosus. Results of a double-blind, placebo-controlled, randomized clinical trial. *Arthritis Rheum.* 1995;38:1826–1831.
28. van Vollenhoven RF, Morabito LM, Engleman EG, et al. Treatment of systemic lupus erythematosus with dehydroepiandrosterone: 50 patients treated up to 12 months. *J Rheumatol.* 1998;25:285–289.
29. Christeff N, Gherbi N, Mammes O, et al. Serum cortisol and DHEA concentrations during HIV infection. *Psychoneuroendocrinology.* 1997;22(Suppl 1):S11-S18.
30. Dyner TS, Lang W, Geaga J, et al. An open-label, dose-escalation trial of oral dehydroepiandrosterone tolerance and pharmacokinetics in patients with HIV disease. *J Acquir Immune Defic Syndr.* 1993;6:459–465.
31. Villareal DT, Holloszy JO. Effect of DHEA on abdominal fat and insulin action in elderly women and men. *JAMA.* 2004;292:2243–2248.
32. Barnhart KT, Freeman E, Grisso JA, et al. The effect of dehydroepiandrosterone supplementation to symptomatic perimenopausal women on serum endocrine profiles, lipid parameters, and health-related quality of life. *J Clin Endocrinol Metab.* 1999;84: 3896–3902.

Dong quai *(Angelica sinensis)*

Dong quai, also known as dang guei or *Angelica sinensis,* is a medicinal herb used for more than 2,000 years in traditional Chinese medicine. It is produced from the plant's root, after the plant is grown for 1 year and then been harvested and dried. According to Chinese classification, dong quai is considered a "tonifying herb" that strengthens or supplements an area or body process that is insufficient or weakened. Dong quai is one of the most widely used herbs in China as part of a formula for gynecological ailments such as menstrual cramps, menstrual irregularity, and weakness during the menstrual period; and menopausal symptoms. In the United States, dong quai is most often used as a single-herb preparation, which some suggest to be less effective than when the plant is used in traditional Chinese multiple-herb formulas. Although the exact mechanism of action has not been determined, a few theories about how dong quai might affect menopause have been proposed. Some speculate that dong quai might support endogenous estrogen production, contain estrogenic compounds, or alleviate signs of estrogen deficiency without altering estrogen levels (1,2).

Media and Marketing Claims	Efficacy
Reduces menopausal symptoms	NR
Reduces PMS symptoms	NR

Safety

♦ Controlled studies testing the safety of dong quai supplementation in humans have not lasted more than 24 weeks. The safety of long-term use (more than 6 months) and high doses is not known.

♦ Dong quai is not recommended during pregnancy because of its potential estrogenic stimulating effects on the uterus.

♦ Dong quai should not be used by individuals with hormone-sensitive cancers (breast, uterine, ovarian) or conditions (endometriosis, uterine fibroids) until the mechanism of action is understood.

♦ Dong quai contains psoralens, which may cause photosensitivity and photodermatitis.

Drug/Supplement Interactions

Dong quai should not be combined with blood-thinning medications or supplements such as warfarin (Coumadin), heparin, aspirin, garlic, ginkgo, vitamin E, or fish oil (3,4).

Key Points

♦ Limited controlled evidence exists to support using single preparations of dong quai to manage menopausal symptoms. In China, dong quai is typically used with four or more herbs, which together have been reported to reduce hot flashes. However, most of this research, which is not available in English, consists of primarily in vitro, animal, and uncontrolled human studies. One controlled study reported no effect of dong quai on menopausal complaints. Clearly, much more controlled research is needed, using single and multiherb preparations to determine the efficacy and safety of dong quai.

♦ Although there is a long history of dong quai use in traditional Chinese medicine for premenstrual syndrome and dysmenorrhea, controlled clinical trials are needed to evaluate the use of dong quai for these conditions.

♦ Whether dong quai has estrogenic properties is debatable, but the proliferative effects of estrogen receptor–positive breast cancer cells in culture suggests that it does. Therefore, those at risk or previously diagnosed with hormone-sensitive cancers should avoid dong quai supplementation (5).

Food Sources

None

Dosage Information/Bioavailability

Dong quai is available in capsules, tablets, tinctures, and teas. The recommended dosage is 1 to 2 g, or 10 to 40 drops of tincture, three times daily (3 to 6 g total). The extract is also used in many combination herbal supplements marketed for women's health, and it is often combined with black cohosh. (*See* Black Cohosh.)

Relevant Research

Dong quai and Menopause

- In a double-blind, placebo-controlled study, 71 postmenopausal women were randomly assigned to receive 4.5 g dong quai root in capsules or a placebo daily for 24 weeks. The subjects had elevated follicle stimulating hormone levels and complained of hot flashes. At the end of the study, endometrial thickness was measured by ultrasonography, vaginal cells were evaluated for cellular maturation, and menopausal symptoms were assessed by the Kupperman index and diary of vasomotor flushes. Although not significantly different, endometrial thickness increased 2.3 mm in the placebo group compared with 0.3 mm in the dong quai group, suggesting that dong quai had no estrogenic effects. The authors could not explain why endometrial thickness would have increased in the placebo group. There were also no significant differences in menopausal symptoms, or in the number of hot flashes (both groups reported significant improvements). Serum levels of estradiol, estrone, sex hormone–binding globulin, blood pressure, and weight did not differ between groups. The authors concluded that dong quai administered alone does not produce estrogen-like responses in vaginal cells or endometrial thickness and was no more helpful than placebo in relieving menopausal symptoms (2).

Dong quai and PMS

- A review of research in Chinese medical journals describes reports of animal experiments using intravenous injection of water or alcohol extraction of dong quai root into female rabbits, cats, and dogs. All studies showed increased excitability of the uterus, and the contractive rhythm of smooth muscle of the uterus changed from fast, irregular, and weak to slow, regular, and strong. The reviewer suggested that this is the pharmacological basis for using dong quai for dysmenorrhea (6).

References

1. Noe JE. Angelica sinensis: a monograph. *J Naturopathic Med.* 1997;(7)66–72.
2. Hirata JD, Swiersz LM, Zell B, et al. Does dong quai have estrogenic effects in postmenopausal women? A double blind, placebo-controlled trial. *Fertil Steril.* 1997;68:981–986.
3. Fugh-Berman A. Herb-drug interaction. *Lancet.* 2000;355:134–138.
4. Heck AM, DeWitt BA, Lukes AL. Potential interactions between alternative therapies and warfarin. *Am J Health Syst Pharm.* 2000;57:1221–1227.

5. Amato P, Christophe S, Mellon PL. Estrogenic activity of herbs commonly used as remedies for menopausal symptoms. *Menopause.* 2002;9:145–150.
6. Zhu DP. Dong quai. *Am J Chin Med.* 1987;15:117–125.

Echinacea

The echinacea plant, known as the purple coneflower herb, was originally used by Native Americans to treat a variety of ailments. Although echinacea is indigenous to the United States, most clinical research on this plant has been done in Germany. In Germany, *Echinacea purpurea* (above-ground parts) and *Echinacea pallida* (root) are approved by the government's expert committee, the German Commission E, for use as supportive therapy for colds and chronic infections of the respiratory tract and lower urinary tract. Commission E has not approved the above-ground parts of *E. pallida* or any part (root or leaves) of *E. angustifolia* because their efficacy has not been substantiated.

Of the nine existing echinacea species, the roots and the flowering leaves of *E. purpurea*, *E. pallida*, and *E. angustifolia* are the most commonly used in dietary supplements. Several polysaccharides, volatile oil, caffeic acid derivatives, isobutylamides, polyenes, and polyines have been identified in the plant, although the active ingredient(s) are not entirely known (1,2).

Media and Marketing Claims	Efficacy
Boosts immune function in healthy individuals	↓
Protects against common cold virus, upper respiratory infections	↔

Safety

- Oral echinacea seems to be well-tolerated, although the safety of long-term use is unknown (2). Symptoms of immunostimulation (eg, shivering, fever, and muscle weakness) have been observed after parenteral administration, but not with oral use (3).

- In rare cases, echinacea may cause fever, nausea, vomiting, heartburn, constipation, abdominal pain, diarrhea, unpleasant taste, dry mouth, sore throat, tingling sensation and numbness of the tongue, mouth ulcers, headache, dizziness, insomnia, or disorientation.

- According to a case report, one woman had an anaphylactic reaction after taking 5 mL of a commercial extract of echinacea (equivalent to 150 mg dry root of *E. purpurea* and 3,825 mg dried extract *E. angustifolia*). Hypersensitivity to the plant was confirmed by skin-prick tests and radioallergosorbent testing. Individuals with asthma, atopy, or allergies to grass pollens should be cautioned about the risk of severe allergic reactions to echinacea (4).

♦ Echinacea is not recommended for individuals with autoimmune disorders including lupus, HIV, tuberculosis, multiple sclerosis, or scleroderma.

♦ Preliminary evidence in animals suggests that high doses of echinacea may reduce male and female fertility; this effect has not been demonstrated in humans.

Drug/Supplement Interactions

♦ Echinacea may decrease the effectiveness of immune-suppressing drugs, including cyclosporine, azathioprine, basiliximab, daclizumab, muromonab-CD3, mycophenolate, tacrolimus, sirolimus, prednisone and other corticosteroids (5) and other medications metabolized through CYP3A4 enzymes, such as lovastatin, ketoconazole, itroconazole, fexofenadine, triazolam, midazolam, and many others.

♦ Echinacea may interact negatively with hepatotoxic medications (anabolic steroids, amiodarone, methotrexate, ketoconazole).

Key Points

♦ Clinical studies have reported conflicting results on the role of echinacea in preventing or reducing symptoms of upper respiratory infections. However, more recent placebo-controlled trials generally have not supported use of echinacea for reducing the symptoms or duration of the common cold. One key issue is whether the study population is healthy or not at the time supplementation is started. Additional well-controlled research is needed to evaluate the claim that echinacea protects the immune system against upper respiratory tract infections and influenza viruses, especially in healthy individuals.

♦ Because there are many varieties of echinacea with varying levels of potentially active compounds, future studies must control for these variables to provide accurate information about the efficacy, dosage, administration, and preparation of supplements.

Food Sources

None

Dosage Information/Bioavailability

Echinacea extract prepared from the fresh expressed juice of the flowering plant or root is available in tinctures, capsules, or tablets. It is also sold in herbal teas and throat lozenges. A few studies have used 6 to 9 mL of *E. purpurea* herb juice. Most supplements provide echinacea from the fresh flower, roots, or a combination of the whole plant equivalent to 300 to 900 mg dried extract.

Relevant Research

Echinacea and Immunity

◆ There is some evidence that echinacea does not improve immunity in healthy volunteers (6). It has been suggested that using echinacea continually for cold prevention may not be efficacious, and that long-term use may actually reduce its efficacy in preventing colds. A potentially more efficacious approach is to initiate supplementation at the onset of cold symptoms. More research is needed to clarify this issue.

◆ In individuals with reduced immunity (older adults, cancer patients, people with HIV, etc), a 1- to 2-week hiatus every 8 weeks may enhance long-term efficacy, although this approach has not been tested in long-term trials (7).

◆ Peripheral blood mononuclear cells from healthy individuals or subjects with either chronic fatigue syndrome or AIDS were treated ex vivo with extracts of either *E. purpurea* or *Panax ginseng*. Echinacea and ginseng at concentrations equal to or greater than 0.1 or 10 µg/kg, respectively, both resulted in a statistically significant enhancement of natural killer cell function and antibody-dependent cellular toxicity in all cells (8).

◆ In a study designed to test the efficacy of daily echinacea in modulating immune response, 40 healthy men were recruited to consume freshly expressed *E. purpurea* juice or placebo juice daily for 2 weeks, followed by a 4-week washout when no juice was consumed, and then a crossover to the alternate juice. Although the study was reportedly blinded, the distinct flavor and smell of echinacea make it difficult to blind studies of this nature. Numerous endpoints for immune assessment were used. No stimulation of immunity, including phagocytic activity, or TNF-α and IL-1 ß production was shown (6). This study suggests that efficacy may be limited in less healthy volunteers. However, a challenge with a viral infection or the recruitment of subjects with mildly suppressed immune function may have provided different results.

Echinacea and Common Cold/Respiratory Infection

◆ Four hundred thirty-seven young, healthy adults participated in a placebo-controlled, randomized, double-blinded clinical trial to assess the efficacy of echinacea in reducing viral load in those susceptible and exposed to rhinovirus type 39 (9). Three echinacea preparations with specific phytochemical profiles were created, and subjects were assigned to one of these preparations or to placebo, which were used either as prophylaxis (beginning 7 days before the virus challenge) or as treatment (beginning at the time of the challenge). No significant differences were shown across treatment groups in: (*a*) rates of infection, (*b*) severity of reported symptoms, (*c*) volume of nasal secretions, (*d*) leukocyte concentration in nasal secretions, (*e*) IL-8 concentrations in nasal secretions, or (*f*) virus titer levels.

◆ The *Cochrane Database of Systematic Reviews* published an assessment of echinacea for common cold in 2000. Sixteen trials were included in the analysis, including eight prevention and eight treatment-related studies. The overall assessment was that studies support the efficacy of this supplement in prevention and treating colds (10).

◆ In a randomized, placebo-controlled, double-blind study of 282 adults with reported colds during the previous 12 months, a specially formulated echinacea supplement (Echinilin) with 0.25 mg alkamides, 2.5 mg cichoric acid, and 25 mg polysaccharides per tablet was used to determine whether supplementation could reduce frequency or symptoms of colds. Subjects were randomly assigned to Echinilin or placebo and were asked to take 10 tablets on the first day that symptoms started and 4 tablets for the next 7 days. One hundred twenty-eight of 282 participants reported cold symptoms during the study period, including 49% of placebo group subjects and 42% of Echinilin group subjects. This difference was not significant. However, the echinacea group had significantly lower symptom scores than the placebo group (11).

◆ In a randomized, double-blind, placebo-controlled clinical trial of 128 adults with new onset cold symptoms, 100 mg three times per day of echinacea (vs placebo) was not shown to reduce symptom scores or duration of the common cold. However, this study has been criticized because the specific constitutive components of the plant in the supplement were not assessed or monitored, and because of, the low dosage and the lack of biomarkers of immune response (12).

◆ In a double-blind, placebo-controlled study of whole-plant echinacea,148 college students with common colds of recent onset were randomly assigned to use placebo or 6 g echinacea supplement on day 1 of symptoms and 3 g for the following days of illness up to 10 days. There was no difference in cold severity, symptoms, or duration for supplementation vs placebo group. However, subjects were allowed to take other medications for cold symptoms; this was controlled for in the analysis (13).

◆ In a double-blind, placebo-controlled study, 108 subjects with a history of more than three colds or respiratory infections in the preceding year were randomly assigned to receive 4 mL fluid extract of *E. purpurea* (above-ground plant) or a placebo twice daily. The incidence and severity of colds and respiratory infections were determined during 8 weeks of treatment, based on subject-reported symptoms together and findings on physical exam. During the study, 35 of 54 of subjects in the echinacea group and 40 of 54 in the placebo group had at least one infection. There were no significant differences between groups in incidence, duration, or severity of colds and respiratory infections (14).

◆ In a double-blind, placebo-controlled study, symptoms of a common cold developed in 246 of 559 recruited healthy volunteers. These 246 were randomly assigned to one of four treatments daily: (*a*) 6.78 mg crude extract of *E. purpurea* tablets (95% above-ground plant, 5% root); (*b*) 48.2 mg crude extract of *E. purpurea* tablets (seven times higher concentration than group A); (*c*) 29.6 mg crude extract of *E. purpurea* radix (root) tablets; or (*d*) a placebo. Subjects were instructed to take the preparations until they felt healthy again, but not longer than 7 days. The primary endpoint was the relative reduction of the complaint index, defined by 12 symptoms during common cold, according to the physician's record. Sixty-five of 246 cases (27%) were excluded from analysis because of dropouts and protocol violations such as co-medication and late start of treatment. With regard to the relative reduction of the complaint index by the doctor's record, echinacea supplementation in the two groups taking supplements from the above-ground part of the plant was significantly more effective than the echinacea root extract or a placebo. With respect to the complaint index according to the subject's diary, the two supplements from the above-ground part of the plant were also significantly more effective than the root extract or the placebo. According to subjective assessments by the doctor and subjects, the two supplements from the above-ground part of the plant were judged as more effective than placebo. The frequency of adverse effects (mainly gastrointestinal symptoms) was similar for all groups (15).

- In a double-blind, placebo-controlled study, 95 subjects with early symptoms of cold or flu were randomly assigned to receive Echinacea Plus tea or a placebo in 5 to 6 cups daily for 1 to 5 days. Fourteen days after starting the study, subjects completed a self-scoring questionnaire that measured the efficacy of the treatment, number of days the symptoms lasted, and number of days before change. There was a significant difference between the groups, with the subjects taking echinacea reporting more effective and faster relief of symptoms (16).

- In a double-blind, placebo-controlled trial, 160 subjects with upper respiratory infections were randomly assigned to receive 900 mg (or 90 drops) *E. pallida* root extract or a placebo for 8 to 10 days. The presence of infection was confirmed by blood tests (increased differential lymphocyte count indicating viral infection and increased differential neutrophil count indicating a bacterial infection). Symptoms (weakness, sweating, increased tear flow, burning eyes, sore throat), were recorded at day 3 or 4 and at days 8 and 10 of the study. The duration of illness was significantly reduced from 13 to 9.8 days in bacterial infections and 9.1 days in viral infections with echinacea supplementation. The clinical findings correlated with the lymphocytosis and differential neutrophil count; as subjects were treated, both of these decreased back to normal, but at a faster rate in subjects taking echinacea than in those taking placebo (statistical significance not reported). There was a significant improvement in overall symptom scores with echinacea compared with the placebo (17).

- In a double-blind, placebo-controlled trial, 180 subjects visiting a general medicine clinic for flu-type or feverish infections of the upper respiratory tract were randomly assigned to receive one of three treatments: (*a*) 450 mg (90 drops) of *E. purpurea* radix in unstandardized liquid extract (1:5, 55% ethanol); (*b*) 900 mg (180 drops) *E. purpurea* radix in unstandardized ethanol extract; or (*c*) a placebo. Physician and subject assessments were obtained at the beginning of treatment, after 3 to 4 days, and after 8 to 10 days of treatment. The low-dose echinacea did not differ statistically from the placebo in relieving symptoms and duration of flu-like infections at all periods of measurement. Compared with the placebo, the 900-mg dosage resulted in a significant improvement in symptoms (inflamed nose, frontal sensitivity, coated tongue) after 3 to 4 days; after 8 to 10 days only one symptom (inflamed nose) remained significantly improved (5).

References

1. Hobbs C. Echinacea: a literature review. *HerbalGram*. 1994;30:33–48.
2. Blumenthal M, ed. *The Complete German Commission E Monographs Therapeutic Guide to Herbal Medicines*. Austin, Tex: American Botanical Council; 1998.
3. Miller LG. Herbal medicinals. Selected clinical considerations focusing on known or potential drug-herb interactions. *Arch Intern Med*. 1998;158:2200–2211.
4. Mullins RJ. Echinacea-associated anaphylaxis. *Med J Aust*. 1998;168:170–171.
5. Braunig B, Dorn M, Limburg E, et al. *Echinacea purpureae* radix for strengthening the immune response in flu-like infections [in German]. *Z Phytother*. 1992;13:7–12.
6. Schwarz E, Metzler J, Diedrich JP, et al. Oral administration of freshly expressed juice of Echinacea purpurea herbs fail to stimulate the nonspecific immune response in healthy young men: results of a double-blind, placebo-controlled crossover study. *J Immunother*. 2002;25:413–420.
7. Pepping J. Echinacea. *Am J Health Syst Pharm*. 1999;56:121–3.
8. See DM, Broumand N, Sahl L, et al. In vitro effects of echinacea and ginseng on natural killer and anti-body dependent cell cytotoxicity in healthy subjects and chronic fatigue syndrome or acquired immunodeficiency syndrome patients. *Immunopharmacology*. 1997;35:229–235.
9. Turner RB, Bayer R, Woelkart K, et al. An evaluation of Echinacea angustifolia in experimental rhinovirus infections. *New Engl J Med*. 2005;353:341–348.
10. Melchart D, Linde K, Fischer P, et al. Echinacea for preventing and treating the common cold. *Cochrane Database Syst Rev*. 2000;2:CD000530.
11. Goel V, Lovlin R, Barton R, et al. Efficacy of a standardized echinacea preparation (Echinilin) for the treatment of the common cold: a randomized, double-blind, placebo-controlled trial. *J Clin Pharm Ther*. 2004;29:75–83.
12. Yale SH, Liu K. Echinacea purpurea therapy for the treatment of the common cold: a randomized, double-blind, placebo-controlled clinical trial. *Arch Intern Med*. 2004;164:1237–1241.
13. Barrett BP, Brown RL, Locken K, et al. Treatment of the common cold with unrefined echinacea. A randomized, double-blind, placebo-controlled trial. *Ann Intern Med*. 2002;137:939–946.
14. Grimm W, Muller HH. A randomized controlled trial of the effect of fluid extract of *Echinacea purpurea* on the incidence and severity of colds and respiratory infections. *Am J Med*. 1999;106:138–143.
15. Brinkeborn RM, Shah DV, Degenring FH. Echinaforce and other echinacea fresh plant preparations in the treatment of the common cold. A randomized, placebo-controlled, double-blind clinical trial. *Phytomedicine*. 1999;6:1–5.
16. Lindenmuth GF, Lindenmuth EB. The efficacy of Echinacea compound herbal tea preparation on the severity and duration of upper respiratory and flu symptoms: a randomized, double-blind, placebo-controlled study. *J Altern Complement Med*. 2000;6:327–334.
17. Dorn M, Knick E, Lewith G. Placebo-controlled, double-blind study of *Echinacea pallidae* radix in upper respiratory tract infections. *Complement Ther Med*. 1997;3:40–42.

Eicosapentaenoic Acid (EPA). *See* Fish Oil.

Enzymes. *See* Bromelain; Pancreatin.

Ephedra. *See* Ma Huang *(Ephedra sinica).*

Evening Primrose Oil *(Oenothera biennis).*

See Gamma Linolenic Acid.

Fenugreek *(Trigonella foenum-graecum)*

Fenugreek is the small stony seed from the pod of a bean-like annual plant native to India and southern Europe. The seeds are small and hard with a yellowish brown hue. The use of fenugreek has been documented as long ago as ancient Egypt, where it was used to treat fevers and embalm mummies. Today, fenugreek is mainly used in curry powders. Egyptians also use it as a supplement in wheat and corn flour, and in India it is used as a lactation aid. Current research indicates fenugreek may be effective in the treatment of diabetes and hypercholesterolemia.

Media and Marketing Claims	Efficacy
Helps control blood glucose in diabetes	NR
Reduces blood cholesterol levels in people with hypercholesterolemia	↑?
Prevents cancer	NR

Safety

- Individuals allergic to peanuts are likely to be allergic to fenugreek. Allergic reactions to fenugreek can include cough, nasal congestion, difficulty breathing, and loss of consciousness. Reactions can occur with both oral and topical fenugreek (1,2). Fenugreek is Generally Recognized as Safe in the United States (3).

- In a study of the toxicity of fenugreek seed extract with 40% 4-hydroxyisoleucine (beyond use as a flavoring agent), the supplement was not shown to be genotoxic at dosages compatible for use in clinical trials of blood glucose control (4).

Drug/Supplement Interactions

Exercise care when taking fenugreek with anticoagulant/antiplatelet or diabetes drugs because fenugreek may have an additive effect; dosages of these drugs may need to be altered by a physician.

Key Points

- A review of the therapeutic applications of fenugreek suggests that the herb has potential hypoglycemic and lipid-lowering properties (5). Limited human studies have shown fenugreek to be effective in reducing serum glucose levels.
- There have been promising results in the treatment of hypercholesterolemia with fenugreek. More research is needed before any recommendations can be made for use to treat diabetes or lipid disorders.
- Data regarding the possible cancer preventive effects of fenugreek are limited to experimental data that generally focused on mechanisms of anticancer action; human intervention studies are lacking.

Food Sources

Fenugreek seeds can be cooked in a variety of ways, such as curry preparations. The taste has been likened to celery, maple syrup, or burnt sugar. There are no other food sources.

Dosage Information/Bioavailability

Fenugreek is available in tablet, topical tea, or tincture formulations. Currently fenugreek supplements are standardized based on 4-hydroxyisoleucine concentration. Recommended dosages are based on studies assessing the efficacy of fenugreek in reducing blood glucose levels and range from 2.5 g twice daily to 5 to 7 g taken with each meal (3 times/day). For hypercholesterolemia, doses of 0.6 to 2.5 g twice per day have been reported.

Relevant Research

Fenugreek and Blood Glucose Control

- A case-control study evaluated whether a polyphenol-rich extract from fenugreek seeds had a protective effects on human erythrocytes subjected to hydrogen peroxide–induced oxidation. Red blood cells were isolated from 10 subjects with type 1 diabetes and 10 age-matched controls for in vitro studies of oxidation. Pre-incubation of red blood cells with polyphenol-rich extracts of fenugreek significantly and dose-dependently reduced both hemolysis and lipid peroxidation in both subject groups both with and without diabetes (6).

◆ A study of the effects of fenugreek vs placebo on blood glucose levels included two separate study groups: (*a*) healthy adults and (*b*) individuals with type 2 diabetes. Fenugreek supplementation at a dosage of 2.5 g twice a day was associated with different responses depending on the severity of diabetes (7). In the 20 subjects with severe type 2 diabetes (mean baseline glucose = 219.8 mg/dL), 1 month of fenugreek supplementation reduced mean glucose levels to 200.0 mg/dL, a change that was not significant. However, in the 20 individuals with mild type 2 diabetes (mean baseline glucose = 174.4 mg/dL), fasting mean blood glucose levels decreased to 142.0 mg/dL, a significant change ($P = .01$). Postprandial glucose levels also decreased significantly in subjects with mild type 2 diabetes who received fenugreek for a 1-month time period. It is not clear whether subjects or investigators were blinded to the interventions.

Fenugreek and Blood Cholesterol Levels

◆ In the Bordia et al study described earlier, a separate analysis was conducted on the efficacy of 2.5 g fenugreek vs placebo twice daily for 6 weeks in subjects with coronary artery disease (CAD) as well as in healthy volunteers (7). In healthy subjects (n = 30), fenugreek had no clinical efficacy in terms of reduced total or LDL cholesterol or increased HDL cholesterol. However, after 3 months, subjects with CAD (n = 30) had a significant reduction in total cholesterol and triglycerides as compared with baseline levels (from 240.2 to 225.0 mg/dL and 160.5 to 135.3 mg/dL, respectively). HDL cholesterol was not changed with fenugreek supplementation in the subjects with CAD. It is not clear whether subjects or investigators were blinded to the interventions.

◆ To determine whether consumption of fenugreek seed powder has an effect on blood lipid levels in human subjects, 20 vegetarian volunteers with hypercholesterolemia (baseline mean serum total cholesterol = 280.1 mg/dL; HDL = 66.8 g/dL; LDL = 184.1 mg/dL) consumed 12.5 or 18 g of fenugreek powder daily for 30 days. Serum cholesterol and triglycerides were determined at baseline and at the study's end. Consumption of fenugreek seed powder significantly reduced total cholesterol and LDL levels in a dose-dependent manner. No effect was seen in levels of HDL, VLDL, or triglycerides (8). This study did not include a control group or a placebo assignment and therefore results should be considered preliminary.

Fenugreek and Cancer

◆ The chemopreventive activities of fenugreek have been tested in a rat mammary cancer model (9). In this study, 200 mg/kg body weight of fenugreek, purchased from commercial sources, was given to Wistar rats 7 days before exposure to 7,12-dimethylbenz-alpha-anthracene (to induce mammary cancer). Compared with rats given no treatment, rats given fenugreek showed reduced tumor progression and hyperplasia. These results are preliminary and need to be replicated in other murine tumor models and human studies.

♦ To determine the effects of fenugreek seed extracts on the activities of β-glucuronidase and mucinase in a rat colon carcinogenesis model, rats were treated with the carcinogen 1,2-dimethylhydrazine (DMH) and fed a diet supplemented with fenugreek seed powder for 30 weeks. Rats with fenugreek supplementation had significantly lower incidence of colon tumors induced by DMH when compared with DMH-exposed rats given a normal diet. Rats supplemented with fenugreek also showed significant reduction in β-glucuronidase activity and mucinase activity in colon tissues, which suggests a protective effect of fenugreek with regard to cancer proliferation in the colon (10).

References

1. Patil SP, Niphadkar PV, Bapat MM.. Allergy to fenugreek (Trigonella foenum graecum). *Ann Allergy Asthma Immunol.* 1997;78:297–300.
2. Fenugreek. Available at: http://www.drugdigest.com. Accessed May 25, 2005.
3. Food and Drug Administration. Center for Food Safety and Applied Nutrition, Office of Premarket Approval. EAFUS: a food additive database. Available at: http://vm.cfsan.fda.gov/~dms/eafus.html.
4. Flammang AM, Cifone MA, Erexson GL, et al. Genotoxicity testing of a fenugreek extract. *Food Chem Toxicol.* 2004;42:1769–1775.
5. Basch, E, Ulbricht C, Kuo G, et al. Therapeutic applications of fenugreek. *Altern Med Rev.* 2003;8:20–27.
6. Kaviarasan S, Vijayalakshmi K, Anuradha CV. Polyphenol-rich extract of fenugreek seeds protect erythrocytes from oxidative damage. *Plant Foods Hum Nutr.* 2004;59:143–147.
7. Bordia A, Verma SK, Srivastava KC. Effect of ginger *(Zingiber officinale Rosc)* and fenugreek *(Trigonella foenumgraecum L.)* on blood lipids, blood sugar and platelet aggregation in patients with coronary artery disease. *Prostaglandins, Leukot Essent Fatty Acids.* 1997;56:379–384.
8. Sowmya P, Rajyalakshmi P. Hypocholesterolemic effect of germinated fenugreek seeds in human subjects. *Plant Foods Hum Nutr.* 1999;53:359–365.
9. Amin A, Alkaabi A, Al-Falasi S, et al. Chemopreventive activities of *trigonella foenum graecum* (fenugreek) against breast cancer. *Cell Biol Int.* 2005;29:687–694.
10. Devasena T, Menon VP. Fenugreek affects the activity of β-glucuronidase and mucinase in the colon. *Phytother Res.* 2003;17:1088–1109

Feverfew *(Tanacetum parthenium)*

The name "feverfew" is derived from the Latin *febrifugia,* meaning "to reduce fever." Feverfew has been used for thousands of years, not only to reduce fever, but also to treat migraines, allergies, and infertility. A member of the chrysanthemum family, feverfew has feathery green leaves and bright yellow and white blossoms.

Currently, feverfew is a popular remedy to treat and prevent migraines. Lactone parthenolide was once widely considered to be the primary active ingredient in feverfew, but this is no longer the case. Although not all the primary active components of feverfew have not been identified, research suggests that one constituent, parthenolide, inhibits the production and secretion of prostaglandins and may reduce inflammation and decrease secretion of histamines. This action is thought to play a role migraine treatment.

Media and Marketing Claims	Efficacy
Prophylaxis of migraine	↑?

Safety

+ No serious side effects have been reported in clinical trials with short- or long-term use (1–4).

+ Withdrawal symptoms known as "post–feverfew syndrome" can include headache, anxiety, and insomnia. These symptoms are typically seen in individuals taking feverfew for several weeks (5). Dosing should be tapered gradually to avoid withdrawal symptoms.

+ Feverfew is contraindicated in individuals allergic to members of the *Asteracae compositae* family, which includes marigolds, chrysanthemums, daisies, and others.

Drug/Supplement Interactions

+ Individuals taking drugs that are cytochrome p450 substrates should use caution when taking feverfew because it may change the metabolism and effectiveness of these drugs.

+ There is theoretical pharmacological evidence that feverfew may adversely effect anticoagulants such as warfarin or aspirin. This has not been studied specifically or reported in clinical trials to date.

Key Points

+ Some clinical trials have shown that feverfew, when taken regularly for migraine prevention, decreases the severity and frequency of migraines (1). Limited evidence suggests that feverfew may ease the pain once a migraine has begun. Most studies have been limited by high dropout rates. More research is needed.

Food Sources

None

Dosage Information/Bioavailability

Feverfew is available in tincture, tablet, fresh herb, dried herb (tea), or capsule forms. Supplement labels suggest taking 50 to 200 mg every morning to prevent migraine. Although optimal doses of feverfew have not been definitively established, studies suggest that feverfew must be taken regularly for 3 to 5 weeks before individuals who get migraines notice an improvement in their symptoms.

Relevant Research

Feverfew and Migraines

- In a double-blind, randomized, placebo-controlled trial to determine the efficacy of combined riboflavin, magnesium, and feverfew supplementation in migraine prophylaxis, 49 subjects with a history of migraines were randomly assigned to (*a*) a combination of 400 mg riboflavin, 300 mg magnesium, and 100 mg feverfew or (*b*) 25 riboflavin as a placebo daily for 3 months after a 1-month run-in. Number and severity of migraines were assessed. Analysis of the first 48 subjects who completed the trial suggested that the number of migraines was not significantly less in the experimental group compared with the placebo group (6).

- In a double-blind, randomized, placebo-controlled trial to determine the safety and efficacy of a new stable extract from feverfew (MIG-99) in migraine prophylaxis, 147 subjects received 2.08 mg, 6.25 mg, or 18.75 mg of feverfew extract three times per day for 12 weeks. The number of migraines during the final 4 weeks of the study was compared with the subjects' baseline. There was a significant dose-dependent reduction in the number of migraines in subjects receiving MIG-99, compared with placebo. In a global assessment of efficacy, it was found that the 6.25-mg dose was the most effective compared with placebo (7).

- In a double-blind, randomized, placebo-controlled trial to investigate the efficacy of feverfew in migraine prophylaxis, 57 subjects received 100 mg feverfew daily for 60 days. In the second phase, half of the subjects continued to receive feverfew while the other half received a placebo for 30 days. In the third phase, the subjects switched groups and continued for an additional 30 days. There were no washout periods. Reduction in pain intensity and associated symptoms such as nausea, vomiting, or sensitivity to light and sound were evaluated. Feverfew led to a significant reduction in pain intensity vs placebo; this was reversed after the switch to placebo. There was also a significant reduction in migraine-associated symptoms in subjects taking feverfew. Resuming feverfew supplementation after placebo treatment resulted in improved migraine prophylaxis (2).

- In a randomized, double-blind, placebo-controlled study that enrolled 284 patients with a history of migraine headaches, 218 subjects completed a 4-week no-treatment phase followed by a 16-week treatment phase that included either 6.25 mg feverfew (MIG-99) three times daily or placebo three times daily. Patients maintained a study log of migraine frequency, duration, and severity, including associated symptoms such as nausea and emesis, throughout the study. The mean number of migraines during the no-treatment phase was 4.8 during the 4 weeks. On follow-up, the number of migraines decreased to 2.9 during 7 weeks in the feverfew group and 3.5 during 7 weeks in the placebo group. This difference in migraine frequency was significant ($P = .0456$). However, the total duration of migraine attacks was not different across groups. Differences in symptoms were not reported (8).

◆ To investigate the antinociceptive (analgesic) and anti-inflammatory effects of feverfew extracts, an aqueous extract was given orally in various doses to rodents 30 minutes before nociceptive or inflammatory tests. Anti-inflammatory effects were assessed using the carrageenan-induced paw edema model. Feverfew extracts had a significant and dose-dependent antinociceptive and anti-inflammatory effect in rodents. The parthenolide constituent of the extract alone had a similar effect (9).

References

1. Pittler MH, Ernst E. Feverfew for preventing migraine. *Cochrane Database Syst Rev.* 2004;(1):CD002286.
2. Palevitch, D, Earon G, Carasso R. Feverfew (*Tanacetum parthenium*) as a prophylactic treatment for migraine: a double-blind, placebo-controlled study. *Phytother Res.* 1997;11: 508–511.
3. Johnson, ES, Kadam NP, Hylands DM, et al. Efficacy of feverfew as prophylactic treatment of migraine. *BMJ.* 1985;291:569–573.
4. Curry EA, Murry DJ, Yoder C, et al. Phase I dose escalation trial of feverfew with standardized doses of parthenolide in patients with cancer. *Invest New Drugs.* 2004;22: 299–305.
5. Feverfew. Available at: http://www.drugguide.com/monograph_library/natural_products/feverfew.htm. Accessed May 25, 2005.
6. Maizels M, Blumenfeld A, Burchette R. A combination of riboflavin, magnesium, and feverfew for migraine prophylaxis: a randomized trial. *Headache.* 2004;44:885–890.
7. Pfaffenrath V, Diener HC, Fischer M, et al. The efficacy and safety of *Tanacetum parthenium* (feverfew) in migraine prophylaxis—a double-blind, multicentre, randomised placebo-controlled dose-response study. *Cephalalgia.* 2002;22:523–532.
8. Diener HC, Pfaffenrath V, Schnitker J, et al. Efficacy and safety of 6.25 mg t.i.d. feverfew CO2-extract (MIG-99) in migraine prevention—a randomized, double-blind, multicentre, placebo-controlled study. *Cephalalgia.* 2005;25:1031–1041.
9. Jain NK, Kulkarni SK. Antinociceptive and anti-inflammatory effects of *Tanacetum parthenium L.* extract in mice and rats. *J Ethnopharmacol.* 1999;68:251–259.

Fish Oil

Fish consumption is associated with lower rates of coronary artery disease in many, but not all, epidemiological studies. Because fish oil is a rich source of the essential n-3 fatty acids eicosapentaenoic acid (EPA) and docosahexaenoic acid (DHA), this cardioprotective effect has been attributed to the n-3 fatty acids. n-3 fatty acids are essential polyunsaturated fatty acids necessary for normal growth and development.

There has been interest in fish oil because EPA and DHA are precursors to eicosanoids, which have antiatherogenic and anti-inflammatory effects. Specifically, n-3 fatty acids have beneficial effects on several precipitating factors involved in the development of inflammatory diseases (cardiovascular, arthritis, etc), including the production of thromboxane A_2, leukotriene B_4, and prostaglandin E_2 (PGE_2), interleukin 1, tumor necrosis factor, platelet-derived growth factor-like protein, triglycerides, lipoprotein(a), and fibrinogen. Additionally, fish oil has been shown to inhibit platelet aggregation, intimal hyperplasia, and monocyte and macrophage functions, and to possibly reduce blood pressure. n-3 fatty acids also increase the formation of protective factors including prostacyclin, leukotriene B_5, interleukin 2, and endothelial-derived relaxing factor, and HDL cholesterol (1–3).

In 2000, the FDA approved a limited health claim for labeling of n-3 fatty acid supplements regarding coronary heart disease (CHD). Fish oil supplement labels can state that the evidence is "suggestive, but not conclusive" and that it is not known whether diets or n-3 fatty acids in fish reduce risk of CHD in the general population (4).

Media and Marketing Claims	Efficacy
Reduces serum triglyceride levels	↑
Reduces risk for atherosclerosis/heart disease	↑?
Improves glucose levels in people with diabetes	NR
Improves lipid levels in people with diabetes	↑? (triglyceride levels)
	↓? (LDL or HDL cholesterol levels)
Reduces blood pressure	↔
Reduces inflammation and pain of arthritis	↑?
Reduces bowel inflammation in colitis or inflammatory bowel disease	↑?
Helps reduce severity of symptoms of psoriasis	↓?
Helps treat depression	NR
Helps treat attention deficit/hyperactivity disorder	NR
Prevents continued weight loss in people with cancer cachexia	NR
Reduces risk of cancer	↓?

Safety

◆ The safety of n-3 fatty acids from Menhaden oil was reviewed by the FDA in 1997. After evaluating more than 2,600 articles, the FDA concluded that dietary intakes of up to 3 g of EPA and DHA from Menhaden oil per day are Generally Recognized as Safe (5).

♦ Some fish oils (halibut and shark liver oils) contain high levels of vitamin A; pregnant women should avoid fish oil supplements high in vitamin A because of that vitamin's teratogenic effects (6,7). However, most commercial fish oil products do not contain vitamin A.

♦ Fish oils, specifically EPA, prolong bleeding time and decrease thromboxane A$_2$ production (1). It has been suggested that fish oil supplements should be avoided before surgery (8). Fish oil should not be used before surgery (7 to 14 days) to avoid a potential increase in bleeding. However, no clinically significant bleeding was observed in coronary artery bypass patients given 4.3 g n-3 fatty acids for 28 days before surgery (9).

♦ Individuals taking anticoagulant medication and those with clotting disorders should be monitored while using fish oil.

♦ Fish oil is highly susceptible to lipid peroxidation, even more so than vegetable oils. One study reported that the addition of vitamin E protected against lipid peroxidation (10), whereas another study supplementing 900 IU vitamin E per day did not suppress oxidation (11). Fish oil and n-3 fatty acid supplements should be stored in the refrigerator, where they are protected from light and high temperatures that could contribute to rancidity.

♦ In a long-term, open, prospective study of 295 subjects ages 18 to 76 years, consumption of 10 to 20 mL refined fish oil providing 1.8 g to 3.6 g EPA/day for 7 years was not associated with any serious adverse effects (12).

♦ Dosages of fish oil up to 3 g/day are considered safe; dosages more than 3 g/day may suppress immune system function and may increase risk of hemorrhagic stroke.

♦ Fish oil may cause belching, halitosis, heartburn, or gastrointestinal upset.

♦ Hypomania may develop in individuals with bipolar or major depressive disorders who take fish oil.

♦ Fish oil may increase risk of cancer in individuals with familial adenomatous polyposis.

Drug/Supplement Interactions

♦ In theory, fish oil may increase bleeding/clotting time when taken with other blood-thinning drugs or supplements (warfarin [Coumadin], garlic, ginger, ginkgo, vitamin E, flaxseed, bromelain, dong quai); use should be monitored by a physician.

♦ Fish oil supplementation may reduce vitamin E levels, although the mechanism is unknown.

♦ Fish oil may have an additive effect on reducing blood pressure when used with antihypertensive agents.

♦ Oral contraceptives may interfere with the triglyceride-reducing effect of fish oil.

Key Points

- The typical American diet provides approximately 1.6 g/day of n-3 fatty acids. The amount of n-3 fatty acids in the Western diet has decreased over time, whereas the amount of n-6 fatty acids in the diet has increased, resulting in a much higher ratio of n-6 to n-3 fatty acids. Some researchers hypothesize that a low intake of n-3 fatty acids contributes to the etiology of many chronic diseases (3).

- Many studies have shown that intake of dietary fish oil seems to inhibit or decrease the risk of precipitating factors in the development of inflammatory diseases, including cardiovascular diseases.

  - *Atherosclerosis*: Studies have not shown a clear pattern of whether fish oil supplementation reduces atherosclerosis or restenosis after angioplasty.

  - *Heart attack:* There is conflicting evidence about whether fish oil reduces the risk of myocardial infarction, cardiovascular disease progression, and/or death in individuals with CHD.

  - *Blood lipids:* Considerable evidence suggests that fish oil (more than 3 g of n-3 fatty acids/day) reduces plasma triglycerides, which may be accompanied by an increase in total and LDL cholesterol in individuals with hypertriglyceridemia.

  - *Blood lipids in diabetes*: A meta-analysis of studies in individuals with diabetes reported favorable effects of fish oil on triglyceride levels. However, fish oil also appears to increase LDL cholesterol levels in people with diabetes. It does not seem to have a beneficial effect on glucose or A1C in people with type 2 diabetes.

  - *Blood pressure*: A meta-analysis reported that fish oil may produce a small reduction in blood pressure, especially in subjects with hypertension. However, not all studies show a blood pressure lowering effect.

  - *American Heart Association (AHA) recommendations*: The AHA recognizes the benefits of consuming fish rich in n-3 fatty acids for heart health, and recommends consuming fish at least two times per week along with increasing other food sources of alpha linolenic acid. The 2002 AHA guidelines regarding fish consumption, fish oil, n-3 fatty acids, and CVD also support the use of 1 g of high-quality, mercury-free n-3 fatty acid supplements daily in individuals with coronary artery disease and 2 to 4 g/day in individuals with hypertriglyceridemia (13).

- There is evidence that fish oil can have mild beneficial effects (reduction of tender joints and morning stiffness) for individuals with rheumatoid arthritis.

- Evidence suggests that fish oil provides modest improvements in clinical symptoms such as pain in individuals with ulcerative colitis, Crohn's disease, and, possibly, inflammatory bowel disease. More research is needed to determine the potential role of fish oil in inflammatory intestinal diseases.

- Limited data are available to test the efficacy of fish oil for psoriasis; to date, studies do not support this clinical application.

♦ There is some evidence that individuals with mood disorders have reduced plasma n-3 fatty acid concentrations. Controlled trials are needed to determine the role of fish oil supplements in depression, schizophrenia, bipolar disorder, dementia, and other psychiatric conditions. A 2005 evidence report from the Agency for Healthcare Research and Quality also recommends more and better-designed research (14).

♦ Preliminary evidence suggests that nutritional formulas enriched in n-3 fatty acid and fish oil/n-3 fatty acid supplements may play a role in reducing the wasting associated with cancer cachexia. However, more controlled research is needed.

♦ A systematic review of n-3 fatty acids and cancer risk found no evidence to support the use of n-3 supplements for cancer prevention.

♦ Several other clinical applications for fish oil or n-3 fatty acid supplementation have been proposed, including treatment for retinitis pigmentosa, lupus, cystic fibrosis, asthma, and atrial fibrillation, hyperactivity, and for improving pregnancy outcomes. Review papers are available for several of these applications.

♦ An evidence report summarizing the state of the evidence for n-3 fatty acid effects on lipids, glucose, inflammatory bowel disease, arthritis, renal disease, lupus, and osteoporosis is available through the Agency for Healthcare Research and Quality (15).

♦ Individuals with conditions shown to benefit from n-3 fatty acid supplementation should discuss this option with their physicians. Eating two to three servings of fatty fish per week while limiting intake of foods high in saturated fat will increase the n-3 fatty acid content of the diet. In addition, n-3 fatty acids may also be consumed in EPA- and DHA-fortified foods such as eggs, margarine, milk, yogurt, and bread. (*See also* Flaxseed.)

Food Sources

Although not a direct source of EPA and DHA, foods such as flaxseed and walnuts are rich in alpha-linolenic acid, the precursors to EPA and DHA. (*See* Flaxseed.) Consumption of a 3.5-oz (100-g) serving of fatty fish two or three times per week provides approximately 3 g fish oil (3). Farm-raised fish contain less n-3 fatty acids than fish found in oceans, rivers, and lakes (3). The fattier the fish, the higher the content of n-3 fatty acids. However, the lipid content can vary depending on water temperature and place and season of capture (1). Several functional foods enriched in n-3 fatty acids are available on the market, such as fish, cereals, breads, and cheeses.

An excess of n-6 fatty acids (vegetable oils) reduces the metabolism of long-chain n-3 fatty acids (2).

Food*	EPA, g	DHA, g
Mackerel	0.90	1.40
Salmon, Chinook	0.79	0.57
Herring	0.71	0.86
Anchovy	0.54	0.91
Tuna	0.28	0.89
Blue fish	0.25	0.52
Swordfish	0.11	0.53
Cod liver oil	6.90	10.97
Egg enriched with n-3 fatty acids, from hens fed flaxseed	—	0.15 g per egg

Serving size for all types of fish is 100 g (raw).
Source: Data are from reference 2.

Dosage Information/Bioavailability

Fish oil supplements are usually derived from sardine, salmon, tuna, menhaden, or anchovy fish and are sold as liquid oil or in softgel capsules. Concentrated EPA and DHA are also available as supplements. Before packaging, oils must be refined to remove moisture, impurities, sulfur, halogen and nitrogen compounds, toxic metals, trace metals, sterols, and other contaminants. Supplements typically provide approximately 180 to 300 mg EPA and 120 to 200 mg DHA per capsule, with manufacturers suggesting a total intake ranging from 1 to 10 g/day. In a bioavailability study, 4 g of highly purified EPA or DHA administered with a high-fat meal to healthy subjects increased EPA and DHA levels in chylomicrons, peaking 6 hours after supplementation (16).

The Food and Nutrition Board of the Institute of Medicine has set dietary guidelines for α-linolenic acid intake. The Board recommends 1.6 g α-linolenic acid daily for men and 1.1 g/day for women. (α-linolenic acid can be converted into EPA and DHA in the body.)

Relevant Research

Because of the large number of studies of fish oil, only recent trials and review articles are discussed here.

Fish Oil and Blood Lipids/Atherosclerosis

- Numerous studies have reported that fish oil supplementation reduces plasma triglyceride levels approximately 30%, and as much as 50% in individuals with severe hypertriglyceridemia (17). However, the triglyceride-reducing effects can be accompanied by increases in LDL cholesterol, especially in individuals with low baseline

LDL levels (18,19). It has been suggested that the increase in LDL cholesterol may not necessarily increase atherosclerosis risk in light of the antithrombotic, anti-inflammatory, and antivasoconstrictive actions of n-3 fatty acids (3). Whether an increase in LDL cholesterol from fish oil is, in fact, atherogenic is unknown. Recent data suggest that DHA may be the primary modulator of triglyceride levels and that DHA may positively affect HDL particle size (20).

- A meta-analysis of seven trials testing fish oil supplements in individuals who underwent angioplasty reported that in the four studies using angiography there was a reduction in restenosis (reconstriction of blood vessels) with fish oil intake. In the three studies that used stress-testing to evaluate re-stenosis, there was no benefit from fish oil consumption. There was a significant positive relationship between the dosage and the absolute difference in re-stenosis rates (21).

- The randomized, double-blinded, placebo-controlled ESPRIT (Esapent for Prevention of Restenosis Italian) study tested the effects of fish oil supplementation on restenosis prevention after percutaneous transluminal coronary angioplasty (PTCA). The 339 subjects were given of 2.1 g DHA and 3 g EPA or a placebo daily for 1 month before and after PTCA and then continued at a half dose for 6 months. Two hundred fifty-seven subjects matched for risk factors underwent PTCA. The investigators concluded that n-3 fatty acid supplementation was associated with a small but significant decrease in the re-stenosis rate compared with placebo (22).

- Repeated coronary angiography and carotid artery intima-media thickness were assessed in 223 subjects with known coronary artery disease to determine the effect of 2 years of daily supplementation with 1.65 g of n-3 fatty acids. One hundred seventy-one subjects completed the trial. At the end of 2 years, there were no significant differences in these clinical outcome markers over time or between the n-3 fatty acid and placebo groups (the mean intima-media thickness increased 0.07 mm in the supplemented group vs 0.05 mm in the placebo group). This suggests that the progression of disease continues at the predicted rate regardless of n-3 supplementation (23). Mortality data was not presented, and the completion rate is a concern because intent-to-treat analysis was not used. In addition, the dosage of n-3 fatty acids may have been too low to expect modulation of intima-media thickness, especially because triglyceride levels also were not lowered as has been shown in the majority of published research.

- In a controlled study, 610 subjects undergoing coronary artery bypass grafting were randomly assigned to receive 4 g concentrated fish oil per day or no supplement (control) for 1 year. All subjects in the fish oil and control groups were also assigned to antithrombotic treatment using either aspirin or warfarin. Compared with the control group, the fish oil group had significantly fewer occluded vein grafts (24).

Fish Oil and Cardiovascular Morbidity or Mortality

- A meta-analysis (10 randomized, controlled trials with a total of 14,727 subjects) of morbidity and mortality from CVD in association with fish oil intake in subjects with CVD showed that all-cause mortality was significantly reduced (16%) with exposure to daily n-3 fatty acid supplementation for a mean of 37 months. Mortality from myocardial infarction was reduced by 24%; however, concern about study designs was cited as rationale not to implement routine n-3 supplementation in clinical practice (25).

♦ A case-control study nested within the Cardiovascular Health Study has shown a significant reduction in fatal ischemic heart disease associated with increased plasma n-3 levels, but no association was shown for nonfatal myocardial infarction. This study is strengthened by the fact that it relies on biomarkers of intake (plasma n-3 levels) rather than self-reported dietary intake (26).

♦ In a large-scale, open label, Italian study (GISSI Prevenzione Study), 11,324 subjects surviving recent (≤ 3 months) myocardial infarction were randomly assigned to one of four groups for 3.5 years: (*a*) 1 g/day n-3 supplements; (*b*) 300 mg/day vitamin E; (*c*) both supplements; or (*d*) neither supplement. The main endpoint was the combined occurrence of death, nonfatal myocardial infarction, and nonfatal stroke. n-3 treatment significantly reduced the risk of the primary endpoint by 10% to 15%. Total mortality in subjects treated with n-3 fatty acid supplements was 20% less (a significant difference) than subjects not receiving n-3 fatty acids. There was no additional benefit from the combined vitamin E and n-3 supplements. The results of this study would have been strengthened if it had been double-blinded (27).

♦ In a double-blind, placebo-controlled study in India, 360 subjects with suspected myocardial infarction were randomly assigned to receive fish oil (1.08 g EPA per day), mustard oil (2.9 g alpha-linolenic acid per day), or placebo for 1 year. Treatments were administered approximately 18 hours after symptoms of myocardial infarction in all three groups. The extent of cardiac disease, increase in cardiac enzymes, and levels of lipid peroxides were similar among the groups at entry. After 1 year, the fish oil and mustard oil groups had significantly fewer total cardiac events compared with the group using the placebo (24.5% and 28% vs 34.7%, respectively). Nonfatal infarctions were also significantly fewer in the fish oil and mustard oil groups compared with the group using the placebo (13% and 15% vs 25.4%, respectively). Fish oil supplementation was significantly correlated with fewer cardiac deaths compared with placebo (11.4% vs 22.0%). Mustard oil had no effect on total cardiac death rate. Both the fish oil and mustard oil groups showed a significant reduction in the incidence of total cardiac arrhythmias, left ventricular enlargement, and angina pectoris compared with the placebo group (28).

♦ Evidence from the Iowa Women's Health Study suggested that in postmenopausal women, fish intake is associated with reduced overall mortality, but no independent protective associations for cardiovascular disease mortality were demonstrated. However, participants in this study generally demonstrated low fish intake, and n-3 supplementation was not evaluated because this cohort did not use n-3 supplements (29).

Fish Oil and Blood Lipids and Glucose Levels in Diabetes

♦ A Cochrane Review evaluated the role of fish oil supplementation in cardiovascular disease, lipid levels, and glycemic control in subjects with type 2 diabetes. In 18 trials with more than 800 participants, triglyceride levels were significantly reduced with supplementation, whereas LDL levels increased, particularly among subjects who had hypertriglyceridemia and also with higher doses of n-3 fatty acids. No effect on fasting glucose or A1C were found (30).

♦ In a randomized intervention trial conducted in 51 subjects with type 2 diabetes and treated hypertension, subjects were randomly assigned to receive either 4 g EPA, 4 g DHA, or olive oil (placebo) daily for 6 weeks. Outcome measures included lipid panel, serum glucose, fasting insulin, and C-reactive protein. Results showed that the n-3 fatty acids were not effective in improving serum lipid levels, with the exception of serum triglyceride levels, which were lowered in response to the intervention. HDL-3 cholesterol was decreased in the EPA group only. Blood pressure was not changed in either group. Glycemic response worsened in the intervention groups— fasting glucose levels increased mildly with both DHA and EPA (A1C and fasting insulin levels remained stable). This challenges the efficacy of such an approach to reduce lipid levels in individuals with type 2 diabetes (31).

♦ A meta-analysis of 26 trials testing fish oil administration on lipid levels in subjects with type 1 or type 2 diabetes revealed a significant 25% to 30% decrease in mean triglyceride concentrations and a slight but statistically significant increase in serum LDL cholesterol. Both findings were more prominent in subjects with type 2 diabetes. Fasting blood glucose levels were significantly lower in subjects with type 1 diabetes but increased insignificantly in subjects with type 2 diabetes (32).

♦ A review of n-3 fatty acids in type 2 diabetes was recently published in *Journal of the American Dietetic Association* with the goal of clarifying the role of fish or fish oil intake among individuals with type 2 diabetes (33). Literature to date points to the benefit of fish intake in improving dyslipidemia, but the evidence of the impact of fish to treat some other cardiovascular complications, such as metabolic syndrome, is poor. For the most part, the literature is favorable for the role of fish oil in reducing cardiovascular risks in individuals with type 2 diabetes; the authors state that "favorable effects outweigh the modest increase in low-density lipoprotein levels that may result from increased n-3 LC PUFA intake."

Fish Oil and Blood Pressure

♦ A meta-analysis of 31 placebo-controlled trials (total n = 1,356 subjects) reported a small but significant reduction in blood pressure (−3.0 mm Hg systolic, −1.5 mm Hg diastolic) associated with fish oil consumption. n-3 fatty acids (mean daily dosage 4.2 g) had no effect on blood pressure in eight studies of healthy, normotensive subjects. Dosages of 5.6 g/day resulted in a significant blood pressure–lowering effect in studies of subjects with hypertension or hypercholesterolemia. The authors concluded that "there is a dose response effect of fish oil on blood pressure of ↓0.66/↓0.35 mm Hg/g omega-3 fatty acids. The hypotensive effect may be strongest in hypertensive subjects and those with clinical atherosclerotic disease or hypercholesterolemia" (34).

♦ In a placebo-controlled, multicenter trial, 350 subjects (ages 30 to 54 years) with normal blood pressure were randomly assigned to receive 6 g purified fish oil daily

(3 g n-3 fatty acids) or a placebo for 6 months. At baseline, the mean differences in blood pressure changes between groups were not significant. There was no tendency for fish oil to reduce blood pressure more in subjects with baseline blood pressure in the upper (132/87 mm Hg) vs lower quartile (114/75 mm Hg), or with low habitual fish consumption (0.4 vs 2.9 times/week), or with low baseline plasma n-3 fatty acids (35).

Fish Oil and Rheumatoid Arthritis

♦ A meta-analysis of 10 double-blind, placebo-controlled, randomized trials (total n = 395 subjects; mean age 54 years) reported that fish oil supplementation for 3 months was associated with a significant reduction in occurrence of subjective assessment of joint tenderness and morning stiffness as compared with use of placebo oils, but there were no significant improvements in joint swelling, grip strength, subject and physician assessment, or erythrocyte sedimentation rate (marker of inflammation). A meta-analysis of the data using primary data from each study (the previous meta-analysis used only summary data), confirmed the results. The dosages of fish oil used in the studies were not given. The authors noted that most of the studies did not report disease duration, rheumatoid factor seropositivity, and functional status of subjects (36).

♦ In a double-blind, placebo-controlled study, 66 subjects with rheumatoid arthritis were randomly assigned to receive 130 mg/kg/day n-3 fatty acids (approximately 9 g fish oil per day) or a placebo (corn oil) while taking diclofenac for pain. Placebo diclofenac was substituted at week 18 or 22, and fish oil supplements were continued for 8 weeks (week 26 or 30). In subjects taking fish oil, there was a significant decrease from baseline in the mean number of tender joints, duration of morning stiffness, physician and subject evaluation of global arthritis activity, and physician's evaluation of pain. Subjects taking the placebo showed no change from baseline. Interleukin-1 beta (a marker of inflammation) decreased significantly from the baseline through weeks 18 and 22 in subjects consuming fish oil. The authors concluded that "some individuals who take fish oil are able to discontinue NSAIDs without experiencing a disease flare" (37).

♦ In a double-blind, placebo-controlled study, 50 subjects with rheumatoid arthritis whose usual background diets were naturally low in n-6 fatty acids (less than 10 g/day) were randomly assigned to receive fish oil supplements (40 mg/kg) or placebo daily for 15 weeks. Clinical evaluations—consisting of tender joint count, swollen joint count, duration of early morning stiffness, visual analog scale of pain, subject and physician global assessment of arthritis activity, Health Assessment Questionnaire, erythrocyte sedimentation rate (ESR), and C-reactive protein (CRP)—were assessed at baseline and at weeks 4, 8, and 15. Twenty-four hour food recalls at each clinical assessment evaluated whether subjects' dietary intake continued to contain less than 10 g n-6 fatty acids per day. Plasma and monocyte EPA levels increased significantly in the subjects taking fish oil supplements. By week 12, subjects receiving supplements achieved a significant improvement from baseline in all clinical variables except total joint count, ESR, and CRP. The control group had no significant changes from baseline (38).

Fish Oil and Inflammatory Bowel Disease

♦ In a double-blind, placebo-controlled trial, 78 subjects with Crohn's disease in remission and a high risk of relapse were randomly assigned to receive nine fish oil capsules (2.7 g n-3 fatty acids) or nine placebo capsules daily for 1 year. A special coating protected the capsules against gastric acidity for at least 30 minutes. Subjects in the fish oil group had significantly fewer relapses than subjects receiving the placebo (28% vs 69%). Fifty-nine percent of the subjects treated with fish oil remained in remission compared with 26% of the subjects in the placebo group; this difference was statistically significant. Logistic-regression analysis revealed that fish oil, but not gender, age, previous surgery, duration of disease, or smoking status, affected the incidence of relapse (39).

♦ In a double-blind, placebo-controlled trial, 87 subjects with ulcerative colitis were randomly assigned to receive, in addition to standard drug therapy, 20 mL EPA-concentrated fish oil (4.5 g EPA) or a placebo (olive oil) daily for 1 year. Fish oil use resulted in a significant increase in EPA content of rectal mucosa (at 6 months), increased synthesis of leukotriene B_5, and suppression of leukotriene B_4 synthesis by ionophore-stimulated neutrophils (at 2 months). For subjects entering the trial in relapse (n = 53), there was a significant reduction in corticosteroid requirements after 1 and 2 months of fish oil supplementation. There was an insignificant trend toward achieving remission (off the use of steroids) faster with fish oil. For subjects in remission (n = 69) at entry or during the trial, there were no significant differences in rate of relapse. The authors concluded that "fish oil supplementation produces a modest corticosteroid-sparing effect in active disease, but there is no benefit in maintenance therapy" (40).

♦ In a double-blind, placebo-controlled, crossover trial, 18 subjects with ulcerative colitis received 18 fish oil capsules (3.24 g EPA, 2.16 g DHA) or an isocaloric placebo daily, each in random order for 4 months, with a 1-month washout period. Monthly assessments of clinical symptoms, sigmoidoscopies and biopsies, and rectal dialysates for leukotriene B_4 were measured at the baseline and at the end of each treatment. Fish oil supplementation resulted in a statistically significant increase in weight gain, improved histology, and a decrease in rectal dialysate leukotriene B_4 levels. In contrast, there were no differences from baseline during placebo administration. The mean prednisone dosage decreased during fish oil ingestion, but this change did not reach statistical significance (41).

Fish Oil and Psoriasis

♦ In a double-blind, placebo-controlled study, 38 subjects with psoriatic arthritis were randomly assigned to receive a combination of fish oil and evening primrose oil (total of 12 capsules/day) or a placebo for 9 months. All subjects received placebo capsules for another 3 months. At month 3, subjects were asked to reduce their

NSAID intake and maintain this level if tolerable. Clinical assessments were done at baseline and every 3 months thereafter. All measures of skin and joint disease activity, including severity, percentage of body affected, and itch were not changed by fish oil and evening primrose oil supplementation. There was also no difference in NSAID requirements between groups or arthritis activity as measured by morning stiffness, Ritchie articular index, and number of active joints. However, in the subjects who had been taking fish oil/primrose oil, thromboxane B_2 increased significantly during the 3 months of placebo treatment. In addition, leukotriene B_4 production decreased significantly during fish oil/evening primrose treatment, followed by an increase during the 3 months of placebo treatment, which the authors noted as suggestive of an anti-inflammatory effect. They concluded that fish oil/evening primrose oil supplements may alter prostaglandin metabolism in subjects with psoriatic arthritis, although it did not produce clinical improvements and did not allow reduction in NSAID requirements (42). This study design does not address whether the effects on prostaglandin metabolism resulted from fish oil, evening primrose oil, or a combination of both.

◆ In a double-blind, placebo-controlled, multicenter study, 145 subjects with moderate to severe psoriasis were randomly assigned to receive 6 g highly purified fish oil (5 g EPA and DHA) or an isocaloric placebo (corn oil) for 4 months. All subjects were advised to reduce their saturated fat intake. In the fish oil group, n-3 fatty acids in serum phospholipids increased significantly, and the ratio of arachidonic acid to EPA, the level of n-6 fatty acids, and serum triglyceride levels all decreased significantly. In the corn oil–supplemented group, only DHA in serum phospholipids increased significantly. The score on the Psoriasis Area and Severity Index, as evaluated by the physicians, did not change in either group. The subjective score also did not change, but a selected area of skin in the corn oil group showed a significant reduction in clinical signs. There were no notable differences in clinical manifestations between groups. In the fish oil group, an increase in the concentration of n-3 fatty acids in serum phospholipids was not accompanied by clinical improvement, whereas in the corn oil group there was a statistically significant correlation between clinical improvement and an increase in EPA and total n-3 fatty acids. The authors concluded that "dietary supplementation with very-long-chain n-3 fatty acids was no better than corn oil supplementation in treating psoriasis" (43).

◆ A review article cited research suggesting that fish oil (1.5 g/day) may minimize the increase in triglycerides associated with retinoid therapy for psoriasis (44).

Fish Oil and Mental Illness

◆ Individuals with major depression seem to have significantly lower levels of n-3 fatty acids (specifically DHA) in erythrocyte phospholipids compared with healthy control subjects. However, whether low levels of n-3 causes depression is unclear (45–47).

◆ A population-based study of more than 29,000 middle-aged men conducted in Finland showed that there was no association between dietary n-3 fatty acid intake and self-reported depression. This study was limited by its use of self-reported data for both diet and depression (48).

+ Review articles note that there is some evidence that n-3 fatty acids may reduce severity of bipolar disorder and schizophrenia, but well designed studies are needed (45–47).

Fish Oil and Attention Deficit/Hyperactivity Disorder

+ Data are limited, but in a randomized double-blind, placebo-controlled study of 41 children with attention deficit/hyperactivity disorder, 12 weeks of n-3 fatty acid supplementation (186 mg EPA, 480 mg DHA, plus 96 mg γ-linolenic acid and 864 mg *cis*-linoleic acid) significantly reduced behavior and cognitive problems compared with placebo. Additional research is warranted (49).

Fish Oil and Cancer Cachexia

+ Most studies in this area have been poorly designed or use supplements that not only offer n-3 fatty acids but other cachexia-modulating nutrients as well.

+ A Phase II study administered high-dose n-3 fatty acid supplements (7.5 g EPA plus DHA for a 75-kg person) for a median time of 1.2 months to 36 subjects with cancer cachexia. Twenty-four subjects showed weight stabilization (a gain of ≤ 5% body weight or a loss of < 5% body weight), six subjects gained more than 5% body weight, and six subjects lost 5% or more of body weight. There was a significant correlation between duration of supplementation and weight gain for the subjects who could tolerate the supplements for at least 1 month (many subjects could not) (50).

Fish Oil and Cancer

+ In a systematic review of 38 published and unpublished studies from 1996 to 2006, the effect of n-3 fatty acids on cancer risk in prospective cohort studies was examined. Across 20 cohorts from 7 countries for 11 different types of cancer and using up to 6 methods to classify n-3 fatty acid consumption, 65 estimates of the association between n-3 fatty acid intake and cancer risk were reported. Of these, only eight were significant. For breast cancer, one significant estimate was reported showing increased risk and three were reported with decreased risk. There was no significant association for seven other estimates. For colorectal cancer, there was one estimate of significant decreased risk and 17 estimates without association. For lung cancer, one of the significant associations was for increased cancer risk, another was for decreased risk, and four other estimates were not significant. For prostate cancer, there was one estimate of significant decreased risk and one of increased risk for advanced prostate cancer; whereas 15 other estimates showed no significant association. One study assessing skin cancer found a significant increased risk. There were no significant associations between n-3 fatty acid intake and incidence of aerodigestive cancer, bladder cancer, lymphoma, ovarian cancer, pancreatic cancer, or stomach cancer. The authors concluded: "A large body of literature spanning numerous cohorts from many countries and with different demographic characteristics does not provide evidence to suggest a significant association between omega-3 fatty acids and cancer incidence. Dietary supplementation with omega-3 fatty acids is unlikely to prevent cancer" (51).

References

1. Uauy-Dagach R, Valenzuela A. Marine oils: the health benefits of n-3 fatty acids. *Nutr Rev.* 1996;54(11 pt 2):S102-S108.
2. Jones PJ, Kubow S. Lipids, sterols, and their metabolites. In: Shils ME, Olson JA, Shike M, et al, eds. *Modern Nutrition in Health and Disease.* 9th ed. Baltimore, Md: Williams & Wilkins; 1999:67–94.
3. Simopoulos AP. Omega-3 fatty acids in health and disease and growth and development. *Am J Clin Nutr.* 1991;54:438–463.
4. Food and Drug Administration. Center for Food Safety and Applied Nutrition, Office of Premarket Approval. EAFUS: a food additive database. Available at: http://vm.cfsan.fda.gov/~dms/eafus.html. Accessed May 2, 2005.
5. FDA Final Rule. Substances Affirmed as Generally Recognized as Safe: Menhaden Oil. *Fed Regist.* 1997;62:30,751–757.
6. Increasing fish oil intake—any net benefits? *Drug Ther Bull.* 1996;34:60–62.
7. Rothman KJ, Moore LL, Singer MR, et al. Teratogenicity of high vitamin A intake. *N Engl J Med.* 1995;333:1369–1373.
8. Petry JJ. Surgically significant nutritional supplements. *Plast Reconstr Surg.* 1996;97:233–240.
9. DeCaterina R, Giannessi D, Mazzone A, et al. Vascular prostacyclin is increased in patients ingesting omega-3 polyunsaturated fatty acids before coronary artery bypass graft surgery. *Circulation.* 1990;82:428–438.
10. Harris WS. Fish oils and plasma lipid and lipoprotein metabolism in humans: a critical review. *J Lipid Res.* 1989;30:785–807.
11. Allard JP, Kurian R, Aghdassi E, et al. Lipid peroxidation during n-3 fatty acid and vitamin E supplementation in humans. *Lipids.* 1997;32:535–541.
12. Saynor R, Gillott T. Changes in blood lipids and fibrinogen with a note on safety in a long term study on the effects of n-3 fatty acids in subjects receiving fish oil supplements and followed for seven years. *Lipids.* 1992;27:533–538.
13. Kris-Etherton PM, Harris WS, Appel LJ; American Heart Association. Nutrition Committee. Fish consumption, fish oil, omega-3 fatty acids, and cardiovascular disease. *Circulation.* 2002;106:2747–2757.
14. MacLean CH, Issa AM, Newberry SJ, et al. *Effects of Omega-3 Fatty Acids on Cognitive Function With Aging, Dementia, and Neurological Diseases.* Summary, Evidence Report/Technological Assessment No. 114. Rockville, Md: Agency for Healthcare Research and Quality; 2005. AHRQ Publication No. 05-E011-1.
15. Agency for Healthcare Research and Quality. Available at: http://www.ahrq.gov. Accessed May 25, 2005.
16. Hansen JB, Grimsgaard S, Nilsen H, et al. Effects of highly purified eicosapentaenoic acid and docosahexaenoic acid on fatty acid absorption, incorporation into serum phospholipids and postprandial triglyceridemia. *Lipids.* 1998;33:131–138.

17. Harris WS, Ginsberg HN, Arunakul N, et al. Safety and efficacy of Omacor in severe hypertriglyceridemia. *J Cardiovasc Risk.* 1997;4:385–392.

18. Harris WS. N-3 fatty acids and serum lipoproteins: human studies. *Am J Clin Nutr.* 1997;65(5 Suppl):S1645-S1654.

19. Kris-Etherton PM, Etherton TD, Yu S. Efficacy of multiple dietary therapies in reducing cardiovascular disease risk factors. *Am J Clin Nutr.* 1997;65:560–561.

20. Buckley R, Shewring B, Turner R, et al. Circulating triacylglycerol and apoE levels in response to EPA and docosahexaenoic acid supplementation in adult human subjects. *Br J Nutr.* 2004;92:477–483.

21. Gapinski JP, VanRuiswyk JV, Heudebert GR, et al. Preventing restenosis with fish oils following coronary angioplasty. A meta-analysis. *Arch Intern Med.* 1993;153:1595–1601.

22. Maresta A, Balduccelli M, Varani E, et al. Prevention of postcoronary angioplasty restenosis by omega-3 fatty acids: main results of the Esapent for Prevention of Restenosis Italian Study (ESPRIT). *Am Heart J.* 2002;143:E5.

23. Angerer P, Kothny W, Stork S, et al. Effect of dietary supplementation with omega-3 fatty acids on progression of atherosclerosis in carotid arteries. *Cardiovasc Res.* 2002;54:183–190.

24. Eritsland J, Arnesen H, Gronseth K, et al. Effect of dietary supplementation with n-3 fatty acids on coronary artery bypass graft patency. *Am J Cardiol.* 1996;77:31–36.

25. Yzebe D, Lievre M. Fish oils in the care of coronary heart disease patients: a meta-analysis of randomized controlled trials. *Fundam Clin Pharmacol.* 2004;18:581–592.

26. Lemaitre RN, King IB, Mozaffarian D, et al. n-3 Polyunsaturated fatty acids, fatal ischemic heart disease, and nonfatal myocardial infarction in older adults: the Cardiovascular Health Study. *Am J Clin Nutr.* 2003;77:319–325.

27. Gruppo Italiano per lo Studio della Sopravvivenza nell'Infarto Miocardico. Dietary supplementation with n-3 polyunsaturated fatty acids and vitamin E after myocardial infarction: results of the GISSI-Prevenzione trial. *Lancet.* 1999;354:447–455.

28. Singh RB, Niaz MA, Sharma JP, et al. Randomized, double-blind, placebo-controlled trial of fish oil and mustard oil in patients with suspected acute myocardial infarction: the Indian experiment of infarct survival—4. *Cardiovasc Drugs Ther.* 1997;11:485–491.

29. Folsom AR, Demissie Z. Fish intake, marine omega-3 fatty acids, and mortality in a cohort of postmenopausal women. *Am J Epidemiol.* 2004;160:1005–1010.

30. Farmer A, Montori V, Dinneen S, et al. Fish oil in people with type 2 diabetes mellitus. *Cochrane Database Syst Rev.* 2001;(3)CD003205.

31. Woodman RJ, Mori TA, Burke V, et al. Effects of purified eicosapentaenoic and docosahexaenoic acids on glycemic control, blood pressure, and serum lipids in type 2 diabetic patients with treated hypertension. *Am J Clin Nutr.* 2002;76:1007–1015.

32. Friedberg CE, Janssen MJ, Heine RJ, et al. Fish oil and glycemic control in diabetes. A meta-analysis. *Diabetes Care.* 1998;21:494–500.

33. Nettleton JA, Katz R. n-3 long change polyunsaturated fatty acids in type 2 diabetes: a review. *J Am Diet Assoc.* 2005;105:428–440.

34. Morris MC, Sacks F, Rosner B. Does fish oil lower blood pressure? A meta-analysis of controlled trials. *Circulation.* 1993;88:523–533.

35. Sacks FM, Hebert P, Appel LJ, et al. The effect of fish oil on blood pressure and high density lipoprotein-cholesterol levels in phase I of the Trials of Hypertension Prevention. Trials of Hypertension Prevention Collaborative Research Group. *J Hypertens.* 1994;12(suppl):S23-S31.
36. Fortin PR, Lew RA, Liang MH, et al. Validation of a meta-analysis: the effects of fish oil in rheumatoid arthritis. *J Clin Epidemiol.* 1995;48:1379–1390.
37. Kremer JM, Lawrence DA, Petrillo GF, et al. Effects of high-dose fish oil on rheumatoid arthritis after stopping nonsteroidal antiinflammatory drugs. Clinical and immune correlates. *Arthritis Rheum.* 1995;38:1107–1114.
38. Volker D, Fitzgerald P, Major G, et al. Efficacy of fish oil concentrate in the treatment of rheumatoid arthritis. *J Rheumatol.* 2000;27:2305–2307.
39. Belluzzi A, Brignola C, Campieri M, et al. Effect of an enteric-coated fish-oil preparation on relapse in Crohn's disease. *N Engl J Med.* 1996;334:1557–1560.
40. Hawthorne AB, Daneshmend TK, Hawkey CJ, et al. Treatment of ulcerative colitis with fish oil supplementation: a prospective 12 month randomized controlled trial. *Gut.* 1992;33:922–928.
41. Stenson WF, Cort D, Rodgers J, et al. Dietary supplementation with fish oil in ulcerative colitis. *Ann Intern Med.* 1992;116:609–614.
42. Veale DJ, Torley HI, Richards IM, et al. A double-blind placebo controlled trial of Efamol Marine on skin and joint symptoms of psoriatic arthritis. *Br J Rheumatol.* 1994;33:954–958.
43. Soyland E, Funk J, Rajka G, et al. Effect of dietary supplementation with very-long-chain n-3 fatty acids in patients with psoriasis. *N Engl J Med.* 1993;328:1812–1816.
44. Frati C, Bevilacqua L, Apostolico V. Association of etretinate and fish oil in psoriasis therapy. Inhibition of hypertriglyceridemia resulting from retinoid therapy after fish oil supplementation. *Acta Derm Venereol Suppl (Stockh).* 1994;186:151–153.
45. Mischoulon D, Fava M. Docosahexanoic acid and omega-3 fatty acids in depression. *Psychiatr Clin North Am.* 2000;23:785–794.
46. Maidment ID. Are fish oils effective therapy in mental illness—an analysis of the data. *Acta Psychiatr Scand.* 2000; 102:3–11.
47. Freeman MP. Omega-3 fatty acids in psychiatry: a review. *Ann Clin Psychiatry.* 2000;12:159–165.
48. Hakkarainen R, Partonen T, Haukka J, et al. Is low dietary intake of omega-3 fatty acids associated with depression? *Am J Psychiatry.* 2004;161:567–569.
49. Richardson AJ, Puri BK. A randomized double-blind, placebo-controlled study of the effects of supplementation with highly unsaturated fatty acids on ADHD-related symptoms in children with specific learning difficulties. *Prog Neuropsychopharmacol Biol Psychiatry.* 2002;26:233–239.
50. Burns CP, Halabi S, Clamon G, et al. Phase II study of high-dose fish oil capsules for patients with cancer-related cachexia. *Cancer.* 2004;101:370–378
51. MacLean CH, Newberry SJ, Mojica WA, et al. Effects of omega-3 fatty acids on cancer risk: a systematic review. *JAMA.* 2006;295:403–415.

Flaxseed

Cultivated for more than 5,000 years, flaxseed originated in Central Asia and is now found throughout North America, Asia, and Europe. Flaxseed is approximately 35% fat, 28% to 30% protein, 35% fiber, and 6% ash. Supplementing the diet with flaxseed products is thought to be beneficial because of compounds found in the seed: n-3 fatty acids and lignans.

α-Linolenic Acid (n-3)

It has been suggested that humans evolved on diets providing a linoleic (n-6) to linolenic (n-3) fatty acid ratio of 1:1 to 2:1. However, because of changes in the food supply and production, the typical US diet currently provides a much higher ratio of 10:1 to 30:1 (1). The essential fatty acid ratio is important because it affects the type of prostaglandins formed in the body. More than half of the fat content of flaxseed is α-linolenic acid as opposed to some other oils that comprise only 1% to 11% of the total (2). Biochemically, some of the α-linolenic acid from flaxseed can be converted into eicosapentaenoic acid (EPA), and to a lesser extent, docosahexaenoic acid (DHA) (3,4). Diets rich in linoleic acid or high in saturated fat reduce the conversion of α-linolenic acid to its long-chain metabolites. Because increased cellular levels of EPA and DHA are precursors to anti-inflammatory and antiatherogenic prostaglandins, flaxseed has been studied for its potential preventive role in heart disease and inflammatory disorders.

Lignans

Flaxseed contains 100 to 800 times more plant lignans (a type of phytoestrogen) than do other major seeds (2). Lignans are digested by colonic bacteria to mammalian lignans, enterolactone, and enterodiol, which enter hepatic circulation (5). These lignans are thought to protect against cancer because of their antimitotic, antioxidant, antitumor, and antiestrogenic properties (6). Mammalian lignans are hypothesized to bind to estrogen receptors to prevent the cancer promoting effects of estrogen. Additionally, lignans may regulate sex-hormone–binding globulin, a protein that binds estrogen, reducing its bioavailability.

Media and Marketing Claims	Efficacy
Improves blood lipids	↔
Reduces risk for heart disease and stroke	NR
Improves symptoms of lupus, eczema, and other inflammatory diseases	NR
Reduces risk of estrogen-related and other cancers	NR
Reduces inflammation in individuals with arthritis	NR
Relieves constipation	↑

Safety

◆ Flaxseed contains cyanogenic glycosides, a naturally occurring toxicant found in foods such as almonds, peaches, apricots, cherries, and plums. Baking eliminated these compounds from muffins made with flaxmeal. A letter to the editor of *Lancet* questioned the safety of cyanogenic glycosides from high doses (> 60 g) of ground flaxseed, which could theoretically increase blood thiocyanate levels (7).

◆ Doses more than 45 g flaxseed powder are associated with laxative effects (8).

◆ Because n-3 fatty acids favor production of the prostaglandins that increase bleeding time, it may be advisable for individuals undergoing surgery or individuals with clotting disorders to avoid consuming flaxseed.

◆ To prevent intestinal blockage, at least 150 mL of liquid is required for every 10 g of whole or cracked flaxseed intake.

◆ Flaxseed supplements can cause allergic and anaphylactic reactions.

◆ Flaxseed is bulk forming; avoid use in individuals with bowel obstruction, esophageal stricture, or acute intestinal inflammation.

◆ No specific safe intake levels for flaxseed have been published for women with hormone-sensitive cancers (breast, uterine, ovarian) or conditions (endometriosis, uterine fibroids); therefore, flaxseed use in these women should be considered with caution.

Drug/Supplement Interactions

◆ The fiber content of ground flaxseed can interfere with the absorption of other nutrients and some medications that are affected by fiber intake (digoxin, lovastatin, and metformin).

◆ Theoretically, flaxseed may increase bleeding/clotting time when taken with other blood-thinning drugs or supplements (ie, warfarin [Coumadin], garlic, ginger, ginkgo biloba, vitamin E, flaxseed, bromelain, dong quai, fish oil, aspirin); use should be monitored by a physician.

◆ Flaxseed may have additive effect with antidiabetes drugs; monitor blood glucose.

Key Points

◆ Flaxseed may increase serum triglycerides in individuals with hypertriglyceridemia.

◆ At this time, there is insufficient research to support the claim that flaxseed reduces the risk of stroke and heart attack. Flaxseed appears to raise cellular EPA levels under certain conditions but has not consistently lowered serum LDL cholesterol and triglycerides. Larger controlled human trials are needed to delineate the effects of flaxseed supplementation in cardiovascular disease. A review of the topic and postulated mechanisms of action has been published (9).

◆ Some evidence from experimental studies in animals suggests that flaxseed inhibits tumor growth, specifically mammary tumors. Flaxseed supplementation seems to increase urinary excretion of estrogen metabolites associated with a reduced breast cancer risk in postmenopausal women. Larger, long-term trials are needed in humans (including those at risk or previously treated for estrogen-related cancers) to determine the role of flaxseed in cancer prevention.

◆ Although flaxseed has been shown to inhibit mediators of inflammation, clinical trials are needed to determine the effects of flaxseed on rheumatoid arthritis and other inflammatory disorders such as psoriasis, multiple sclerosis, and lupus.

◆ Several researchers have suggested that the low ratio of n-3 to n-6 fatty acids in the average American diet creates an imbalance that is linked to several conditions, including coronary heart disease, hypertension, lupus, eczema, and inflammatory disorders. Consuming flaxseed products is one way to increase the n-3 content of the diet. Other food sources of n-3 fatty acids include walnuts, soybean and canola oil (not partially hydrogenated), fatty fish (salmon, swordfish, mackerel, herring), and eggs from hens fed special diets rich in flaxseed.

◆ Consumption of flaxseed products can increase the fiber (ground flaxseed) and n-3 fatty acid (ground flaxseed and/or oil) content of the diet and thus may be effective in treating constipation. However, tolerance may be poor unless adequate fluid/water is taken along with flaxseed to avoid gastrointestinal distress.

◆ Individuals supplementing with flaxseed oil while following a weight-control diet should allow for approximately 140 kcal and 14 g fat per tablespoon of oil. Flaxseed oil, ground flaxseed, and flaxseed powder supplements are unstable and must be refrigerated or stored in the freezer in airtight, opaque containers to prevent oxidation of fatty acids (2). or beyond the expiration date on the label. Flaxseed oil can be added to hot foods (eg, soups, casseroles) after cooking or flaxseed can be mixed with foods during cooking. It should not be used in high-temperature frying.

Food Sources

Whole flaxseed, flaxseed oil, margarine made from flaxseed oil, flax cereals, and breads made with ground flaxseed flour.

Dosage Information/Bioavailability

Flaxseed is available in liquid, capsule, or powder form. Manufacturers suggest 1 tablespoon of flaxseed oil daily, which provides approximately 7 g of α-linolenic acid and 2 g linoleic acid. The Food and Nutrition Board of the Institute of Medicine has set dietary guidelines for α-linolenic acid intake. The Board recommends 1.6 g α-linolenic acid daily for men and 1.1 g/day for women. (α-linolenic acid can be converted into EPA and DHA in the body.)

A study testing the bioavailability of 50 g flaxseed flour and 20 g flaxseed oil in healthy subjects found that plasma n-3 fatty acids increased only after 2 and 4 weeks of supplementation, respectively (10). Furthermore, it has been reported that a diet rich in linoleic acid may negatively affect the conversion of α-linolenic acid in flaxseed to EPA (11). In one study, EPA levels were maximized by reducing intake of n-6 fatty acids from vegetable oils and increasing intake of n-3–rich flaxseed oil (11). Consumption of raw ground flaxseed (5 to 25 g) for 7 days increased urinary lignan (enterolactone and enterodiol) levels in a dose-dependent manner in healthy, young women. There were no differences in total urinary lignan excretion with the raw compared with the processed forms of flaxseed at an intake of 25 g (12). To increase the availability of lignans to the gut microflora, flaxseed should be consumed freshly ground (not whole). Note: lignans are only found in the fiber portion of the plant, not the oil.

Relevant Research

Flaxseed and Cardiovascular Disease

♦ In a trial of flaxseed vs wheat germ supplementation, 199 postmenopausal women were randomly selected to supplement their diets with 40 g flaxseed/day (n = 101) or wheat germ placebo (n = 98) for 12 months. Serum lipids and bone mineral density were evaluated at baseline and after 12 months of supplementation. Using intent-to-treat analysis, flaxseed was shown to reduce total cholesterol (P = .01) and HDL (P = .03). Given the small change in serum cholesterol levels, the authors suggest that the clinical efficacy of this approach may be limited. Flaxseed did not seem to significantly reduce menopausal symptoms (13).

♦ In a randomized, double-blind parallel study of 58 postmenopausal women, supplementation with 40 g ground flaxseed daily for 3 months was associated with significant decreases in total cholesterol (6%), apolipoprotein A-1 (6%), and apolipoprotein B (7.5%), as well as nonsignificant reductions in LDL, HDL, and triglycerides (14). However, attrition rates were high, with six subjects dropping out of the study in the flaxseed group and 10 in the control group (who took a wheat-based supplement). Laxative effects/gastrointestinal distress was reported in five subjects in the flaxseed group.

♦ In a double-blind, comparative, crossover study, 29 subjects with hyperlipidemia received (in random order) muffins that contributed approximately 20 g fiber per day from either flaxseed (50 g partially defatted flaxseed per day) or wheat bran (control) for 3 weeks each while they consumed self-selected National Cholesterol Education Program Step II diets. Treatment phases were separated by a 2-week washout period. During the flaxseed phase, total cholesterol decreased significantly by 4.6%, LDL cholesterol by 7.6%, apolipoprotein B by 5.4%, and apolipoprotein A-I by 5.8%, but there was no effect on serum lipoprotein ratios at week 3 compared with the control. Neither treatment had a significant effect on serum HDL cholesterol, possibly due to an insufficient time period of supplementation (15).

Flaxseed and Lupus

♦ In a randomized, crossover study with 23 subjects with lupus nephritis, subjects were randomly assigned to receive 30 g ground flaxseed daily or placebo for 1 year. This was followed by a 12-week washout period and then a switch to the alternate group for an additional 12 months. Of the 23 who started the study, eight dropped out and only nine of the remaining 15 demonstrated compliance to the flaxseed intervention. Although flaxseed supplementation improved serum creatinine levels compared with placebo, the effect did not reach statistical significance ($P = .08$), probably because of the low sample size. Comparison of compliant subjects with those who selected not to participate (n = 17) showed a significant reduction in serum creatinine levels associated with flaxseed use ($P = .05$). This study demonstrates a key issue with the clinical application of flaxseed for lupus: the lack of long-term compliance (16).

Flaxseed and Cancer

- Several animal studies have shown that flaxseed inhibits tumor growth in experimentally induced mammary cancer (8,17,18).

- In a pilot study exploring the effect of daily (30 g) flaxseed supplementation on prostate tissue proliferation in 15 men undergoing repeat prostate biopsies for elevated prostate specific antigen (PSA) and benign disease, daily flaxseed combined with a low-fat eating plan resulted in significant reductions in proliferation rates ($P = .017$) (19). Serum total cholesterol and PSA also decreased significantly, whereas serum testosterone levels were unresponsive to flax supplementation.

- In a randomized, crossover design trial, 28 postmenopausal women were studied for three 7-week feeding periods. Subjects ate their usual diets plus ground flaxseed (0 g, 5 g, or 10 g per day). Urinary excretion of estrogen metabolites 2-hydroxyestrogen and 16 α-hydroxyetrone, as well as their ratio (2:16α-OHE1 ratio) were measured (biomarkers for breast cancer risk). Flaxseed supplementation significantly increased urinary 2-hydroxyestrogen and the 2:16α-OHE1 ratio in a dose-dependent way. Women with elevated ratios of these metabolites are believed to have a decreased risk of breast cancer, and the authors hypothesized that flaxseed may have chemoprotective effects (20). A similar study by the same researchers compared flaxseed with wheat bran use and found that flaxseed significantly increased the 2:16α-OHE1 ratio, whereas wheat bran had no effect (21). Similar increases in 2-hydroxyestrone concentrations were demonstrated in a randomized study of postmenopausal women (n = 46) receiving 25 g of flaxseed or soy flour daily (22).

- In a cross-sectional study of 121 French women with breast cancer, low breast tissue levels of a-linolenic acid were associated with a significant increased risk of metastases but not tumor size or mitotic index. The authors hypothesized that in women with breast cancer flaxseed supplementation to replenish n-3 fatty acids in adipose stores may delay or even prevent the appearance of tumors (23).

Flaxseed and Inflammatory Disorders

- In a parallel group study, 30 healthy male subjects were instructed to consume a diet low in n-6 fatty acids by using flaxseed oil in food preparation or a diet high in n-6 fatty acids by using sunflower oil (control) for 2 months. At 1 month, all subjects took fish oil capsules (9 g/day). Subject's diet diaries indicated that dietary α-linolenic acid was 13.7 (± 5.5) g/day in the flaxseed oil group and 1.1 (± 0.5) g/day in the sunflower oil group. The total fat intake was not different between the two groups (mean = 29.4% of total energy intake). There were no significant differences in BMI during the course of the study. Unlike sunflower oil, flaxseed oil increased cellular EPA concentrations, which increased more after fish oil intake. Proinflammatory markers (tumor necrosis factor α[TNF-α] and interleukin 1ß [IL-1ß]) decreased significantly by a mean of 30% in the flaxseed oil group compared with the sunflower oil group. These markers are hypothesized to aggravate the pathology occurring in rheumatoid arthritis and atherosclerosis (24).

- In a double-blind, placebo-controlled study, 22 subjects with rheumatoid arthritis were randomly assigned to receive 30 g flaxseed powder or 30 g sunflower oil powder (prepared identical in taste and appearance) for 3 months. Subjects were instructed not to change their dietary habits or antirheumatic medications during the study. At the study end, the flaxseed group had an increased bleeding time but experienced no effect on the clinical, subjective (global assessment, classification of functional status, joint score index, visual analogue scale, pain tenderness score), or laboratory parameters. Despite serum increases in α-linolenic acid, there was no change in arachidonic acid, EPA, or DHA concentrations. The authors suggested that the low conversion of a-linolenic acid to EPA and DHA, together with a low α-linolenic acid:linoleic acid body ratio, may explain the lack of clinical benefit (25).

Flaxseed and Constipation

- In a randomized, controlled, crossover design study in which 10 healthy subjects were asked to consume muffins containing 25 g of flaxseed or control muffins twice per day for 4 weeks. Bowel movement frequency increased by 30% in the flaxseed group in a weekly time period. The stimulatory effects of flaxseed on bowel movements have led to its use for subjects with chronic laxative abuse and colitis (26).

References

1. Simopoulos AP. Essential fatty acids in health and chronic disease. *Am J Clin Nutr.* 1999;70(suppl):S560–S569.
2. Carter JF. Potential of flaxseed and flaxseed oil in baked goods and other products in human nutrition. *Cereal Foods World.* 1993;10:753–759.
3. Mantzioris E, James MJ, Gibson RA, et al. Differences exist in the relationships between dietary linoleic and alpha-linolenic acids and their respective long-chain metabolites. *Am J Clin Nutr.* 1995;61:320–324.
4. Gerster H. Can adults adequately convert alpha-linolenic acid (18:3n-3) to eicosapentaenoic acid (20:5n-3) and docosahexaenoic acid (22:6n-3)? *Int J Vitam Nutr Res.* 1998;68:159–173.
5. Lampe JW, Martini MC, Kurzer MS, et al. Urinary lignan and isoflavonoid excretion in premenopausal women consuming flaxseed powder. *Am J Clin Nutr.* 1994;60:122–128.
6. Serraino M, Thompson LU. The effect of flaxseed supplementation on early risk markers for mammary carcinogenesis. *Cancer Lett.* 1991;60:135–142.

7. Rosling H. Cyanide exposure from linseed [letter]. *Lancet.* 1993;341:177.
8. Serraino M, Thompson LU. The effect of flaxseed supplementation on the initiation and promotional stages of mammary tumorigenesis. *Nutr Cancer.* 1992;17:153–159.
9. Bloedon LT, Szapary PO. Flaxseed and cardiovascular risk. *Nutr Rev.* 2004;62:18–27.
10. Cunnane SC, Ganguli S, Menard C, et al. High a-linolenic acid flaxseed (*Linum usitatissimum*): some nutritional properties in humans. *Br J Nutr.* 1993;69:443–453.
11. Mantzioris E, James MJ, Gibson RA, et al. Dietary substitution with alpha-linolenic acid-rich vegetable oil increases eicosapentaenoic acid concentrations in tissues. *Am J Clin Nutr.* 1994;59:1304–1309.
12. Nesbitt PD, Lam Y, Thompson LU. Human metabolism of mammalian lignan precursors in raw and processed flaxseed. *Am J Clin Nutr.* 1999;69:549–555.
13. Dodin S, Lemay A, Jacques H, et al. The effects of flaxseed dietary supplement on lipid profile, bone mineral density, and symptoms in menopausal women: a randomized, double-blind, wheat germ placebo-controlled clinical trial. *J Clin Endocrinol Metab.* 2005;90:1390–1397.
14. Lucas EA, Wild RD, Hammond LJ, et al. Flaxseed improves lipid profile without altering biomarkers of bone metabolism in postmenopausal women. *J Clin Endocrinol Metab.* 2002;87:1527–1532.
15. Jenkins DJ, Kendall CW, Vidgen E, et al. Health aspects of partially defatted flaxseed, including effects on serum lipids, oxidative measures, ex vivo androgen, and progestin activity: a controlled crossover trial. *Am J Clin Nutr.* 1999;69:395–402.
16. Clark WF, Kortas C, Heidenheim P, et al. Flaxseed in lupus nephritis: a 2-year non-placebo-controlled crossover study. *J Am Coll Nutr.* 2001;20:143–148.
17. Thompson LU, Rickard SE, Orcheson LJ, et al. Flaxseed and its lignan and oil components reduce mammary tumor growth at a late stage of carcinogenesis. *Carcinogenesis.* 1996;17:1373–1376.
18. Thompson LU, Seidl MM, Rickard SE, et al. Antitumorigenic effect of a mammalian lignan precursor from flaxseed. *Nutr Cancer.* 1996;26:159–165.
19. Demark-Wahnefried W, Robertson CN, Walther PJ, et al. Pilot study to explore effects of low-fat, flaxseed-supplemented diet on proliferation of benign prostatic epithelium and prostate specific antigens. *Urology.* 2004;63:900–904.
20. Haggans CJ, Hutchins AM, Olson BA, et al. Effect of flaxseed consumption on urinary estrogen metabolites in postmenopausal women. *Nutr Cancer.* 1999;33:188–195.
21. Haggans CJ, Travelli EJ, Thomas W, et al. The effect of flaxseed and wheat bran consumption on urinary estrogen metabolites in premenopausal women. *Cancer Epidemiol Biomarkers Prev.* 2000;9:719–725.
22. Brooks JD, Ward WE, Lewis JE, et al. Supplementation with flaxseed alters estrogen metabolism in postmenopausal women to a greater extent than does supplementation with an equal amount of soy. *Am J Clin Nutr.* 2004;79:318–325.
23. Bougnoux P, Koscielny S, Chajes V, et al. Alpha-linolenic acid content of adipose breast tissue: a host determinant of the risk of early metastasis in breast cancer. *Br J Cancer.* 1994;70:330–334.
24. Caughey GE, Mantzioris E, Gibson RA, et al. The effect on human tumor necrosis factor alpha and interleukin 1 beta production of diets enriched in n-3 fatty acids from vegetable oil or fish oil. *Am J Clin Nutr.* 1996;63:116–122.

25. Nordstrom DC, Honkanen VE, Nasu Y, et al. Alpha-linolenic acid in the treatment of rheumatoid arthritis. A double-blind placebo controlled and randomized study: flaxseed vs safflower seed. *Rheumatol Int.* 1995;14:231–234.

26. Cunnane SC, Hamadeh MJ, Liede AC, et al. Nutritional attributes of traditional flaxseed in healthy young adults. *Am J Clin Nutr.* 1995;61:62–68.

Folate/Folic Acid

Folate is the general term used to refer to a group of compounds structurally similar to folic acid. Folic acid, also referred to as "pteroylmonoglutamate," is formed by the linkage of pteridine and para-aminobenzoic acid (PABA) conjugated to a molecule of glutamic acid. Folic acid is the synthetic form of the vitamin that is used as a supplement. Natural food forms of folate are chemically reduced, frequently have one-carbon substitutions in the pteridine ring, and may have up to 10 additional glutamate residues linked to the proximal glutamic acid moiety. Folate functions in the body as a coenzyme in reactions involving the transfer of one-carbon units. In this role, folate is involved in amino acid and purine metabolism, and in nucleic acid synthesis. About half of the total body folate is stored as polyglutamate by the liver. When it functions as a coenzyme in various reactions, it is reduced to the active form tetrahydrofolic acid (THFA) (1).

A dietary deficiency or inadequate absorption of folate impairs DNA synthesis and cell division, and results in megaloblastic anemia among other clinical symptoms. In 1996, because of significant evidence showing that folic acid intake reduces the risk of neural tube defects, the FDA mandated that beginning in June 1998 all breads, pastas, rice, and cereal products be fortified with folic acid at levels ranging from 0.43 to 1.4 mg per pound of food (95 to 309 µg/100 g) (2). Folic acid is also being investigated for its potential role in cardiovascular disease, particularly its effect on reducing homocysteine levels.

Media and Marketing Claims	Efficacy
Prevents neural tube defects in newborns	↑
Reduces homocysteine levels	↑
Prevents heart disease	↓?
Reduces cancer risk	↔
Reduces symptoms of depression	NR
Improves cognition in elderly	NR

Safety

♦ Doses up to 15 mg (15,000 µg) folic acid in healthy humans without convulsive disorders have not been associated with any reported serious adverse effects (1).

- The Tolerable Upper Intake Level (UL) is 1 mg (1,000 µg) in adults older than 19 years (3).
- Supplementation with folic acid at levels exceeding 400 µg/day can mask pernicious anemia caused by a vitamin B-12 deficiency, which could lead to permanent nerve damage (1). Some researchers have suggested that adding 0.5 to 1.0 mg of vitamin B-12 to folic acid supplements would prevent this potential problem (except in patients who are deficient in vitamin B-12 due to pernicious anemia) (4,5).
- There have been some studies suggesting that intakes greater than the UL may negatively affect zinc status (1). However, other studies show no adverse effects (6,7).
- Dosages equal to or greater than 5 mg folic acid per day may cause abdominal cramps, diarrhea, and rash.
- Dosages equal to or greater than 15 mg folic acid per day can alter sleep patterns or cause vivid dreaming, irritability, excitability, overactivity, confusion, impaired judgment, exacerbation of seizure frequency and psychotic behavior, nausea, abdominal distention, flatulence, bitter taste, allergic skin reactions, and zinc depletion.
- Large doses exacerbate neuropathy in individuals with vitamin B-12 deficiency.
- Some evidence suggests that high amounts folate from diet and/or supplements may worsen cognitive decline people older than 65 years; more research is needed.

Drug/Supplement Interactions

- Dosages more than 1 mg/day interfere with anticonvulsant medications (eg, diphenyhdantoin, carbamazepine, valproic acid, phenytoin, phenobarbital).
- The absorption or activity of folate can be affected by some drugs, including oral contraceptives, aspirin, indomethacin (NSAID), methotrexate (chemotherapeutic), famotidine (antacid), some antibiotics (tetracycline, isoniazid, cycloserine, erythromycin, sulfonamides), and cholestyramine.
- Folate may decrease the effectiveness of methotrexate in treatment of lymphoblastic leukemia; consult oncologist before use.
- Folate may decrease side effects of long-term, low-dose methotrexate treatment of rheumatoid arthritis.
- Folate can antagonize antiparisitic effects of pyrimethamine against toxoplasmosis and pneumocystis carinii; folate is not an antagonist in the treatment of malaria.
- Data about folate effects on dietary zinc absorption are conflicting; adverse effects are unlikely with adequate dietary zinc and normal doses of supplemental folate.

Note

Folate fortification of all cold cereals and baking flour (includes breads, pastas, bakery items, cookies, crackers, etc) has been required in the United States since 1998; the estimated mean increase in folic acid intake after fortification is 200 µg/day.

Key Points _____

- Populations at risk for inadequate folate nutriture include pregnant and lactating women, individuals who abuse alcohol, those with malabsorption, people on hemodialysis, and those with hepatic disease.

- There is compelling evidence that women who take folic acid supplements in the months before conception and during the first trimester of pregnancy reduce the risk of having a child with neural tube defects. The FDA mandates fortification of certain food products and permits these foods and dietary supplements containing folic acid to carry a health claim acknowledging this protective effect against neural tube defects in conjunction with a varied diet. The Institute of Medicine recommends that all women of childbearing age consume 400 µg of folic acid per day from fortified foods and/or supplements in addition to eating folate-rich foods from a varied diet (3).

- There is also compelling evidence that folic acid supplements reduce blood homocysteine concentrations, considered by some researchers as a risk factor for cardiovascular disease. However, the American Heart Association currently does not recognize an elevated level of homocysteine as an independent risk factor for CVD. A large-scale, open-label, randomized study of folic acid suggests that supplementation, while modulating homocysteine levels, does not alter cardiovascular morbidity or mortality (8).

- Epidemiological studies show an inverse relationship of folic acid supplements to colon cancer; however, controlled, prospective intervention trials are needed to provide more definitive evidence that folic acid supplementation confers a protective effect. In addition, the impact of food fortification with folic acid on cancer risk over time has not been evaluated. The efficacy of folic acid in reducing cancer risk may depend on whether the tumor (or premalignant lesion) is hypo- or hypermethylated, but that information is not currently used clinically in the diagnostic process.

- A polymorphism in the gene for methylenetetrahydrofolate reductase (MTHFR) has been associated with the risk of several types of cancer, and may also contribute to the risk for CVD through increases in serum homocysteine (9). Approximately 10% of the population has this defective folate metabolizing enzyme. Supplementing the diet with folic acid may reduce the risk of colon and breast cancer in women who consume alcohol (10), and possibly the risk of CVD in those with the polymorphism.

- Studies testing the efficacy of supplemental folic acid in women with cervical dysplasia are conflicting. The relationship between human papilloma virus (associated with cervical cancer risk) and folate status must also be explored.

- Poor folate status has been reported in a few studies of subjects having depression and in elderly individuals with cognitive impairment. However, controlled clinical trials are needed to determine whether supplementation improves symptoms of depression or cognitive function in the elderly.

Food Sources

Folic acid is only available in supplements. Folate is found naturally in some foods.

Food	Folate, µg/serving
Spinach (raw, 1 cup)	108
Orange (1 medium)	44
Romaine lettuce (1 cup)	38
Peanut butter (2 Tbsp)	29
Milk, nonfat (1 cup)	13
Beef, ground (3.5 oz)	9
Raisin bran cereal (1 cup)	181

Source: Data are from reference 11.

Dosage Information/Bioavailability

In 1998 the Institute of Medicine increased the RDA for adults from 180 to 400 µg Dietary Folate Equivalent (DFE) (3). The RDA during pregnancy is 600 µg DFE. Women of child-bearing age should consume 400 µg as synthetic folic acid from supplements and/or forti-fied foods in addition to intake of food from the diet. The UL for adults is 1,000 µg/day of folic acid, exclusive of food folate. Folic acid supplements are available in single prepara-tions or multivitamin/mineral supplements providing up to 400 µg/serving. Prescription prenatal vitamins may contain up to 1,000 µg.

According to the Institute of Medicine, DFE adjust for nearly 50% lower bioavailabil-ity of food folate compared with that of synthetic folic acid. One microgram of food folate equals 0.5 µg of folic acid taken on an empty stomach equals 0.6 µg folic acid with meals (3). Food folate is absorbed less efficiently because it is primarily in the polyglutamate form and requires intestinal enzymes to split off excess glutamates before absorption can occur. In contrast, folic acid (supplemental form) is in the monoglutamate form and does not require hydrolysis to be absorbed (1). Intervention trials have shown similar improved serum responsiveness associated with folic acid over food sources of folate (12).

Several medications alter folate bioavailability, including anticonvulsant medications, metformin, sulfasalazine, triamterene, methotrexate, and barbiturates (13).

Relevant Research

Folate and Neural Tube Defects

◆ In 1996, the FDA reviewed numerous studies showing a relationship between folic acid intake and neural tube defects. The FDA concluded that there was substantial research to permit foods and supplements containing folic acid to carry the health claim that "healthful diets with adequate folic acid may reduce a woman's risk of hav-ing a child with a brain or spinal cord birth defect." Four years earlier, the Centers for Disease Control and Prevention issued had recommended daily consumption of a 400 µg folic acid supplement by all women of childbearing age to reduce the risk of neural tube defects (14).

- In 1998, the Institute of Medicine recommended that to reduce the risk of neural tube defects, all women capable of becoming pregnant should consume 400 µg of synthetic folic acid daily from fortified foods and/or supplements, in addition to consuming food folate from a varied diet (3).

- A national study examining the occurrence of neural tube defects before and after folic acid food fortification reported a 19% reduction in the incidence of these defects after fortification (37.8 cases per 100,000 live births compared with 30.5 cases per 100,000 live births) (15).

Folate and Cardiovascular Disease, Homocysteine Levels

- In a randomized, prospective, open-label study, 593 subjects with stable coronary artery disease were provided either 0.5 mg folic acid daily or placebo for a mean of 24 months. Folic acid supplementation was associated with a significant 18% reduction in plasma homocysteine levels; however, all-cause mortality and cardiovascular events were not significantly different between study groups (8). Thus, while modulation of homocysteine levels occurred, the relevance to clinical disease progression remains unsupported and needs further research. The findings from this study would have been strengthened if it was double-blinded.

- A randomized, double-blind, controlled intervention study investigated the role of daily high-dose vs low-dose supplementation with folic acid and vitamins B-12 and B-6 in reducing recurrent stroke in 3,680 adults with nondisabling cerebral infarction. The high dose included 2.5 mg folic acid, 25 mg vitamin B-6, and 0.4 mg vitamin B-12, whereas the low dose provided 20 µg folic acid, 200 µg vitamin B-6, and 6 µg vitamin B-12. Mean reduction in plasma homocysteine levels was significantly greater in the high-dose group after 2 years of supplementation. However, risk for recurrent stroke, coronary heart disease events, and death were not different across intervention groups. Lower baseline homocysteine levels were associated with reduced risk for recurrent disease including stroke, cardiovascular events, and death (16).

- In a prospective cohort study, 80,082 women from the Nurses' Health Study with no history of cardiovascular disease, cancer, hypercholesterolemia, or diabetes were followed up from 1980 to 1994. In those 14 years, 658 cases of nonfatal myocardial infarction and 281 cases of fatal coronary heart disease occurred. After controlling for cardiovascular risk factors, the relative risk of developing coronary heart disease was 0.55 (45% risk reduction) in women in the highest quintile of both folate and vitamin B-6 intake compared with women in the lowest quintiles. After excluding vitamin users, coronary heart disease risk was also reduced in subjects with higher dietary intakes of folate and vitamin B-6 (17).

- A meta-analysis of 12 randomized trials (total n = 1,114 subjects) assessed the effects of folic acid supplementation on blood homocysteine concentrations. Blood homocysteine decreased more among subject with higher pretreatment blood homocysteine concentrations and at lower pretreatment blood folate concentrations. Researchers found that dietary folate significantly reduced blood homocysteine (by

25%), with similar effects in the range of 0.5 to 5 mg folic acid daily (18). Similar findings were reported in a meta-analysis of 27 studies relating homocysteine to vascular disease and 11 studies of folic acid effects on homocysteine levels (19).

- In a retrospective cohort study, serum folate levels were measured between 1970 to 1972 in 5,056 subjects with no history of coronary heart disease. These subjects were assessed retrospectively through 1985. A total of 165 deaths from coronary heart disease occurred after 15 years. There was a significant association between low serum folate levels and risk of fatal coronary heart disease, but no association between dietary folate (estimated by 24-hour food recall) and fatal coronary heart disease. Folic acid from supplements was not measured. The authors noted the limitations of using a food recall questionnaire to classify subjects because of within-individual variation in diet (20).

- Folic acid supplementation has also been shown to reduce total homocysteine (tHcy) levels in subjects receiving hemodialysis or after renal transplant. Although significant reductions were shown either with 15 mg folic acid or with 17 mg methyltetrahydrofolate, tHcy levels did not normalize in hemodialysis or renal transplant patients, although renal transplant patients were more responsive. Whether reductions in plasma tHcy levels in this population with end-stage renal disease translates to reduced cardiovascular events remains to be tested (21).

Folate and Cancer

- It has been hypothesized that increased folic acid intake may increase cancer risk in the US population, particularly in those with undiagnosed premalignant or malignant lesions (22). This hypothesis is based on premise that folic acid may contribute to hypermethylation of CPG islands in the genetic material and hypermethylation of abnormal cells is associated with cancer development. Epidemiological and clinical trial data are lacking at this time.

- In a prospective cohort study, 88,756 women from the Nurses' Health Study who did not have cancer in 1980 were followed up until 1994. A total of 442 new cases of colon cancer were reported during the 14-year period. The study controlled for age, family history of colon cancer, aspirin use, smoking, body mass index, physical activity, and intakes of red meat, alcohol, methionine, and fiber. A higher energy-adjusted folate intake (> 400 μg vs < 200 μg from food and supplements), assessed by food-frequency questionnaires in 1980, was related to a lower risk of colon cancer. Women who used multivitamins containing folic acid for more than 15 years had a significantly lower risk of developing colon cancer compared with users of the same type of supplements for 14 years or less. There was no benefit associated with 4 years or less of supplement use, and only an insignificant trend toward reduced colon cancer risk with supplement use for 5 years to 14 years. Folate from diet alone was related to a modest reduction in colon cancer risk (4).

- A subgroup analysis of women with a reported family history of colorectal cancer from the same cohort showed a protective relationship between folic acid supplementation (in multivitamins) and colon cancer risk. Higher dietary folate intake showed a trend for protection, but this trend did not reach statistical significance (23).

- In a prospective cohort study, 751 subjects with at least one recent large-bowel adenoma underwent colonoscopy 1 and 4 years after their qualifying colon exam. A food-frequency questionnaire was administered at the beginning and end of the study. After adjusting for energy intake, estimated dietary folate had a significant protective association with the risk of recurrence of adenoma. However, this effect diminished after adjusting for fiber and fat intake. Reported use of folic acid supplements was not associated with a reduction in risk (24).

- In a double-blind, placebo-controlled, ex vivo study, 24 subjects with ulcerative colitis (in remission for at least 1 month) were randomly assigned to receive 15 mg folic acid (as calcium folate) or placebo for 3 months. Cell proliferation was analyzed in rectal biopsies before and after treatment. Compared with the baseline, subjects treated with supplements had a significant reduction in the frequency of occurrence of labeled cells (measure of cell proliferation) in the upper 40% of the crypts (the area typically associated with the development of colon cancer). No significant changes were seen in the placebo group. The authors concluded that "these results suggest that folate supplementation contributes to regulating rectal cell proliferation in subjects with long-standing ulcerative colitis. These findings may be significant for chemoprevention of colon cancer in these patients" (25).

- Twenty subjects with adenomas were randomly assigned to receive 5 mg folic acid or placebo daily for 1 year after polypectomy. At baseline, 6 months, and 1 year, systemic and colonic measures of folate status were obtained, along with biomarkers of colon cancer (DNA methylation and DNA strand breaks in exons 5–8 of the p53 gene of the colonic mucosa). Serum, red blood cell, and colonic mucosal folate levels were significantly increased in to the group taking folic acid supplements and significantly increased the extent of genomic DNA methylation and reduced DNA strand breaks at 6 months and 1 year. Significant effects on these molecular markers were also observed in the placebo group, but only at the 1-year mark. The authors noted that improvement in the placebo group indicated that confounding factors other than folate supplementation were involved (26).

- In a placebo-controlled study, 235 subjects with cervical dysplasia were randomly assigned to receive 10 mg folic acid or a placebo daily for 6 months. Clinical status, human papillomavirus Type 16 infection, and blood folate levels were monitored every 2 months. The baseline incidence of human papillomavirus infection was significantly greater among subjects in the lower tertile of red blood cell folate. However, there were no significant differences among the groups regarding dysplasia status, biopsy results, or prevalence of human papillomavirus. The authors concluded that "folate deficiency may be involved as a co-carcinogen during the initiation of cervical dysplasia, but folic acid supplements do not alter the course of established disease" (27).

- In a double-blind, placebo-controlled trial, 47 women using oral contraceptives with mild or moderate cervical dysplasia were given 10 mg folic acid or a placebo daily for 3 months. Mean biopsy scores from subjects taking folate supplements were significantly better (rated by a single observer without knowledge of treatment status using a scoring system) than those taking the placebo. Final vs initial cytology scores were also significantly improved in supplemented subjects and unaffected in the placebo group. Compared with control subjects, subjects with dysplasia has lower mean red cell folate concentrations and had morphological features of megaloblastosis. The authors concluded that "these studies indicate that either a reversible, localized derangement in folate metabolism may sometimes be misdiagnosed as cervical dysplasia, or else such a derangement is an integral component of the dysplastic process that may be arrested or in some cases reversed by oral folic acid supplementation" (28).

♦ A review of relevant research on the association of cancer risk and intake of folate and other methyl-related nutrients, alcohol, and the methyltetrahydrofolate receptor (MTHFR) 677C→T polymorphism demonstrated that adequate intake of folate (folic acid) is important for women at higher risk for breast and colorectal cancer. Moderate alcohol consumption, especially for women with the homozygous genotype for the MTHFR 677C→T polymorphism, in the presence of low folate intake/folic acid deficiency is associated with increased risk for these cancers. The summary of recommendations included consumption of folate-dense fruits and vegetables and foods that are fortified with folic acid (29).

♦ A population-based, case-control study (1,481 case subjects and 1,518 control subjects) identified significant inverse associations between B vitamin and folate intake and breast cancer risk. Study participants with the MTHFR 677C→T polymorphism had an increased risk of breast cancer. The associations between MTHFR and breast cancer were more prominent among women who did not use multivitamin supplements compared with the MTHFR-breast cancer individuals with high folate intake. Breast cancer risk was most evident among MTHFR-breast cancer women with the lowest dietary folate intake (odds ratio [OR] = 1.83; 95% CI = 1.13–2.96) or total folate intake (OR = 1.71; 95% CI = 1.08–2.71) (30).

Folate and Cognitive Impairment

♦ Several studies suggest an association between low serum folate and red cell folate levels and depression (31,32). One study found that low folate levels were linked to poorer response to antidepressant treatment (33). One review article reported that low folate status has been detected in 15% to 38% of adults diagnosed with depressive disorders (34). However, because many depressed individuals are also alcohol consumers and vice versa, alcohol intake may be a confounder in testing the relationship between folate and depression (alcohol intake reduces folate stores).

♦ In a placebo-controlled, multicenter trial, 127 men and women with major depression were randomly assigned to receive 500 μg folic acid or a placebo daily in addition to treatment with the antidepressant fluoxetine for 10 weeks. Depressive symptoms were assessed using the Hamilton Rating Scale at baseline and at weeks 2, 4, 6, and 10. Folic acid significantly increased plasma folate in all subjects, and homocysteine levels were reduced significantly only in female subjects. Overall, there was a significant improvement in depressive symptoms in the group taking folic acid supplements. However, when subjects were divided by gender, symptoms improved only female subjects receiving folic acid and fluoxetine. The authors concluded that folic acid is a simple method that may enhance the action of antidepressants, and that dosages should be given in amounts sufficient to decrease plasma homocysteine. They also noted that men may require a higher dosage of folic acid than women do to achieve this decrease (35).

◆ A Cochrane Database Review conducted in 2003, which included three studies with a total of 247 subjects, concluded that the limited available evidence suggest that folic acid supplementation may have a potential role as a complement to other treatments for depression, but that benefits may differ depending on baseline folate status (36).

◆ In a double-blind multicenter study, 96 subjects with reduced cognitive function and elevated depression scores were randomly assigned to receive 5'-methyltetrahydrofolic acid or trazodone therapy, in addition to psychiatric medications, for 8 weeks. Both approaches resulted in significant improvements in cognitive function and depression scores at 4 weeks and again at 8 weeks (37).

References

1. Herbert V. Folic acid. In: Shils ME, Olson JA, Shike M, Ross AC, eds. *Modern Nutrition in Health and Disease.* 9th ed. Baltimore, Md: Williams & Wilkins; 1999:433–446.
2. Food and Drug Administration. Food standards: amendment of standards of identity for enriched grain products to require addition of folic acid. *Fed Regist.* 1996;61: 8781–8807.
3. Institute of Medicine. *Dietary Reference Intakes for Thiamin, Riboflavin, Niacin, Vitamin B-6, Folate, Vitamin B-12, Pantothenic Acid, Biotin, and Choline.* Washington, DC: National Academy Press; 1998.
4. Giovannucci E, Stampfer MJ, Colditz GA, et al. Multivitamin use, folate, and colon cancer in women in the Nurse's Health Study. *Ann Intern Med.* 1998;129:517–524.
5. Herbert V, Bigaouette J. Call for endorsement of a petition to the Food and Drug Administration to always add vitamin B12 to any folate fortification or supplement. *Am J Clin Nutr.* 1997;65:572–573.
6. Kauwell GP, Bailey LB, Gregory JF, et al. Zinc status is not adversely affected by folic acid supplementation and zinc intake does not impair folate utilization. *J Nutr.* 1995;125:66–72.
7. Keating JN, Wada L, Stokstad EL, et al. Folic acid: effect on zinc absorption in humans and in the rat. *Am J Clin Nutr.* 1987;46:835–839.
8. Liem A, Reynierse-Buitenwerf GH, Zwinderman AH, et al. Secondary prevention with folic acid: effects on clinical outcomes. *J Am Coll Cardiol.* 2003;41:2105–2113.
9. Willett WC. Balancing lifestyle and genomics research for disease prevention. *Science.* 2002;296:695–698. Available at: http://www.sciencemag.org. Accessed July 19, 2005.
10. Bailey LB. Folate, methyl-related nutrients, alcohol, and the MTHFRv677C→T polymorphism affect cancer risk: intake recommendations. *J Nutr.* 2002;133(11 Suppl 1):S3748-S3753.
11. Pennington JA. *Bowes and Church's Food Values of Portions Commonly Used.* 17th ed. Philadelphia, Pa: Lippincott; 1998.
12. Riddell LJ, Chisholm A, Williams S, Mann JI. Dietary strategies for lowering homocysteine concentrations. *Am J Clin Nutr.* 2000;71:1448–1454.

13. Office of Dietary Supplements Web site. Available at: http://dietary-supplements. info.nih.gov. Accessed May 25, 2005.

14. Centers for Disease Control and Prevention. Recommendations for the use of folic acid to reduce the number of cases of spina bifida and other neural tube defects. *MMWR Morb Mortal Wkly Rep.* 1992;41(RR-14):1–7.

15. Honein MA, Paulozzi LJ, Mathews TJ, et al. Impact of folic acid fortification on the US food supply on the occurrence of neural tube defects. *JAMA.* 2001;285:2981–2986.

16. Toole JF, Malinow MR, Chambless LE, et al. Lowering homocysteine in patients with ischemic stroke to prevent recurrent stroke, myocardial infarction, and death: the Vitamin Intervention for Stroke Prevention (VISP) randomized controlled trial. *JAMA.* 2004;291:565–575.

17. Rimm EB, Willett WC, Hu FB, et al. Folate and vitamin B-6 from diet and supplements in relation to risk of coronary heart disease among women. *JAMA.* 1998;279:359–364.

18. Homocysteine Lowering Trialists' Collaboration. Lowering blood homocysteine with folic acid-based supplements: meta-analysis of randomized trials. *BMJ.* 1998;316:894–898.

19. Boushey CJ, Beresford SA, Omenn GS, et al. A quantitative assessment of plasma homocysteine as a risk factor for vascular disease. Probable benefits of increasing folic acid intakes. *JAMA.* 1995;274:1049–1057.

20. Morrison HI, Schaubel D, Desmeules M, et al. Serum folate and risk of fatal coronary heart disease. *JAMA.* 1996;275:1893–1896.

21. Bostom AG, Shemin D, Gohh RY, et al. Treatment of hyperhomocysteinemia in hemodialysis patients and renal transplant recipients. *Kidney Int Suppl.* 2001;59:S246–S252.

22. Kim YI. Will mandatory folic acid fortification prevent or promote cancer? *Am J Clin Nutr.* 2004;80:1123–1128.

23. Fuchs CS, Willett WC, Colditz GA, et al. The influence of folate and multivitamin use on the familial risk of colon cancer in women. *Cancer Epidemiol Biomarkers Prev.* 2002;11:227–234.

24. Baron JA, Sandler RS, Haile RW, et al. Folate intake, alcohol consumption, cigarette smoking, and risk of colorectal adenomas. *J Natl Cancer Inst.* 1998;90:57–62.

25. Biasco G, Zannoni U, Paganelli GM, et al. Folic acid supplementation and cell kinetics of rectal mucosa in patients with ulcerative colitis. *Cancer Epidemiol Biomarkers Prev.* 1997;6:469–471.

26. Kim YI, Baik HW, Fawaz K, et al. Effects of folate supplementation on two provisional molecular markers of colon cancer: a prospective, randomized trial. *Am J Gastroenterol.* 2001;96:184–194.

27. Butterworth CE, Hatch KD, Soong SJ, et al. Oral folic acid supplementation for cervical dysplasia: a clinical intervention trial. *Am J Obstet Gynecol.* 1992;166:803–809.

28. Butterworth CE, Hatch KD, Gore H, et al. Improvement in cervical dysplasia associated with folic acid therapy in users of oral contraceptives. *Am J Clin Nutr.* 1982;35: 73–82.

29. Bailey LB. olate, methyl-related nutrients, alcohol and MTHFR 677C→T polymorphisms affect cancer risk: intake recommendations. J Nutr 2003;133(11 suppl):3748S–53S.

30. Chen J, Gammon MD, Chan W, et al. One-carbon metabolism, MTHFR polymorphisms, and risk of breast cancer. Cancer Res. 2005;65:1606–1614.

31. Ortega RM, Manas LR, Andres P, et al. Functional and psychic deterioration in elderly people may be aggravated by folate deficiency. *J Nutr.* 1996;126:1992–1999.
32. Wesson VA, Levitt AJ, Joffe RT. Change in folate status with antidepressant treatment. *Psychiatry Res.* 1994;53:313–322.
33. Fava M, Borus JS, Alpert JE, et al. Folate, vitamin B12, and homocysteine in major depressive disorder. *Am J Psychiatry.* 1997;154:426–428.
34. Alpert JE, Fava M. Nutrition and depression: the role of folate. *Nutr Rev.* 1997;55: 145–149.
35. Coppen A, Bailey J. Enhancement of the antidepressant action of fluoxetine by folic acid: a randomized, placebo-controlled trial. *J Affect Disord.* 2000;60:121–130.
36. Taylor MJ, Carney S, Geddes J, et al. Folate for depressive disorders. *Cochrane Database Syst Rev.* 2003;2:CD003390.
37. Passeri M, Cucinotta D, Abate G, et al. Oral 5'-methyltetrahydrofolic acid in senile organic mental disorders with depression: results of a double-blind multicenter study. *Aging (Milano).* 1993;5:63–71.

Fructo-oligosaccharides (FOS)

Fructo-oligosaccharides (FOS) are a class of oligosaccharides made up of glucose linked to multiple fructose units. Depending on their chain length, FOS are classified as either oligofructose(OF) (2, 3, or 4 fructose units) or inulin (3 to 60 units). The chemical structure of FOS does not permit digestion by intestinal enzymes. Instead, FOS travel past the upper gastrointestinal tract and are selectively used as fuel by beneficial bacteria in the colon (see Acidophilus/*Lactobacillus Acidophilus* [LA]). Once fermented by bacteria, the energy value provided to the host ranges between 1.5 to 2.4 kcal per gram of FOS ingested. Because they selectively stimulate the growth and activity of beneficial colonic bacteria (*Bifidobacterium, Lactobacillus*), FOS are termed "prebiotics" and have been investigated for their potential role in intestinal health (1–3).

Media and Marketing Claims	Efficacy
Supports healthy digestive tract/reduces constipation	↑?
Reduces risk for colon cancer	NR
Reduces blood glucose levels in individuals with diabetes	NR
Reduces cholesterol levels	NR

Safety

- The effects of long-term, concentrated, daily use of FOS have not been evaluated.
- One study testing the safety of 15 g FOS per day in enteral formulas for 14 days in healthy subjects reported no clinically significant differences in serum chemistry

(glucose, blood urea nitrogen, total cholesterol, triglycerides, total protein, albumin, globulin, alkaline phosphatase, liver function measures, calcium, sodium, potassium chloride, iron, inorganic phosphorus, and gamma-glutamyl transpeptidase) compared with placebo (4).

◆ Several researchers have given dosages up to 20 g FOS per day with few adverse effects other than mild flatulence (1). Doses more than 50 g/day have been associated with bloating, cramps, and osmotic diarrhea (5,6).

◆ Supplemental FOS (15 g/day) did not interfere with calcium and nonheme-iron absorption in healthy, male subjects (7). Several animal studies have reported that FOS positively affect calcium absorption (8–10).

Drug/Supplement Interactions

◆ There have been no reported adverse interactions.

◆ FOS may enhance calcium absorption.

Key Points

◆ Eating a minimum of five servings of fruits and vegetables daily (focusing on the foods lists in the "Food Sources" section that follows) will help increase FOS in the diet.

◆ FOS supplementation seems to specifically increase bifidobacteria in the colon, which is beneficial to intestinal health. An increase in bifidobacteria is accompanied by a reduction in the number of bacteria reported to have pathogenic potential.

◆ FOS seem to have stool-bulking properties that may help prevent constipation. More controlled clinical trials are needed in humans to test the role of FOS on intestinal conditions and diseases.

◆ Some preliminary animal studies suggest that FOS may have anticarcinogenic properties in the colon. However, there are no human studies testing FOS supplementation in the prevention and treatment of colon cancer, nor are there reliable data on the influence of FOS on biomarkers or enzymes involved in colon carcinogenesis.

◆ More research is needed on the role of FOS in reducing blood glucose and lipid levels in healthy subjects, those with diabetes, and those with hyperlipidemia. Preliminary trials did not find a beneficial effect of FOS on blood sugars and serum lipids.

Food Sources

◆ FOS are found naturally in onions, asparagus, jerusalem artichokes, garlic, bananas, tomatoes, wheat, rye, honey, beer, chicory root, and leeks. Because of their mild sweetness and stability, FOS are used in commercial confections and pastries (3). FOS concentrations in foods tend to vary depending on harvest time and storage time. The average American diet provides 2 to 8 g FOS/day (11).

Food	FOS, mg/serving
Artichoke, jerusalem (½ cup)	4,380
Onion powder (1 Tbsp)	293
Banana, ripe (1 medium)	236
Chicory root, raw (½ cup)	189
Shallot (1 Tbsp)	85
Peach (½ cup)	34
Garlic (1 clove)	12

Source: Data are from reference 11.

Dosage Information/Bioavailability

FOS supplements are sold in powders and capsules. On a commercial scale, FOS are produced from sucrose using a fungal enzyme or by partial hydrolysis using endoglycosidases made from chicory inulin (12). Labels suggest starting with 1 g (¼ tsp) and gradually increasing up to 4 g/day. In the powdered form, FOS can be used to mildly sweeten cereals, fruit, and drinks. Other products combine FOS with probiotic bacteria (*see* Acidophilus/ *Lactobacillus Acidophilus* [LA]). FOS are also included in some enteral formulas. In one study, approximately 90% of a 20-g dose of FOS was not absorbed and none was excreted in the stools, indicating that FOS were completely fermented by colonic flora (1).

Relevant Research

FOS and Intestinal Health

♦ A multicenter, randomized, placebo-controlled study tested the efficacy of FOS combined with other nondigestible carbohydrates and oral rehydration therapy in 144 boys with acute non-cholera diarrhea. The boys were randomly assigned to receive either standard oral rehydration therapy (ORT) or ORT plus nondigestible carbohydrate solution (18.5% FOS, 25% soy polysaccharide, 9% alpha cellulose, 19% arabic gum, 21.5% inulin, and 7% resistant starch) until diarrhea resolved. Outcomes, which included duration of diarrhea, length of hospital stay, and unscheduled IV rehydration, were not significantly different across treatment groups (13).

♦ In a double-blind, placebo-controlled, multicenter trial, 119 subjects with diagnosed irritable bowel syndrome (IBS) were randomly assigned to receive 20 g FOS powder or placebo daily for 12 weeks. Before the study, all subjects received a placebo for a 2-week, single-blind phase to wash out any effects of medication or dietary supplements previously used for IBS symptoms. Efficacy (based on subjects overall response to treatment and severity of abdominal distension, rumbling, pain and abnormal flatulence), tolerability, and compliance were assessed at baseline (end of first 2 weeks) and weeks 4, 6, 8, and 12. Twenty-three subjects dropped out of the study (14 subjects in the FOS group and 9 subjects in the placebo group). After weeks

4 and 6, there was a nonsignificant trend toward a greater improvement in IBS symptoms in the placebo group, but not the FOS group. By weeks 8 and 12, there were no differences in symptoms between the groups. The authors concluded that although symptoms worsened at the onset of FOS ingestion, continuous treatment resulted in no deterioration of IBS symptoms (14).

♦ Eight subjects were fed a controlled diet while living in a metabolic unit for 15 days, followed by 15 g oligofructose (OF) per day for 15 days in place of dietary sucrose, followed by a final 15 days on the control diet again. This was followed by 5 days on a free diet for stool collection. Four subjects completed an additional study of 15 g inulin per day for 15 days. OF and inulin were administered with breakfast in free form, with the remaining 10 g given in biscuits. Both OF and inulin resulted in a significant increase in bifidobacteria in the stool compared with the sucrose control periods. There was a significant increase in stool wet matter and nitrogen excretion with OF compared to sucrose controls. The numbers of potentially pathogenic bacteria (*bacteroides, clostridia,* and *fusobacteria*) were significantly lowered in subjects fed OF. The authors concluded that "small changes in diet can alter the balance of colonic bacteria towards a potentially healthier microflora" (15).

FOS and Colon Cancer

♦ In a double-blind, placebo-controlled study, 20 healthy subjects were supplemented with 12.5 g FOS per day or a placebo in addition to their usual diet for 12 days. Although colonic bifidobacteria increased with FOS supplementation, there were no changes in fecal pH, concentrations of bile acids, or neutral sterols. Furthermore, there was no reduction in bacterial enzymes such as nitroreductase, azoreductase, and beta-glucuronidase, which are potential indices of colon carcinogenesis (16).

♦ A study of mice with intramuscularly implanted tumors reported that a 15% FOS diet inhibited tumor growth compared to a control diet (17).

♦ Preneoplastic lesions (aberrant crypt foci [ACF]) were chemically induced in the colons of male rats prior to feeding a control diet or OF- or inulin-supplemented diets. OF and inulin significantly inhibited ACF formation and the crypt multiplication in the colon, although inulin had a more pronounced effect. The authors hypothesized that this result may be caused by butyrate production by fermentation of FOS and that butyrate may have anticarcinogenic properties (18).

FOS and Blood Glucose and Cholesterol

♦ In a single-blind, placebo-controlled, crossover study, 20 subjects with type 2 diabetes were randomly assigned to receive 15 g FOS per day or a placebo (4 g glucose per day) for 20 days each. Mean daily intakes of energy, macronutrients, and fiber were similar with both treatments. FOS had no significant effects on total, HDL, and LDL cholesterol, serum triglycerides, serum free fatty acids, serum acetate, or blood glucose (19).

♦ In a double-blind, crossover design study, 12 healthy male subjects were randomly assigned to ingest 20 g FOS per day or a placebo in cookies for 4 weeks at a time, with a 2-week washout period. Basal hepatic glucose decreased significantly during FOS intake; however, there was no change in insulin-stimulated glucose metabolism, serum triglycerides, total and HDL cholesterol, apolipoproteins A-I and B, or lipoprotein(A) (20). In a follow-up double-blind, placebo-controlled, crossover study, the same researchers investigated the effects of 20 g FOS powder per day in 12 subjects with type 2 diabetes. After 4 weeks, FOS had no effect on fasting plasma glucose or insulin concentrations or basal hepatic glucose production. There was also no change in serum lipids or plasma glucose response to a fixed insulin bolus (21).

References

1. Gibson GR, Roberfroid MB. Dietary modulation of the human colonic microbiota: introducing the concept of prebiotics. *J Nutr.* 1995;125:1401–1412.
2. Oku T. Oligosaccharides with beneficial health effects: a Japanese perspective. *Nutr Rev.* 1996;54(11 pt 2):S59-S66.
3. Molis C, Flourie B, Ouarne F, et al. Digestion, excretion and energy value of fructooligosaccharides in healthy humans. *Am J Clin Nutr.* 1996;64:324–328.
4. Garleb KA, Snook JT, Marco MJ, et al. Effect of fructooligosaccaride containing enteral formulas on subjective tolerance factors, serum chemistry profiles, and fecal bifidobacteria in healthy adult male subjects. *Microbial Ecology Health Dis.* 1996;9: 279–285.
5. Briet F, Achour L, Flourie B, et al. Symptomatic response to varying levels of fructooligosaccharides consumed occasionally or regularly. *Eur J Clin Nutr.* 1995;49:501–507.
6. Stone-Dorshow T, Levitt MD. Gaseous response to ingestion of a poorly absorbed fructo-oligosaccharide sweetener. *Am J Clin Nutr.* 1987;46:61–65.
7. van den Heuvel EG, Schaafsma G, Muys T, et al. Nondigestible oligosaccharides do not interfere with calcium and nonheme-iron absorption in young, healthy men. *Am J Clin Nutr.* 1998;67:445–451.
8. Ohta A, Motohashi Y, Sakai K, et al. Dietary fructooligosaccharides increase calcium absorption and levels of mucosal calbindin-D9k in the large intestine of gastrectomized rats. *Scand J Gastroenterol.* 1998;33:1062–1068.
9. Morohashi T, Sano T, Ohta A, et al. True calcium absorption in the intestine is enhanced by fructooligosaccaride feeding in rats. *J Nutr.* 1998;128:1815–1818.
10. Ohta A, Motohashi Y, Ohtsuki M, et al. Dietary fructooligosaccharides change the concentration of calbindin-D9k differently in the mucosa of the small and large intestine of rats. *J Nutr.* 1998;128:934–939.
11. Campbell JM, Baurer LL, Fahey GC, et al. Selected fructooligosaccharides (1-Ketose, Nystose and 1F-ß-Fructofuranosylnystose) composition of foods and feeds. *J Agri Food Chem.* 1997;45:3076–3082.
12. Roberfroid MB. Health benefits of non-digestible oligosaccharides. *Adv Exp Med Biol.* 1997;427:211–219.
13. Hoekstra JH, Szajewska H, Zikri MA, et al. Oral rehydration solution containing a mixture of non-digestible carbohydrates in the treatment of acute diarrhea: a multicenter randomized placebo-controlled study on behalf of the ESPGHAN Working Group on Intestinal Infections. *J Pediatr Gastroenterol Nutr.* 2004;39:239–245.

14. Olesen M, Gudmand-Hoyer E. Efficacy, safety, and tolerability of fructooligosaccharides in the treatment of irritable bowel syndrome. *Am J Clin Nutr.* 2000;72:1570–1575.
15. Gibson GR, Beatty ER, Wang X, et al. Selective stimulation of bifidobacteria in the human colon by oligofructose and inulin. *Gastroenterology.* 1995;108:975–982.
16. Bouhnik Y, Flourie B, Riottot M, et al. Effects of fructo-oligosaccharides ingestion on fecal bifidobacteria and selected metabolic indexes of colon carcinogenesis in healthy humans. *Nutr Cancer.* 1996;26:21–29.
17. Taper HS, Delzenne NM, Roberfroid MB. Growth inhibition of transplantable mouse tumors by nondigestible carbohydrates. *Int J Cancer.* 1997;71:1109–1112.
18. Reddy BS, Hamid R, Rao CV. Effect of dietary oligofructose and inulin on colonic preneoplastic aberrant crypt foci inhibition. *Carcinogenesis.* 1997;18:1371–1374.
19. Alles MS, de Roos NM, Bakx JC, et al. Consumption of fructooligosaccharides does not favorably affect blood glucose and serum lipid concentrations in patients with type 2 diabetes. *Am J Clin Nutr.* 1999;69:64–69.
20. Luo J, Rizkalla SW, Alamowitch C, et al. Chronic consumption of short-chain fructooligosaccharides by healthy subjects decreased basal hepatic glucose production but had no effect on insulin-stimulated glucose metabolism. *Am J Clin Nutr.* 1996;63:939–945.
21. Luo J, Van Yperselle M, Rizkalla SW, et al. Chronic consumption of short-chain fructooligosaccharides does not affect basal hepatic glucose production or insulin resistance in type 2 diabetes. *J Nutr.* 2000;130:1572–1577.

Gamma-Linolenic Acid

Gamma-linolenic acid (GLA) is an essential n-6 fatty acid found naturally in evening primrose oil (*Oenothera biennis*, 8% to 10% GLA), borage oil (*Borago officinalis*, 23% to 26% GLA), and black currant oil (*Ribes nigrum,* 15% to 20% GLA). In addition to GLA, the remaining fatty acid content of these plant oils is primarily linoleic acid (LA) and a small amount of alpha-linolenic acid (n-3) and other fatty acids. In the body, GLA is synthesized from LA by the rate-limiting enzyme delta-6 desaturase. GLA can then be elongated into dihomo-GLA (DGLA). DGLA can be directed into three pathways: (*a*) conversion into 1-series (anti-inflammatory) prostaglandin (PGE_1); (*b*) conversion into 15-(S)-hydroxy-8, 11, 13-eicosatrienoic acid (15-HETrE), which inhibits the biosynthesis of pro-inflammatory arachidonic acid (AA) metabolites; or (*c*) conversion into AA by delta-5 desaturase. However, due to the limited activity of delta-5 desaturase, only a small fraction of DGLA is converted to AA. It is estimated that only 5% to 10% of the daily intake of LA is converted into GLA and its metabolites (1,2).

Media and Marketing Claims	Efficacy
Reduces PMS symptoms	↔
Reduces inflammation in rheumatoid arthritis	↔
Reduces atopic dermatitis	↔

Media and Marketing Claims	Efficacy
Reduces acne	NR
Improves diabetic neuropathy	NR
Reduces cardiovascular disease risk	NR
Reduces risk for breast cancer; improves response of anti-estrogen medications in breast cancer	↔

Safety

- Long-term human trials have shown that up to 2,800 mg GLA per day are well-tolerated (1). It has been estimated that dosages less than 100 mg GLA/kg/day likely are not toxic (2).

- Borage seed contains low concentrations of unsaturated pyrrolizidine alkaloids that may be hepatotoxic (3). Manufacturers state that these alkaloids are removed by washing before packaging.

- Potential side-effects include belching, bloating, nausea, vomiting, flatulence, soft stools, and diarrhea.

Drug/Supplement Interactions

- Evening primrose oil may reduce seizure threshold when used with tricyclic antidepressants and anticonvulsant medications (3).

- Borage seed should not be taken with hepatotoxic drugs (anabolic steroids, phenothiazines, ketoconazole) (3).

- GLA could potentially increase bleeding time; use should be monitored by a physician if the individual is taking anticoagulant drugs or supplements. GLA should be avoided prior to surgery.

- There is preliminary evidence in animal models that GLA may enhance the therapeutic efficacy of the breast cancer drug tamoxifen. However, more research is needed before clinical recommendations can be made.

Key Points

- Evidence is conflicting concerning the effect of GLA supplementation on mastalgia and other symptoms of PMS. According to one reviewer, many of the clinical trials, especially those in PMS, resulted in a large placebo response, making it difficult to show any true response (2).

- The research on the potential benefits of GLA supplements in rheumatoid arthritis is also conflicting. Some studies have been criticized for large numbers of dropouts and for failing to control concomitant use of medications. In addition, studies shorter than 1 year offer limited information about the efficacy of pharmacologic agents in the treatment of rheumatoid arthritis (4). Furthermore, the results from GLA studies may be confounded by the use of olive oil as the placebo because one author reported that it is conceivable that olive oil itself may alleviate symptoms of rheumatoid arthritis (5). One study reported that the reduction in EPA associated with supplementation may actually have adverse clinical effects in rheumatoid arthritis because EPA is a precursor to anti-inflammatory prostaglandins (6).

♦ Evidence from a meta-analysis suggests that GLA from evening primrose oil may reduce symptoms in individuals with atopic dermatitis; however, other individual studies show no benefit.

♦ There is no evidence at this time that GLA supplements clear acne blemishes.

♦ Animal and preliminary human studies suggest a benefit of GLA-rich oils for individuals with diabetic neuropathy. Additional controlled trials in humans are needed.

♦ Overall, there is insufficient human research to draw definite conclusions about the role of GLA oils in heart disease including CVD mortality. Preliminary evidence from animal studies suggest that GLA-rich oil may reduce blood pressure. Existing human studies are underpowered statistically to test these hypotheses. GLA oils do not seem to affect triglyceride levels, and their effect on LDL cholesterol is inconsistent.

♦ There are preliminary data that GLA supplements may enhance the action of the breast cancer drug tamoxifen. Cell culture studies also indicate that GLA may enhance docetaxel cytotoxicity as well as tamoxifen and fulvestrant efficacy. Clinical trial research is needed.

♦ Although the role of GLA in human health has been proposed in several literature reviews (1,2,7), additional controlled research on the efficacy, safety, dose, and duration of treatment with GLA oils in humans is needed before specific recommendations can be made.

Food Sources

No significant typical food sources. Human breastmilk contains approximately 100 to 400 mg GLA plus DGLA per liter (2).

Dosage Information/Bioavailability

Evening primrose, borage, and black currant oils are available in softgels or as liquid oils. Dosages of GLA range from 45 to 300 mg per softgel, with a total suggested daily intake ranging from 500 to 3,000 mg (10 to 15 large capsules/softgels) taken with food. Almost all the studies of evening primrose oil have used SP116, an extract selected because it is consistent in its composition and is used in commercial products (2).

Normal human endogenous production of GLA is approximately 250 to 1,000 mg/day (2). Acute administration of 280 mg GLA from 3 g evening primrose oil (SP116) in healthy volunteers resulted in a significant increase in plasma GLA concentrations, which reached maximum levels in 2.7 to 4.4 hours. There was no significant effect on DGLA and AA levels (8).

Relevant Research

GLA and PMS, Mastalgia, and Menopause

♦ Some researchers have suggested that symptoms of PMS may be associated with defective metabolism of n-6 fatty acids. In a cross-sectional observational study, serum samples from 250 women with PMS, cyclic mastalgia, and noncyclic mastalgia were analyzed for fatty acid content. LA levels were normal for all subjects with symptoms; however, DGLA and AA levels were significantly lower in subjects with mastalgia compared with control subjects. Subjects with PMS had significantly lower AA levels than control subjects did. Subjects with noncyclic mastalgia had significantly lower docosahexaenoic acid levels compared with control subjects. The authors concluded that these results suggest a defect in the conversion of linoleic acid to other n-6 fatty acids in this population (9). Another study reported significantly reduced DGLA and AA levels in women with cyclic mastalgia (n = 36), and significantly reduced AA in subjects with noncyclic mastalgia (n = 6), but no differences in plasma fatty acids in subjects with breast cysts (n = 200) when compared with blood samples from control subjects (10).

♦ In a systematic review of seven placebo-controlled trials testing evening primrose oil in the treatment of PMS, the authors noted that the two best controlled studies failed to show beneficial effects, although the trials were small and only five of seven trials reported randomization. (11).

♦ In a double-blind, placebo-controlled, crossover study, 38 women with PMS were randomly assigned to receive 360 mg GLA from evening primrose oil or a placebo daily for three menstrual cycles each. There were no significant differences in PMS symptoms (psychological, fluid retention, breast) between evening primrose oil and placebo, although both groups reported improvement in subjective symptoms (12).

♦ In a double-blind, placebo-controlled study, 200 women with breast cysts were randomly assigned to receive 270 mg GLA from evening primrose oil or a placebo daily for 1 year. Follow-up continued for 1 year after therapy. Recurrent cyst formation was slightly lower in the evening primrose group than the placebo group, but this change did not reach statistical significance (13).

♦ In a double-blind, placebo-controlled study, 56 women in menopause experiencing hot flashes at least three times per day were randomly assigned to receive 500 mg evening primrose oil (approximately 45 mg GLA) with 10 mg natural vitamin E or a placebo daily for 6 months. Only 18 women in the treatment group and 17 women in the placebo group completed the trial. Both groups had reductions in the mean number of hot flashes, with a greater significant overall improvement in the placebo group. The only significant improvement in the evening primrose group over the placebo group was a reduction in the maximum number of self-reported nighttime hot flashes. The authors concluded that evening primrose oil should not currently be recommended for the treatment of menopausal hot flashes (14).

GLA and Rheumatoid Arthritis

♦ In a double-blind, placebo-controlled trial, 34 subjects (mean age 55 years) with rheumatoid arthritis and active synovitis were randomly assigned to receive 10.5 g black currant oil in 15 capsules (providing approximately 2,000 mg GLA) or a placebo daily for 24 weeks. Subjects continued stable dosages of NSAIDs and corticosteroids 1 month before the study and were instructed to maintain their pre-entry dosages during the study. There were no significant differences in medication use between groups. Clinical assessment of disease activity was completed every 6 weeks. At 24 weeks, subjects taking black currant oil had significantly reduced signs and symptoms of disease activity compared with baseline, but not significantly different from placebo (15). Twenty patients dropped out of the study, and this high dropout rate makes the results of this study difficult to evaluate.

♦ In a double-blind, placebo-controlled study, 37 individuals with rheumatoid arthritis and active synovitis were randomly assigned to receive 1,400 mg GLA in borage seed oil or a placebo (cottonseed oil) daily for 24 weeks. Physician and subject global assessments of disease activity, joint tenderness, joint swelling, duration of morning stiffness, grip strength, and ability to do daily activities were completed before and after the study. In the group taking GLA, signs and symptoms of disease activity were significantly reduced compared with the placebo group. Further trials of GLA oils in rheumatoid arthritis are warranted (16).

♦ In a double-blind, placebo-controlled study, 40 individuals with rheumatoid arthritis with gastrointestinal lesions associated with NSAID use were randomly assigned to receive 540 mg GLA from 6 g evening primrose oil plus 120 mg vitamin E or a placebo (6 g olive oil) daily for 6 months. Subjects were assessed at baseline and every 3 months for pain on a visual analogue scale, analgesic use, blood samples, and the Ritchie articular index. NSAID use did not stop during the study, but three subjects in each group reduced their dosages. Evening primrose oil was associated with a statistically significant reduction in morning stiffness at 3 and 6 months. Olive oil was associated with a significant reduction in pain and articular index at 6 months. There were no changes in blood parameters of inflammation. The authors concluded: "While gamma-linolenic acid may produce mild improvement in rheumatoid arthritis, olive oil may itself have unrecognized benefits" (5).

♦ In a double-blind, placebo-controlled study, 49 subjects with rheumatoid arthritis were randomly assigned to receive one of three treatments daily for 12 months: (*a*) 540 mg GLA from evening primrose oil, (*b*) 240 mg eicosapentaenoic acid (EPA) plus 450 mg GLA, or (*c*) a placebo. At the end of the study, all subjects were given a placebo for an additional 3 months. There was a statistically significant subjective improvement of symptoms in subjects receiving GLA and EPA plus GLA compared with the placebo group at 12 months. GLA and EPA plus GLA were also associated with a statistically significant decrease in NSAID use. After 3 months of placebo, those who had received active treatment relapsed. The authors concluded that evening primrose oil alone or in combination with fish oil produced a subjective improvement that allowed some patients to reduce or stop treatment with NSAIDs (17).

GLA and Skin Disorders

- ◆ A meta-analysis of placebo-controlled clinical trials of oral fatty acid supplementation for atopic dermatitis that included a separate analysis of 11 studies using GLA found no significant clinical benefit from GLA supplementation (18). In relaying the clinical relevance of the GLA effect size in terms of Costa score (a standard clinical scoring scale of atopic dermatitis ranging from 0 to 100 points), the authors concluded that daily supplementation with GLA would reduce Costa symptom scores by only 1.5 points. This suggests minimal clinical significance for GLA supplementation for this condition.

- ◆ In a double-blind, randomized, placebo-controlled study of the role of GLA in reducing atopic dermatitis in infants with a strong family history of the disease, van Gool and colleagues randomly assigned 118 infants at high risk for atopic dermatitis to borage oil (103 mg GLA) or sunflower oil (placebo) daily for the first 6 months of life. The dosage of GLA was determined from data regarding the upper end of the standard amounts in human milk. All infants were formula-fed. SCORAD (SCORing Atopic Dermatitis) was used to quantify disease severity/symptoms. Increases in plasma phospholipids GLA levels were associated with significantly reduced severity scores at year 1, but did not modulate serum IgE levels (19). In addition, the intention-to-treat analysis showed that GLA was associated with a trend toward lower SCORAD scores, but this association was not significant ($P = .09$).

- ◆ In a double-blind, placebo-controlled, multicenter trial,160 subjects with atopic eczema of moderate severity were randomly assigned to receive 500 mg borage oil (naturally contains 23% GLA) or a placebo daily for 24 weeks. Use of a topical diflucotolone-21-valerate cream was permitted as a "rescue" medication if symptoms became intolerable, with amount used until response being defined as the primary endpoint, and clinical improvement as a secondary efficacy criterion. Although several clinical symptoms improved, compared with the placebo group, the overall response to borage oil was not significant (20).

- ◆ In a double-blind, placebo-controlled trial, 39 subjects with chronic hand dermatitis were randomly assigned to receive 600 mg GLA from evening primrose oil or a placebo daily for 16 weeks, and observation continued for another 8 weeks. Subjects were assessed monthly for clinical changes using a visual analogue scale. Plasma and red blood cell lipograms, and skin biopsies were taken before therapy, after 16 weeks and at week 24. Tissue was used for histologic evaluation, electronmicroscopic assessment, and epidermal lipid analysis. Both groups improved in clinical parameters, with no statistical difference between the groups (21).

- ◆ A meta-analysis of nine controlled trials (four parallel, five crossover design) of evening primrose oil (standardized extract SP116) to treat atopic dermatitis reported a statistically significant improvement over baseline in patient and physician symptom scores of inflammation, dryness, scaliness, pruritus, and overall skin involvement compared with the placebo groups in the parallel studies. Analysis of the crossover trials yielded similar results, but the difference between evening primrose oil and the placebo groups in the physicians' global scores did not reach statistical significance. However, there was a significant improvement in pruritus in the primrose oil groups compared with the placebo groups in the crossover studies. There was also a positive association between clinical improvement and plasma levels of DGLA and AA (22).

GLA and Diabetes

◆ In a double-blind, placebo-controlled, multicenter trial, 111 individuals with mild diabetic neuropathy were randomly assigned to receive 480 mg GLA from 12 evening primrose capsules or a placebo daily for 1 year. Neurophysiological responses to hot and cold thresholds, sensation, tendon reflexes, and muscle strength were assessed by standard tests in upper and lower limbs at 3, 6, and 12 months. For all 16 parameters measured, the change during 1 year in response to GLA was more favorable than the change with the placebo, and for 13 parameters this difference was significant. Specifically, GLA supplementation significantly improved 8 of 10 neurophysiological parameters and 5 of 6 neurological assessments. Gender, age, and type of diabetes did not affect the results, although treatment with GLA was more effective among subjects with relatively well-controlled diabetes than among those with poorly controlled diabetes, as defined by A1C (23).

◆ Several studies supplementing diabetic animals with GLA-rich oils have demonstrated improvement in nerve blood flow and nerve function (24–26).

GLA and Cardiovascular Disease

◆ In a dietary intake/linolenic acid exposure cross-sectional study of blood samples from 4,440 white subjects who participated in the National Heart, Lung, and Blood Institute Family Heart Study, subjects in the upper quintile of dietary intake of linolenic acid demonstrated significantly reduced serum triglyceride levels, which may play a role in CVD risk reduction (27). Total linolenic acid intake was estimated from a food frequency questionnaire.

◆ In a double-blind, placebo-controlled trial, 27 men with borderline hypertension were randomly assigned to receive 6 g black currant oil or a placebo (safflower oil) for 8 weeks. Weekly blood pressure readings were recorded and blood pressure and heart reactivity were measured before and at the end of the study during a mental arithmetic test. There was a significant decrease in diastolic blood pressure in subjects taking black currant oil compared with those in the placebo group (28).

◆ Evening primrose oil reduced platelet hyperaggregability in rabbits fed atherogenic diets compared with rabbits on atherogenic diets not supplemented with evening primrose oil (29).

♦ Rats with spontaneous hypertension that were fed diets containing evening primrose, black currant, borage, or fungal oils for 7 weeks had significant reductions in blood pressure (30).

GLA and Cancer

♦ In a pilot study (not randomized or blinded) of 38 elderly breast cancer patients, those receiving 2.8 g/day of GLA with tamoxifen were compared with matched control subjects who took tamoxifen alone. Tumor biopsies were taken to assess changes in estrogen receptor and bcl-2 expression during treatment. GLA plus tamoxifen was associated with a significantly faster clinical response than tamoxifen alone by 6 weeks. There were significant reductions in estrogen receptor expression in both treatments, but a greater reduction was observed in subjects in the GLA supplement group (31). The lack of both randomization and blinding weakens the results of this trial.

♦ Cell culture studies support a role for GLA in breast cancer prevention, including inhibition of oncogenic antigen 519 (32); enhanced taxotere cytotoxicy against MCF-7 cells (33) as well as MDA-MB-231 cells (34); and selective estrogen receptor modulation and tamoxifen enhancement as well as blocking of the expression of HER-2/neu oncogene expression (35,36). However, these findings warrant replication by other investigators.

References

1. Fan YY, Chapkin RS. Importance of dietary gamma-linolenic acid in human health and nutrition. *J Nutr.* 1998;128:1411–1414.
2. Horrobin DF. Nutritional and medical importance of gamma-linolenic acid. *Prog Lipid Res.* 1992;31:163–194.
3. Miller LG. Herbal medicinals. Selected clinical considerations focusing on known or potential drug-herb interactions. *Arch Intern Med.* 1998;158:2200–2211.
4. Joe LA, Hart LL. Evening primrose oil in rheumatoid arthritis. *Ann Pharmacother.* 1993;27:1475–1477.
5. Brzeski M, Madhok R, Capell HA. Evening primrose oil in patients with rheumatoid arthritis and side-effects of nonsteroidal anti-inflammatory drugs. *Br J Rheumatol.* 1991;30:370–372.
6. Jantti J, Nikkari T, Solakivi T, et al. Evening primrose oil in rheumatoid arthritis: changes in serum lipids and fatty acids. *Ann Rheum Dis.* 1989;48:124–127.
7. Gamma-linolenic acid (GLA). Monograph. *Altern Med Rev.* 2004;9:70–78.
8. Martens-Lobenhoffer J, Meyer FP. Phamacokinetic data of gamma-linolenic acid in healthy volunteers after the administration of evening primrose oil (Epogam). *Int J Clin Pharmacol Ther.* 1998;36:363–366.
9. Horrobin DF, Manku MS, Brush M, et al. Abnormalities in plasma essential fatty acid levels in women with premenstrual syndrome and with nonmalignant breast disease. *J Nutr Med.* 1991;2:259–264.

10. Gateley CA, Maddox PR, Pritchard GA, et al. Plasma fatty acid profiles in benign breast disorders. *Br J Surg.* 1992;79:407–409.
11. Budeiri D, Li Wan Po A, Dornan JC. Is evening primrose oil of value in the treatment of premenstrual syndrome? *Control Clin Trials.* 1996;17:60–68.
12. Khoo SK, Munro C, Battistutta D. Evening primrose oil and treatment of premenstrual syndrome. *Med J Aust.* 1990;153:189–192.
13. Mansel RE, Harrison BJ, Melhuish J, et al. A randomized trial of dietary intervention with essential fatty acids in patients with categorized cysts. *Ann N Y Acad Sci.* 1990;586:288–294.
14. Chenoy R, Hussain S, Tayob Y, et al. Effect of oral gamolenic acid from evening primrose oil on menopausal flushing. *BMJ.* 1994;308:501–503.
15. Leventhal LJ, Boyce EG, Zurier RB. Treatment of rheumatoid arthritis with black currant seed oil. *Br J Rheumatol.* 1994;33:847–852.
16. Leventhal LJ, Boyce EG, Zurier RB. Treatment of rheumatoid arthritis with gamma-linolenic acid. *Ann Intern Med.* 1993;119:867–873.
17. Belch JJ, Ansell D, Madhok R, et al. Effects of altering dietary essential fatty acids on requirements for nonsteroidal anti-inflammatory drugs in patients with rheumatoid arthritis: a double blind placebo controlled study. *Ann Rheum Dis.* 1988;47:96–104.
18. van Gool CJ, Zeegers MP, Thijs C. Oral essential fatty acid supplementation in atopic dermatitis—a meta-analysis of placebo-controlled trials. *Br J Dermatol.* 2004;150: 728–740.
19. van Gool CJ, Thijs C, Henquet CJ, et al. Gamma-linolenic acid supplementation for prophylaxis of atopic dermatitis—a randomized controlled trial in infants at high familial risk. *Am J Clin Nutr.* 2003;77:943–951.
20. Henz BM, Jablonska S, Van De Kerkhof PC, et al. Double-blind, multi-center analysis of the efficacy of borage oil in patients with atopic eczema. *Br J Dermatol.* 1999;140:685–688.
21. Whitaker DK, Cilliers J, de Beer C. Evening primrose oil (Epogam) in the treatment of chronic hand dermatitis: disappointing therapeutic results. *Dermatology.* 1996;193: 115–120.
22. Morse PF, Horrobin DF, Manku MS, et al. Meta-analysis of placebo-controlled studies of the efficacy of Epogam in the treatment of atopic eczema. Relationship between plasma essential fatty acid changes and clinical response. *Br J Dermatol.* 1989;121: 75–90.
23. Keen H, Payan J, Allawi J, et al. Treatment of diabetic neuropathy with gamma-linolenic acid. The Gamma Linolenic Acid Multicenter Trial Group. *Diabetes Care.* 1993;16:8–15.
24. Horrobin DF. Essential fatty acids in the management of impaired nerve function in diabetes. *Diabetes.* 1997;46(Suppl 2):S90-S93.
25. Julu PO. Latency of neuroactivity and optimum period of treatment with evening primrose oil in diabetic rats. *J Lipid Mediat Cell Signal.* 1996;13:99–113.
26. Cameron NE, Cotter MA, Robertson S. Essential fatty acid diet supplementation. Effects on peripheral nerve and skeletal muscle function and capillarization in streptozocin-induced diabetic rats. *Diabetes.* 1991;40:532–539.

27. Djousse L, Hunt SC, Arnett DK, et al. Dietary linolenic acid is inversely associated with plasma triacylglycerol: the National Heart, Lung, and Blood Institute Family Heart Study. *Am J Clin Nutr.* 2003;78:1098–1102.

28. Deferne JL, Leeds AR. Resting blood pressure and cardiovascular reactivity to mental arithmetic in mild hypertensive males supplemented with black currant seed oil. *J Hum Hypertens.* 1996;10:531–537.

29. De La Cruz JP, Martin-Romero M, Carmona JA, et al. Effect of evening primrose oil on platelet aggregation in rabbits fed an atherogenic diet. *Thromb Res.* 1997;87:141–149.

30. Engler MM. Comparative study of diets enriched with evening primrose, black currant, borage, or fungal oils on blood pressure and pressor responses in spontaneously hypertensive rats. *Prostaglandins Leukot Essent Fatty Acids.* 1993;49:809–814.

31. Kenny FS, Pinder SE, Ellis IO, et al. Gamma linolenic acid with tamoxifen as primary therapy in breast cancer. *Int J Cancer.* 2000;85:643–648.

32. Mendez JA, Ropero S, Mehmi I, et al. Overexpression and hyper activity of breast cancer-associated fatty acids synthase (oncogenic antigen-519) is insensitive to normal arachidonic fatty acid-induced suppression in lipogenic tissues but it is selectively inhibited by tumoricial alpha-linolenic and gamma-linolenic fatty acids: a novel mechanism by which dietary fat can alter mammary tumorigenesis. *Int J Oncol.* 2004;24:1369–1383.

33. Mendez JA, Ropero S, Lupu R, et al. Omega-6 polyunsaturated fatty acid gamma-linolenic acid (18:3n9–6) enhances docetaxel (Taxotere) cytotoxicity in human breast carcinoma cells: Relationship to lipid peroxidation and HER-2/neu expression. *Oncol Rep.* 2004;11:1241–1252.

34. Menendez JA, del Mar Barbacid M, Montero S, et al. Effects of gamma-linolenic acid and oleic acid on paclitaxel cytotoxicity in human breast cancer cells. *Eur J Cancer.* 2001;37:402–413.

35. Kenny FS, Gee JM, Nicholson RI, et al. Effect of dietary GLA+/-tamoxifen on the growth ER expression and fatty acid profile of ER positive human breast cancer xenografts. *Int J Cancer.* 2001;92:342–347.

36. Meneddez JA, Vellon L, Colomer R, et al. Effect of gamma-linolenic acid on the transcriptional activity of the Her-2/neu (erbB-2) oncogene. *J Natl Cancer Inst.* 2005;97:1611–1615.

Gamma-Oryzanol

Gamma-oryzanol is a lipid fraction derived from rice-bran oil. Oryzanol was first isolated from rice-bran oil in the 1950s. Several lipid fractions were isolated from the oil. The third (gamma) fraction isolated was oryzanol (1). It is made up of a mixture of ferulic acid esters and plant sterols (2). Similar in structure to cholesterol, the phytosterols and triterpenes that comprise oryzanol include campesterol, stigmasterol, beta sitosterol, cycloartanol, and cycloartenol (1). Because phytosterols are poorly absorbed, it has been suggested that they may reduce blood cholesterol by inhibiting intestinal cholesterol absorption. In contrast, the ferulic acid portion of gamma-oryzanol is easily absorbed into the body's tissues. Ferulic acid also has demonstrated antioxidant properties in vitro (3–8).

Media and Marketing Claims	Efficacy
Reduces cholesterol levels	NR
Helps build muscle; anabolic agent	NR
Reduces oxidative stress during exercise	NR

Safety

♦ A study of B6C3F1 mice (mice who are bred to develop tumors in response to toxic substances and are commonly used to study the carcinogenicity of toxic substances) fed 0, 200, 600, or 2,000 mg gamma-oryzanol/kg body weight/day for 78 weeks showed no adverse events on general condition, body weight, food consumption, mortality, organ weight, or hematology. There were no differences in tumor incidence (9).

♦ There are no long-term studies on the safety of gamma-oryzanol supplementation in humans. No serious adverse effects have been reported in human studies lasting up to 16 weeks at doses ranging from 300 to 500 mg daily.

♦ Gamma-oryzanol may decrease serum TSH in individuals with primary hypothyroidism.

Drug/Supplement Interactions

No reported adverse interactions

Key Points

♦ Preliminary evidence from uncontrolled human trials and animal studies suggest that gamma-oryzanol has a potential beneficial effect on serum lipids. However, well-controlled clinical trials of gamma-oryzanol or ferulic acid supplements in humans are required before recommendations can be made.

♦ There is no evidence that gamma-oryzanol builds muscle by acting as an anabolic agent. In fact, one review suggested that it has the opposite effect (1). However, because absorption of phytosterols is limited, it is unlikely to have a detrimental effect on body mass.

♦ Although gamma-oryzanol has demonstrated antioxidant potential in vitro (3–8), there is no research specifically testing whether gamma-oryzanol supplements reduce oxidative stress in vivo caused by exercise in humans.

Food Sources

Gamma-oryzanol is found in rice-bran oil, which is commercially available in Japan for use in salad oils and frying. Crude rice-bran oil contains approximately 1.56% oryzanol. Of the 180 mg of plant sterols found in the typical American diet, about 4% is gamma-oryzanol (1). One cup of brown rice provides 18 mg gamma-oryzanol, whereas white rice provides 4 mg (1). The ferulic acid portion of gamma-oryzanol is naturally found in the bran of cereals, and in fruits and vegetables. Ferulic acid is also a metabolite of caffeic acid found in coffee (2).

Dosage Information/Bioavailability

Gamma-oryzanol supplements are sold in capsules or tablets in doses ranging from 100 to 500 mg. Ferulic acid and rice-bran oil concentrate capsules are also available as separate supplements. Phytosterols are poorly absorbed, with less than 5% taken up by the intestinal tract after ingestion (1).

Relevant Research

Gamma-Oryzanol and Cholesterol

- ◆ A review article of mechanistic studies and animal and human research found evidence to support the anti-hyperlipidemic effects of rice-bran oil and gamma-oryzanol (10).

- ◆ In an uncontrolled study, 80 subjects with hyperlipidemia were given 300 mg gamma-oryzanol daily for 6 months. In subjects with type IIa and IIb hypercholesterolemia, plasma cholesterol decreased by 12% and 13%, respectively, in the first month. The decrease was significant only after 3 months. Plasma triglycerides decreased significantly in all subjects after 3 months (11). The results of this study should be viewed with caution because the design was not double-blinded or placebo-controlled.

Gamma-Oryzanol and Muscle Mass

- ◆ In a double-blind, placebo-controlled study, 22 weight-trained men were supplemented with 500 mg gamma-oryzanol or a placebo for 9 weeks. Strength tests were taken before the study and after 4 and 9 weeks of a resistance exercise program. There were no significant differences between groups in one-repetition maximum muscular strength (bench press and squat) and vertical jump power; or in testosterone, cortisol, estradiol, growth hormone, insulin, beta-endorphin, or blood lipids and resting cardiovascular variables (12).

- ◆ One review article cites several animal studies that suggest an antianabolic or catabolic effect of gamma-oryzanol, including suppression of luteinizing hormone release, reduced growth hormone synthesis and release, and increased release of catecholamines, dopamine, and norepinephrine in the brain (1).

References

1. Wheeler KB, Garleb KA. Gamma-oryzanol-plant sterol supplementation: metabolic, endocrine, and physiologic effects. *Int J Sport Nutr.* 1991;1:170–177.
2. de Deckere EA, Korver O. Minor constituents of rice bran oil as functional foods. *Nutr Rev.* 1996;54(11 pt 2):S120–S126.
3. Graf E. Antioxidant potential of ferulic acid. *Free Radic Biol Med.* 1992;13:435–448.
4. Garica-Conesa MT, Plumb GW, Waldron KW, et al. Ferulic acid dehydrodimers from wheat bran: isolation, purification, and antioxidant properties of 8-O-4-diferulic acid. *Redox Rep.* 1997;3:319–323.
5. Kim SJ, Han D, Moon KD, et al. Measurement of superoxide dismutase-like activity of natural antioxidants. *Biosci Biotechnol Biochem.* 1995;59:822–826.
6. Ohta T, Nakano T, Egashira Y, et al. Antioxidant activity of ferulic acid beta-glucuronide in the LDL oxidation system. *Biosci Biotechnol Biochem.* 1997;61:1942–1943.
7. Bourne LC, Rice-Evans CA. The effect of the phenolic antioxidant ferulic acid on the oxidation of low density lipoprotein depends on the pro-oxidant used. *Free Radic Res.* 1997;27:337–344.
8. Castelluccio C, Bolwell GP, Gerrish C, et al. Differential distribution of ferulic acid to the major plasma constituents in relation to its potential as an antioxidant. *Biochem J.* 1996;316(pt 2):691–694.
9. Tamagawa M, Otaki Y, Takahashi T, et al. Carcinogenicity study of gamma-oryzanol in B6C3F1 mice. *Food Chem Toxicol.* 1992;30:49–56.
10. Cicero AF, Gaddi A. Rice bran oil and gamma-oryzanol in the treatment of hyperlipoproteinaemias and other conditions. *Phytother Res.* 2001;15:277–289.
11. Yoshino G, Kazumi T, Amano M, et al. Effects of gamma-oryzanol and probucol on hyperlipidemia. *Curr Ther Res.* 1989;45:975–982.
12. Fry AC, Bonner E, Lewis DL, et al. The effects of gamma-oryzanol supplementation during resistance exercise training. *Int J Sport Nutr.* 1997;7:318–329.

Garlic

Garlic *(Allium sativum),* one of the best-selling herbal supplements in the United States, has been cultivated for medicinal and culinary purposes for 5,000 years. In Germany, garlic supplements are approved as a nonprescription medicine to reduce blood cholesterol and other cardiovascular risk factors. Of recent interest are the sulfur-containing compounds (S-allyl cysteine [SAC], S-allyl mercaptocysteine [SAMC], allicin, alliin, and diallyl polysulfides) that are considered to be the primary active agents in garlic. Other active components such as ajoene (produced from the combination of allicin and diallyl disulfide) also have been examined. Numerous studies have focused on the effect of garlic on hyperlipidemia, hypertension, platelet aggregation, cancer, and bacterial and fungal diseases (1–3).

Media and Marketing Claims	Efficacy
Reduces cholesterol levels	↑?
Reduces blood pressure	↑?
Improves circulation	↑?
Reduces cancer risk	NR
Improves immune function	NR

Safety

◆ Garlic supplements are relatively well-tolerated with the only reported adverse effects being mild gastrointestinal discomfort at high doses. One harmless side effect is the presence of undesirable body odor, even from some odor-free varieties (4).

◆ Different garlic preparations have different effects on intestinal mucosa. One animal study reported that dried raw garlic powder caused significant damage to gut mucosa, dried boiled garlic powder caused reddening of the mucosa, and aged garlic extract had no deleterious effects (5).

◆ The safety of enteric-coated garlic products (designed to pass through the stomach and deposit garlic compounds in the intestine) is questionable. In one study, enteric-coated garlic supplements caused a loss of epithelial cells at the top of crypts in the ileum and reddening of the gut mucosa (5).

◆ An increase in bleeding time was reported in 50 young, healthy subjects supplemented with 10 g raw garlic (approximately three cloves) daily for 2 months (6).

◆ Some researchers have cautioned that patients should discontinue garlic supplements or dietary use of garlic 7 days before surgery. Data from in vitro and in vivo studies indicate that the effects of garlic on platelet function "is undesirable in the surgical patient, especially if taking other antiplatelet agents" (7,8).

Drug/Supplement Interactions

◆ Garlic taken as a food or supplement may increase bleeding time when taken with other blood-thinning drugs or supplements (eg, warfarin [Coumadin], ginger, ginkgo, vitamin E, flaxseed, bromelain, dong quai, eicosapentaenoic acid and fish oil, aspirin, angelica, clove, danshen, red clover, turmeric). Use should be monitored by a physician (7).

◆ Garlic supplements may decrease the concentration of the HIV drug saquinavir (Fortovase).

◆ Garlic supplements may interfere with the effectiveness of oral contraceptives.

◆ Garlic supplements may decrease the effectiveness of drugs that are cytochrome P450 3A4 (CYP3A4) enzyme substrates, including cyclosporine, some calcium channel blockers (diltiazem, nicardipine, verapamil), chemotherapeutic agents (etoposide, paclitaxel, vinblastine, vincristine, vindesine), antifungals (ketoconazole, itraconazole), glucocorticoids, alfentanil, cisapride, fentanyl, lidocaine, losartan, fexofenadine, midazolam, and others. Avoid using garlic supplements with these medications until more information is available.

- Garlic may decrease plasma concentration of non-nucleoside reverse transcriptase inhibitors (NNRTIs) and the protease inhibitor saquinavir (Fortovase, invirase); until more information is available, avoid use of garlic with NNRTI antiretroviral drugs, including nevirapine (Viramune), delavirdine (Rescriptor), efavirenz (Sustiva), and protease inhibitors saquinavir (Fortovase, invirase), amprenavir (Agenerase), nelfinavir (Viracept), ritonavir (Norvir) and other HIV medications in the protease inhibitor family.

Key Points

- According to a recent report from the Agency for Healthcare Research and Quality (AHRQ) the evidence for garlic and cardiovascular disease risk reduction is not strong. Although garlic does appear to lower serum LDL and triglyceride levels, "there are insufficient data to draw conclusions regarding garlic's effects on clinical cardiovascular outcomes such as claudication and myocardial infarction." The AHRQ brought together national experts in science of garlic and health to review the evidence, focusing on clinical trials in humans that lasted longer than 4 weeks (n = 37 randomized trials) (9). Compared with placebo, garlic supplementation accounts for small reductions in serum lipids, with total cholesterol dropping by 1.2 to 25.4 mg/dL. LDL and triglycerides decreased proportionally to total cholesterol, and HDL levels tended to remain stable during garlic supplementation (9). Efforts to complete longer-term trials in at-risk populations and to differentiate effects associated with different supplement formulations are warranted.

- Limited meta-analyses and systemic reviews (10) have suggested that garlic supplements reduce cholesterol and blood pressure compared with placebo. However, the authors of the meta-analyses criticized the methodological limitations of several of the studies. For example, comparing the various garlic formulations (fresh, dried, powdered, oil, aged) and dosages is difficult. Additionally, blinding is difficult because of the characteristic smell of garlic supplements, even in "odor-free" preparations. Additional well-controlled, larger clinical trials are needed before garlic supplements are considered adjunctive treatment for cardiovascular disease.

- One meta-analysis reported that standardized dried garlic powder supplements resulted in a mild blood pressure reduction. The authors of the meta-analysis concluded: "There is insufficient evidence at present to recommend garlic as an effective antihypertensive agent for routine clinical use. However, there is equally no evidence to suggest it is harmful, and the currently available data strongly support the likelihood of dried garlic powder therapy being beneficial for the lowering of lipid levels, and possibly against mild hypertension, at least in the short term" (11). Additional well-controlled trials are needed to verify the results of these studies.

- There is evidence that garlic (aged extract and dried powder) may reduce platelet aggregation and improve microcirculation in subjects with arterial disease. Preliminary evidence from studies with small numbers of subjects suggests that garlic enhances microcirculation in healthy individuals. More research with larger sample sizes is needed.

- Epidemiological studies are conflicting regarding the cancer-protective effects of garlic. Some observational studies show that raw or cooked garlic may reduce cancer risk, with the strongest evidence for stomach and colorectal cancers. Allium vegetables as a group may protect against prostate cancer. Although animal and in vitro studies demonstrate anticarcinogenic effects, large-scale prospective intervention studies are needed to determine the effectiveness of garlic supplements against cancer in human subjects.

- Garlic has been used worldwide for centuries as both a topical and oral antibacterial, antifungal, and antiviral agent. Human studies are limited. Controlled human studies testing the effectiveness of garlic supplements in treating the common cold, flu, or herpes virus are needed.

- The amount of garlic (equivalent to one to two raw cloves) used in most studies can be easily consumed in the diet. However, cooking garlic may destroy some of its active compounds.

Food Sources

Garlic cloves and powder (one raw clove ≈ 3 g). Most studies have used the equivalent of 2 to 5 g raw garlic (12). To optimize the therapeutic effects, some research suggests crushing raw garlic and then allowing it to sit for 10 minutes to help retain some of the biologically active compounds that are normally destroyed when heated (13).

Dosage Information/Bioavailability

Garlic powder, oil, and garlic aged in aqueous-alcoholic extract are available in capsules or enteric-coated pills. Garlic is also sold in "deodorized," "odor-free," or "odor-controlled" preparations. Most studies have used 40 to 1,200 mg dried powder (equivalent to approximately 2 to 5 g raw garlic [one to two cloves]) or 1 to 7.2 g aged garlic extract. Some garlic manufacturers state that their supplements are standardized to 1.3% or 10 mg allicin or have "allicin potential." There has been some controversy regarding whether allicin must be present for supplements to be biologically active. Numerous sulfur-containing compounds, as well as some nonsulfur compounds, seem to contribute to the potential beneficial effects of garlic. Although some suggest that allicin activity may be important for reducing cholesterol, it may not be important for anticarcinogenic activity (14–16). Allicin does not seem to be absorbed by the gastrointestinal tract and has been shown to break down rapidly when administered intravenously (15,17).

Relevant Research

Garlic and Cholesterol Control and Atherogenesis

- In a double-blind, placebo-controlled study of garlic supplementation, 62 adults with normal blood lipid levels were randomly assigned to take dried garlic powder tablets (10.8 mg allicin) or a placebo daily for 12 weeks. The primary outcome was modulation of serum cholesterol levels. Supplementation was not associated with a significant difference in total cholesterol, LDL or HDL cholesterol, or triglyceride levels, as compared with the placebo group. However, the study population presented with normal lipid levels and thus the likelihood of a significant response in a population of 62 people is low (18).

- Null results were shown in a randomized, controlled, double-blind study of 136 subjects with hypercholesterolemia living in Thailand who were randomly assigned to take 5.6 mg allicin or placebo nightly after the evening meal for 12 weeks (19). Subjects had a mean age of 47 years; one third were men, two thirds were women; mean BMI was 24.6 in the intervention group and 24.3 in the placebo group.

- A meta-analysis of 13 randomized, double-blind, placebo-controlled trials of the effects of garlic on lipids (n = 796 subjects with hypercholesterolemia) found that garlic significantly reduced total cholesterol levels from baseline compared with placebo. Six diet-controlled trials with the highest scores for methodological quality revealed a nonsignificant difference between garlic and placebo groups (20).

- A meta-analysis of 16 trials (n = 952 subjects) compared the pooled mean difference in the change of total serum cholesterol, triglycerides, and HDL cholesterol among subjects treated with garlic therapy (powder, fresh, oil, or aged extract) and those treated with a placebo or another agent in trials lasting a minimum of 4 weeks. The analysis revealed a statistically significant 12% mean reduction in total cholesterol (−0.77 mmol/L) with garlic therapy (dried powder, fresh, oil, aged extract) beyond the levels achieved with placebo. In the dried garlic powders, there were no significant differences in the size of reduction across the dosage range of 600 to 900 mg (estimated to be equivalent to 1.8 to 2.7 g fresh garlic) daily. Dried garlic powders also significantly reduced triglyceride levels (−0.3 mmol/L) compared with the placebo. The authors acknowledged that many of the trials had methodological shortcomings (failure to provide information about randomization or use an intention-to-treat analysis) (21).

- In a double-blind, placebo-controlled trial, 115 subjects with hypercholesterolemia were randomly assigned to receive 900 mg of dried garlic powder or a placebo daily for 6 months. Compared with the placebo, garlic had no significant effect on cholesterol (total, LDL, HDL), triglycerides, lipoproteins, or apolipoprotein A1 or B (22). Similar results were shown in a study using 900 mg garlic powder for 12 weeks conducted among 50 subjects with hypercholesterolemia (23).

- In a double-blind, placebo-controlled, crossover study, 41 moderately hypercholesterolemic men were given (in random order) 7.2 g aged garlic extract or a placebo daily for 6 months before switching treatments for 4 additional months. All subjects were advised to follow a Step I cholesterol-reducing diet during the study. Vital signs, body weight, blood chemistry, and liver function tests were monitored throughout the study. Aged garlic extract resulted in a statistically significant 6.1% to 7.0% reduction in serum total cholesterol compared with the placebo phase and baseline evaluation, and LDL cholesterol decreased 4.6% compared with the placebo. In addition, the garlic extract produced a significant 5.5% decrease is systolic blood pressure compared with placebo and baseline. There were no significant changes in HDL cholesterol, triglycerides, or diastolic blood pressure (24).

Garlic and Blood Pressure and Cardiac Elasticity

◆ Efficacy was demonstrated in a randomized, double-blind study of 20 individuals with essential hypertension, age- and gender-matched to 20 control subjects, each receiving a 250-mg garlic tablet (Ranbaxy Laboratories Ltd, Mumbai, India) daily for 2 months. Reductions in systolic and diastolic blood pressure were demonstrated in the garlic-supplemented group as compared with baseline, whereas the control group showed no change over time. In the garlic-treated group, the lower blood pressure levels were accompanied by significantly reduced levels of lipid peroxidation biomarkers at the end of 8 weeks, a change not demonstrated in control group subjects (25).

◆ A meta-analysis assessed eight randomized controlled trials testing the effect of garlic on blood pressure (n = 415 subjects) lasting at least 4 weeks. Only three of eight studies included subjects with hypertension, and all studies used the same dried garlic powder preparation in dosages ranging from 600 to 900 mg daily (equivalent to 1.8 to 2.7 g fresh garlic). Three of seven trials that were placebo-controlled reported a statistically significant reduction in systolic blood pressure with garlic. The overall pooled mean difference in systolic blood pressure (7.7 mm Hg) was greater in subjects taking garlic than those treated with placebo. For diastolic blood pressure, four of seven trials reported significant reductions with garlic therapy compared with the placebo. The pooled mean difference between garlic and placebo was 5.0 mm Hg for this measure (11).

◆ In a cross-sectional, observational study, 101 healthy older adults (ages 50 to 80 years) with normal blood pressure who were taking more than 300 mg/day standardized garlic powder for 2 or more years were paired with 101 age- and sex-matched control subjects. Blood pressure, heart rate, and plasma lipids were similar between groups. Measures of aortic stiffness (pulse wave velocity and pressure-standardized elastic vascular resistance) were lower in the garlic group (26).

Garlic and Circulation and Platelet Function

◆ In a double-blind, placebo-controlled study, 80 subjects with peripheral arterial occlusive disease, stage II, were randomly assigned to receive 800 mg garlic powder or a placebo for 12 weeks. The use of other therapeutic drugs was not permitted. Garlic intake resulted in a significant increase in walking distance (+31 meters) when compared with the placebo group. The effect appeared at the fifth week of the study.

There was a significant decrease in diastolic blood pressure, spontaneous thrombo-cyte aggregation, plasma viscosity, and blood cholesterol levels with garlic therapy. The authors concluded: "Garlic may be an appropriate agent especially for the long-term treatment of incipient intermittent claudication" (27).

- In a double-blind, placebo-controlled study, 60 subjects with cerebrovascular risk factors including increased platelet aggregation were randomly assigned to receive 800 mg enteric-coated powdered garlic or a placebo daily for 4 weeks. Garlic inges-tion led to a significant inhibition of the increased ratio of circulating platelet aggre-gates and of spontaneous platelet aggregation. There were no significant changes in the placebo group. After a 4-week washout phase, the ratio of circulating platelet aggregates and spontaneous platelet aggregation increased to initial values (run-in phase prior to garlic supplementation). The authors concluded: "Since garlic is well tolerated it would be worthwhile testing it in a controlled clinical trial for usefulness in preventing disease manifestations associated with platelet aggregation" (28).

- In a study of the effects of garlic on peripheral blood flow, 13 healthy young women (ages 23 to 33 years) took 600 mg garlic tablet (1,800 µg allicin) daily for 7 days whereas 13 age- and BMI-matched control subjects received no treatment. Calf blood flow was measured using the Filtrass strain gauge plethysmograph system. Over time, there was a significant increase in calf blood flow and IL-6 (known to increase vasodilation) among participants receiving garlic, but not in the control group subjects (29).

Garlic and Cancer

- Few studies using garlic supplementation in humans to reduce cancer risk have been published; however, several epidemiological studies on garlic consumption and can-cer risk provide conflicting results regarding garlic's anticarcinogenic potential. Stomach cancer risk was 13 times less for Chinese subjects consuming 20 g garlic/day than for those who ate less than 1 g/day. In the Iowa Women's Health Study, colon cancer risk was less in women who ate garlic more than once a week as compared with those who ate no garlic (30).

- In a large-scale, prospective cohort epidemiological study in the Netherlands, self-reported intake of garlic supplements was not associated with a reduced risk of breast (31), colon (32), or lung cancer (33). US epidemiological studies regarding the role of garlic in cancer risk reduction are limited by the fact that data on garlic supple-mentation is almost never collected.

- A review of epidemiological studies reported that dietary garlic (not supplemental) consumption is most strongly associated with a reduction in stomach and colorectal cancers, but that garlic pills do not seem to reduce cancer risk at any site. However, the researchers noted limitations of observational studies and emphasized the need for intervention trials (34).

- An epidemiological study of 238 prostate cancer cases and 471 age-matched controls in Shanghai, China, showed that high intake of allium vegetables (the major biologically active constituent in garlic) were associated with an almost 50% reduction in prostate cancer risk (OR = 0.51; 95% CI = 0.34–0.76). The highest tertile of garlic intake was associated with a 53% reduction in risk (35) and was stronger in men with localized disease, independent of body weight.

◆ One review article cited several animal and in vitro studies showing a protective effect of garlic on breast, uterine, esophageal, skin, colon, stomach, bladder, prostate, and lung cancer cell lines. The author noted that the benefits of garlic were not limited to a specific species, tissue, or carcinogen. Overall, S-allyl cysteine (SAC), a water-soluble compound, was effective in reducing the risk of chemically induced tumors in experimental animals but had no effect on established tumors. In contrast, oil-soluble compounds such as diallyl disulfide were effective in reducing the proliferation of neoplasms (30). Similarly, ajoene—a garlic-derived compound—has demonstrated anti-carcinogenic effects against basal cell skin cancer and leukemia cell lines (36).

Garlic and Immune Function

◆ A randomized, placebo-controlled study of 146 healthy British adult volunteers was conducted to determine the effect of daily allicin-containing garlic supplementation for 12 weeks, during winter months, on common cold incidence and severity. Subjects were randomly assigned to garlic supplementation, using one capsule daily of a proprietary product containing only stabilized allicin (no specific dosage provided) or placebo. The 73 subjects in each group were matched on age, gender, and dietary garlic consumption pattern. Subjects recorded health status in a daily log using a 5-point, Likert-like scale, ranging from well to full cold symptoms (headache, sneezing, runny nose, and fatigue). Allicin supplementation resulted in approximately 40% fewer self-reported colds (24 vs 65) and shortened duration of symptoms (37). Larger studies with objective rather than subjective endpoints are needed before conclusions can be made.

◆ There are several cell culture and animal model studies that lend preliminary evidence to the idea that garlic may inhibit the growth (replication) of select viral and bacterial pathogens. For example, the growth of *Candida albicans* yeast cells was inhibited by the presence of garlic extract in an in vitro study (38). In addition, garlic has been shown to inhibit the growth of *Pseudomonas aeruginosa* infection (a common lung infection among patients with cystic fibrosis) by reducing the drug resistance of the bacteria in vitro (39). Similar growth inhibition effects have been shown in vitro for *Bacillus anthracis* (40).

References

1. Blumenthal M, ed. *The Complete German Commission E Monographs Therapeutic Guide to Herbal Medicines*. Austin, Tex: American Botanical Council; 1998.
2. Abdullah TH, Kandil O, Elkadi A, et al. Garlic revisited: therapeutic for the major diseases of our time? *J Natl Med Assoc*. 1988;80:439–445.

3. Birt DF, Shull JD, Yaktine AL. Chemoprevention of cancer. In: Shils ME, Olson JA, Shike M, et al, eds. *Modern Nutrition in Health and Disease*. 9th ed. Baltimore, Md: Williams & Wilkins; 1999:1263–1295.

4. Farrell AM, Straughton RC. Garlic burns mimicking herpes zoster. *Lancet*. 1996;347: 1195.

5. Hoshino T, Kashimoto N, Kasuga S. Effects of garlic preparations on the gastrointestinal mucosa. *J Nutr*. 2001;131(3 Suppl):S1109-S1113.

6. Gadkari JV, Joshi VD. Effect of ingestion of raw garlic on serum cholesterol level, clotting time, and fibrinolytic activity in normal subjects. *J Postgrad Med*. 1991;37:128–131.

7. Petry JJ. Surgically significant nutritional supplements. *Plast Reconstr Surg*. 1996;97: 233–240.

8. Ang-Lee MK, Moss J, Yuan CS. Herbal medicines and perioperative care. *JAMA*. 2001;286:208–216.

9. Garlic: Effects on Cardiovascular Risks and Disease, Protective Effects Against Cancer, and Clinical Adverse Effects. Rockville, Md: Agency for Healthcare Research and Quality; 2000. AHRQ Publication No. 01-E023. Available at: http://www.ahrq.gov/ clinic/garlicinv.htm. Accessed March 6, 2006.

10. Alder R, Lookinland S, Berry JA, et al. A systematic review of the effectiveness of garlic as an anti-hyperlipidemic agent. *J Am Acad Nurse Pract*. 2003;15:120–129.

11. Silagy CA, Neil HA. A meta-analysis of the effect of garlic on blood pressure. *J Hypertens*. 1994;12:463–468.

12. Pennington JA, ed. *Bowes & Church's Food Values of Portions Commonly Used*. 17th ed. Philadelphia, Pa: Lippincott; 1998.

13. Song K, Milner J. The influence of heating on the anticancer properties of garlic. *J Nutr*. 2001;131(3 Suppl):S1054-S1057.

14. Cavallito CJ, Bailey JH. Allicin, the antibacterial principle of *Allium sativum*. Isolation, physical properties, and antibacterial action. *J Am Chem Soc*. 1944;66:1950–1951.

15. Egen-Schwind C, Eckard R, Kemper FH. Metabolism of garlic constituents in the isolated perfused rat liver. *Planta Med*. 1992;58:301–305.

16. Lawson LD, Ransom DK, Hughes BG. Inhibition of whole blood platelet-aggregation by compounds in garlic clove extracts and commercial garlic products. *Thromb Res*. 1992;65:141–156.

17. Freeman F, Kodera Y. Garlic chemistry: stability of s-(2-propenyl)-2-propene-1-sulfinothioate (allicin) in blood, solvents, and simulated physiological fluids. *J Agric Food Chem*. 1995;43:2332–2338. Available at: http://www.ahrq.gov. Accessed May 1, 2005.

18. Turner B, Molgaard C, Marckmann P. Effect of garlic (Allium sativum) powder tablets on serum lipids, blood pressure and arterial stiffness in normo-lipidaemic volunteers: a randomized, double-blind, placebo-controlled trial. *Br J Nutr*. 2004;92:701–706.

19. Satitvipawee P, Rawdaree P, Indrabhakti S, et al. No effect of garlic extract supplement on serum lipid levels in hypercholesterolemic subjects. *J Med Assoc Thai*. 2003;86: 750–757.

20. Stevinson C, Pittler MH, Ernst E. Garlic for treating hypercholesterolemia: a meta-analysis of randomized clinical trials. *Ann Int Med*. 2000;133:420–429.

21. Silagy C, Neil A. Garlic as a lipid lowering agent—a meta-analysis. *J R Coll Physicians Lond.* 1994;28:39–45.

22. Neil HA, Silagy CA, Lancaster T, et al. Garlic powder in the treatment of moderate hyperlipidaemia: a controlled trial and meta-analysis. *J R Coll Physicians Lond.* 1996;30:329–334.

23. Isaachsohn JL, Moser M, Stein EA, et al. Garlic powder and plasma lipids and lipoproteins: a multicenter, randomized, placebo-controlled trial. *Arch Intern Med.* 1998;158: 1189–1194.

24. Steiner M, Khan AH, Holbert D, et al. A double-blind crossover study in moderately hypercholesterolemic men that compared the effect of aged garlic extract and placebo administration on blood lipids. *Am J Clin Nutr.* 1996;64:866–870.

25. Dhawan V, Jain S. Effect of garlic supplementation on oxidized low density lipoproteins and lipid peroxidation in patients of essential hypertension. *Mol Cell Biochem.* 2004;266:109–115.

26. Breithaupt-Grogler K, Ling M, Boudoulas H, et al. Protective effect of chronic garlic intake on elastic properties of aorta in the elderly. *Circulation.* 1997;96:2649–2655.

27. Kiesewetter H, Jung F, Jung EM, et al. Effects of garlic coated tablets in peripheral arterial occlusive disease. *Clin Investig.* 1993;71:383–386.

28. Kiesewetter H, Jung F, Jung EM, et al. Effect of garlic on platelet aggregation in patients with increased risk of juvenile ischemic attack. *Eur J Clin Pharmacol.* 1993;45: 333–336.

29. Anim-Nyame N, Sooranna SR, Johnson MR, et al. Garlic supplementation increases peripheral blood flow: a role for interleukin-6? *J Nutr Biochem.* 2004;15:30–36.

30. Milner JA. Garlic: its anticarcinogenic and antitumorgenic properties. *Nutr Rev.* 1996;54(11 pt 2):S82-S86.

31. Dorant E, van den Brandt PA, Goldbohm RA. Allium vegetable consumption, garlic supplement intake, and female breast carcinoma incidence. *Breast Cancer Res Treat.* 1995;33:163–170.

32. Dorant E, van den Brandt PA, Goldbohm RA. A prospective cohort study on the relationship between onion and leek consumption, garlic supplement use and the risk of colorectal carcinoma in The Netherlands. *Carcinogenesis.* 1996;17:477–484.

33. Dorant E, van den Brandt PA, Goldbohm RA. A prospective cohort study on allium vegetable consumption, garlic supplement use, and the risk of lung carcinoma in The Netherlands. *Cancer Res.* 1994;54:6148–6153.

34. Fleischauer AT, Arab L. Garlic and cancer: a critical review of the epidemiologic literature. *J Nutr.* 2001;131(3 Suppl):S1032–S1040.

35. Hsing AW, Chokkalingam AP, Gao YT, et al. Allium vegetables and risk of prostate cancer: a population-based study. *J Natl Cancer Inst.* 2002;94:1648–1651.

36. Hassan HT. Ajoene (natural garlic compound): a new anti-leukaemia agent for AML therapy. *Leuk Res.* 2004;28:667–671.

37. Josling P. Preventing the common cold with a garlic supplement: a double-blind, placebo-controlled survey. *Adv Ther.* 2001;18:189–193.

38. Ghannoum MA. Studies on the anticandidal mode of action of *Allium sativum* (garlic). *J Gen Microbiol.* 1988;134(pt 11):2917–2924.

39. Bjarnsholt T, Jensen PO, Rasmussen TB, et al. Garlic blocks quorum sensing and promotes rapid clearing of pulmonary *Pseudomonas aeruginosa* infections. *Microbiology.*
2005;151:3873–3880.
40. Sasaki J, Kita J. Bacteriocidal activity of garlic powder against Bacillus anthracis. *J Nutr
Sci Vitaminol (Tokyo).* 2003;49:297–299.

Ginger *(Zingiber officinale)*

Ginger is a natural spice widely revered for its healing properties. Since ancient Greece, ginger has been used to improve circulation, aid digestion, and ease nausea and other gastrointestinal troubles. A close relative of turmeric and marjoram, ginger is native to coastal India and is also commonly grown in Africa, China, and Jamaica.

Ginger grows as a shoot-like plant with a large rhizome, which contains the usable part of the herb. A rhizome is similar to a root but botanically is considered a large stem. The biologically active components in the rhizome of ginger are gingerols and shogaols. These constituents give ginger its pungent odor and are also responsible for its anti-nausea and anti-vomiting effects. Because ginger is thought to act directly on the gastrointestinal system to reduce nausea, it does not cause drowsiness as traditional anti-nausea medications do, which work through the central nervous system (1).

Media and Marketing Claims	Efficacy
Treats morning sickness in pregnancy	↑?
Treats nausea associated with chemotherapy	NR
Treats postsurgery nausea	↔

Safety

- Ginger has a Generally Recognized as Safe (GRAS) status in the United States (2).
- Clinical data conflict about whether taking ginger before surgery is safe for patients taking anticoagulation medications. Individuals who will undergo surgery should consult with their physicians before taking ginger as there is some limited evidence that ginger may have antiplatelet effects.

Drug/Supplement Interactions

- Caution should be exercised when taking ginger with anticoagulant/antiplatelet (eg, warfarin) drugs. Theoretically, ginger may have an additive effect.
- Ginger may reduce blood glucose levels; patients with diabetes taking glucose-lowering drugs should monitor blood glucose even more closely when taking ginger.

Key Points _____

- ◆ In April 2004, the American College of Obstetrics and Gynecologists issued an endorsement of ginger stating, "treatment of nausea and vomiting of pregnancy with ginger has shown beneficial effects and can be considered as a nonpharmacologic option." While no specific dose is recommended, the review cites a controlled trial that tested the efficacy of ginger in pregnancy-related nausea and vomiting using a dose of 350 mg taken three times daily (3).

- ◆ Ginger had no effect on chemotherapy-induced nausea in one study. More research is needed to determine whether ginger may benefit individuals with nausea from chemotherapy.

- ◆ Results from a small number of controlled trials using ginger to treat postoperative nausea are conflicting.

Food Sources

Ginger root can be purchased in a variety of forms, including, fresh, dried, pickled, preserved, candied, and powdered. Extracts of ginger are used in a variety of foods, condiments, candies, and beverages. It is difficult to extrapolate the amount of food-based ginger required to see the clinical efficacy associated in some research with supplement use, especially because it remains unclear which ginger constituents are the most biologically relevant. However, fresh ginger is thought to be more effective than other forms.

Dosage Information/Bioavailability

Ginger is available in tablets and capsules with the standardized dry extract, capsules containing powdered ginger, fluid extracts, tinctures, fresh ginger root, ginger tea, ginger ale, and crystallized ginger. Dosages vary widely based on the form of ginger used and condition being treated. For morning sickness, research has used 250 mg (made from ground fresh ginger root) four times/day (4). To prevent postoperative nausea and vomiting, 1 g of powdered ginger root rhizome administered 1 hour before surgery has been used, but doses vary widely (5).

Relevant Research

Ginger and Morning Sickness

- ◆ In a systematic review of the randomized, controlled, double-blind studies of the effectiveness and safety of oral ginger supplementation for the treatment of morning sickness, researchers concluded that ginger may ease nausea and vomiting in pregnancy and that it appears to be safe to use during pregnancy (6). A total of 27 studies were considered, but only 6 included pregnant women with reported nausea that was not associated with other clinical conditions, such as inflammation or concurrent medications. A total of 675 pregnant women with morning sickness were included overall in the 6 studies, which used doses ranging from 125 mg four times daily to 500 mg three times daily. Specifics regarding ginger formulations were not provided. More studies are needed to confirm this report.

♦ A randomized, double-blind, placebo-controlled trial assessing the efficacy of ginger for reducing pregnancy-related nausea was conducted among 70 Chinese women. Subjects were within 17 weeks of gestation, complained of pregnancy-associated nausea, and attended a central maternity clinic (4). In this study, women were randomly assigned to 1 g (250 mg in four doses) ground fresh ginger (n = 32) or placebo (n = 38) daily for four days. Assessment of efficacy was determined by self-reported nausea symptoms during the last 24 hours on treatment and included two scales, a visual analog scale of nausea severity and a Likert scale ranging from 0 for no nausea to 10 for the worst nausea could be. Results showed that the change in nausea scores between groups was significantly greater for the ginger group than the placebo, using intent-to-treat analysis. However, all subjects reported at least one vomiting episode in the same 24-hour period, regardless of group assignment.

♦ In a randomized, double-blind, controlled trial to compare the efficacy of ginger vs vitamin B-6 in the treatment of nausea and vomiting in pregnancy, 291 pregnant Australian women with self-reported morning sickness who were less than 16 weeks' gestation, received 350 mg ginger three times a day or 25 mg vitamin B-6 three times daily for 3 weeks. Weekly assessments of nausea and vomiting were compared with baseline in both groups. Ginger and vitamin B-6 were equally effective in reducing the frequency of nausea, vomiting, and dry retching as compared with baseline: 53% of those taking ginger and 55% of those taking vitamin B-6 reported an improvement in symptoms from baseline (7).

♦ To determine the safety and efficacy of ginger in the treatment of nausea and vomiting in pregnancy, 187 women who had called the Motherisk program to query about the use of ginger during pregnancy and retrospectively reported ginger use during the first trimester of pregnancy were contacted after delivery to ascertain tolerance or self-reported efficacy of ginger. Data from those women were compared with data from an additional 187 women who did not report using ginger. Outcome and subjective scoring of nausea and vomiting during pregnancy were assessed. The only significant difference between the groups was that more infants weighing less than 2,500 g were born to women in the comparison group. Ginger may have a mild effect on the reduction of nausea and vomiting during pregnancy, but the study design allowed for only subjective, nonstatistical evaluation (8).

♦ In a double-blind, randomized, placebo-controlled trial to investigate the effect of ginger extract on nausea during pregnancy, 120 women with pregnancy-related nausea and vomiting lasting greater than 7 days and who were at less than 20 weeks' gestation received either 125 mg ginger extract or placebo four times daily for 4 days. Effectiveness was evaluated using the Rhodes Index of Nausea, Vomiting, and Retching. Compared with the placebo group, in the ginger extract group both nausea and retching decreased significantly after the first study day and continued throughout the 4-day trial. However, there was no significant difference in vomiting (9). A sub-sample analysis of pregnancy outcomes among 81 women who had taken ginger showed unfavorable outcomes at a level equal to the overall obstetric population, indicating no clear safety concerns evolved as a result of ginger supplementation during pregnancy.

Ginger and Chemotherapy-Induced or Postoperative Nausea

◆ In a systematic review of six randomized, double-blind, placebo-controlled clinical trials that used ginger for a variety of illness that are associated with nausea such as morning sickness, seasickness, chemotherapy, or gynecological surgery, investigators found that collectively the studies favored the use of ginger over placebo for the treatment of nausea and vomiting. In two of the studies that include prescription anti-nausea medication, ginger was as effective as the prescription drug. A total of 439 subjects were included in the analysis, with ginger dosages in all studies set at 1 g/day (some as single dosage, others as divided dosages) (10).

◆ In a double-blind, randomized, crossover study to evaluate the efficacy of ginger as an antiemetic agent, 48 women with gynecologic cancer (ages 36–56 years) received 1 g ginger root powder per day for 5 days starting with the first day of the first chemotherapy cycle or placebo on the first day of the cycle and metoclopramide for the next 4 days. All subjects received standard antiemetics on the first day of chemotherapy. Subjects switched to the alternate treatment for their second cycle. In the 43 women who completed both cycles of chemotherapy, there was no difference in nausea and vomiting between the two groups. Addition of ginger to an antiemetic regimen had no effect on chemotherapy-induced nausea and vomiting (11).

◆ In a randomized, placebo-controlled double-blind study to evaluate the efficacy of ginger in preventing postoperative nausea and vomiting, 184 women undergoing gynecologic laparoscopic procedures were given (*a*) placebo capsules, (*b*) 300 mg ginger extract plus placebo capsules, or (*c*) 600 mg ginger extract capsules preoperatively and at 3 hours and 6 hours postoperatively. Subjects were asked to rate nausea and quantify emesis. No significant difference in postoperative nausea and vomiting among the three groups was detected at any point in the study (12).

◆ A randomized, controlled, blinded trial among 120 women scheduled for elective gynecological surgery randomly assigned subjects to one of three groups: (*a*) 10 mg metoclopramide (n = 40); (*b*) 1 g powdered ginger root (n = 36); or (*c*) 1 g lactose (n = 40), which served as placebo. Women took the assigned pills 1 hour before anesthesia was applied. Standardized anesthesia protocols were used and were based on dose per kg body weight. Nurses who were unaware of the study documented patient progress postoperatively. Compared with placebo, ginger supplementation was associated with a significant 50% reduction in postoperative nausea ($P = .006$). Findings for subjects treated with ginger were not statistically different from the findings for the metoclopramide group (5).

References

1. Holtmann S, Clarke AH, Scherer H, et al. The anti-motion sickness mechanism of ginger. A comparative study with placebo and dimenhydrinate. *Acta Otolaryngol.* 1989;108: 168–174.
2. Food and Drug Administration. Center for Food Safety and Applied Nutrition, Office of Premarket Approval. EAFUS: A food additive database. Available at: http://vm.cfsan.fda.gov/~dms/eafus.html. Accessed May 22, 2005.
3. American College of Obstetricians and Gynecologists. ACOG (American College of Obstetrics and Gynecology) Practice Bulletin: nausea and vomiting of pregnancy. *Obstet Gynecol.* 2004;103:803–814.
4. Vutyavanich T, Kraisarin T, Ruangsri R. Ginger for nausea and vomiting in pregnancy: randomized, double-masked, placebo-controlled trial. *Obstet Gynecol.* 2001;97: 577–582.
5. Phillips B, Ruggier R, Hutchinson SE. *Zingiber officinale* (ginger)—an antiemetic for day case surgery. *Anaesthesia.* 1993;48:715–717.
6. Borrelli F, Capasso R, Aviello G, et al. Effectiveness and safety of ginger in the treatment of pregnancy-induced nausea and vomiting. *Obstet Gynecol.* 2005;105:849–856.
7. Smith C, Crowther C, Willson K, et al. A randomized controlled trial of ginger to treat nausea and vomiting in pregnancy. *Obstet Gynecol.* 2004;103:639–645.
8. Portnoi G, Chng LA, Karimi-Tabesh L, et al. Prospective comparative study of the safety and effectiveness of ginger for the treatment of nausea and vomiting in pregnancy. *Am J Obstet Gynecol.* 2003;189:1374–1377.
9. Willetts KE, Ekangaki A, Eden JA. Effect of a ginger extract on pregnancy-induced nausea: a randomized controlled trial. *Aust N Z J Obstet Gynaecol.* 2003;43:139–144.
10. Ernst E, Pittler MH. Efficacy of ginger for nausea and vomiting: a systematic review of randomized clinical trials. *Br J Anaesth.* 2000;84:367–371.
11. Manusirivithaya S, Sripramote M, Tangjitgamol S, et al. Antiemetic effect of ginger in gynecologic oncology patients receiving cisplatin. *Int J Gynecol Cancer.* 2004;14: 1063–1069.
12. Eberhart LH, Mayer R, Betz O, et al. Ginger does not prevent postoperative nausea and vomiting after laparoscopic surgery. *Anesth Analg.* 2003;96:995–998.

Ginkgo Biloba

The leaves of the ginkgo tree have been used in China for centuries. It is one of the most frequently prescribed herbs for cognitive disorders in Germany and is one of the top-selling herbs in the United States (1). *Ginkgo biloba* leaves contain flavonoids, sesquiterpenes, and diterpenes (ginkgolides) that have been identified as possible active ingredients. The flavonoids are thought to act as free-radical scavengers and the ginkgolides may be platelet-activating factor (PAF) antagonists that reduce clotting time (2). Many studies have been conducted in Europe using a standardized extract of *Ginkgo biloba* (EGb 761), but not all studies were well-controlled.

Media and Marketing Claims	Efficacy
Improves memory in individuals with Alzheimer's disease or dementia	↔
Improves memory in healthy individuals	↔
Improves symptoms of reduced circulation in individuals with intermittent claudication	↑?
Relieves tinnitus (ringing in ears)	↓
Prevents mountain or altitude sickness	↓

Safety

- Different safety and clinical application profiles exist for ginkgo seed and ginkgo leaf.

- Consumption of ginkgo seeds can be fatal and is associated with convulsions and repetitive seizures in children (3,4). Roasting may reduce toxicity.

- In a 7-day blinded, placebo-controlled study, 50 healthy men were randomly assigned to 120 mg *Ginkgo biloba* extract EGb 761 (dry extract of ginkgo leaves; manufactured by Schwabe Pharmaceuticals, Karlsruhe, Germany) or placebo twice daily. Subjects showed no significant changes in 29 parameters of coagulation or bleeding time, which indicates that purified extract forms of *Ginkgo biloba* are likely safe. However, select over-the-counter forms may have anti-platelet aggregation effects (5).

- Ginkgo should be avoided at least 36 hours prior to surgery due to potential increased bleeding time (6).

- Ginkgo has been used safely in studies of several weeks to 1 year in duration.

- Ginkgo should not be taken with trazodone (Desyrel); this combination has been associated with induction of coma.

- Avoid all fresh ginkgo plant parts because they may contain more than 5 ppm of the toxic ginkgolic acid (ginkgotoxin) and cause severe allergic reaction; antidote for ginkgotoxin poisoning is pyridoxine (7).

- Consumption of more than 10 roasted seeds per day or long-term use of ginkgo may cause difficulty breathing, weak pulse, seizures, loss of consciousness, and shock. In general, ginkgo plant parts should be avoided due to potential toxicity at doses above 5 ppm.

- Ginkgo can cause mild gastrointestinal upset, headache, dizziness, palpitations, constipation, and allergic skin reactions.

- Large doses (estimated to be more than 600 mg/day) of ginkgo may cause restlessness, diarrhea, nausea, vomiting, lack of muscle tone, and weakness.

- Ginkgo leaf products should be avoided by individuals with seizure disorders and those taking drugs or supplements that lower the seizure threshold (see list in Drug/Supplement Interactions section).

♦ Evidence in animals suggests that fertility may be reduced by high concentrations of ginkgo; this has not yet been demonstrated in humans.

Drug/Supplement Interactions

♦ Ginkgo may increase clotting when taken with other blood-thinning drugs or supplements (warfarin [Coumadin], clopidogrel, dalteparin, enoxaparin, heparin, indomethacin, ticlopine, garlic, ginger, vitamin E, flaxseed, bromelain, dong quai, fish oil, aspirin, angelica, clove, danshen, Panax ginseng, and others). This is related to the effect of ginkgolides on P450 2C9 enzyme activity. People on these medications should be monitored by a physician and may be advised to discontinue ginkgo.

♦ Ginkgo may increase seizure risk when used with seizure threshold–lowering herbs and supplements (butanediol, cedar leaf, Chinese club moss, folate, gamma butyrolactone, gamma hydroxybutyrate, glutamine, huperzine A, hydrazine sulfate, hyssop oil, juniper, L-carnitine, melatonin, rosemary, sage, wormword, and others), and anticonvulsant/antiepileptic drugs (phenobarbital, primidone, valproic acid, gabapentin, carbamazepine, phenytoin, and others). Avoid ginkgo with these products.

♦ Ginkgo should not be taken with fluoxentine (Prozac) because it has been associated with hypomania.

♦ Ginkgo may interact with CYP1A2 enzymes, leading to a slight increase in levels of medications metabolized through this pathway, but no clear clinical problems have been identified.

♦ Preliminary and conflicting evidence suggests that ginkgo may also interfere with the clearance/levels of medications metabolized through the P450 2D6 enzymes, such as amitriptyline, clozapine, meperidine, and metoprolol, as well as medications metabolized through the P450 CYP3A4 enzyme, such as lovastatin, fexofenadine, and triazolam.

♦ Individuals with diabetes, and particularly those on insulin therapy, should monitor blood glucose levels closely while on ginkgo as it has been shown to stimulate beta cell function in the pancreas, which may lead to hypoglycemia.

♦ Ginkgo can reduce efficacy of thiazide diuretics in controlling blood pressure.

Key Points

♦ Several studies suggest that ginkgo may slow the progression of dementia, particularly in Alzheimer's disease. However, the positive effect of ginkgo seems to be small. Further, not all studies reported improvements. A physician should be involved in deciding whether to supplement with ginkgo for dementia.

♦ Research in healthy individuals suggests that ginkgo supplementation may enhance some aspects of memory. More research is needed to clarify ginkgo's effect on cognitive function in healthy people. A large study (n = 1,570) suggests that daily ginkgo may enhance mood and increase participation in activities of daily living (ADLs) in healthy older volunteers (8). However, not all studies have shown improvements in memory with ginkgo in healthy people.

♦ Preliminary evidence suggests that ginkgo increases walking time and reduces pain in individuals with peripheral vascular disease and can increase forearm blood flow in healthy adults.

♦ Meta-analyses and clinical trials do not support a protective effect of ginkgo on tinnitus or mountain/altitude sickness.

Food Sources

None

Dosage Information/Bioavailability

Ginkgo biloba is available in tincture, infusions, capsule, or tablet form. The majority of research used a 50:1 concentrated leaf extract standardized to 24% ginkgo flavonoid glycosides and 6% terpenes (EGb 761). Manufacturers recommend taking 40 to 80 mg extract three times daily.

Relevant Research

Ginkgo and Alzheimer's Disease/Dementia

♦ Researchers summarized the effects of ginkgo on cognitive function in patients with Alzheimer's disease in a meta-analysis of randomized, placebo-controlled, double-blind studies. Of 50 articles reviewed, most did not meet inclusion criteria, primarily because of a lack of clear diagnosis. Of the four studies selected (total subjects = 212, lasting 3 to 6 months, using 120 to 230 mg ginkgo), there was a significant effect in favor of ginkgo that translated into a modest 3% difference in the Alzheimer's Disease Assessment Scale-cognitive subtest (9).

♦ In a double-blind, placebo-controlled, multicenter trial, 214 subjects with mild to moderate dementia (either Alzheimer's dementia or vascular-related dementia) were randomly assigned to receive a placebo or *Ginkgo biloba* EGb 761 (160 or 240 mg) for 12 weeks. After 12 weeks, the initial ginkgo users were randomly assigned again to either continued treatment or to a placebo for another 12 weeks. Outcome measures included neuropsychological testing, clinical assessment, self-perceived health and memory status, and self-reported level of daily life activities. An intention-to-treat analysis showed no effect on each of the outcome measures for subjects taking ginkgo compared with the placebo after 12 or 24 weeks. After 12 and 24 weeks, the combined ginkgo dose groups performed slightly, but significantly, better on self-reported activities of daily life. However, they performed slightly worse in regard to self-perceived health. No beneficial effects of the higher ginkgo dose were observed. Additionally, no subgroups seemed to benefit from ginkgo treatment. No negative side-effects were reported (10).

◆ In a double-blind, placebo-controlled, multicenter trial, 309 patients (older than 45 years) with Alzheimer's disease or multi-infarct dementia were randomly assigned to receive 120 mg *Ginkgo biloba* extract tablets (EGb 761) or a placebo daily for 52 weeks. Only 202 subjects completed the study (main reasons for dropout were non-compliance of subjects, caregiver request, and ineffective intervention). At weeks 12, 24, and 52, cognitive impairment, daily living and social behavior, and changes in psychopathology were assessed by the Alzheimer's Disease Assessment Scale (ADAS-Cog), Geriatric Evaluation by Relative's Rating Instrument (GERRI), and the Clinical Global Impression of Change (CGIC), respectively. Cognitive function decreased significantly in the placebo group, whereas no significant cognitive change was observed in the ginkgo group. Regarding daily living and social behavior as assessed by GERRI, a mild improvement was observed for ginkgo subjects, while the placebo group scores decreased, resulting in a significant difference between groups. There were no differences between groups in psychopathology as measured by CGIC, or in reported side effects (not specified). The authors concluded that ginkgo was safe and capable of stabilizing, and in some cases improving, cognitive performance and social function of patients with dementia for 6 months to 1 year (11).

◆ In a double-blind, placebo-controlled study, 216 patients with mild to moderate Alzheimer's disease or multi-infarct dementia were randomly assigned to receive 240 mg *Ginkgo biloba* extract (EGb 761) or a placebo for 24 weeks after a 4-week run-in period. Only 156 patients completed the trial. Psychopathological changes, attention and memory, and ADLs were variables measured by CGIC, Syndrom-Kurztest (SKT), and Nurnberger Alters-Beobachtungsskala, respectively. Clinical efficacy was defined as a response in at least two of the three variables. A significant clinical response was seen in 28% of the ginkgo group compared with 10% of the placebo group. When patients were analyzed by diagnosis, a greater benefit of ginkgo was seen for Alzheimer's patients than multi-infarct dementia patients (12). This data set was reanalyzed using modernized measurement and modified intent-to-treat analysis, resulting in a consistent finding for a beneficial effect of *Ginkgo biloba* in the treatment of dementia (13).

◆ A randomized trial in 214 elderly subjects with dementia was conducted in the Netherlands using placebo or *Ginkgo biloba* supplementation (160 or 240 mg/day) for 12 weeks, followed by a randomized crossover to *Ginkgo biloba* or placebo. Results showed no improvement in dementia scores (SKT) with *Ginkgo biloba*, regardless of dose or duration of treatment (14).

◆ A Cochrane Database Systematic Review that pooled adult subjects from randomized, controlled studies assessing the efficacy of *Ginkgo biloba* for cognitive impairment and dementia supported the use of less than 200 mg *Ginkgo biloba* daily for up to 12 weeks to improve clinical global improvement scores (OR = 15.3; 95% CI = 5.9–39.8). Significant, but less pronounced associations were demonstrated between *Ginkgo biloba* use at dosages of more than 200 mg/day and clinical global improvement scores as scored by physicians at 24 weeks (OR = 2.16; 95% CI = 1.11–4.20). There was also an overall significant improvement in cognition at 12 weeks as compared to placebo which persisted through 52 weeks of follow-up. Furthermore, activities of daily living (ADLs) also improved significantly by 12 weeks as compared with placebo. However, the authors acknowledge that more recent studies with improved design (double-blinded) have not been consistent in their findings, and a large, prospective, randomized, controlled trial with an intent-to-treat analysis is needed (15).

Ginkgo for Memory and Concentration in Healthy People

- A 6-week, randomized, double-blind, placebo-controlled, parallel group trial of ginkgo extract (EGb 761) vs placebo was conducted in 262 healthy elderly adults who showed baseline Mini-Mental State Examination scores more than 26 (indicating normal cognitive function). After 6 weeks of daily supplementation with 180 mg ginkgo biloba, there was a significant improvement in Selective Reminding Test (SRT) and Weschler Memory Scale Faces II scores when changes in scores over time were compared between ginkgo and placebo groups (16).

- In a double-blind, placebo-controlled study, 256 healthy, middle-aged subjects were randomly assigned to receive a placebo or a combination of ginkgo and *Panax ginseng* in two dosing regimens (60 mg ginkgo + 100 mg ginseng or 120 mg ginkgo + 200 mg ginseng) for 14 weeks. At baseline and at weeks 4, 8, 12, and 14, subjects performed a series of tests of attention and memory from the CDR computerized assessment system prior to morning dosing and again at 1, 3, and 6 hours later. Subjects also completed questionnaires about mood, quality of life, and sleep quality. The ginkgo-ginseng mixture yielded significantly improved results on an Index of Memory Quality. However, the design of the study does not identify whether the ginkgo, the ginseng, or the combination of both herbs is responsible for the improvement in memory (17).

- A randomized, double-blind, placebo-controlled, parallel group design study of over-the-counter ginkgo (120 mg/day) in 98 male and 132 female healthy, elderly community-dwelling volunteers has shown that ginkgo supplementation, when analyzed using intent-to-treat analysis, was not associated with improved performance on standardized neuropsychological tests of learning, memory, attention, or concentration (18).

- In a double-blind, placebo-controlled study, 48 healthy subjects (ages 55 to 86 years) with normal cognitive function were randomly assigned to receive 180 mg ginkgo extract (EGb 761) or a placebo daily for 6 weeks. Cognitive function was evaluated by a series of neuropsychological tests at baseline and at 6 weeks. Compared with placebo, ginkgo treatment was associated with significant improvement on a task assessing speed of processing abilities (eg, Stroop Color and Word Test color-naming task). There was a trend favoring improved performances in the ginkgo group in three of the four remaining tasks that involved a timed speed of processing component, but this did not reach statistical significance. In contrast, no improvements were observed with ginkgo in relation to any of the objective memory measures. The subjects' self-assessment of memory significantly improved with use of ginkgo compared with the placebo (19).

- In a double-blind, placebo-controlled study, 31 subjects older than 50 years with mild to moderate memory impairment were randomly assigned to receive 120 mg *Ginkgo biloba* extract (EGb 761) divided into three doses or a placebo daily for 6 months. At weeks 0, 12, and 24, subjects were assessed with a range of psychometric tests. In the ginkgo group, cognitive function improved significantly compared with baseline on the digit copying subtest of the Kendrick battery at weeks 12 and 24, and improved significantly on the median response speed on a classification task than the placebo at week 24. However, subjects taking ginkgo performed worse over time on the digit recall task compared with the placebo group (20).

- A systematic review of 40 European trials testing ginkgo extract to improve cerebral insufficiency (characterized by symptoms of concentration and memory difficulties, confusion, fatigue, depression, and anxiety) found that only eight of the trials were well-controlled. The authors noted that all 40 trials reported positive results and suggested there may have been a publication bias (21).

Ginkgo and Peripheral Vascular Disease

- A meta-analysis of eight randomized, placebo-controlled, double-blinded trials evaluated the efficacy of ginkgo extract for intermittent claudication. There was a significant difference in the increase in pain-free walking distance in favor of ginkgo (+33 meters). The authors concluded that ginkgo "is superior to placebo in the symptomatic treatment of intermittent claudication. However, the overall treatment effect is modest and of uncertain clinical relevance" (22).

- In a double-blind, placebo-controlled, multicenter trial, 111 subjects with peripheral occlusive arterial disease (mean age 61 years) were randomly assigned to receive 120 mg *Ginkgo biloba* extract (EGb 761) or a placebo for 24 weeks. The distance of pain-free walking on a treadmill was measured after weeks 0, 8, 16, and 24. Pain-free walking distance and maximal walking distance were significantly greater in the ginkgo subjects. Doppler studies measuring blood flow were unchanged in both groups. Subjective assessment showed an amelioration of symptoms in both groups (23).

- In a placebo-controlled trial, 37 subjects with stage 2 peripheral vascular disease were randomly assigned to receive *Ginkgo biloba* extract (EGb 761) or a placebo daily for 6 months. Subjects who took ginkgo had a significant improvement in walking distance compared with the placebo group. Doppler studies did not show any improvement in the perfusion of the ischemic leg (24).

- A randomized, double-blind, placebo-controlled, crossover design study of ginkgo vs placebo was conducted to determine changes in hemodynamics of forearms (forearm vascular resistance) of healthy young adults (n = 16; mean age 32 years). Eight subjects were randomly assigned to 9.6 mg ginkgoflavonglucoside and 2.4 mg terpenlactones, whereas the other eight were assigned to placebo for a period of 6 weeks. Forearm vascular resistance was assessed at 3, 6, 9, and 12 weeks. Subjects were switched to the alternate treatment after 6 weeks of treatment. The results demonstrated that blood flow was significantly greater during treatment with ginkgo (at both 3 and 6 weeks) while systemic blood pressure remained unchanged (25).

Ginkgo and Tinnitus

◆ In a randomized, double-blind, placebo-controlled trial in 66 subjects with tinnitus, use of 120 mg of sustained release ginkgo daily for 12 weeks (n = 31) showed no significant improvement in Tinnitus Handicap Inventory, Glasgow Health Status Inventory, or hearing threshold as compared with baseline or change demonstrated by the placebo group subjects (26). This article included a meta-analysis of six published randomized, placebo-controlled human studies in which the dosage of ginkgo ranged from 29.2 to 160 mg daily. Using a pooled analysis, it was found that ginkgo treatment provided no benefit for tinnitus above placebo.

◆ A 2004 Cochrane Database meta-analysis of research on ginkgo for tinnitus reviewed 12 trials and determined that none had adequate scientific methodology for inclusion. The authors concluded that "the limited evidence did not demonstrate that GB [*Ginkgo biloba*] was effective for tinnitus" (27).

Ginkgo and Mountain Sickness

◆ The effect of ginkgo on acute mountain sickness was tested in 57 subjects who were randomly assigned in a double-blind fashion to receive a single 120-mg dose of ginkgo, standard medication (acetazolamide), or placebo before ascent to an elevation of 3,800 meters. The medication resulted in a significant reduction in Lake Louise Acute Mountain Sickness (LLAMS) score, whereas subjects receiving ginkgo had LLAMS scores equivalent to the placebo group, which indicates that ginkgo was not effective in reducing altitude sickness in this group (28).

◆ In a separate study of 614 healthy male trekkers, 487 of whom completed the Himalayan trek (approximate elevation of 4,300 meters) and were between the ages of 18 and 65 years, participated in a randomized, double-blind, placebo-controlled study testing the efficacy of ginkgo for altitude sickness. For 1.5 to 2 full days prior to ascent, participants took 3 to 4 doses of (*a*) ginkgo (120 mg twice daily), (*b*) ginkgo plus acetazolamide (250 mg twice daily), (*c*) acetazolamide alone, or (*d*) placebo. Among subjects taking ginkgo alone, 35% showed symptoms of acute mountain sickness, compared with 34% in the placebo group and 12% of those receiving acetazolamide alone and 16% receiving the combined therapy. None of these differences were statistically significant across groups or as compared with baseline (29).

References

1. Blumenthal M, ed. *The Complete German Commission E Monographs Therapeutic Guide to Herbal Medicines*. Austin, Tex: American Botanical Council; 1998.
2. Smith PF, Maclennan K, Darlington CL. The neuroprotective properties of the *Ginkgo biloba* leaf: a review of the possible relationship to platelet-activating factor (PAF). *J Ethnopharmacol*. 1996;50:131–139.
3. Arenz A, Kelin M, Flehe K, et al. Occurrence of neurotoxic 4'-O-methylpyridoxine in ginkgo biloba leaves, ginkgo medications and Japanese ginkgo food. *Planta Med*. 1996;62:548–551.

4. Kajiyama Y, Fuji K, Takeuchi H, et al. Ginkgo seed poisoning. *Pediatrics.* 2002;109: 325–327.
5. Kohler S, Funk P, Kieser M. Influence of a 7-day treatment with Ginkgo biloba special extract EGb 761 on bleeding time and coagulation: a randomized, placebo-controlled, double-blind study in healthy volunteers. *Blood Coagul Fibrinolysis.* 2004;15:303–309.
6. Ang-Lee, Moss J, Yuan CS. Herbal medicines and perioperative care. *JAMA.* 2001;286:208–216.
7. Siegers CP. Cytotoxicity of alkylphenols from Ginkgo biloba. *Phytomedicine.* 1999;6: 281–283.
8. Trick L, Boyle J, Hindmarch I. The effects of Ginkgo biloba extract (LI 1370) supplementation and discontinuation on activities of daily living and mood in free living older volunteers. *Phytother Res.* 2004;18:531–537.
9. Oken BS, Storzbach DM, Kaye JA. The efficacy of *Ginkgo biloba* on cognitive function in Alzheimer disease. *Arch Neurol.* 1998;55:1409–1415.
10. van Dongen MC, van Rossum E, Kessels AG, et al. The efficacy of ginkgo for elderly people with dementia and age-associated memory impairment: new results of a randomized clinical trial. *J Am Geriatr Soc.* 2000;48:1183–1194.
11. Le Bars PL, Katz MM, Berman N, et al. A placebo-controlled, double-blind, randomized trial of an extract of *Ginkgo biloba* for dementia. *JAMA.* 1997;278:1327–1332.
12. Kanowski S, Herrmann WM, Stephan K, et al. Proof of efficacy of the *Ginkgo biloba* special extract EGb 761 in outpatients suffering from mild to moderate primary degenerative dementia of the Alzheimer type or multi-infarct dementia. *Pharmacopsychiatry.* 1996;29:47–56.
13. Kanowski S, Hoerr R. Ginkgo biloba extract EGb761 in dementia: intent-to-treat analyses of a 24-week, multi-center, double-blind, placebo-controlled, randomized trial. *Pharmacopsychiatry.* 2003;36:297–303.
14. Van Dongen M, van Rossum E, Kessels A, et al. Ginkgo for elderly people with dementia and age-associated memory impairment: a randomized clinical trial. *J Clin Epidemiol.* 2003;56:367–376.
15. Birks J, Grimley EV, van Dongen M. Ginkgo biloba for cognitive impairment and dementia. *Cochrane Database Syst Rev.* 2002;(4):CD003120.
16. Mix JA, Crews WD Jr. A double-blind, placebo-controlled, randomized trial of Ginkgo biloba extract EGb 761 in a sample of cognitively intact older adults: neuropsychological findings. *Hum Psychopharmacol.* 2002;17:267–277.
17. Wesnes KA, Ward T, McGinty A, et al. The memory enhancing effects of *Ginkgo biloba*/Panax ginseng combination in healthy middle-aged volunteers. *Psychopharmacology (Berl).* 2000;152:353–361.
18. Solomano PR, Adams F, Silver A, et al. Ginkgo for memory enhancement: a randomized controlled trial. *JAMA.* 2002;288:835–840.
19. Mix JA, Crews WD. An examination of *Ginkgo biloba* extract EGb 761 on the neuropsychological functioning of cognitively intact older adults. *J Altern Complement Med.* 2000;6:219–229.
20. Rai GS, Shovlin C, Wesnes KA. A double-blind, placebo-controlled study of *Ginkgo biloba* extract ("tanakan") in elderly outpatients with mild to moderate memory impairment. *Curr Med Res Opin.* 1991;12:350–355.

21. Kleijnen J, Knipschild P. *Ginkgo biloba* for cerebral insufficiency. *Br J Clin Pharmacol.* 1992;34:352–358.
22. Pittler MH, Ernst E. *Ginkgo biloba* extract for the treatment of intermittent claudication: a meta-analysis of randomized trials. *Am J Med.* 2000;108:276–281.
23. Peters H, Kieser M, Holscher U. Demonstration of the efficacy of *Ginkgo biloba* special extract EGb 761 on intermittent claudication—a placebo-controlled, double-blind multicenter trial. *Vasa.* 1998;27:106–110.
24. Thomson GJ, Vohra RK, Carr MH, et al. A clinical trial of *Ginkgo biloba* extract in patients with intermittent claudication. *Int Angiol.* 1990;9:75–78.
25. Mehlsen J, Drabeck H, Wiinberg N, et al. Effects of a Ginkgo biloba extract on forearm haemodynamics in healthy volunteers. *Clin Physiol Funct Imaging.* 2002;22: 375–378.
26. Rejali D, Sivakumar A, Balaji N. Ginkgo biloba does not benefit patients with tinnitus: a randomized placebo-controlled double-blind trial and meta-analysis of randomized trials. *Clin Otolaryngol Allied Sci.* 2004;29:226–231.
27. Hilton M, Stuart E. Ginkgo biloba for tinnitus. *Cochrane Database Syst Rev.* 2004;(2):CD003852.
28. Chow T, Browne V, Heilson HL, et al. Ginkgo biloba and acetazolamide prophylaxis for acute mountain sickness: a randomized, placebo-controlled trial. *Arch Intern Med.* 2005;165:296–301.
29. Gertsch JH, Basnyat B, Johnson EW, et al. Randomised, double-blind, placebo controlled comparison of ginkgo biloba and acetazolamide for prevention of acute mountain sickness among Himalayan trekkers: the prevention of high altitude illness trial (PHAIT). *BMJ.* 2004;328:797.

Ginseng

Ginseng is the collective term used to describe several species of plants belonging to the genus *Panax*. Asian ginsengs (*Panax ginseng* C.A. Meyer and *Panax japonicus* C.A. Meyer) have been used medicinally for more than 2,000 years in China, Japan, and Korea. American ginseng (*Panax quinquefolius L*) grows in North America and is largely exported to Asia. Siberian/Russian ginseng (*Eleutherococcus senticosus*) is not considered a true "ginseng" because it is not in the genus *Panax*. (Although Siberian ginseng *[E. senticosus]* is not related botanically to Asian or American ginseng, it is included here because it is often sold alongside *Panax ginseng* products.)

The bioactive compounds in the *Panax* plant are believed to be the saponins (or ginsenosides) found in the roots. Several ginsenosides that have been identified are labeled ginsenoside R_x, (where x is a, b_1, b_2, c, d, e, f, g_1, g_2, g_3, h_1, h_2, or o). Eleutherosides, which are believed to be the active agents in Siberian ginseng, have different chemical structures than do ginsenosides. Ginseng plants contain varying levels of several different saponins that seem to exert opposing pharmacologic effects. This natural variation may explain the conflicting results in ginseng studies reported in the literature. Other reasons for differing results may be related to time of harvest; lack of standardization of bioactive compounds; and variability in dosage, administration, and type of ginseng used (1–3).

Media and Marketing Claims	Efficacy
Improves exercise performance	↓
Improves quality of life, energy, mood, cognition	↔
Improves sexual function; aphrodisiac	NR
Helps control blood glucose levels in diabetes	NR
Reduces risk for cancer	NR

Safety

- No serious adverse effects have been reported in the research in subjects consuming ginseng for short periods of time.

- Reports of hypertension, nervousness, sleeplessness, acne, edema, headache, and diarrhea have been associated with ingestion of more than 3 g ginseng root per day (equivalent to approximately 600 mg ginseng extract) (4).

- According to the German Commission E monographs, Siberian ginseng root, but not *Panax* ginseng root, is contraindicated for those with hypertension (5).

- Ginsenosides may inhibit platelet aggregation and increase bleeding time; therefore, one review suggested that ginseng be discontinued at least 7 days before surgery (6).

- Although ginseng may slow coagulation, in one case report ginseng was associated with the opposite effect: it decreased the efficacy of warfarin (7). A recent pharmacokinetic study did not support changes in prothrombin time or platelet aggregation or warfarin pharmacokinetics or pharmacodynamics in 12 healthy male subjects (8).

- Animal data suggest that American ginseng may be teratogenic; therefore, it should not be taken during pregnancy (9) or lactation.

- Ginseng should not be taken by individuals at risk or previously treated for estrogen-related cancer (breast, ovarian, etc) because it has been shown to have estrogenic effects (10).

- Some studies have shown ginseng to have a potential hypoglycemic effect; individuals with diabetes should monitor their blood glucose levels.

Drug/Supplement Interactions

- Ginseng may interfere with phenelzine (a monamine oxidase inhibitor), corticosteroids, digoxin, diabetes medications, and estrogen therapy.

- Ginseng may increase bleeding time when taken with other blood-thinning drugs or supplements (warfarin, garlic, ginger, ginkgo, vitamin E, flaxseed, bromelain, dong quai, fish oil, aspirin); use should be monitored by a physician.

◆ Use of ginseng with caffeine may stimulate hypertension.

◆ Use of Siberian ginseng was associated with elevated digoxin levels in a 74-year-old man on digoxin therapy. Digoxin levels returned to the therapeutic range after ginseng was discontinued (11).

◆ Ginseng has been reported to have mild hormonal effects similar to those of estrogen and therefore may interact with hormone replacement, oral contraceptives, or select estrogen receptor modulators. Cases of both postmenopausal bleeding and premenopausal amenorrhea have been documented with ginseng use (12).

◆ One review article summarized research suggesting that ginseng blocks the analgesic effects of opioids (morphine) and inhibits the tolerance to and dependence on opioids and psychostimulants (13).

Key Points

◆ Although hundreds of ginseng studies have been conducted in Asia, most of the research has not been translated into English and thus is difficult to review. Furthermore, confusion is exacerbated by the difference in Eastern compared with Western interpretations of the effects of ginseng. For instance, Eastern traditional medicine practitioners would suggest that the actions of opposing ginsenosides "adapt" to meet the individual's individual mental or physical state. Western practitioners would assume that the differing actions of the ginsenosides neutralize each other (14). The results from the research are insufficient to support or refute either argument.

◆ Controlled studies do not support ginseng use to enhance exercise performance or reduce fatigue in humans. There are several studies that purportedly show an ergogenic benefit, but they have been criticized for lacking sufficient controls and blinding (1,2).

◆ Although animal trials suggest some benefit to ginseng in boosting energy, there is little comparable research in humans.

◆ Scientists have suggested a hypothesis for the possible aphrodisiac effect of ginseng involving the production of nitric oxide, which may enhance penile blood flow. However, sufficient data to support this hypothesis are lacking.

◆ Animal data and a few small studies of individuals with diabetes suggest that ginseng may exert a hypoglycemic effect; however, more controlled clinical research is needed to verify this effect.

◆ Epidemiological evidence from Korea suggests a possible reduced risk of cancer associated with ginseng consumption. Ginseng has also exhibited potential anticancer effects in animal and in vitro studies.

◆ Because of the complex chemical composition of the ginseng root and lack of controlled studies, it is not surprising that evidence is inconclusive regarding its clinical impact. Variations in harvest time/maturity of plant roots, different methods of preparation, lack of standardized preparation, and varying dosages and administrations of ginseng complicate research about the efficacy of this herb. Animal studies have also been criticized for using very high doses to achieve short-term effects ("forced pharmacology") and for administering intravenous as opposed to oral ginseng (14). Overall, there have been few placebo-controlled, double-blind clinical studies using ginseng preparations with known ginsenoside contents.

Food Sources

Fresh ginseng root is available at health food stores and Asian markets.

Dosage Information/Bioavailability

Ginseng (Asian, American, or Siberian/Russian) is available in capsules, tablets, tinctures, powders, and teas. Products usually provide 100 to 400 mg of dried extract equivalent to 0.5 to 2.0 g of ginseng root. Ginseng roots are air-dried, producing white ginseng, or steam treated, yielding red ginseng. Although products claim to be standardized with 4% to 7% ginsenosides, a survey of 50 commercial ginseng products sold in 11 countries found the ginsenoside concentrations varied greatly, with some products containing no ginseng compounds at all (15). Several studies have used G115, a *Panax ginseng* CA Meyer *(P. ginseng)* extract standardized to contain 13 ginsenosides at a level of 4%. Animal studies have shown a rapid absorption of ginsenoside Rg_1 following an oral dose (16).

The American Botanical Council's Ginseng Evaluation Program (GEP) reported the results of a 7-year study that examined 500 commercial ginseng products for content and consistency. One component of the program was an encoded, blinded study of 13 Asian ginseng products for lot-to-lot consistency assessed by (*a*) frequency of acceptable R_{b1}/R_{g1} value; (*b*) percentage of lots (within a product) that met claim for total ginsenoside content; and (*c*) percent relative standard deviation of total ginsenoside content. Overall, most products were reasonably consistent. However, GEP found that the term "standardized" on labels was frequently inappropriate, confusing, or misleading (17).

Relevant Research

Ginseng and Exercise Performance

- In a randomized, controlled, double-blind study of 92 adults diagnosed with chronic obstructive pulmonary disease (COPD), subjects were randomly assigned to receive either ginseng at a dosage of 100 mg twice/day (n = 49) or placebo (n = 43) for 3 months. Pulmonary function tests (PFTs), maximal voluntary ventilation (MVV), and maximal inspiratory pressure (MIP) were assessed every 2 weeks throughout the study period. Exercise test and maximum oxygen consumption (VO_{2max}) were tested at baseline, and at 6 and 12 weeks. Comparison of change in performance from baseline to 6 and 12 weeks as measured by PFTs, MVV, MIP and VO_{2max} showed that the intervention group demonstrated significant improvements while the placebo group did not (18). However, there was wide variability in disease severity, which was not clearly controlled for. Further research is needed before use of ginseng in COPD can be advocated.

◆ In a double-blind, placebo-controlled study, 28 nonathlete subjects were randomly assigned to receive 200 mg *P. ginseng* (7% standardized ginsenosides) or a placebo daily for 3 weeks. Before and at the end of the study period, subjects completed a maximal exercise test on a cycle ergometer. There were no significant effects of ginseng administration on exercise time, workload, VO_{2max}, heart rate, plasma lactate, or hematocrit at peak; or in rate of perceived exertion at 150 watts, 200 watts, or peak. The authors concluded: "This study does not support an ergogenic effect on peak aerobic exercise performance following a 3-week supplementation period in healthy, young adults with moderate exercise capacities and unrestricted diets" (19).

◆ In a double-blind, placebo-controlled trial, 36 young, healthy men (not athletes) were randomly assigned to receive 200 or 400 mg of a standardized ginseng extract capsules (G115) or a placebo daily for 8 weeks. This dosage was equivalent to 1 to 2 g *P. ginseng* root. Thirty-one subjects completed the study. Submaximal and maximal aerobic exercise parameters were measured before and after the trial. Ginseng had no effect on oxygen consumption, respiratory exchange ratio, minute ventilation, blood lactic acid, heart rate, or rate of perceived exertion (20).

◆ In a double-blind, placebo-controlled, crossover study, 50 male gym teachers received in random order (*a*) capsules containing an unspecified amount of *P. ginseng* extract (G115) in combination with dimethylamino-ethanol bitartrate (choline complex), vitamins, and minerals, or (*b*) a placebo daily for 6 weeks each, separated by a 1-week washout period. The ginseng-choline complex significantly enhanced total workload and maximal oxygen uptake during maximal exercise tests compared with the placebo. The ginseng-choline complex also resulted in statistically significant lower oxygen consumption, plasma lactate levels, ventilation, CO_2 production, and heart rates during exercise. The effects of the ginseng-choline supplement were more pronounced in subjects with lower VO_{2max} capacities (21). In this study, the potential effects of ginseng could not be separated from those of the other ingredients in the combined supplement regimen.

◆ In a double-blind, placebo-controlled study, 20 elite distance runners were randomly assigned in matched pairs (matched by gender, body weight, and 10-km race pace) to receive 60 drops (3.4 mL) of *E. senticosus L* (Siberian ginseng) extract containing eleutherosides B and E or a placebo daily for 6 weeks. Every 2 weeks, and 2 weeks after the study's end, subjects completed a 10-minute treadmill run at their 10-km pace and a maximal treadmill test. Siberian ginseng had no effect on time to exhaustion, heart rate, VO_{2max}, rate of perceived exertion, respiratory exchange ratio, or serum lactate (22).

◆ Although some studies have suggested that ginseng or its active components may prolong survival to physical or chemical stress in animals, a comprehensive review found that there is lack of compelling evidence demonstrating the ability of ginseng to consistently enhance physical performance in humans (1,2).

Ginseng for Mood and Cognitive Function

◆ In a double-blind, placebo-controlled, parallel design, randomized study using a combined *Panax* ginseng—*Ginkgo biloba* supplement that contained 100 mg ginseng, 256 healthy adults randomly assigned to the combined supplement (160 mg twice a day or 320 mg daily) or placebo. Seventeen cognitive tests were applied to determine the overall Index of Memory Quality score for each participant. The group receiving the ginseng-ginkgo combination supplement, regardless of dosage approach (single or divided dose), had significantly greater memory index as compared with those receiving placebo at each timepoint throughout the 12-week intervention and 2 weeks postintervention (23).

◆ In a double-blind, placebo-controlled study, 83 healthy men and women (mean age 27 years) were randomly assigned to receive one of three treatments for 8 weeks: (*a*) a placebo; (*b*) 200 mg *P. ginseng* (G115); or (*c*) 400 mg *P. ginseng* (G115). Prior to intervention and after 56 to 60 days of supplementing, subjects' positive and negative affect was assessed by the 20-item Positive Affect Negative Affect Scale and the 65-item Profile of Mood States Inventory, which measured total mood disturbance. Ginseng had no effect on psychological well-being (affect or mood) at either dose compared with the placebo (24).

◆ In a double-blind, placebo-controlled (not randomized) trial, 60 geriatric subjects received a commercial product containing 40 mg *P. ginseng* extract (G115) and vitamins and minerals or a placebo daily for 8 weeks. Length of stay in the hospital, activities of daily living, cognitive function (measured using the Mini-Mental State Examination, Kendrick Object Learning test, and the Trail Making test) and symptoms of depression and anxiety were assessed. Forty-nine subjects finished the study (25 in the placebo group, 24 in the ginseng group). Reasons for dropping out included lack of motivation; difficulty swallowing the capsules; and clinical events unrelated to treatment (one hip fracture and one death in the placebo group). There were no differences between groups, except the placebo group had a significant improvement on one cognitive function test (Kendrick Object Learning Test). The authors concluded that there was no identifiable benefit of the ginseng complex as adjuvant to treatment and rehabilitation of geriatric patients (25). The potential effects of ginseng could not be separated from those of other ingredients in the combined supplement regimen. In addition, the lack of randomization weakens the findings of this study.

Ginseng and Sexual Function

◆ Traditional Chinese medicine has long used ginseng as an aphrodisiac. It has been hypothesized that ginseng may act as an aphrodisiac by enhancing nitric oxide (NO) production, which plays a potential role in stimulating penile erection (3,26).

◆ A randomized, double-blind, placebo-controlled crossover-design trial of Korean red ginseng (900 mg three times/day) given to 45 subjects with erectile dysfunction for 8 weeks, followed by a 2-week washout, and a crossover to the alternate treatment for an additional 8 weeks, showed that the ginseng supplement was able to modulate erectile function. While receiving ginseng, subjects reported significantly higher mean International Index of Erectile Function (IIEF) scores ($P = .01$). Penile tip rigidity was also used as an objective measure of improved function, and this measure also showed significantly greater function for subjects while on ginseng vs placebo (27).

- In a placebo-controlled (not blinded) study, 90 subjects with erectile dysfunction (not because of organic causes) were randomly assigned to one of three groups for 3 months: (*a*) 300 mg *P. ginseng*/day; (*b*) trazodone (antidepressant)/day; or (*c*) placebo. Changes in frequency of intercourse, premature ejaculation, and morning erections after treatment were not changed in any group. However, improvements in early detumescence, penile rigidity and girth, libido, and patient satisfaction were greater in the ginseng group compared with the placebo or trazodone-treated groups. None of the treatments resulted in complete remission of erectile dysfunction (28). The lack of blinding in this study may have introduced bias.

Ginseng and Diabetes

- In a double-blind, placebo-controlled study, 36 individuals newly diagnosed with type 2 diabetes were treated with 100 or 200 mg ginseng extract daily (species and percent ginsenosides were not identified) or a placebo for 8 weeks. Subjective tests of mood, vigor, memory, sleep, physical activity, and well-being were self-rated on linear analog scales. Psychophysical performance was evaluated by time to complete a numbered diagram. Fasting blood glucose, serum lipids, A1C, serum aminoterminal propetide (PIIINP), and fasting serum immunoreactive insulin (IRI) and C-peptide were also measured. Subjects were given individual and group-based instruction on diabetes management including diet and glucose monitoring. Ginseng therapy resulted in a significant reduction in fasting blood glucose, elevation in mood, and improvement of psychophysical performance, but it had no effect on memory, sleep, serum lipids, or IRI. The 200-mg dosage resulted in a significant improvement in A1C and PIIINP and increased physical activity. The authors speculated that ginseng improved subjects' mood, which may have improved self-care and physical activity, and thus led to improved glucose balance (29).

- Evidence from a study comparing the hypoglycemic effects of eight different types of ginseng (American, American wild, Asian, Asian red, Vietnamese wild, Siberian, Japanese rhizome, and Sanchi ginsengs) that contain variable types and concentrations of ginosenosides indicates that variance in constituents may account for the variability in results (blood glucose modulation) shown across studies (30). In this study, which used a randomized, double-blind, multiple-crossover design, 12 (6 men and 6 women) of the 14 nondiabetic adults recruited were able to complete the trial. Subjects were between the ages of 18 and 53 years and had BMIs ranging from 18.8 to 33.9. In each stage of the trial, subjects took a 3-g dosage of one type of ginseng or a placebo 40 minutes before a 75-g oral glucose tolerance test. There were a total of ten stages (ie, all subjects took each type of ginseng and two placebos). Glucose and insulin levels were evaluated at baseline (40 minutes prior) and at 0 (at time of ginseng dose), 15, 30, 45, 60, 90, and 120 minutes. American and Vietnamese ginsengs tended to significantly lower plasma glucose as compared with placebo whereas Asian, American wild, and Siberian ginseng elevated plasma glucose at variable time points as compared with placebo.

Ginseng and Cancer

◆ *Panax ginseng* has been postulated as a likely chemotherapeutic agent. A recent review paper described the potential role of ginseng in cancer prevention. The article provides evidence of the antioxidant, anti-inflammatory, apoptotic, and gene-modulating effects of this compound, which may account for any anticarcinogenic effects (31).

◆ In a study among 49 patients who had undergone resection of gastric cancer lesions in Korea, individuals with stage III gastric cancer were treated with *Panax* (red) ginseng (4.5 g/day) or placebo for 6 months postoperatively, during 5-FU chemotherapy. The red ginseng was associated with a significant reduction in mortality (7/22 vs 13/20 for placebo) as well as significantly greater mean survival time (44.4 months vs 33.5 months for placebo) (32). Although favorable, these results seem so pronounced that replication of these findings is needed in larger study populations with longer follow-up. A large symposium on this topic was held in Korea in 2001 and published in the *Journal of Korean Medical Science* (33).

◆ A case-control study of 905 pairs of case and control subjects matched by age, sex, and date of admission to the Korea Cancer Center Hospital reported a statistically significant decrease in cancer cases with increasing frequency of *P. ginseng* CA Meyer intake. Ginseng extract and powder seemed to be associated with a lower risk of cancer than did fresh sliced ginseng, ginseng juice, or ginseng tea (34). A second case-control study of 1,987 pairs of subjects reported similar results. On the site of cancer, the odds ratios were 0.47 for cancer of the lip, oral cavity, and pharynx; 0.20 for esophageal cancer; 0.36 for stomach cancer; 0.42 for colorectal cancer; 0.48 for liver cancer; 0.22 for pancreatic cancer; 0.18 for laryngeal cancer; 0.55 for lung cancer; and 0.15 for ovarian cancer. In cancers of the female breast, uterine cervix, urinary bladder, and thyroid gland, however, there was no association with ginseng intake (35). Recall data of ginseng intake were used rather than plasma levels of ginsenosides.

◆ According to one review, a 5-year prospective cohort study of 4,587 Korean subjects older than age 40 reported a significant decreased risk of cancer incidence in ginseng consumers (relative risk of 0.48) compared with nonconsumers. The risk decreased as the frequency of ginseng intake increased, demonstrating a significant dose-responsive effect (36).

◆ The same review summarized animal and in vitro research on ginseng and cancer. The author noted that ginsenosides have demonstrated in vitro antimutagenic activity, inhibition of tumor cell lines in mice and humans, and immunmodulating activity. Other constituents of ginseng (polysaccharides, polyacetylenes) have also exhibited potential cancer-protective effects (36).

References

1. Bahrke MS, Morgan WR. Evaluation of the ergogenic properties of ginseng. *Sports Med.* 1994;18:229–248.
2. Bahrke MS, Morgan WR. Evaluation of the ergogenic properties of ginseng: an update. *Sports Med.* 2000;29:113–133.
3. Gillis CN. *Panax ginseng* pharmacology: a nitric oxide link? *Biochem Pharmacol.* 1997;54:1–8.
4. Siegel RK. Ginseng abuse syndrome: problems with the panacea. *JAMA.* 1979;241: 1614–1615.
5. Blumenthal M, ed. *The Complete German Commission E Monographs Therapeutic Guide to Herbal Medicines.* Austin, Texas: American Botanical Council; 1998.
6. Ang-Lee, Moss J, Yuan CS. Herbal medicines and perioperative care. *JAMA.* 2001;286: 208–216.
7. Yuan CS, Wei G, Dey L, et al. American ginseng reduces warfarin's effect in healthy patients: a randomized, controlled trial. *Ann Intern Med.* 2004;141:23–27.
8. Jiang X, Williams KM, Liauw WS, et al. Effect of St John's wort and ginseng on the pharmacokinetics and pharmacodynamics of warfarin in healthy subjects. *Br J Clin Pharmacol.* 2004;57:592–599.
9. Chan LY, Chiu PY, Lau TK. An in-vitro study of ginsenoside Rb(1)-induced teratogenicity using a whole rat embryo culture model. *Human Reprod.* 2003;18:2166–2168.
10. Amato P, Christophe S, Mellon PL. Estrogenic activity of herbs commonly used as remedies for menopausal symptoms. *Menopause.* 2002;9:145–150.
11. McRae S. Elevated serum digoxin levels in patient taking digoxin and Siberian ginseng. *CMAJ.* 1996;155:293–295.
12. Greenspan EM. Ginseng and vaginal bleeding. *JAMA.* 1983;249:2018.
13. Takahashi M, Tokuyama S. Pharmacological and physiological effects of ginseng on actions induced by opioids and psychostimulants. *Methods Find Exp Clin Pharmacol.* 1998;20:77–84.
14. Sonnenborn U, Proppert Y. Ginseng (Panax ginseng CA Meyer). *Br J Phytother.* 1991; 2:3–14.
15. Cui J, Garle M, Eneroth P, et al. What do commercial ginseng preparations contain? *Lancet.* 1994;344:134.
16. Odani T, Tanizawa H, Takino Y. Studies on the absorption, distribution, excretion and metabolism of ginseng saponins: the absorption, distribution, and excretion of ginsenoside R_{g1} in the rat. *Chem Pharm Bull (Tokyo).* 1983;31:292–298.
17. Hall T, Lu ZZ, Yat PN, et al. Evaluation of consistency of standardized Asian ginseng products in the ginseng evaluation program. *HerbalGram.* 2001;52:31–45.
18. Gross D, Shenkman Z, Bleiberg B, et al. Ginseng improves pulmonary functions and exercise capacity in patients with COPD. *Monaldi Arch Chest Dis.* 2002;57:225–226.
19. Allen JD, McLung J, Nelson AG, et al. Ginseng supplementation does not enhance healthy young adults' peak aerobic exercise performance. *J Am Coll Nutr.* 1998;17: 462–466.
20. Engels HJ, Wirth JC. No ergogenic effects of ginseng (*Panax ginseng* CA Meyer) during graded maximal aerobic exercise. *J Am Diet Assoc.* 1997;97:1110–1115.

21. Pieralisi G, Ripari P, Vecchiet L. Effects of a standardized ginseng extract combined with dimethylaminoethanol bitartrate, vitamins, minerals, and trace elements on physical performance during exercise. *Clin Ther.* 1991;13:373–382.

22. Dowling EA, Redondo DR, Branch JD, et al. Effect of *Eleutherococcus senticosus* on submaximal and maximal exercise performance. *Med Sci Sports Exerc.* 1996;28: 482–489.

23. Wesnes KA, Ward T, McGinty A, et al. The memory enhancing effects of a Ginkgo biloba/Panax ginseng combination in healthy middle-aged volunteers. *Psychopharmacology.* 2000;152:353–361.

24. Cardinal BJ, Engels HJ. Ginseng does not enhance psychological well-being in healthy, young adults: results of a double-blind, placebo-controlled randomized clinical trial. *J Am Diet Assoc.* 2001;101:655–660.

25. Thommessen B, Laake K. No identifiable effect of ginseng (Gericomplex) as an adjuvant in the treatment of geriatric patients. *Aging (Milano).* 1996;8:417–420.

26. Chen X. Cardiovascular protection by ginsenosides and their nitric oxide releasing action. *Clin Exp Pharmacol Physiol.* 1996;23:728–732.

27. Hong B, Ji YH, Hong JH, et al. A double-blind crossover study evaluating the efficacy of Korean red ginseng in patients with erectile dysfunction: a preliminary report. *J Urol.* 2002;168:2070–2073.

28. Choi HK, Seong DH, Rha KH. Clinical efficacy of Korean red ginseng for erectile dysfunction. *Int J Impot Res.* 1995;7:181–186.

29. Sotaniemi EA, Haapakoski E, Rautio A. Ginseng therapy in non-insulin-dependent diabetic patients. *Diabetes Care.* 1995;18:1373–1375.

30. Sievenpiper JL, Arnason JT, Leiter LA, Vuksan V. Decreasing, null and increasing effects of eight popular types of ginseng on acute postprandial glycemic indices in healthy humans: the role of ginsenosides. *J Am Coll Nutr.* 2004;23:248–258.

31. Helms S. Cancer prevention and therapeutics: Panax ginseng. *Altern Med Rev.* 2004;9:259–274.

32. Suh SO, Kroh M, Kim NR, et al. Effects of red ginseng upon postoperative immunity and survival in patients with stage III gastric cancer. *Am J Chin Med.* 2002;30:483–494.

33. Cancer chemoprevention of INSAM (ginseng). Proceedings of a symposium. *J Korean Med Sci.* 2001;16(suppl):S1–86.

34. Yun TK, Choi SY. A case-control study of ginseng intake and cancer. *Int J Epidemiol.* 1990;19:871–876.

35. Yun TK, Choi SY. Preventive effect of ginseng intake against various human cancers: a case control study on 1,987 pairs. *Cancer Epidemiol Biomarkers Prev.* 1995;4:401–408.

36. Yun TK. Experimental and epidemiological evidence of the cancer-preventive effects of *Panax ginseng* CA Meyer. *Nutr Rev.* 1996;54(11 pt 2):S71–S81.

Glucosamine

Glucosamine is an amino-monosaccharide that is synthesized in the body from glucose and glutamine by chrondrocytes (cells that form cartilage). It functions as a building block in substances found in articular cartilage (1). Glucosamine supplements have gained popularity as an alternative to nonsteroidal anti-inflammatory drugs (NSAIDS) for arthritis relief. NSAIDs, while effective in decreasing pain and inflammation, have been associated with serious adverse effects including gastrointestinal complications and cartilage degeneration (2,3). In contrast, glucosamine is thought to have a good safety record and may have potential chondroprotective effects (4).

Some researchers suggest that supplying exogenous glucosamine provides the extra raw materials needed to keep joints healthy. Glucosamine seems to stimulate the production of molecules that provide strength and elasticity to the joint. Specifically, in vitro and animal studies report that glucosamine sulfate enhances production of collagen, glycosaminoglycans (GAGs), and proteoglycans in the joint matrix. Collagen is a thick protein that physically connects cartilage to tissue for tensile strength. GAGs are large polysaccharides that include chondroitin sulfate, keratan sulfate, and hyaluronic acid. Proteoglycans are made up of chains of GAGs arranged on a protein core. They function by attracting water to produce an elastic layer, thereby cushioning and protecting cartilage from mechanical stress (1,5).

Media and Marketing Claims	Efficacy
Relieves osteoarthritis pain in knee, hip, etc	↔

Safety

♦ Because glucosamine is a derivative of shellfish, it is possible for a reaction to occur in individuals allergic to shellfish.

♦ There is controversy regarding the effect of glucosamine on blood glucose control (1,6–9). To be safe, individuals with diabetes should have glucose levels monitored. Newer evidence has not found changes in blood glucose with glucosamine use.

♦ A 3-year study of glucosamine sulfate reported no serious adverse effects (6).

♦ Preliminary and theoretical evidence suggests that glucosamine may contribute to chemotherapy resistance for select chemotherapeutic agents, including VP16, VePesid, VM26, and doxorubicin (adriamycin) by reducing the inhibition of topoisomerase II in tumor cells.

Drug/Supplement Interactions

No reported adverse interactions

Key Points

♦ Preliminary evidence suggests that glucosamine may improve symptoms of osteoarthritis compared with a placebo, or improve symptoms at least as effectively as

NSAIDs. A meta-analysis (10) suggested that glucosamine and chondroitin combinations provided significant pain relief. However, some of these studies have been criticized for poor methodology, and not all have reported a benefit. A large (n = 1,588), 24-week, controlled multicenter US trial of glucosamine plus chondroitin found these supplements to be safe but ineffective in treating osteoarthritis of the knee (11).

♦ Researchers and clinicians are calling for new, more objective measures of clinical efficacy for agents proposed to reduce osteoarthritis pain or improve clinical status, including, at minimum, measures of joint space narrowing (12).

♦ Although previous research supported the clinical efficacy of glucosamine in osteoarthritis, a few more recent trials have been negative. A review of the evidence by EULAR (the European League Against Rheumatism) suggests, that glucosamine sulphate, chondroitin sulphate, ASU, diacerein, and hyaluronic acid have symptomatic effects and may modify the joint space and surrounding structures so as to reduce pain and inflammation to the tissue (13).

♦ A few controlled studies using radiological evidence suggest that glucosamine may have a structure-modifying effect on osteoarthritis by slowing knee joint degeneration and reducing narrowing of knee joint width over time. Further studies are needed to confirm these results.

♦ Although glucosamine is part of the structure that makes up tendons, ligaments, and cartilage, there is currently little evidence demonstrating that supplementation repairs damaged tendons and ligaments from sports-related injuries.

Food Sources

None

Dosage Information/Bioavailability

Glucosamine is available in tablets, capsules, or powders as glucosamine sulfate, glucosamine hydrochloride, or N-acetyl-D-glucosamine (NAG). Glucosamine supplements are derived from the exoskeleton of the crustacean chitin. It is often combined with chondroitin sulfate (*see* Chondroitin). Manufacturers' labels suggest taking 1,500 mg glucosamine/day divided into three doses.

In one human study, 90% of orally ingested glucosamine sulfate was absorbed and diffused into bone and articular cartilage (14). Another study supplemented human subjects with 1 g polymeric (sustained-release) NAG or nonpolymeric NAG and found that both forms are absorbed and increase serum glucosamine levels (15). There is no evidence that topical applications simulate oral dosages in terms of bioavailability or efficacy.

Relevant Research

Glucosamine Sulfate and Osteoarthritis

♦ A large (n =1,583 subjects with osteoarthritis of the knee), double-blind, placebo-controlled, randomized trial tested the efficacy of glucosamine (1,500 mg/day) vs chondroitin (1,200 mg/day) vs both vs 200 mg celecoxib vs placebo for 24 weeks. Mean age of subjects was 58 years; more than 60% of them were women, and the majority were white. The mean BMI for subjects was greater than 30. Efficacy was measured using the Western Ontario and McMasters University Osteoarthritic (WOMAC) Index. No significant differences between WOMAC pain score, stiffness score, function score, or Alternate Disability score was seen between any of the dietary supplements and placebo (11).

♦ A Cochrane Database Systematic Review of evidence from 16 randomized, controlled trials of glucosamine sulfate (GS) was published in 2001. Although most studies (15 of 16) were overwhelmingly positive, there was concern regarding efficacy of all glucosamine preparations given that the majority of studies used the Rotta product and had industry funding support (16). In addition, there is evidence that market products may vary considerably in the glucosamine content in terms of label values and analytical quantification (17).

♦ A 2004 article reported findings from two studies that included both subjective pain scores (WOMAC) and joint narrowing. In these two studies, 414 subjects (including 319 postmenopausal women) with osteoarthritis of the knee were randomly assigned to receive 1,500 mg GS or placebo daily for 3 years. Although the interventions were the same in both studies, each identified a different rescue medication for subjects to take for symptom relief as needed during the trial: one study used 500 mg acetaminophen; the other used 500 mg acetaminophen and select NSAIDs. In the 319 postmenopausal women enrolled, knee joint narrowing stopped in the glucosamine group vs a narrowing of 0.33 mm in the placebo group at the end of the 3-year period (18). WOMAC scores also improved in the glucosamine group and showed a trend toward worsening in the placebo group. Both findings support a role for GS in treatment of osteoarthritis.

♦ In a study in which all subjects were recruited and followed entirely over the Internet, 205 subjects with symptomatic osteoarthritis of the knee (confirmed by medical record review) were provided 1.5 g GS daily for 12 weeks. The glucosamine was found to be no more effective than placebo in reducing pain scores or analgesic use (19). The key limitation of this study is the lack of objective clinical measures of disease.

♦ In a double-blind, placebo-controlled study, 212 Belgian subjects with knee osteoarthritis were randomly assigned to receive 1,500 mg glucosamine sulfate or a placebo daily for 3 years. Disease progression was assessed by x-rays of knee joint-space width at baseline and after 1 and 3 years. Subjects assigned to placebo had significant progressive joint-space narrowing. In contrast, there were no significant losses in joint space in subjects taking glucosamine. Symptoms worsened in patients taking placebos compared with an improvement in symptoms in subjects taking glucosamine. Treatment was well-tolerated with no differences in safety or early withdrawal between the groups. The authors concluded that glucosamine may have a positive structure-modifying effect on osteoarthritis of the knee (6).

♦ In a double-blind, placebo-controlled study, 98 men (age range 34 to 81 years, mean age 63 years) being treated for osteoarthritis pain of the knee were randomly assigned to receive 1,500 mg glucosamine sulfate or placebo daily for 2 months. Pain intensity both at rest and while walking was assessed by a visual analog scale at baseline, and after 30 days and 60 days. There were no differences in pain between groups at baseline or at any point of the study. The authors noted that results contrast most other studies of glucosamine. They suggested that the lack of benefit could be due to the fact that their subjects tended to be older, heavier, and had more severe arthritis than other trials (20).

♦ In a double-blind, placebo-controlled trial, 49 subjects with temporomandibular joint (TMJ) osteoarthritis were randomly assigned to receive 1,500 mg glucosamine sulfate or 1,200 mg ibuprofen daily for 90 days. TMJ pain and function, pain-free and voluntary maximum mouth opening, Brief Pain Inventory questionnaire, and masticatory muscle tenderness were assessed after a 1-week washout period and at day 90. Additionally, acetaminophen (500 mg) use for breakthrough pain was evaluated every 30 days until day 120. Within-group analysis reported significant improvements in all variables in both treatment groups, with no differences in acetaminophen use. There were no significant differences in positive clinical responses between the groups. However, between days 90 and 120 (after discontinuation of treatment), the glucosamine group had significantly greater reductions in TMJ pain during function and, pain associated with performing daily activities. A decrease in acetaminophen use for break-through symptoms was also reported in the glucosamine group as compared with the group of subjects who had taken ibuprofen. The authors suggested that glucosamine seems to have a carryover effect (21).

♦ In a double-blind, parallel study, 200 hospitalized patients with clinically documented knee osteoarthritis were randomly assigned to receive 1,200 mg GS divided into three doses or 1,200 mg ibuprofen divided into three doses for 4 weeks. Only occasional use of NSAIDs (type, dose, and amount not specified) as a rescue therapy were permitted. Patients were not permitted to exercise or apply heat or cold therapy to the knees during the trial. The treatments were equally effective as assessed by improvement on Lesquesne's Index (which assesses functional status and quality of life), although there was an insignificant trend for the ibuprofen group to respond sooner. The ibuprofen group had significantly more adverse effects, such as gastrointestinal discomfort, than did the glucosamine group (35% vs 6%). The authors did not report information on NSAID use (22).

♦ A randomized, double-blind, placebo-controlled study of 80 individuals with osteoarthritis of the knee conducted in the United Kingdom showed that 1,500 mg glucosamine daily for 6 months compared with placebo had no significant improvement in global assessment of pain (23). There was a statistically significant improvement in knee flexion (13 degrees); however, the author suggests that the difference was so small that it was unlikely to be of clinical irrelevance.

Glucosamine Hydrochloride (HCL) and Chondroitin Combinations in Arthritis

♦ A meta-analysis examined 15 trials of glucosamine and chondroitin preparations. Studies were selected if they were double-blinded, controlled, and randomized, and lasted for 4 or more weeks' duration. In addition, studies were only included if subjects had knee or hip osteoarthritis. The pooled results suggested that glucosamine and chondroitin significantly improved osteoarthritis symptoms with moderate (glucosamine) to large effects (chondroitin). The researchers noted that the benefits might be exaggerated due to issues of quality and publication bias. Specifically, important demographic details including age, sex, radiological stage of arthritis, duration of disease, and use of analgesics and NSAIDs were not provided in many of the studies (24).

◆ In a double-blind, placebo-controlled study, 93 subjects with knee osteoarthritis were randomly assigned to receive a placebo or 2,000 mg glucosamine HCL plus 1,600 mg sodium chondroitin sulfate for 6 months. The treatment group had a significantly greater improvement in scores on the Lesquesne's Index compared with placebo. There was also a significant drop in pain medication used in the treatment group compared with the placebo group (25).

◆ In a double-blind, placebo-controlled study, 118 subjects with knee osteoarthritis were randomly assigned to receive 1,500 mg glucosamine HCL plus 1,200 mg sodium chondroitin sulfate plus 228 mg manganese ascorbate or a placebo daily for 8 weeks. Two weeks before the study, subjects were examined and instructed to take only prescribed acetaminophen for pain. At baseline, patients were examined and prescribed acetaminophen and given either glucosamine, chondroitin, and manganese, or placebo. At week 4, the prescriptions for acetaminophen were renewed. At weeks 4 and 8, patients returned diaries and unused medications, and were examined. The WOMAC questionnaire was given before, at baseline and the end of the study. Ninety-eight subjects completed the study. Reasons for dropout included scheduling conflicts, violating study protocol, etc. The primary endpoint (difference in WOMAC pain score from baseline to week 8) was not significant in either group. However, during weeks 5 through 8, there was a significant improvement in the knee exam and in the response to daily diary pain question ("How much pain do you have today compared with yesterday?") in the glucosamine group. There was no difference between responses to "Are you better than at the start of the trial?" (40% of the placebo and 49% of glucosamine subjects answered yes). The authors concluded that although the primary endpoint was not met, sufficient positive trends in favor of glucosamine suggest the need for larger trials (26).

◆ In a double-blind, placebo-controlled, crossover study, 34 Navy SEALs and divers with degenerative joint disease of the knee or back (mean age 43 years) were given in random order 1,500 mg glucosamine HCL plus 1,200 mg sodium chondroitin sulfate plus 228 mg manganese ascorbate or a placebo for 8 weeks each. Subjects were not permitted NSAIDs but were allowed acetaminophen for pain during the study. Subjects were assessed at the baseline and at week 7 to 8 for each treatment period. A summary disease score incorporated results of pain and functional questionnaires, physical examination scores, and running times (time to run 100 yards and to run up and down a tower with 80 stairs, touching every stair). Glucosamine plus chondroitin supplementation was associated with a significant improvement in the overall summary disease score compared with the placebo. Specifically, significant improvements were seen in the patients' assessment of treatment result and the visual analogue score (VAS) for pain. However, trends in physical examination scores, acetaminophen use, disability scores of Lesquesne and Roland, patient assessment of handicap, and physician assessment of severity were not different between treatments. There was also no change in running times or range of motion. When the knee data were separated from back data, the improvements in summary disease scores, patient self-assessment, and VAS for pain were mainly attributable to improvements in knee symptoms. None of the trends for low-back pain reached significance. Treatment had no adverse effects on vital signs, occult blood testing, or hematologic parameters. The authors concluded that the combination of glucosamine and chondroitin relieved symptoms of knee osteoarthritis, but that a larger data set is needed to determine the value of this therapy for spinal degenerative joint disease (27).

References

1. Barclay TS, Tsourounis C, McCart GM. Glucosamine. *Ann Pharmacother*. 1998;32:574–579.
2. Gabriel SE, Jaakkimainen L, Bombardier C. Risk for serious gastrointestinal complications related to use of nonsteroidal anti-inflammatory drugs: a meta-analysis. *Ann Intern Med*. 1991;115:787–796.
3. Palmoski MJ, Brandt KD. Effects of some nonsteroidal anti-inflammatory drugs on proteoglycan metabolism and organization in canine articular cartilage. *Arthritis Rheum*. 1980;23:1010–1020.
4. de los Reyes GC, Koda RT, Lien EJ. Glucosamine and chondroitin sulfates in the treatment of osteoarthritis: a survey. *Prog Drug Res*. 2000;55:81–103.
5. da Camara CC, Dowless GV. Glucosamine sulfate for osteoarthritis. *Ann Pharmacother*. 1998;32:580–587.
6. Reginster JY, Deroisy R, Rovai LC, et al. Long-term effects of glucosamine sulfate on osteoarthritis progression: a randomized, placebo-controlled clinical trial. *Lancet*. 2001;357:247–248.
7. Monauni T, Zenti MG, Cretti A, et al. Effects of glucosamine infusion on insulin secretion and insulin action in humans. *Diabetes*. 2000;49:926–935.
8. Pouwels MJ, Jacobs JR, Span PN, et al. Short-term glucosamine infusion does not affect insulin sensitivity in humans. *J Clin Endocrinol Metab*. 2001;86:2099–2103.
9. Scroggie DA, Albright A, Harris MD. The effect of glucosamine-chondroitin supplementation on glycosylated hemoglobin levels in patients with type 2 diabetes mellitus: a placebo-controlled, double-blinded, randomized clinical trial. *Arch Intern Med*. 2003;163:1587–1590.
10. Biggee BA, McAlindon T. Glucosamine for osteoarthritis: part I, review of the clinical evidence. *Med Health R I*. 2004;87:176–179.
11. Clegg D, Reda DJ, Harris CL, et al. Glucosamine, chondroitin sulfate, and the two in combination for painful knee osteoarthritis. *N Engl J Med*. 2006;354:795–808.

12. Abadie E, Ethgen D, Avouac B, et al. Recommendations for the use of new methods to assess the efficacy of disease-modifying drugs in the treatment of osteoarthritis. *Osteoarthritis Cartilage.* 2004;12:263–268.
13. Jordan KM, Arden NK, Doherty M, et al. EULAR Recommendations 2003: an evidence based approach to the management of knee osteoarthritis: Report of a Task Force of the Standing Committee for International Clinical Studies Including Therapeutic Trials ESCISIT. *Ann Rheum Dis.* 2003;62:1145–1155.
14. Setnikar I, Palumbo R, Canali S, et al. Pharmacokinetics of glucosamine in man. *Arzneimittelforschung.* 1993;43:1109–1113.
15. Talent JM, Garcy RW. Pilot study of oral polymeric N-acetyl-D-glucosamine as a potential treatment for patients with osteoarthritis. *Clin Ther.* 1996;18:1184–1190.
16. Towheed TE, Anastassiades TP, Shea B, et al. Glucosamine therapy for treating osteoarthritis. *Cochrane Database Syst Rev.* 2001;1:CD002946.
17. Towheed TE. Current status of glucosamine therapy in osteoarthritis. *Arthritis Rheum.* 2003;49:601–604.
18. Bruyere O, Pavelka K, Rovati LC, et al. Glucosamine sulfate reduces osteoarthritis progression in postmenopausal women with knee osteoarthritis: evidence from two 3-year studies. *Menopause.* 2004;11:138–143.
19. McAlindon T, Formica M, LaValley M, et al. Effectiveness of glucosamine for symptoms of knee osteoarthritis: results from an internet-based randomized double-blind controlled trial. *Am J Med.* 2004;117:643–649.
20. Rindone JP, Hiller D, Collacott E, et al. Randomized, controlled trial of glucosamine for treating osteoarthritis of the knee. *West J Med.* 2000;172:91–94.
21. Thie NM, Prasad NG, Major PW. Evaluation of glucosamine sulfate compared to ibuprofen for the treatment of temporomandibular joint osteoarthritis: a randomized double-blind controlled 3 month clinical trial. *J Rheumatol.* 2001;28:1347–1355.
22. Muller-Fassbender H, Bach GL, Haase W, et al. Glucosamine sulfate compared to ibuprofen in osteoarthritis of the knee. *Osteoarthritis Cartilage.* 1994;2:61–69.
23. Hughes R, Carr A. A randomized, double-blind, placebo-controlled trial of glucosamine sulphate as an analgesic in osteoarthritis of the knee. *Rheumatology.* 2002:41: 279–284.
24. McAlindon TE, LaValley MP, Gulin JP, et al. Glucosamine and chondroitin for treatment of osteoarthritis: a systematic quality assessment and meta-analysis. *JAMA.* 2000;283:1469–1475.
25. Das AK, Eitel J, Hammad T. Efficacy of a combination of FCHG49 glucosamine hydrochloride, TRH122 low molecular weight sodium chondroitin sulfate and manganese in the treatment of osteoarthritis of the knee. *Osteoarthritis Cartilage.* 2000;8: 343–350.
26. Houpt JB, McMillan R, Wein C, et al. Effect of glucosamine hydrochloride in the treatment of pain of osteoarthritis of the knee. *J Rheumatol.* 1999;26:2423–2430.
27. Leffler CT, Philippi AF, Leffler SG, et al. Glucosamine, chondroitin, and manganese ascorbate for degenerative joint disease of the knee or low back: a randomized, double-blind, placebo-controlled pilot study. *Mil Med.* 1999;164:85–91.

Glutamine

Glutamine, a nonessential amino acid, is the most abundant free amino acid in skeletal muscle and plasma. It is a fuel source for the gut mucosal cells, lymphocytes, macrophages, endothelial cells, and renal tubular cells. Body stores of glutamine decrease during trauma, infection, surgery, acidosis, and physical stress. Increased gluconeogenesis and hepatic, gut, and renal uptake of glutamine during catabolic states may account for the depletion of plasma glutamine. Because the demands for muscle glutamine exceed the supply during stress, many researchers consider glutamine to be conditionally essential (1–3).

There is considerable scientific evidence that glutamine is effective for certain disease states in the acute care setting when administered by a qualified health professional. For more details about the effects of glutamine supplementation on catabolic states, cancer, intestinal function, organ transplants, and burn injuries, see reference 3. This section will only review non–acute care marketing claims for glutamine.

Media and Marketing Claims	Efficacy
Improves immune response during exercise	↓?
Induces muscle mass repletion among people with HIV/AIDS who have experienced undesirable weight loss	NR
Relives mouth sores associated with chemotherapy	↑?

Safety

- In the cited studies, glutamine was well-tolerated. However, there are no long-term studies testing the safety of high-dose glutamine supplementation.
- No reported serious adverse effects are associated with glutamine.
- Orally, glutamine is well-tolerated at dosages of 40 g/day in adults and 0.65 mg/kg/day in children.
- Individuals with bipolar disorder should be monitored by a physician when taking glutamine; mania has been reported.

Drug/Supplement Interactions

No reported adverse interactions.

Key Points

- Research suggests that strenuous exercise is associated with reduced plasma glutamine levels and impaired immune function.
- The limited research on the role of glutamine supplements on immunity after intensive activity yielded inconsistent results and used only small numbers of subjects,

and thus is difficult to interpret. Laboratory studies have not shown improvements in immune parameters with glutamine ingestion, whereas field studies suggest glutamine supplementation after endurance exercise may reduce the incidence of *self-reported* infection. Published studies are weak in design, lacking sufficient sample size and controls. More controlled research is needed to determine the efficacy, dosage, and timing before recommendations can be made (4).

♦ One strategy to maintain plasma glutamine levels may be to consume carbohydrate between repeated exercise bouts. Carbohydrate may not only attenuate glutamine levels from decreasing, but a large body of research (not discussed here) has shown that carbohydrate ingestion also enhances exercise performance by replenishing glycogen stores (5).

♦ Although limited in numbers, a few initial reports suggest glutamine may retard wasting in patients with HIV/AIDS.

♦ Glutamine supplementation may reduce the severity of mucositis associated with high-dose chemotherapy used in cancer patients receiving bone marrow transplantation; however, a standard of care to provide glutamine in this setting has not been established.

Food Sources

Glutamine is a nonessential amino acid found predominantly in protein-rich foods. It is also synthesized in the body from glutamic acid.

Dosage Information/Bioavailability

Glutamine is available in capsules, pills, and sport beverages in the form of L-glutamine. It is also found in protein powder supplements. Products provide from 0.5 to 20 g glutamine per serving. Plasma glutamine increases approximately 2 hours after eating, especially protein-rich foods (6).

Relevant Research

Plasma Glutamine Levels and Immunity During Exercise Training

♦ Research reviews suggest that there is a transient decrease in plasma glutamine after acute exercise and from chronic overtraining (7,8).

♦ Athletes with overtraining syndrome (OTS) have been reported to have low plasma glutamine levels. In one study, 40 athletes diagnosed with OTS had significantly lower plasma glutamine levels than did a group of control subjects (9).

♦ Decreased plasma glutamine levels and an impairment in the number and activity of CD4+ T cells were observed in untrained subjects after an 8-week anaerobic exercise program (10).

♦ Serum glutamine levels decreased and natural killer and lymphokine activated killer cell activities were suppressed in triathletes after a half-ironman race (11).

Glutamine Supplementation and Immunity During Exercise

♦ In a placebo-controlled, crossover study, eight male subjects performed three bouts of ergometer cycle exercise lasting 60, 45, and 30 minutes at 75% maximum oxygen consumption (VO_{2max}) separated by 2 hours. Each subject randomly underwent two trials separated by 30 days: (*a*) 9 equal doses of 100 mg glutamine/kg body weight 30 minutes before, at the end, and 30 minutes after exercise session; or (*b*) a placebo. The authors chose this dosage regimen based on pilot studies showing that this regimen maintained plasma glutamine levels. Plasma glutamine levels were less during placebo administration compared with the glutamine phase. Circulating lymphocytes, phytohemagglutinin-stimulated lymphocyte proliferative response, and lymphokine-activated killer (LAK) cell activity decreased 2 hours after each bout of exercise in both groups. However, glutamine supplementation had no effect on these immune responses to exercise (12).

♦ Data were summarized from eight double-blind, placebo-controlled studies of a total of 151 athletes (middle-distance, marathon, and ultramarathon runners and elite rowers) who took a placebo or 5 g glutamine dissolved in 330 mL water immediately after and 2 hours after a marathon, ultramarathon, or intensive rowing (total glutamine = 10 g). The incidence of infection was self-reported for 7 days after exercise. Significantly more athletes in the glutamine group reported no infection (81%) compared with the placebo group (49%). However, whether an oral beverage containing glutamine can be "blinded" (13) is questionable.

Glutamine and Glycogen Stores

♦ Eighteen subjects were randomly assigned to receive an infusion of glutamine, alanine plus glycine, or saline, 30 minutes after completing glycogen-depleting exercise (90 minutes cycling at 70% to 140% maximal oxygen capacity). Muscle glutamine increased 16% during glutamine infusion, but it decreased or remained unchanged during alanine plus glycine and saline infusions, respectively. Two hours after exercise, muscle glycogen in the glutamine-infused group increased significantly compared with the other two groups (14).

♦ Seven male distance runners with depleted glycogen stores performed a 60-minute treadmill run after a 14-hour fast or after a high-carbohydrate meal. Plasma glutamine did not change in response to exercise when runners fasted, but it increased when they had eaten. The authors stressed the importance of dietary carbohydrate intake between repeated bouts of exercise to lessen the decrease in plasma glutamine (15).

♦ Three studies assessing the effect of oral glutamine supplementation on muscular strength, endurance, resistance training performance and/or weight lifting performance have been published. All involved small numbers of subjects and showed that the training improvements that occurred were not different across glutamine and placebo groups (16–18).

Glutamine and HIV Wasting

♦ In Clark et al's randomized, double-blind, placebo-controlled study, 68 individuals with HIV who had documented weight loss of more than 5% of usual body weight in the previous 3 months were recruited to receive an oral beverage containing glutamine (14 g), arginine, and beta-hydroxy beta-methylbutyrate, or a isocaloric maltodextrin nutrient mixture for 8 weeks. Forty-three subjects completed the study (21 in placebo group and 22 in the supplemented group), setting attrition at approximately 30%—a major limitation to the study. Weight gain in the glutamine group averaged 3 kg, whereas in the control group mean weight gain was significantly lower (0.37 kg) (19). The weight gain demonstrated was predominantly lean body mass for the glutamine group while the control group showed a significant increase in fat mass of 1.07 kg, despite the net increase in weight of 0.37 kg. Changes in mass were measured using displacement plethysmography and abdominal slice computed tomography. Of interest, CD3 and CD8 cell counts increased while viral load decreased in response to supplementation. However, improvements cannot be solely attributed to glutamine because the beverage contained other nutrients, including arginine. The article also did not describe whether there may have been other confounders that may have yielded study findings.

♦ In a randomized, double-blind, controlled glutamine supplementation trial, 26 individuals with HIV were blocked to balance gender, age, antiviral treatment, nutritional status, and mode of contracting the disease. Subjects received 40 g glutamine per day or glycine for 12 weeks. Weight gain was similar to the study by Clark et al, with glutamine supplementation resulting in a mean change in weight of +2.2 kg in 12 weeks and the control group gaining a mean 0.3 kg (20). All subjects received weekly nutrition counseling throughout the trial, and it is unclear whether the diet counselors were blinded to the intervention (investigators were given the double-blind design). Dropout rate in this study was approximately 22%.

♦ In a double-blind placebo-controlled pilot study testing the effect of glutamine supplementation on intestinal permeability, 24 patients with AIDS were randomly assigned to receive placebo or 4 or 8 g glutamine daily for 28 days. Intestinal permeability was estimated using urinary excretion of lactulose and mannitol. Seventeen subjects also underwent small bowel biopsies as clinical indicators of disease. Results showed no significant effect on intestinal permeability at these doses or for this duration. The author recommends longer term studies in more subjects (21).

Glutamine and Mucositis from Chemotherapy

♦ A retrospective analysis of medical records from 21 patients receiving bone marrow transplant (BMT) with the same chemotherapy regimen showed that swish-and-swallow glutamine administration every 4 hours for 24 days (day −7 through +16) was associated with fewer days of mucositis, delayed onset of mucositis, lower maximum grade of mucositis, and more immediate return to liquid oral food as compared to no glutamine treatment in this population at risk for chemotherapy-induced mucositis

(22). The study lacked scientific rigor in that it was retrospective and was not placebo-controlled.

♦ A randomized, double-blind, crossover trial by Anderson et al in 24 patients treated for cancer used glutamine swish-and-swallow (or placebo glycine) on chemotherapy days plus an additional 2 weeks after chemotherapy. Duration and severity of mouth pain was significantly less in the glutamine-treated group (23). However, outcome measures were generally subjective in nature. Given the simplicity of the approach, the author suggests that oral glutamine should be used to reduce mucositis in cancer patients undergoing BMT.

References

1. Lacey JM, Wilmore DW. Is glutamine a conditionally essential amino acid? *Nutr Rev.* 1990;48:297–309.
2. Walsh NP, Blannin AK, Robson PJ, et al. Glutamine, exercise and immune function. Links and possible mechanisms. *Sports Med.* 1998;26:177–191.
3. Abcouwer SF, Souba WW. Glutamine and arginine. In: Shils ME, Olson JA, Shike M, et al, eds. *Modern Nutrition in Health and Disease.* 9th ed. Baltimore, Md: Williams & Wilkins; 1999:559–569.
4. Shephard RJ, Shek PN. Heavy exercise, nutrition, and immune function: is there a connection? *Int J Sports Med.* 1995;16:491–497.
5. Coleman EJ. Carbohydrate—the Master Fuel. In: Berning JR, Steen SN, eds. *Nutrition for Sport and Exercise.* 2nd ed. Gaithersburg, Md: Aspen Publishers; 1998:21–44.
6. Castell LM, Liu CT, Newsholme EA. Diurnal variation of plasma glutamine in normal and fasting humans. *Proc Nutr Soc.* 1995;54:118A.
7. Rowbottom DG, Keast D, Morton AR. The emerging role of glutamine as an indicator of exercise stress and overtraining. *Sports Med.* 1996;21:80–97.
8. Keast D, Arstein D, Harper W, et al. Depression of plasma glutamine concentration after exercise stress and its possible influence on the immune system. *Med J Aust.* 1995;162:15–18.
9. Parry-Billings M, Budgett R, Koutedakis Y, et al. Plasma amino acid concentrations in the overtraining syndrome: possible effects on the immune system. *Med Sci Sports Exerc.* 1992;24:1353–1358.
10. Hack V, Weiss C, Friedmann B, et al. Decreased plasma glutamine level and CD4+ T cell numbers in response to 8 wk of anaerobic training. *Am J Physiol.* 1997;272(5 pt 1): E788-E795.
11. Rohde T, MacLean DA, Hartkopp A, et al. The immune system and serum glutamine during a triathlon. *Eur J Appl Physiol.* 1996;74:428–434.
12. Rohde T, MacLean DA, Pedersen BK. Effect of glutamine supplementation on changes in the immune system induced by repeated exercise. *Med Sci Sports Exerc.* 1998;30:856–862.
13. Castell LM, Newsholme EA. The effects of oral glutamine supplementation on athletes after prolonged exhaustive exercise. *Nutrition.* 1997;13:738–742.

14. Varnier M, Leese GP, Thompson J, et al. Stimulatory effect of glutamine on glycogen accumulation in human skeletal muscle. *Am J Physiol.* 1995;269(2 pt 1):E309–E315.
15. Zanker CL, Swaine IL, Castell LM, et al. Responses of plasma glutamine, free tryptophan, and branched-chain amino acids to prolonged exercise after a regime designed to reduce muscle glycogen. *Eur J Appl Physiol.* 1997;75:543–548.
16. Falk DJ, Heelan KA, Thyfault JP, et al. Effects of effervescent creatine, ribose, and glutamine supplementation on muscular strength, muscular endurance, and body composition. *J Strength Cond Res.* 2003;17:810–816.
17. Antonio J, Sanders MS, Kalman D, et al. The effects of high-dose glutamine ingestion on weightlifting performances. *J Strength Cond Res.* 2002;16:157–160.
18. Candow DG, Chilibeck PD, Burke DG, et al. Effect of glutamine supplementation combined with resistance training in young adults. *Eur J Appl Physiol.* 2001;86:142–149.
19. Clark RH, Feleke G, Din M, et al. Nutritional treatment for acquired immunodeficiency virus-associated wasting using beta-hydroxy beta-methylbutyrate, glutamine, and arginine: a randomized, double-blind, placebo-controlled study. *JPEN J Parenter Enteral Nutr.* 2000;24:133–139.
20. Shabert JK, Winslow C, Lacey JM, et al. Glutamine-antioxidant supplementation increases body cell mass in AIDS patients with weight loss: a randomized, double-blind controlled trial. *Nutrition.* 2000;15:860–864.
21. Noyer CM, Simon D, Borczuk A, et al. A double-blind placebo-controlled pilot study of glutamine therapy for abnormal intestinal permeability in patients with AIDS. *Am J Gastroenterol.* 1998;93:972–975.
22. Cockerham MB, Weinberger BB, Lerchie SB. Oral glutamine for the prevention of oral mucositis associated with high-dose paclitaxel and melphalan for autologous bone marrow transplantation. *Ann Pharmacother.* 2000;34:300–303.
23. Anderson PM, Schroeder G, Skubitz KM. Oral glutamine reduces the duration and severity of stomatitis after cytotoxic cancer chemotherapy. *Cancer.* 1998;83:1433–1489.

Glycerol

Glycerol, a three-carbon molecule, makes up the structural core of triglycerides and phospholipids. It is produced endogenously and is present in the body as a component of stored fat and as free glycerol in body fluids. Through gluconeogenesis, glycerol can be converted into glucose in the liver. Intravenous or oral administration of glycerol increases blood osmolarity, resulting in fluid retention in the body, with the exception of the brain and eyes. Because glycerol does not penetrate these areas, it has been prescribed to decrease intracranial pressure in serious clinical conditions such as stroke, Reye's syndrome, meningitis, and encephalitis and to reduce intraocular pressure in glaucoma. Sports scientists are investigating glycerol loading prior to exercise as a possible way to maintain hydration and thus enhance exercise performance (1–3).

Media and Marketing Claims	Efficacy
Improves hydration status during exercise	NR
Controls body temperature during exercise	NR
Enhances exercise performance	NR

Safety

◆ According to a recent review article, several studies have shown no adverse effects with glycerol ingestion, whereas other studies have reported adverse effects in 10% to 25% of the subjects (1). Reported side effects include nausea, headache, and blurred vision, attributed to fluid drawn away from the cranial and ocular regions. Symptoms seem to intensify as the dose increases (4).

◆ Hyperglycemia in individuals with diabetes has been reported with intravenous glycerol (2).

◆ In one small study, glycerol ingestion increased systolic blood pressure but had no effect on diastolic pressure (3).

◆ Because glycerol seems to cause fluid retention, it should be avoided by people with edema, congestive heart failure, renal disease, hypertension, and other conditions that may be exacerbated by fluid retention.

◆ Glycerol is an FDA-approved prescription product for glaucoma therapy.

Drug/Supplement Interactions

No reported adverse interactions.

Key Points

◆ There is mixed evidence that glycerol ingestion results in a state of hyperhydration for exercise lasting less than 2 hours. The limited research and small numbers of subjects used in varying states of physical fitness have led to conflicting conclusions regarding the efficacy of glycerol in enhancing physical performance or improving thermoregulation. Until more studies assess the efficacy, dosage, and timing of glycerol ingestion, the claim that glycerol "enhances sport performance" is unsupported.

◆ Individuals deciding to use glycerol products should be warned that the supplement may produce headache and blurred vision, which could interfere with athletic performance.

◆ Because of the potential for serious adverse effects, individuals with compromised health status (ie, congestive heart failure, diabetes, hypertension, renal disease) should avoid glycerol.

Food Sources

Glycerol or glycerin is a food additive in processed foods, medications, and skin products. Glycerol yields 4.32 kcal/g when oxidized to carbon and water (2).

Dosage Information/Bioavailability

Glycerol is available in drugstores as glycerin or glycerin in oral and topical formulations. It is also sold as glycerate in individual packets and is in some sport beverages. Glycerol products marketed to athletes recommend taking approximately 1 g glycerate per kg to be mixed with a large volume of water ($\approx$ 1.5 liters). For a person weighing 70 kg, manufacturers recommend different doses, ranging from 60 to 177 mL glycerate (2 to 6 oz) consumed with water (1). Researchers have used varying doses of glycerol and water, generally 60 to 90 minutes before exercise. Glycerol is easily absorbed, with plasma levels peaking approximately 60 to 90 minutes after ingestion (2).

Relevant Research

Glycerol and Hydration

♦ In a double-blind, placebo-controlled study, 11 nonexercising male subjects participated in two separate acute trials of hyperhydration and a third control trial without hydration. Subjects drank: (*a*) water plus 1.5 g glycerol per liter of the subject's measured total body water (TBW), or (*b*) plain water matched for taste and color. Change in TBW was calculated by subtracting urine volumes from the volume of liquid ingested. Total ingested volume was equal to 37 mL/L TBW (mean volume was 1,765 mL). Three hours after ingestion, glycerol intake resulted in significantly greater fluid retention (500 mL) than water intake alone (60% water retention with glycerol vs 32% water). Both glycerol and water increased blood and plasma volumes, but there were no differences between the groups. Systolic blood pressure was significantly higher during the final 60 minutes in glycerol-treated subjects compared with subjects receiving the placebo (114 vs 109 mm Hg) (3).

♦ In a double-blind, crossover study, eight competitive cyclists were given either a glycerol solution (1 g/kg body mass) in a diluted carbohydrate drink or a placebo (carbohydrate drink alone) prior to completing a 60-minute cycle ergometer trial (30 minutes fixed workload phase and 30 minutes variable workload phase). The total fluid intake in each trial was 22 mL/kg body mass. Glycerol intake expanded body water by approximately 600 mL more than the placebo. Glycerol also significantly increased performance by 5% compared with the placebo. There were no differences in rectal temperature, sweat rate, or cardiac frequency between treatment phases (5).

Glycerol and Thermoregulation

♦ In a double-blind, controlled, crossover study, eight heat-acclimated male subjects were hydrated in five separate trials in random order prior to 120 minutes of treadmill exercise in the heat (35°C): (*a*) euhydration (determined by plasma osmolality), (*b*) glycerol hyperhydration (1.2 g glycerol/kg lean body mass [LBM]) with water replacement equivalent to sweat loss, (*c*) glycerol hyperhydration with no water replacement, (*d*) hyperhydration with water replacement equivalent to sweat loss, and (*e*) hyperhydration with no water replacement. Hyperhydration was achieved by drinking 3.9 mL/kg lean body mass (LBM) of either a glycerol solution (containing 1.2 g glycerol/kg LBM) or plain water, followed by drinking a large volume of water (25.2 mL/kg LBM). The total volume of fluid consumed during a 30-minute period was 29.1 mL/kg. Glycerol hyperhydration with or without water replacement had no effect on body temperature, whole-body sweating rate, sweating threshold temperature, sweating sensitivity, or heart rate compared with water hyperhydration or euhydration. The authors concluded that neither water nor glycerol hyperhydration provide a thermoregulatory advantage over maintaining euhydration during exercise-heat stress (6).

- In a controlled trial, six untrained subjects followed three different hydration protocols in randomized order on three separate days: (*a*) glycerol (1 g/kg body weight) plus a large volume of water (21.4 mL/kg), (*b*) large volume of water (21.4 mL/kg), or (*c*) limited fluid (3.3 mL/kg). Two and a half hours after fluid intake, subjects performed 90 minutes of treadmill exercise at 60% VO_{2max} in a hot, dry environment (42°C). Urine volume prior to exercise was significantly less with glycerol ingestion when compared with both of the other water ingestion protocols. Glycerol ingestion resulted in a significantly lower rectal temperature and significantly elevated sweat rate during exercise compared with trials with water alone. The authors concluded: "These data support the hypothesis that glycerol-induced hyperhydration reduces the thermal burden of moderate exercise in the heat" (7).

Glycerol and Exercise Performance

- In a double-blind, placebo-controlled, crossover study, 11 trained subjects were randomly assigned to drink a glycerol solution (1.2 g/kg glycerol in 26 mL/kg water) or water (placebo) during a 90-minute period prior to exercise on a cycle ergometer (74% VO_{2max}). A second study (reported in the same article as the first) was completed using the same pre-exercise regimen with the addition of a carbohydrate replacement drink (5% glucose) given to seven subjects during exercise. In both studies, glycerol intake resulted in significantly reduced heart rate and prolonged endurance time. Body temperature (rectal) was not affected by glycerol (4).

- In a placebo-controlled trial, nine subjects completed four trials of cycling for 90 minutes at 50% VO_{2max} while consuming one of four solutions (total = 650 mL) every 15 minutes: 10% glycerol drink, 6% carbohydrate drink, carbohydrate drink plus 4% glycerol, and water (placebo). Glycerol ingestion attenuated the decrease in plasma volume associated with water intake alone. Heart rate, esophageal temperature, sweat rate, ratings of perceived exertion, cortisol, and aldosterone were measured. There were no substantial cardiovascular, metabolic, hormonal, or thermoregulatory advantages associated with glycerol ingestion (8).

References

1. Wagner DR. Hyperhydrating with glycerol: implications for athletic performance. *J Am Diet Assoc.* 1999;99:207–212.
2. Frank MS, Nahata MC, Hilty MD. Glycerol: a review of its pharmacology, pharmacokinetics, adverse reactions, and clinical use. *Pharmacotherapy.* 1981;1:147–160.
3. Freund BJ, Montain SJ, Young AJ, et al. Glycerol hyperhydration: hormonal, renal, and vascular fluid responses. *J Appl Physiol.* 1995;79:2069–2077.
4. Montner P, Stark DM, Riedesel ML, et al. Pre-exercise glycerol hydration improves cycling endurance time. *Int J Sports Med.* 1996;17:27–33.
5. Hitchins S, Martin DT, Burke L, et al. Glycerol hyperhydration improves cycle time trial performance in hot humid conditions. *Eur J Appl Physiol Occup Physiol.* 1999;80: 494–501.
6. Latzka WA, Sawka MN, Montain SJ, et al. Hyperhydration: thermoregulatory effects during compensable exercise-heat stress. *J Appl Physiol.* 1997;83:860–866.
7. Lyons TP, Riedesel ML, Meuli LE, et al. Effects of glycerol-induced hyperhydration prior to exercise in the heat on sweating and core temperature. *Med Sci Sports Exerc.* 1990;22:477–483.
8. Murray R, Eddy DE, Paul GL, et al. Physiological response to glycerol ingestion during exercise. *J Appl Physiol.* 1991;71:144–149.

Goldenseal *(Hydrastis canadensis)*

Originally used orally and topically by Native Americans to treat a variety of conditions such as dyspepsia, diarrhea, whooping cough, mouth sores, anorexia, eye infections, and fever, goldenseal is among the top 20–selling herbs in the United States (1,2). The active constituents in goldenseal are believed to be isoquinoline alkaloids. Berberine (2% to 3%) and hydrastine (2% to 4%) have been identified as the major alkaloids. Although there is a lack of pharmacological and clinical research on goldenseal, several studies have been conducted on the isolated alkaloid berberine (1). Other herbs that contain berberis alkaloids include barberry *(Berberis vulgaris),* Oregon grape *(Mahonia aquifolium),* barberry bush *(Berberis aristata)* and the Chinese herb goldthread *(Coptis chinensis).* Extracts from berberine-containing plants have been used in antidiarrheal medications in Ayurvedic medicine in India and in traditional medicine in China (3).

Media and Marketing Claims	Efficacy
Enhances immune function through antibiotic activity	NR
Reduces risk for infectious diarrhea	NR
Masks drug use in urine drug testing	NR

Safety

- Safety has been demonstrated for short-term use, but long-term use at high doses (500 mg berberine) has been associated with cardiac spasms and death.

- Oral long-term use has also been associated with gastrointestinal upset, hallucinations, and even delirium.

- Preliminary evidence suggests that topical application of goldenseal results in photosensitivity to UVA exposure (4).

- Goldenseal is endangered and extremely expensive; therefore, several adulterated products have entered the market for which no safety data are available.

- There is theoretical evidence that long-term use may reduce B vitamin absorption.

Drug/Supplement Interactions

- No reported adverse interactions in current research. However, as stated in Safety, the potential for reduced absorption of B vitamins has been described. No studies have directly addressed this issue.

- Theoretical evidence suggests goldenseal may alter efficacy of medications metabolized via the P450 3A4 enzyme system, but this has not been demonstrated clinically.

Key Points

- Marketing claims about goldenseal cannot be supported at this time because of a lack of clinical research. A component of goldenseal, berberine, seems to have antibiotic and antiparasitic actions in vitro and in animal studies. However, there is conflicting evidence on the efficacy of berberine sulfate on enterotoxin-induced secretory diarrhea in humans.

- Although some proponents have used anecdotal evidence and historical use to suggest that goldenseal reduces mucous production, soothes sore throats, alleviates dyspepsia, and stimulates menstrual flow, clinical trials have not been done to verify these claims.

- There is no evidence that goldenseal masks drug use in urine tests. Some goldenseal products claiming to "detoxify" the urine also suggest drinking massive quantities of fluid before urine testing, which would dilute urine and decrease drug detection.

Food Sources

None

Dosage Information/Bioavailability

The dried roots and rhizome of the goldenseal plant are available in capsules, tinctures, and teas, often combined with echinacea. Doses range from 500 to 2,000 mg of the dried extract, 1 mL liquid extract, or 2 to 4 mL tincture. It is often recommended for short-term use to help treat infections and promote healing. Some goldenseal products are standardized to contain 5% hydrastine. There are no recent studies on the absorption and bioavailability of goldenseal. In a study published in 1969, berberine was found to be poorly absorbed across the human small intestine (5).

Relevant Research

Goldenseal/Berberine and Antibiotic Activity

◆ No studies have tested the effects of goldenseal on infection. In an in vitro study, berberine sulfate (an alkaloid in goldenseal) had no effect on bacterial growth or the synthesis of major outer membrane proteins of the *Escherichia coli* enterotoxin. However, berberine sulfate did block adhesion of bacteria to host cells. The authors hypothesized that the anti-infectious activity of berberine in *E. coli*–induced urinary tract infections could interfere with the adhesion of uropathogenic organisms to the urinary tract, but this has not been tested in humans (6).

Goldenseal/Berberine and Infectious Diarrhea

◆ No studies have tested goldenseal in digestive disorders. However, studies supplementing with berberine (an alkaloid in goldenseal) are reported here.

◆ In a parallel trial, 165 subjects from Bangladesh with acute diarrhea caused by enterotoxigenic *E. coli* and *Vibrio cholerae* were randomly assigned to receive 400 mg berberine sulfate, 1,200 mg berberine sulfate plus tetracycline in a single oral dose, or no treatment (control). Subjects with *E. coli* infections who received berberine had significantly lower mean stool volumes than control subjects during three consecutive 8 hour periods after treatment. After 24 hours, significantly more subjects treated with berberine stopped having diarrhea compared with control subjects (42% vs 20%). In subjects with cholera who received 400 mg berberine, stool volume significantly decreased during the second 8-hour period after treatment compared with control subjects, but not during the first or third period. Among cholera patients, there were no differences in stool output between patients receiving berberine and tetracycline compared with controls. The authors concluded: "Berberine sulfate is an effective and safe anisecretory drug for ETEC diarrhea, whereas the activity against cholera is slight and not additive with tetracycline" (7).

◆ In a double-blind, placebo-controlled trial, 400 subjects with acute watery diarrhea were randomly assigned to receive 400 mg berberine, 2,000 mg tetracycline, a combination of the two, or a placebo divided into four doses/day. Of 185 patients with cholera, those given tetracycline or tetracycline plus berberine had reduced volume and frequency of diarrhea stools, reduced duration of diarrhea, and reduced requirements for oral rehydration (both volumes and frequency). Berberine alone had no effect. Of the 215 patients with diarrhea not caused by cholera, neither berberine nor tetracycline had any benefit compared with the placebo (3).

◆ Berberine has been shown to inhibit the intestinal secretory response to enterotoxins (*V. cholerae* and *E. coli*) in animal and ex vivo studies (8–11). These effects were apparent when administered before or after enterotoxin binding and when berberine was given either intraluminally or parentally (7).

Goldenseal and Masking of Urinary Drug Tests

◆ It is a popular myth that ingestion of goldenseal before urinary drug testing can mask the detection of illicit drug use. Early urine tests relied on thin-layer chromatography, in which goldenseal may have interfered with the detection of morphine. However, goldenseal would have no effect in current urine analysis techniques (immunoassays and gas chromatography-mass spectrometry) (12).

◆ The effect of goldenseal on urinary drug test results has not been studied.

References

1. Blumenthal M, ed. *The Complete German Commission E Monographs Therapeutic Guide to Herbal Medicines.* Austin, Tex: American Botanical Council; 1998.
2. Foster S. *Botanical Series No. 309—Goldenseal.* Austin, Tex: American Botanical Council; 1996.
3. Khin-Maung-U, Myo-Khin, Nyunt-Nyuny-Wai, et al. Clinical trial of berberine in acute watery diarrhoea. *Br Med J (Clin Res Ed).* 1985;291:1601–1605.
4. Inbaraj JJ, Kukielczak BM, Bilski P, Sandvik SL, Chignell CF. Photochemistry and photocytotoxicity of alkaloids from Goldenseal (Hydrastis Canadensis L) 1. Berberine. *Chem Res Toxicol.* 2001;14:1529–1534.
5. Bhide MB, Chavan SR, Duttak NK. Absorption, distribution, and excretion of berberine. *Indian J Med Res.* 1969;57:2128–2131.
6. Sun D, Abraham SN, Beachey EH. Influence of berberine sulfate on synthesis and expression of Pap fimbrial adhesion in uropathogenic *Escherichia coli. Antimicrob Agents Chemother.* 1988;32:1274–1277.
7. Rabbani GH, Butler T, Knight J, et al. Randomized controlled trial of berberine sulfate therapy for diarrhea due to enterotoxigenic *Escherichia coli* and *Vibrio cholerae. J Infect Dis.* 1987;155:979–984.
8. Sack RB, Froehlich JL. Berberine inhibits intestinal secretory response of *Vibrio cholerae* and *Escherichia coli* enterotoxins. *Infect Immun.* 1982;35:471–475.
9. Zhu B, Ahrens FA. Effect of berberine on intestinal secretion mediated by *Escherichia coli* heat-stable enterotoxin in jejunum of pigs. *Am J Vet Res.* 1982;43:1594–1598.
10. Zhu B, Ahrens F. Antisecretory effects of berberine with morphine, clonidine, L-phenylephrine, yohimbine, or neostigmine in pig jejunum. *Eur J Pharmacol.* 1983;96:11–19.
11. Tai YH, Feser JF, Marnane WG, et al. Antisecretory effects of berberine in rat ileum. *Am J Physiol.* 1981;241:G253-G258.
12. Morgan JP. Urine tests for drug use: are they reliable? *HerbalGram.* 1988;32:46–51,70.

Grape Seed Extract

For thousands of years people have been using grapes not only for eating and drinking, but for medicinal purposes as well. Grape seed extract has been purported to prevent atherosclerosis, prevent cancer, treat hypercholesterolemia, and heal wounds. The extract is produced from the small seeds found in *red* grapes used to make wine. One of the active constituents of grape seed extract is a subclass of flavonoids known as proanthocyanidins. Proanthocyanidins are effective antioxidants and are thought to improve the elasticity of blood vessels as well as increase serum antioxidant activity.

Media and Marketing Claims	Efficacy
Acts as an antioxidant	↑
Promotes cardiovascular health	NR
Reduces cancer risk	NR
Treats chloasma (hyperpigmentation of skin)	NR

Safety

- There have been no serious safety concerns reported with the used of grape seed extract (1).
- Grape seed extract sold under the brand name ActiVin (Dry Creek Nutrition, Inc, Modesto, CA) received Generally Recognized as Safe status for use in the United States.

Drug/Supplement Interactions

None.

Key Points

- Grape seed extract has a strong free radical scavenging effect on radical oxygen species. Its antioxidant activity has been reported to be significantly greater than beta carotene or vitamins C or E.
- Research in humans regarding cardiovascular disease risk associated with grape seed extract is limited. Animal studies have suggested that grape seed extract strengthens collagen in blood vessels, thereby allowing for increased blood flow throughout the body and improved cardiovascular health.
- Early reports from animal and cellular studies indicate that grape seed extract may have potential as a chemopreventive agent. Controlled clinical trials will be necessary to determine if these results can be realized in humans.

- Pilot data in animal and human models have shown grape seed extract may be effective in treating hyperpigmentation of the skin. More research is needed to verify these initial results.

Food Sources

Grape seed extract is derived from the seeds of red grapes used to make wine.

Dosage Information/Bioavailability

Grape seed extract is available in tablet, liquid, or capsule form. Most research has used preparations that contain at least 92% proanthocyanidins, the essential flavonoids in grape seed extract. Most supplement labels suggest taking 100 to 300 mg/day.

Relevant Research

There have been few studies using grape seed extract in human populations. The majority of the studies reported here used animal models or cell culture lines.

Grape Seed Extract and Antioxidant Activity

- In two similar articles, investigators reported that grape seed extract acted as a powerful antioxidant both in vitro and in vivo. Both articles found grape seed extract to be significantly more effective at scavenging free radicals than beta carotene, or vitamins C or E. The extract also increased the growth and viability of normal cells, while being cytotoxic to breast, lung, and gastric cancer cells. Similar results were seen in mouse models (2,3).

Grape Seed Extract and Cardiovascular Health

- A descriptive review of the literature investigating the molecular mechanisms of grape seed extract demonstrated that grape seed extract has several properties that make it an effective cardioprotective agent. First, it is a strong scavenger of free radicals, it is anti-apoptotic and anti-necrotic, and it modulates cardioregulatory genes. The authors recommended clinical trials to determine the effectiveness of grape seed extract as a therapeutic agent in promoting cardiovascular health in humans (4).

Grape Seed Extract and Cancer

- Animal models and cellular studies have shown promising results for grape seed extract as a chemopreventive agent. Grape seed extract supplementation in rats was protective against carcinogen-induced mammary tumorigenesis (5). In a quantitative apoptosis study, grape seed extract and the chemotherapy medication doxorubicin in combination showed a strong synergistic effect for a potential breast cancer treatment (6). Grape seed extract supplementation also inhibited tumor growth in mice implanted with human prostate carcinoma cells (7).

Grape Seed Extract and Chloasma

◆ To determine whether grape seed extract is effective in treatment of chloasma (also known as melasma), a blotchy brown pigmentation typically seen on the face, 12 nonpregnant women with chloasma were given 67 mg grape seed extract orally three times/day for 6 months in an open-label study. The effect on chloasma was evaluated monthly using reflectance spectrophotometric analysis on hyperpigmented skin and normal skin. Grape seed extract improved chloasma in 10 of 12 women in the 6 months as assessed by reflectance spectrophotometric evaluation. Melanin-index was also significantly decreased. There was no further improvement in symptoms beyond what was shown after 6 months of treatment. There was no placebo control group for comparison (8).

◆ Proanthocyanin-rich grape seed extract was fed to 5 guinea pigs, standard guinea pig chow to five others, and vitamin C to the final 5 guinea pigs for 8 weeks. The guinea pigs had previously been irradiated with ultraviolet light twice/day for 3 weeks in order to induce pigmentation (9). Histological evaluation of the exposed skin showed that the presence of affected melanocytes reduced significantly among guinea pigs given grape seed extract. Investigators theorize that the lightening may be related to the reactive oxygen species–related proliferation of melanocytes.

References

1. Schulz V, Hansel R, Tyler VE. *Rational Phytotherapy: A Physicians' Guide to Herbal Medicine*. 3rd ed. Berlin, Germany: Springer Verlag; 1998.
2. Bagchi D, Bagchi M, Stohs S, et al. Cellular protection with proanthocyanidins derived from grape seeds. *Ann N Y Acad Sci*. 2002;957:260–270.
3. Bagchi D, Bagchi M, Stohs SJ, et al. Free radicals and grape seed proanthocyanidin extract: importance in human health and disease prevention. *Toxicology*. 2000;148:187–197.
4. Bagchi D, Sen CK, Ray SD, et al. Molecular mechanisms of cardioprotection by a novel grape seed proanthocyanidin extract. *Mutat Res*. 2003;523–524:87–97.
5. Kim H, Hall P, Smith M, et al. Chemoprevention by grape seed extract and genistein in carcinogen-induced mammary cancer in rats is diet dependent. *J Nutr*. 2004;134:3445S–3452S.
6. Sharma G, Tyagi AK, Singh RP, et al. Synergistic anti-cancer effects of grape seed extract and conventional cytotoxic agent doxorubicin against human breast carcinoma cells. *Breast Cancer Res Treat*. 2004;85:1–12.
7. Singh RP, Tyagi AK, Dhanalakshmi S, et al. Grape seed extract inhibits advanced human prostate tumor growth and angiogenesis and upregulates insulin-like growth factor binding protein-3. *Int J Cancer*. 2004;108:733–740.
8. Yamakoshi J, Sano A, Tokutake S, et al. Oral intake of proanthocyanidin-rich extract from grape seeds improves chloasma. *Phytother Res*. 2004;18:895–899.
9. Yamakoshi J, Otsuka F, Sano A, et al. Lightening effect on ultraviolet-induced pigmentation of guinea pig skin by oral administration of a proanthocyanidin-rich extract from grape seeds. *Pigment Cell Res*. 2003;16:629–638.

Green Tea Extract

Tea *(Camellia sinensis)* is one of the most popular beverages in the world. Of the total tea manufactured worldwide from *Camellia sinensis,* 78% is black, 20% is green, and 2% is oolong tea. Green tea is an integral part of Japanese and Chinese cultures and is consumed at an average of 3 cups per day in those cultures. Although green, oolong, and black teas are made from the same species of tea plant, they each have different chemical compositions. The fresh tea leaf contains flavonoids, a large group of polyphenolic compounds with antioxidant properties. The polyphenols found in green tea, known as catechins, make up 30% to 50% of the dry tea leaf weight. Green tea is produced by steaming and drying the tea leaves, which preserves the polyphenol content. During black tea production, natural fermentation occurs, causing complexation of most of the polyphenols, with the retention of the antioxidant properties. Oolong tea is semifermented and is intermediate in polyphenol composition between green and black teas (1–3).

One cup of green tea provides approximately 100 to 200 mg polyphenols, which include epigallocatechin gallate (EGCG), epicatechin (EC), and epicatechin gallate (ECG). EGCG is present in the highest concentrations and is thought to be the most biologically active ingredient in green tea. Green tea also contains caffeine (3% to 5% dry weight), minerals (6% to 8%), and free amino acids (4%) (1–3). Regular varieties contain caffeine (approximately 10 to 50 mg/cup), but green tea is also available decaffeinated. With decaffeination, the polyphenol content will decrease slightly, but not enough to be of clinical importance.

Media and Marketing Claims	Efficacy
Acts as an antioxidant	↑
Reduces the risk for cancer	↑?
Improves heart health	↔
Assists in blood pressure control	NR
Promotes weight control by increasing energy expenditure	NR

Safety

- Moderate doses of green tea extract used for several years have been demonstrated to be safe. One study examining toxicity and pharmacological effects of green tea extract in cancer patients reported no serious adverse effects with doses of 1 g/m² (three times daily) to 4.2 g/m² (once daily) for 6 months. The 1 g/m² dose corresponds to about 7 to 8 Japanese cups (approximately 24 ounces) of tea three times daily. Side effects (gastrointestinal and neurological) were determined to be caffeine-related (4).

- Green tea as a beverage has been consumed safely in China for more than 4,000 years (3).

- Green tea supplements contain caffeine. Individuals sensitive to caffeine should use caution.

- In one study, green tea extract added to foods reduced dietary nonheme iron absorption in young women (5).

- The most common side effect is nausea if supplements are consumed on an empty stomach.

Drug/Supplement Interactions

- Green tea extract may interfere with iron absorption.

- Green tea should not be used with any medications that have negative interactions with caffeine (amphetamines, clozapine, dipyridamole, disulfiram, theophylline, etc).

- There is controversy about whether green tea alters platelet aggregation—individuals on anticoagulant medications should be monitored until more data are available.

Key Points

- The polyphenols in green tea have demonstrated antioxidant capacities in vitro and in vivo. Human intervention trials show that green tea intake can modulate biomarkers of oxidative stress and that catechin levels in tea correlate with antioxidant capacity (6).

- Although much more research is needed, evidence from in vitro, animal, and epidemiological studies suggest that green tea has anticarcinogenic activity. The National Cancer Institute is currently funding Phase I and II trials to test the safety and efficacy of green tea constituents for future intervention trials. In addition, several independent intervention research studies are on-going.

- Animal arteriosclerosis models support a protective effect for green tea, more controlled intervention trials supplementing with green tea extract are needed. Case-control studies to date generally show a lipid-reduction effect and a reduction in cardiac events among green tea drinkers (> 3 cups/day). Many of these studies are in populations where lifelong exposure to green tea has been substantial.

- Limited evidence suggests green tea may reduce blood pressure; but, data may be confounded by the effects of caffeine on blood pressure.

- There is some evidence in a few small human studies that green tea/extracts can modulate resting energy expenditure and that regular consumption may promote weight control. Further well-designed intervention trials are needed.

- Drinking green and black tea can be part of a healthful diet. More information on the safety and efficacy of green tea extract supplements is needed before recommendations regarding their use can be made.

Food Sources

Infusions made from green tea leaves

Dosage Information/Bioavailability

Green tea extract is sold in capsules providing 100 to 600 mg green tea standardized to 50% catechins (polyphenols). Consumption of 1.5 and 3.0 g green tea solids dissolved in 500 mL water resulted in a maximum plasma concentration of tea catechins within 1.4 to 2.4 hours (4). The half-life of EGCG (5.0 to 5.5 hours) was more than EGC or EC (2.5 to 3.4 hours) (7). Decaffeination of green tea does not substantially change the antioxidant capacity or phytochemical content.

Relevant Research

Green Tea and Antioxidant Activity

◆ In a study by the US Department of Agriculture, a serving of green or black tea brewed for 5 minutes in 5 oz of boiling water had more antioxidant activity (as measured by the Oxygen Radical Absorbance Capacity-ORAC assay) than individual servings of commonly consumed fruits and vegetables (8).

◆ Green tea consumption in smokers decreased oxidative DNA damage (8-OHdG in white blood cells and urine), lipid peroxidation (malondialdehyde in urine), and free radical generation (2,3-DHBA in urine). In nonsmokers, there was also a decrease in overall oxidative stress (9).

◆ In a double-blind, placebo-controlled study, 20 healthy nonsmoking women (ages 23 to 50 years) were randomly assigned to receive 3 g green tea extract (equivalent to 10 cups of tea) or a placebo daily for 4 weeks. The background diet was rich in linoleic acid and contained 27% fat, 14% protein, and 59% carbohydrate. Fasting blood samples and five 24-hour urine specimens were collected from each subject before and at the end of the study. The same samples were taken from 10 control subjects. Green tea extract significantly decreased plasma malondialdehyde concentration (marker of lipid peroxidation) compared with the placebo. There was no effect of green tea on serum lipids; indicators of antioxidant status; urinary 8-isoprostaglandin F2 alpha (marker of oxidative stress); 2,3 dinorthromboxane B_2; nitric oxide metabolites; or coagulation indicators. The authors concluded that green tea extract resulted in a small but significant reduction of lipid peroxidation, but it did not have specific effects on other markers related to cardiovascular disease (10).

Green Tea and Cancer

◆ Several animal studies have demonstrated anticarcinogenic activity of tea polyphenols in carcinogen-induced tumors in the stomach, duodenum, colon, pancreas, mammary glands, liver, lung, skin, and prostate (11–15). In vitro studies have shown that green tea polyphenols increase activity of antioxidant and detoxifying enzymes, block nitrosamines, suppress tumor growth by inhibition of tumor necrosis factor-α release, modulate DNA replication and repair, and inhibit estrogen receptor interaction in mammary cancer (2,16,17).

♦ In a study of the effects of green tea extract (polyphenol E and EGCG) in capsule and ointment forms on chronic cervicitis or progressive stages of cervical dysplagia, the extract significantly reduced cervical lesions in 51 women who received treatment as compared with 39 untreated subjects (18). Three treatment protocols were used: some subjects applied polyphenol E ointment topically twice each week for 12 weeks directly to the cervical lesions; others took 200 mg poly E or EGCG capsule orally every day for 8 to 12 weeks; and a third group received a combined treatment protocol with both topical and oral green tea polyphenols. Response rate was 10% in untreated group, 74% with polyphenol E ointment, 75% with polyphenol E ointment plus capsule, and 50% with polyphenol E capsule alone. A subgroup of patients infected with human papilloma virus demonstrated reduced viral titer counts of 50% to 100%, depending on the stage of cervical dysplagia diagnosed at baseline; advanced lesions (CIN III) were less likely to be responsive to treatment.

♦ A review article summarized 31 epidemiological studies of green tea consumption and cancer risk. Of five studies reporting on colon cancer, three reported an inverse relationship, one reported an insignificant inverse trend, and one found a positive relationship with green tea intake. For rectal cancer, one of four studies reported an inverse relationship, but increased risks were apparent in two studies. Both studies on urinary bladder cancer reported an inverse association. Of the 10 studies on stomach cancer, six suggested an inverse and three reported a positive relationship. Two of three studies report an inverse relationship of green tea and pancreatic cancer. Although studies examining esophageal cancer had mixed results, there was a consistent positive association between cancer risk and temperature of tea (defined as very hot or scalding hot). Of the total studies in the review, 17 demonstrated reduced risk, seven reported increased risk, three showed no association, and five reported an increased risk of cancer with scalding hot temperature (17).

♦ A large case-control study conducted in 1984 evaluated the association between tea consumption and gastric cancer. Tea consumption was assessed in a total of 26,311 Japanese adults older than 40 years, 419 of whom developed gastric cancer. Daily green tea intake of more than 5 cups/day vs less than 1 cup/day was not shown to be protective against gastric cancer for the total study population (OR = 1.4; 95% CI = 1.0–1.9; P for trend = .07 in the multivariant analysis), or for men or women separately (19).

♦ In an epidemiological study conducted among 1,160 Japanese women with newly diagnosed invasive breast cancers, breast cancer recurrence was reduced significantly in Japanese women who reported the highest intake of tea beverage daily. One hundred thirty-three breast cancer recurrences were diagnosed during a 9-year period. The hazards ratio for recurrence was 31% lower in those who consumed green tea regularly before their initial breast cancer event and continued drinking it compared with those who reported no regular green tea intake (20). A study like this has not been done in the United States, where regular green tea intake is much less. Of interest, the tea intake was most likely to be associated with reduced cancer recurrence in women with stage I and II disease and less likely in those with more advanced disease.

◆ In a retrospective study of 472 Japanese subjects with stages I, II, and III breast cancer, green tea consumption of these subjects prior to clinical cancer diagnosis was assessed. Higher levels of green tea intake significantly correlated with decreased numbers of axillary lymph node metastases among premenopausal but not postmenopausal patients with stage I and II cancer. Green tea was also associated with increased expression of progesterone receptors and estrogen receptors among postmenopausal subjects. Higher levels of green tea intake were associated with a significant decrease in recurrence of stage I and II breast cancer after 7 years. Specifically, the recurrence rate was 16.7% among those consuming 5 or more cups/day, and 24.3% among those consuming 4 or more cups/day. No improvement in prognosis was found in individuals with stage III cancer (21).

◆ A case-control study from China of 254 women diagnosed with ovarian cancer and 652 controls, showed an adjusted odds ratio for developing ovarian cancer of 0.39 (95% CI = 0.27–0.57) for daily tea drinkers and 0.23 (95% CI = 0.13–0.41) for those who reported regular tea consumption for more than 30 years. For green tea specifically, adjusted OR was 0.43 (95% CI = 0.30–0.63) for those consuming green tea at least once each day vs those who never or seldom drank green tea, supporting a significant protective effect for green tea intake against ovarian cancer. This study is limited by the case-control design and retrospective nature of the dietary data collection, but it lends promise to a dietary intervention for ovarian cancer risk reduction (22).

Tea and Cardiovascular Disease

◆ Epidemiological studies suggest that tea consumption (green or black) is associated with decreased risk of cardiovascular disease and stroke (23,24).

◆ In a double-blind, placebo-controlled Chinese study using theaflavin-enriched green tea extract, 240 patients with hyperlipidemia and consuming a low-fat diet, were randomly assigned to receive the green tea supplement (375 mg) or placebo for 12 weeks. Green tea extract supplementation was associated with a significant reduction in total cholesterol and LDL, with no significant effect on HDL or triglyceride levels as compared with baseline values (25).

◆ In the Rottenham longitudinal study of 4,807 adults age 50 years or older with no history of CVD, 146 people reported a myocardial infarction (MI) within the first 5.6-year period. In regular tea drinkers (> 375 mL/day), relative risk for MI, particularly those involving fatal events, was significantly less (43%; OR = 0.57; 95% CI = 0.33–0.98) (26).

◆ In a study assessing the role of tea consumption on myocardial mortality within the Determinants of Myocardial Infarction Onset Study, 1,900 patients with a confirmed MI provided focused dietary intake data regarding caffeine-containing beverage intake, including tea intake. Compared with those who did not drink tea, moderate tea consumers (< 14 cups/week) showed a 31% reduction in risk for MI, and heavy tea drinkers (> 14 cups/week) showed a 39% reduction in risk (27). Prospective intervention trials are needed.

+ A 2002 meta-analysis of observational studies of tea intake in association with cardiovascular disease endpoints included 10 cohort studies and 7 case-control studies with a total of 5,878 cardiac cases and approximately 200,000 control subjects. Estimates from the analysis suggest an borderline significant 11% decrease in MI risk with intake of 3 or more cups of tea daily (OR = 0.89; 95% CI = 0.79–1.01) (28). The eight studies conducted among US adults showed a 5% reduction in risk for MI for every 3 cups of tea consumed daily.

+ In a single-blind, placebo-controlled, ex vivo study, 64 healthy smokers were randomly assigned to drink 6 cups black tea, green tea, or water per day; or a supplement of 3.6 g green tea polyphenols/day (equivalent to 18 cups green tea) for 4 weeks. Subjects were instructed by a dietitian to maintain normal eating habits and avoid red wine. Blood samples were taken at the baseline and at the end of the study. Compared with the control, there were no significantly different effects shown by green tea or black tea consumption on plasma cholesterol, triglycerides, HDL or LDL cholesterol, plasma beta carotene or vitamins C or E, or uric acid. There were also no differences found in parameters of LDL oxidation ex vivo. Intake of green tea polyphenol supplements had no significant effect on any of the parameters measured except a decrease in plasma vitamin E concentrations compared with control subjects (29).

+ In a parallel comparison trial, 48 subjects were randomly assigned to drink 6 cups black tea, green tea, or water (control) daily for 4 weeks. Blood samples were taken at the baseline and at the end of the study. Neither green nor black tea affected serum lipid concentrations, resistance of LDL to oxidation ex vivo, or markers of oxidative damage in vivo. However, green tea slightly increased total antioxidant activity of plasma. The in vitro experiment showed a decrease in LDL oxidation only after incubation with very high concentrations of green or black tea, higher than achievable in vivo. The authors concluded: "Future research should focus on mechanisms by which tea flavonoids may reduce the risk of cardiovascular disease other than by increasing the intrinsic antioxidant status of LDL" (30).

+ In a cross-sectional study, green tea intake and lipid levels were assessed in 371 subjects from five regions in Japan. Mean serum concentrations of total cholesterol, triglycerides, and HDL cholesterol were compared with three levels of daily green tea intake (< 1 cup, 1–4 cups, and > 4 cups). After researchers adjusted for dietary and nondietary factors, green tea was not associated with lipid levels (31). However, the baseline lipid levels of generally lean Japanese populations may have reduced the probability of seeing a clinical intervention effect.

+ In a cross-sectional study, green tea consumption and associated lipid levels and liver function were evaluated in 1,371 Japanese men older than age 40. Increased consumption of green tea was significantly associated with decreased serum total cholesterol and triglyceride levels. There was also a significant association of green tea with increases in HDL cholesterol levels together with a decreased proportion of LDL and VLDL cholesterol, which resulted in a lowered atherogenic index (32).

Green Tea and Hypertension

♦ In a case-control epidemiological study of 1,507 subjects with newly diagnosed hypertension, habitual tea consumption was associated with a 46% reduced risk of hypertension if intake ranged between 120 and 600 mL daily as compared with no tea intake (33). Intake of more than 600 mL/day further reduced risk by 65% as compared with no tea consumption. One limitation of this study is that tea intake data was collected retrospectively. Prospective intervention trials are needed to confirm these results.

♦ In a randomized, controlled trial assessing the short-term effects of tea intake vs caffeinated water vs plain water on blood pressure in subjects with normal blood pressure (n = 20 men), green tea increased systolic and diastolic blood pressure at 30 minutes significantly above the effects of caffeinated water and water alone, but the difference between the groups drinking tea and caffeinated water was not significant at 60 minutes. Repeat measures of blood pressure every 24 hours for 7 days showed that ambulatory blood pressure was stable throughout the 1-week measurement period among subjects who continued to consume green tea daily (34).

Green Tea and Weight Control

♦ Several components in green tea, including catechins, caffeine, and theanine, have been associated with potential anti-obesity efficacy. In an obese mouse model, daily intake of green tea powder with varying amounts of these three compounds showed that each played a role in modulating body weight and intraperitoneal adipose tissue (35).

♦ In an intervention study in 10 men conducted in a respiratory chamber, 24-hour energy expenditure and respiratory quotient (RQ) were measured. Subjects were randomly assigned to green tea extract (50 mg caffeine, 90 mg EGCG), caffeine (50 mg), or placebo. Green tea extract was associated with a 4% increase in energy expenditure and a significant decrease in RQ as compared with placebo. Caffeine showed no effect on these markers of energy utilization. Twenty-four-hour norepinephrine levels were also increased with green tea extract as compared with placebo, suggesting a role for green tea in sympathetic activation of thermogenesis (36).

♦ A study using AR25 (Exolise brand) green tea extract to promote weight loss was completed among overweight (mean BMI 28.9; range = 25–32), otherwise healthy adults (n = 70) age 20 to 69 years. Mean body weight decreased by a mean of 4.6% and waist circumference by 4.5%. REE increased significantly during the 12-week intervention (37). Plasma cholesterol levels did not change; however, participants did not present with elevated lipid levels. This study was open-label and not placebo-controlled, thus limiting interpretation of the results. In vitro data collected in this study indicated that the green tea extract inhibited both gastric and pancreatic lipase activity and stimulated thermogenesis.

References

1. Graham HN. Green tea composition, consumption, and polyphenol chemistry. *Prev Med.* 1992;21:334–350.
2. Fujiki H, Suganuma M, Okabe S, et al. Japanese green tea as a cancer preventive in humans. *Nutr Rev.* 1996;54(11 pt 2):S67-S70.
3. Kuroda Y, Hara Y. Antimutagenic and anticarcinogenic activity of tea polyphenols. *Mutat Res.* 1999;436:69–97.
4. Pisters KM, Newman RA, Coldman B, et al. Phase I trial of oral green tea extract in adult patients with solid tumors. *J Clin Oncol.* 2001;19:1830–1838.
5. Samman S, Sandstrom B, Toft MB, et al. Green tea or rosemary extract added to foods reduces nonheme-iron absorption. *Am J Clin Nutr.* 2001;73:607–612.
6. Henning SM, Fajardo-Lira C, Lee HW, et al. Catechin content of 18 teas and a green tea extract supplement correlates with the antioxidant capacity. *Nutr Cancer.* 2003;45:226–235.
7. Yang CS, Chen L, Lee MJ, et al. Blood and urine levels of tea catechins after ingestion of different amounts of green tea by human volunteers. *Cancer Epidemiol Biomarkers Prev.* 1998;7:351–354.
8. Prior RL, Cao G. Antioxidant capacity and polyphenolic components of teas: implications for altering in vivo antioxidant status. *Proc Soc Exp Biol Med.* 1999;220:255–261.
9. Klaunig JE, Xu Y, Han C, et al. The effect of tea consumption on oxidative stress in smokers and nonsmokers. *Proc Soc Exp Biol Med.* 1999;220:249–254.
10. Freese R, Basu S, Hietanen E, et al. Green tea extract decreases plasma malondialdehyde concentration but does not affect other indicators of oxidative stress, nitric oxide production, or hemostatic factors during a high linoleic acid diet in healthy females. *Eur J Nutr.* 1999;38:149–157.
11. Fujiki H, Suganuma M, Okabe S, et al. Cancer inhibition by green tea. *Mutat Res.* 1998;402:307–310.
12. Hibasami H, Komiya T, Achiwa Y, et al. Induction of apoptosis in human stomach cancer cells by green tea catechins. *Oncol Rep.* 1998;5:527–529.
13. Yang CS, Yang GY, Landau JM, et al. Tea and tea polyphenols inhibit cell hyperproliferation, lung tumorigenesis, and tumor progression. *Exp Lung Res.* 1998;24:629–639.
14. Wang ZY, Huang MT, Ferraro T, et al. Inhibitory effect of green tea in the drinking water on tumorigenesis by ultraviolet light and 12-o-tetradecanoylphorbol-13-acetate in the skin of SKH-1 mice. *Cancer Res.* 1992;52:1162–1170.
15. Paschka AG, Butler R, Young CY. Induction of apoptosis in prostate cancer cell lines by the green tea component (-)-epigallocatechin-3-gallate. *Cancer Lett.* 1998;130:1–7.
16. Fujiki H, Suganuma M, Okabe S, et al. Mechanistic findings of green tea as cancer preventive for humans. *Proc Soc Exp Biol Med.* 1999;220:225–228.
17. Bushman JL. Green tea and cancer in humans: a review of the literature. *Nutr Cancer.* 1998;31:151–159.
18. Ahn WS, Yoo J, Huh SW, et al. Protective effects of green tea extracts (polyphenon E and EGCG) on human cervical lesions. *Eur J Cancer Prev.* 2003;12:383–390.
19. Tsubono Y, Nishino Y, Komatsu S, et al. Green tea and the risk of gastric cancer in Japan. *N Engl J Med.* 2001;344:632–636.

20. Inoue M, Tajima K, Mizutani M, et al. Regular consumption of green tea and the risk of breast cancer recurrence: follow-up study from the Hospital-based Epidemiologic Research Program at Aichi Cancer Center (HERPACC), Japan. *Cancer Lett.* 2001;167: 175–182.
21. Nakachi K, Suemasu K, Suga K, et al. Influence of drinking green tea on breast cancer malignancy among Japanese patients. *Jpn J Cancer Res.* 1998;89:254–261.
22. Zhang M, Binns CW, Lee AH. Tea consumption and ovarian cancer risk: a case-control study in China. *Cancer Epidemiol Biomarkers Prev.* 2002;11:713–718.
23. Hertog MG, Feskens EJ, Hollman PC, et al. Dietary antioxidant flavonoids and risk of coronary heart disease: the Zutphen Elderly Study. *Lancet.* 1993;342:1007–1011.
24. Keli SO, Hertog MG, Feskens EJ, et al. Dietary flavonoids, antioxidant vitamins, and incidence of stroke: the Zutphen Study. *Arch Intern Med.* 1996;156:637–642.
25. Maron DJ, Lu GP, Cai NS, et al. Cholesterol-lowering effect of a theaflavin-enriched green tea extract: a randomized controlled trial. *Arch Intern Med.* 2003;163: 1448–1453.
26. Geleijnse JM, Launer LJ, Van der Kuip DA, et al. Inverse association of tea and flavonoid intakes with incident myocardial infarction: the Rotterdam Study. *Am J Clin Nutr.* 2002;75:880–886.
27. Mukamal KJ, Maclure M, Muller JE, et al. Tea consumption and mortality after acute myocardial infarction. *Circulation.* 2002;105:2476–2481.
28. Peters U, Poole C, Arab L. Does tea affect cardiovascular disease? A meta-analysis. *Am J Epidemiol.* 2001;154:495–503.
29. Princen HM, van Duyvenvoorde W, Buytenhek R, et al. No effect of consumption of green and black tea on plasma lipid and antioxidant levels and on LDL oxidation in smokers. *Arterioscler Thromb Vasc Biol.* 1998;18:833–841.
30. van het Hof KH, de Boer HS, Wiseman SA, et al. Consumption of green or black tea does not increase resistance of low-density lipoprotein to oxidation in humans. *Am J Clin Nutr.* 1997;66:1125–1132.
31. Tsubono Y, Tsugane S. Green tea intake in relation to serum lipid levels in middle-aged Japanese men and women. *Ann Epidemiol.* 1997;7:280–284.
32. Imai K, Nakachi K. Cross sectional study of effects of drinking green tea on cardio-vascular and liver disease. *BMJ.* 1995;310:693–696.
33. Yang YC, Lu FH, Wu JS, et al. The protective effect of habitual tea consumption on hypertension. *Arch Intern Med.* 2004;164:1534–1540.
34. Hodgson JM, Puddey IB, Burke V, et al. Effects on blood pressure of drinking green and black tea. *J Hypertens.* 1999;17:457–463.
35. Zheng G, Sayama K, Okubo T, et al. Anti-obesity effects of three major components of green tea, catechins, caffeine and theanine, in mice. *In Vivo.* 2004;18:55–62.
36. Dulloo AG, Duret C, Rohrer D, et al. Efficacy of a green tea extract rich in catechin polyphenols and caffeine in increasing 24-h energy expenditure and fat oxidation in humans. *Am J Clin Nutr.* 1999;70:1040–1050.
37. Chantre P, Lairon D. Recent findings of green tea extract AR25 (Exolise) and its activity for the treatment of obesity. *Phytomedicine.* 2002;9:3–8.

Guarana

Guarana is extracted from the seeds of a South American creeping shrub grown almost exclusively in a small area of northern Brazil. Guarana is named after the Guarani Amazonian tribe that originally used the seeds to brew tea. The tribe also added the crushed seeds to food and beverages to increase alertness and decrease fatigue. Guarana's effectiveness comes from the fact that its seeds contain 4% to 5% caffeine (whereas coffee beans contain only 1% to 2%). Guarana supplements contain as much caffeine as is found in 1 to 2 cups of coffee. Guarana is also being added to many energy drinks and bars. There have been reports of caffeine intoxication, sometimes leading to death, when guarana is taken with other products that contain caffeine. The majority of these cases and most of the fatal events have occurred in young adults with no underlying cardiac disease. In an effort to protect consumers, the Swedish National Food Administration recommends against consuming energy drinks with guarana after exercise or with alcohol. The Australian Food and Drug Administration requires all energy drinks with guarana to carry a warning label.

Media and Marketing Claims	Efficacy
Aids weight loss	NR
Suppresses appetite	NR
Improves athletic performance	NR
Prevents fatigue	NR

Safety

- Guarana should not be taken in combination with ephedrine (ma huang) because potentially fatal irregular heartbeats have been reported (1).

- Guarana has Generally Recognized as Safe (GRAS) status as a food additive in the United States (2).

- A case report of a healthy 54-year-old woman reported the presence of rhabdomyolysis with a peak concentration of creatine kinase of 1,028 IU/L following ingestion of a weight-loss herbal medicine containing guarana. Three hours after ingestion, the woman complained of severe chest pain that gradually resolved within 2 hours (3). The creatine kinase elevation indicates muscle breakdown. More study is needed to determine the effects of guarana on bulk muscle.

- When taken in large doses, guarana can cause insomnia, anxiety, nausea, vomiting, tremors, tinnitus, tachycardia, and arrhythmia (1).

- Due to the high content of caffeine in guarana, individuals with the following conditions should *not* take guarana: heart condition, high blood pressure, bleeding conditions, glaucoma, or anxiety disorders.

- Stopping use of guarana will cause withdrawal symptoms similar to that seen with other products with caffeine. Other side effects of taking guarana include insomnia, heart palpitations, tremor, nausea, diarrhea, and severe dehydration.

Drug/Supplement Interactions

Persons taking *any* medication, even over-the-counter types, should consult their physician before beginning a regimen of guarana. Most guarana supplements contain high levels of caffeine, which may interact with antidiabetic, anticoagulant, antipsychotic and other medications.

Key Points

- There is limited evidence that suggests guarana may have limited efficacy as a short-term weight-loss aid. There have been no studies investigating the efficacy of long-term use.

- Guarana contains caffeine and, as such, acts as a strong stimulant. However, studies have not been conducted regarding the use of guarana for suppressing appetite, increasing athletic performance, or preventing fatigue.

Food Sources

Guarana is added to a variety of weight-loss products and energy drinks.

Dosage Information/Bioavailability

Guarana is available in capsule and tablet form and as an ingredient in many energy drinks and bars. Most tablets contain 500 to 1,000 mg. No more than 3,000 mg/day should be taken because serious side effects could occur (1).

Relevant Research

Guarana and Weight Loss

- In a double-blind, randomized, placebo-controlled trial to investigate the safety and efficacy of an herbal supplement containing ma huang and guarana for weight loss in overweight humans, 67 subjects (24 in each arm completed the study) received placebo or the supplement (72 mg ephedrine, 240 mg caffeine) daily for 8 weeks. Subjects ranged in age from 25 to 55 years, were reportedly weight stable for at least 3 months prior to enrolling in the study, and had a mean BMI of 32.6. Weight loss, percentage body fat, hip and waist circumference, blood pressure, heart rate, and serum lipid profiles were evaluated. The herbal supplement produced a significant reduction in weight and percentage body fat compared with placebo. The active supplement also reduced hip circumference and serum triglycerides. Subjects in the treatment group were more likely to withdraw because of adverse events, which may have been related to the study compounds. The unequal dropout rate makes interpretation of the results suspect. Complaints included dry mouth, insomnia, headache, irritability, and heartburn (4).

◆ A randomized, double-blind, placebo-controlled study was conducted to determine the effect of an herbal supplement containing yerbe mate (112 mg), guarana (95 mg), and damiana (36 mg) on gastric emptying and weight loss. Subjects (7 for gastric emptying and 44 for weight loss) were healthy but slightly overweight. They were randomly assigned to the supplement or placebo, which was taken three times daily before each meal. Gastric emptying was evaluated by ultrasound. Body weight was measured after 10 days, 45 days, and 1 year of treatment. The guarana-containing supplement produced a prolonged gastric emptying time as compared with placebo. The placebo group demonstrated weight loss averaging 0.3 kg over 10 days while the supplement group showed a mean weight loss of 0.8 kg; at 45, days, the mean difference in weight loss between groups was 4.8 kg, but no significant effect was found after 1 year of treatment (5). Given this was a mixed supplement containing three different potentially weight-reducing herbals, the independent effects of any one of these constituents cannot be assessed.

References

1. Cannon ME, Cooke CT, McCarthy JS. Caffeine-induced cardiac arrhythmia: an unrecognized danger of healthfood products. *Med J Aust.* 2001;174:520–521.
2. Food and Drug Administration. Center for Food Safety and Applied Nutrition, Office of Premarket Approval. EAFUS: a food additive database. Available at: http://vm.cfsan.fda.gov/~dms/eafus.html. Accessed May 7, 2006.
3. Mansi IA, Huang J. Rhabdomyolysis in response to weight-loss herbal medicine. *Am J Med Sci.* 2004;327:356–357.
4. Boozer CN, Nasser J, Heymsfield SB, et al. An herbal supplement containing Ma Huang-Guarana for weight loss: a randomized, double-blind trial. *Int J Obes Relat Metab Disord.* 2001;25:316–324.
5. Andersen T, Fogh J. Weight loss and delayed gastric emptying following a South American herbal preparation in overweight patients. *J Hum Nutr Diet.* 2001;14:243–250.

Guggul/Guggulipids

Guggul, also known as guggulipids, is an ethyl acetate extract of the gum resin of the guggul tree *(Commiphora mukul).* Native to India and Pakistan, the gum resin from this tree has been used for centuries to treat ailments ranging from arthritis to sore throats, and even leprosy. In the early 1980s, herbalists began to tout guggulipid as a cholesterol-reducing agent. Although several human studies have investigated the effectiveness of guggulipid on treating hypercholesterolemia as well as other ailments, there is not enough published evidence to support the use of guggulipid for any medical condition (1,2).

Media and Marketing Claims	Efficacy
Treats hypothyroidism	NR
Treats hypercholesterolemia	NR
Treats acne	NR
Aids weight loss	NR

Safety

- Preliminary data suggest that guggul is safe for up to 18 months (3).
- Short-term clinical trials have reported no adverse effects other than mild stomach upset (4).

Drug/Supplement Interactions

- Guggulipids have the potential to stimulate the thyroid gland. Guggulipids should not be taken by individuals being treated for any thyroid disorder or those taking thyroid medications.
- Guggulsterone, the active component of guggul, has been shown to interfere with many prescription drugs (5). Guggul has the potential to change the effectiveness of HIV and cancer medications and even acetaminophen.

Key Points

- A recent study found that guggul may ameliorate hypothyroidism in female mice (6). There is no evidence for this use in humans.
- A small number of studies have reported that guggul is effective in reducing total cholesterol levels. However, in a double-blind, randomized, clinical trial investigating the use of guggulipid for the treatment of hypercholesterolemia, subjects showed no improvement in their cholesterol levels and in fact had a 4% to 5% increase in their LDL levels compared with placebo (3).
- Guggul has been marketed to treat acne and obesity. The studies in these areas have been small and poorly controlled; it is not clear what benefits guggul may offer in these areas.

Food Sources

None

Dosage Information/Bioavailability

Guggul is available in capsules, softgels, and tablets. Guggulipid can be found in a variety of cholesterol-lowering formulations. Most of these contain 500 mg per tablet. Guggul has been safely used at dosages of 1 to 2 g twice/day in an experimental trial (3).

Relevant Research

Guggul and Hypothyroidism

- ◆ To determine the efficacy of guggul treatment for hypothyroidism in mice, four groups of mice were treated with (*a*) normal saline throughout, (*b*) 10 mg/kg/day 6-n-propyl-2-thiouracil (PTU) for 30 days, (*c*) 10 mg/kg/day PTU for 15 days and PTU plus 200 mg/kg/day of guggulu for an additional 15 days, or (*d*) 10 mg/kg/day PTU for 15 days and only guggulu for the final 15 days. Following the 30-day study period, the animals were killed for analysis of LPO, SOP, and CAT activities from liver homogenates, and serum T_3 and T_4 were determined by radioimmunoassay. Guggul increased the level of T_3 in the serum of euthyroid mice as well as in mice rendered hypothyroid by PTU exposure. Guggul may function to enhance conversion of T_4 to T_3 (6).

Guggul and Hypercholesterolemia

- ◆ To determine whether *Commiphora mukul* and guggulsterone increase the resistance of LDL to oxidative modification, purified LDL was subjected to oxidation by either copper ions, free radicals, lipoxygenase, or resident peritoneal macrophages harvested from BALB/c mice in the presence or absence of *Commiphora mukul* and guggulsterone. A dose-dependent decrease in LDL oxidation was found in LDL treated with *Commiphora mukul* and guggulsterone in each of the assays used in this study (7).

- ◆ In a randomized, controlled clinical trial of 103 healthy adults with hypercholesterolemia, investigators studied the safety and efficacy of a standardized guggul extract containing 2.5% guggulsterones. Subjects were randomly assigned to receive placebo, a standard (1,000 mg) dose of guggulipid, or a high (2,000 mg) dose daily. After 8 weeks of treatment, LDL levels increased in participants in the standard- and high-dose guggulipid groups (4% and 5%, respectively) as compared with the placebo group, in which LDL decreased 5%. There were no significant changes for HDL, VLDL, or total cholesterol (3).

- ◆ In a study to determine whether the lipid-lowering effect of guggulipid is mediated through the nuclear receptor FXR, a synthetic FXR–responsive reporter plasmid was transfected into HepG2 cells. Quantitative real-time polymerase chain reaction (PCR) was used to detect SHP mRNA expression in response to chenodeoxycholic acid (CDCA) with or without guggulsterone. Fluorescence resonance energy transfer (FRET)–based coactivator binding assay was used to test whether guggulsterone is an antagonistic ligand of FXR. To determine whether guggulsterone's lipid-lowering effects require FXR, wild-type and FXR-null mice were fed normal or high-cholesterol diets. Supplementation of each diet with guggulsterone occurred for some mice in each group. In these studies, guggulsterone alone had no effect on FXR activity; however, it inhibited FXR activation by a potent activator, CDCA, in a dose-dependent manner. Guggulsterone also inhibited CDCA-induced expression of SHP mRNA is primary mouse hepatocytes. FRET-based testing demonstrated that guggulsterone reduced the hepatic cholesterol of mice fed a high-cholesterol diet. This effect was not seen in FXR-null mice. Guggulsterone had cholesterol-lowering activity mediated through FXR (8).

References

1. Nityanand S, Srivastava JS, Asthana OP. Clinical trials with guggulipid. A new hypolipidaemic agent. *J Assoc Physicians India.* 1989;37:323,328.
2. Singh RB, Niaz MA, Ghosh S. Hypolipidemic and antioxidant effects of *Commiphora mukul* as an adjunct to dietary therapy in patients with hypercholesterolemia. *Cardiovasc Drugs Ther.* 1994;8:659,664.
3. Szapary PO, Wolfe ML, Bloedon LT, et al. Guggulipid for the treatment of hypercholesterolemia: a randomized controlled trial. *JAMA.* 2003;290:765–772.
4. Bhatt AD, Dalal DG, Shah SJ, et al. Conceptual and methodologic challenges of assessing the short-term efficacy of Guggulu in obesity: data emergent from a naturalistic clinical trial. *J Postgrad Med.* 1995;41:5–7.
5. Brobst DE, Ding X, Creech KL, et al. Guggulsterone activates multiple nuclear receptors and induces CYP3A gene expression through the pregnane X receptor. *J Pharmacol Exp Ther.* 2004;310:528–535.
6. Panda S, Kar A. Guggulu (*Commiphora mukul*) potentially ameliorates hypothyroidism in female mice. *Phytother Res.* 2005;19:78–80.
7. Wang X, Greilberger J, Ledinski G, et al. The hypolipidemic natural product *Commiphora mukul* and its component guggulsterone inhibit oxidative modification of LDL. *Atherosclerosis.* 2004;172:239–246.
8. Urizar NL, Liverman AB, Dodds DT, et al. A natural product that lowers cholesterol as an antagonist ligand for FXR. *Science.* 2002;296:1703–1706.

Hawthorn

Hawthorn is derived from the leaf, berries, and flower of the *Crataegus laevigata* and *Crataegus monogyna* tree. Grown in the United States, northern Europe, and Asia, hawthorn has been purported to treat cardiac conditions and anxiety disorders, and to act as a natural sedative. Chinese herbalists have used hawthorn to promote digestive health for centuries. Currently, scientists are investigating the use of hawthorn as a treatment for congestive heart failure (CHF). Early results have been promising, but more clinical trials are needed to determine efficacy and safety.

Media and Marketing Claims	Efficacy
Treats cardiovascular conditions	↑?
Treats anxiety disorders	NR
Sedative	NR

Safety

+ Use of hawthorn may interfere with the treatment of cardiovascular conditions in that it can cause dilation of the smooth muscles and increases blood flow. Because of this, hawthorn may increase heart rate.
+ In clinical trials using hawthorn, side effects were mild, including dizziness, nausea, stomach upset, and increased heart rate (1).

Drug/Supplement Interactions

Hawthorn augments the effect of cardiac medications, such as digoxin or blood pressure drugs. Individuals taking any of these medications should not take hawthorn before consulting their physician.

Key Points

+ In a meta-analysis, researchers concluded that there is a significant benefit from hawthorn extract as an adjunctive treatment for CHF (2).
+ There is no evidence to suggest that hawthorn is effective for the treatment of anxiety or as a sedative.

Food Sources

None

Dosage Information/Bioavailability

Available in tincture, tablet, powder, dried herb/tea, and capsule forms, hawthorn is typically used at 100 to 250 mg three times daily for angina, arrhythmia, CHF, and high blood pressure (3). Given these are significant medical conditions, physician supervision is necessary.

Relevant Research

Hawthorn and Cardiovascular Disease

- Pittler et al used literature searches of several databases to identify double-blind, randomized, and placebo-controlled studies using standardized dosing of hawthorn among patients with chronic heart disease based on the New York Heart Association cardiac symptom score. Authors also contacted researchers and manufacturers to further identify studies for a meta-analysis. A total of eight studies including 311 patients met all a priori inclusion criteria. Although the main outcome assessed was mean change in workload as compared with baseline, results presented are for the significant increase in maximal workload shown in patients receiving hawthorn extract compared with placebo. Meta-analysis also found a significant benefit of hawthorn in the reduction of pressure × heart rate product (a combined measure of systolic blood pressure and heart rate that when reduced is associated with improved clinical status) as well as symptomatic relief of dyspnea and fatigue (2).

- In a double-blind, randomized, placebo-controlled trial to test the safety and efficacy of a Crataegus berry extract in the treatment of congestive heart failure, 143 patients with Class II heart failure received a standardized extract (30 drops or 12.7 mg phenolic compounds) of *Crataegus oxyacantha* L. and *Crataegus monogyna* Jacq. berries (n = 69) or placebo (n = 74) daily for 8 weeks. Patients were equally distributed in terms of gender, smoking status and clinical comorbidities such as leg edema. The mean age of the study population was 64.8 years. Data from a total of 59 subjects in the treatment group and 58 in the placebo group were considered for analysis. Exercise tolerance was assessed using maximal wattage achieved during stationary cycling, which was sustained for at least 2 minutes. Blood pressure × heart rate product and relevant cardiac-associated symptoms (fatigue, quick pulse, etc) as reported by patients were also assessed. All measures were taken at baseline and after 8 weeks. While all subjects showed a significant improvement in exercise tolerance from baseline, subjects receiving the hawthorn extracts also demonstrated a significant increase in exercise tolerance as compared with those in the placebo group. No significant effects on blood pressure × heart rate product or related subjective symptoms were shown. Tolerance for hawthorn was also reportedly good (4).

References

1. Tauchert M. Efficacy and safety of crataegus extract WS 1442 in comparison with placebo in patients with chronic stable New York Heart Association class-III heart failure. *Am Heart J.* 2002;143:910–915.
2. Pittler MH, Schmidt K, Ernst E. Hawthorn extract for treating chronic heart failure: meta-analysis of randomized trials. *Am J Med.* 2003;114:665–674.
3. Rigelsky JM, Sweet BV. Hawthorn: pharmacology and therapeutic uses. *Am J Health Syst Pharm.* 2002;59:417–422.

4. Degenring FH, Suter A, Weber M, et al. A randomised double blind placebo controlled clinical trial of a standardized extract of fresh Crataegus berries (Crataegisan) in the treatment of patients with congestive heart failure NYHA II. *Phytomed.* 2003;10:363–369.

HCA. *See* Hydroxycitric Acid *(Garcinia cambogia).*

HMB. *See* ß-Hydroxy ß-Methylbutyrate (HMB).

Horse Chestnut

The horse chestnut tree *(Aesculus hippocastanum)* has a thick, short trunk and typically grows to approximately 25 to 30 meters in height. The tree produces its fruit every fall, which contains two to four large seeds, or "nuts." In the 19th century, herbalists began to use the seed extract to treat varicose veins, hemorrhoids, arthritis, and menstrual cramps. While native to northern and central Asia, the horse chestnut tree is cultivated all over the world. The active component of the seed, aescin, is thought to be responsible for reducing inflammation and increasing the vascular integrity, or tone, of veins. Horse chestnut seeds are toxic and can cause severe gastrointestinal and neurotoxic reactions if consumed. The toxin aesculin in the unprocessed seeds is removed through a purification process before distribution.

Media and Marketing Claims	Efficacy
Treats chronic venous insufficiency	↑?
Treats hemorrhoids	NR

Safety

♦ The bark, raw seed, leaf, and flower of horse chestnut are extremely toxic. Consuming these constituents can be lethal (1).

♦ Because many of the components of horse chestnut are toxic, the FDA has classified it as an "unsafe herb." However, purified horse chestnut seed extract seems to be safe for short-term use (2).

Drug/Supplement Interactions

Horse chestnut taken with anticoagulant/antiplatelet drugs has an additive effect. Individuals taking anticoagulants may be advised to avoid horse chestnut and should check with their physician before using this supplement.

Key Points

- In a meta-analysis of horse chestnut seed extract for chronic venous insufficiency, investigators found horse chestnut extract to be safe and effective as a short-term treatment (2). Similar conclusions were reached by the same research group in an earlier review of the literature and an alternate research group in 2002 (3); however, authors also noted the need for more clinical trials to fully evaluate the supplement's effectiveness (4).

- There has been no research to support the use of horse chestnut for the treatment of hemorrhoids.

Food Sources

None

Dosage Information/Bioavailability

Horse chestnut is available as powder, ointment, lotion, liquid, gel, cream, and capsule. To see any clinical benefit, it is important to use only products that are standardized to contain 50 mg aescin/dose. Topical formulations are new to the US market and may not be as effective as oral forms. Research studies have used 250 mg twice/day or 1 teaspoon of liquid extract twice/day for the treatment of varicose veins.

Relevant Research

Horse Chestnut and Chronic Venous Insufficiency

- A Cochrane Database review included 17 trials of horse chestnut seed extract as a treatment for chronic venous insufficiency. All studies used extract standardized to aescin, the biologically active constituent in horse chestnut. All but one of these studies were double-blind, and all were placebo-controlled. In six of seven trials (n = 543 patients), leg pain was significantly reduced in the treatment group compared with the control group. Meta-analysis of four of six trials (n = 461 subjects) found that leg edema was significantly reduced with horse chestnut compared with placebo. In four of eight studies (n = 407 subjects), pruritis significantly improved with horse chestnut treatment compared with placebo. Finally, the analysis of six of seven studies (n = 502 subjects) showed that leg volume significantly improved with horse chestnut seed extract supplementation as compared with placebo (2).

◆ The findings of the Cochrane review described in the previous bullet are supported by two criteria-based reviews (3,4) that included double-blind, placebo-controlled studies. Further, four randomized, parallel-group clinical trials that tested the efficacy of horse chestnut supplementation against standard medications suggest that horse chestnut is as effective as o-(ß-hydroxytheyl)-rutosides (3). No data to support horse chestnut flowers, raw seeds, bark, or leaves efficacy were found (4).

◆ A randomized, partially blinded, placebo-controlled study compared the safety and efficacy of dried horse chestnut seed extract vs compression stockings in the reduction of leg edema. Two hundred and forty subjects (194 women and 46 men) with chronic venous insufficiency were treated with compression stockings, horse chestnut seed extract (50 mg aescin), or placebo for 12 weeks. Investigators designed an intention-to-treat protocol that required the partial blinding of the study. Lower-leg edema decreased significantly in subjects in the horse chestnut seed extract and compression stocking groups vs placebo. The efficacy of horse chestnut seed extract and compression stockings were equivalent (5).

◆ A double-blind, randomized, placebo-controlled trial assessed the efficacy of horse chestnut seed extract in the reduction of leg edema in 38 subjects (9 men and 29 women) between the ages of 25 and 65 years (mean age 53 years) who had stage 2 chronic venous insufficiency. Subjects were randomly assigned to horse chestnut seed extract (1 capsule daily, standardized to 75 mg aescin) or placebo. Before and after 6 weeks of supplementation, subjects were evaluated with hydroplethysmography (to measure leg volume) and leg circumference measurements were taken before and after edema provocation. Compared with placebo, horse chestnut seed extract significantly reduced leg edema as measured by hydroplethysmography and measures of leg volume. This finding was also supported by patients' self-reports of leg heaviness, leg fatigue, itching, and paresthesia (6).

References

1. Ellenhorn MJ, Schonwald S, Orgod G, et al. *Ellenhorn's Medical Toxicology: Diagnoses and Treatment of Human Poisoning.* 2nd ed. Baltimore, Md: Williams and Wilkins; 1997.
2. Pittler MH, Ernst E. Horse chestnut seed extract for chronic venous insufficiency. *Cochrane Database Syst Rev.* 2006;(1):CD003230.
3. Pittler MH, Ernst E. Horse-chestnut seed extract for chronic venous insufficiency. A criteria-based systematic review. *Arch Dermatol.* 1998;134:1356–1360.
4. Tiffany N, Booh H, Ulbricht C, et al. Horse chestnut: a multidisciplinary clinical review. *J Herb Pharmacother.* 2002;2:71–85.
5. Diehm C, Trampisch HJ, Lange S, et al. Comparison of leg compression stocking and oral horse-chestnut seed extract therapy in patients with chronic venous insufficiency. *Lancet.* 1996;347:292–294.
6. Diehm C, Vollbrecht D, Amendt K, et al. Medical edema protection—clinical benefit in patients with chronic deep vein incompetence. A placebo controlled double blind study. *Vasa.* 1992;21:188–192.

5-Hydroxy-Tryptophan (5-HTP)

5-Hydroxy-tryptophan, or 5-HTP, is derived from the seed of the African plant *Griffonia simplifica*. 5-HTP supplements should not be confused with L-tryptophan supplements; the latter are currently banned in the United States for safety reasons. 5-HTP is a metabolite of the essential amino acid L-tryptophan, and both are precursors to the neurotransmitter serotonin in the body. Serotonin regulates several processes in the body, including sleep, emotions, pain sensitivity, and addictive cravings. If there is a sufficient supply of L-tryptophan and its metabolite 5-HTP in the body, serotonin will be produced. Scientists believe that low levels or insufficient activity of serotonin and/or norepinephrine may cause depression. In addition, low levels of serotonin may also be involved in sleep disorders, obesity, excessive appetite, and anxiety. In theory, therapeutic use of 5-HTP would result in bypassing the step in which L-tryptophan is converted into 5-HTP by the enzyme tryptophan hydroxylase. The chemical makeup of 5-HTP allows it to cross the blood-brain barrier, whereas L-tryptophan requires a transport molecule to enter the central nervous system. Thus, it is theorized that supplementing 5-HTP would initiate a more immediate and abundant conversion of 5-HTP into the neurotransmitter serotonin (1,2).

Media and Marketing Claims	Efficacy
Reduces depression	↑?
Reduces anxiety disorders such as sleep terrors, panic attacks, and tension-type headaches	NR
Reduces pain of fibromyalgia	NR
Promotes weight control by reducing appetite	NR

Safety

- ◆ 5-HTP may cause gastrointestinal symptoms (nausea, heartburn); may need to start with a low dosage and gradually increase for better tolerability.

- ◆ In 1989, the supplement L-tryptophan was banned due to an outbreak of eosinophilia-myalgia syndrome (EMS) in more than 1,500 people, resulting in 30 deaths. There is some concern about the purity of 5-HTP, because EMS-like symptoms have been reported with its use (3,4).

- ◆ There is one confirmed case of EMS-related syndrome in a mother and her children after taking 5-HTP (3).

- ◆ One study analyzed eight commercially available synthetically and naturally derived 5-HTP supplements and found contamination by an impurity similar to that found in L-tryptophan in all supplements tested (4).

Drug/Supplement Interactions

In theory, 5-HTP should not be combined with other serotonin-enhancing drugs because of the potential risk of serotonin syndrome, which can cause agitation, confusion, blood pressure fluctuations, and diaphoresis. However, this effect has not been reported in the literature.

Key Points

◆ Theoretically, 5-HTP, a precursor to serotonin, may have a variety of beneficial effects because a lack of serotonin seems to be involved in mood disorders, sleep disorders, pain sensitivity, addiction, and satiety.

◆ A recent Cochrane Review of subjects with depression (5) suggests that, although 5-HTP demonstrates a stronger antidepressant effect than placebo, more evidence is needed from long-term, large-scale, controlled trials to determine efficacy. Individuals with moderate or severe depression should be under the care of a mental health professional and should not self-supplement using 5-HTP without physician approval.

◆ Controlled studies are needed to determine whether 5-HTP reduces the perception of pain or reduces anxiety. Small, uncontrolled studies in patients with tension headaches, panic disorder, or sleep terrors provide promising results, but larger well-designed studies are needed.

◆ Evidence is insufficient to determine whether 5-HTP reduces the pain associated with fibromyalgia.

◆ Small, poorly controlled trials report that 5-HTP supplementation reduces appetite, reduces carbohydrate cravings, and stimulates weight loss. It is worth noting that 5-HTP causes mild nausea, which could also have contributed to the reported loss of appetite and weight. Well-controlled research in larger numbers of subjects is needed to validate the claim that 5-HTP is an effective tool for weight reduction.

Food Sources

None

Dosage Information/Bioavailability

5-HTP is available in capsules and tablets in amounts ranging from 50 to 100 mg. Studies have used a range of dosages from 100 to 1,200 mg/day. Some manufacturers recommend taking 100 mg/day on an empty stomach (2). However, because 5-HTP may cause mild nausea in some patients, some researchers recommend taking it with food.

5-HTP seems to be well-absorbed, with approximately 70% reaching the bloodstream (2). Absorption is not affected by ingesting it with other amino acids (2). 5-HTP has been associated with increases in the cerebrospinal fluid levels of 5-hydroxyindolacetic acid, the primary metabolite of serotonin, suggesting that 5-HTP stimulates serotonin release (1).

Relevant Research

5-HTP and Depression

- A Cochrane Review published in 2002 found that only 2 of 108 studies testing 5-HTP for depression were of adequate scientific rigor to support inclusion. These two studies included 64 patients receiving 5-HTP in a placebo-controlled, randomized design. Overall the studies represented a four-fold greater risk for depression in the placebo group vs those taking 5-HTP (5). However, further studies are needed before any clinical recommendations can be made.

- In a double-blind, comparative, multicenter study in Switzerland, 63 patients with severe depression were randomly assigned to receive 300 mg 5-HTP or 150 mg fluvoxamine with meals daily for 6 weeks. No other antidepressant medications were permitted during the study. Subjects were assessed with the Hamilton Rating Scale for Depression (HRSD), Clinical Global Impression (CGI) scale, and their own self-assessment. Both treatment groups showed significant improvements in depressive symptoms as assessed by the HRSD, CGI, and self-assessment; however, there were no significant group differences. Compared with subjects taking fluvoxamine, subjects treated with 5-HTP had less severe adverse events (mostly mild gastrointestinal disturbance, nausea) (6).

- In a double-blind, placebo-controlled study, 26 subjects hospitalized for depression were randomly assigned to receive 300 mg L-5-HTP or placebo plus 50 mg/day chlorimipramine (antidepressant) daily for 28 days. Depressive symptoms were evaluated weekly by the HRSD and at baseline and study end by the CGI scale and Zung's Depression Status Inventory (ZDSI). All subjects improved based on the HRSD, with the L-5-HTP group showing significantly greater improvement. ZDSI scores were also significantly improved in the L-5-HTP group compared with placebo. The parameters that improved more than others were mood, insomnia, work and activities, agitation, anxiety, general and gastrointestinal somatic disturbances, and hypochondriasis (7).

5-HTP and Anxiety-Related Disorders—Tension Headaches, Panic Attacks, and Sleep Terrors

- In a double-blind, placebo-controlled study of 300 mg 5-HTP daily for 8 weeks for the treatment of chronic tension-type headaches conducted among 78 patients in Portugal, 5-HTP neither reduced number of headaches or severity. Fifteen percent of subjects either dropped out of the study or were excluded from analysis due to poor compliance despite the study's short duration making interpretation difficult (8).

- In a study of 32 adult volunteers (14 men, 18 women) who underwent a CCK-4 challenge to induce a panic attack, 5-HTP was no more effective than placebo in treating the panic symptoms. Given the small number of subjects in the trial, the study may have been underpowered in terms of sample size to detect an effect. In addition, the authors noted that women seemed to have greater response rates (lower panic attack rates) with 5-HTP than the men did (9). Results may also have been affected by the selection of healthy volunteers. A separate study that recruited both healthy volunteers and subjects with a history of panic attacks (n = 24 in each group) showed that 200 mg L-5-HTP just after an experimental 35% carbon dioxide panic challenge resulted in lower panic symptom scores (as compared with placebo) only among those with a history of panic disorder, not in healthy volunteers (10). Additional studies are needed.

◆ Preliminary evidence from a small nonrandomized, non–placebo-controlled study of 45 children with sleep terrors, 2 mg/kg/day of 5-HTP for 20 days was given at bedtime to 31 of the children. In 93% of those receiving 5-HTP, sleep terror frequency decreased after 30 days; however, the statistical significance of these data was not provided (11).

5-HTP and Fibromyalgia

◆ In a placebo-controlled, but unblinded study, 200 subjects diagnosed with fibromyalgia and who experienced migraines were randomly assigned to one of four groups for 1 year: (*a*) 400 mg 5-HTP/day; (*b*) tricyclic antidepressants; (*c*) monoamine oxidase inhibitors (MAOIs); or (*d*) 5-HTP plus MAOIs. After an initial 1-month washout period, all subjects were given a placebo for 1 month before beginning the 12 months of treatment. Pain levels were recorded in a daily diary and on a visual analogue scale during the washout, the initial placebo phase, and during the main study. At the end of 12 months, all groups showed significant improvement over measures taken while on the placebo, with the combination of 5-HTP plus MAOIs being the most effective in reducing pain associated with fibromyalgia. The effect of treatment on migraine was not evaluated (7,12).

5-HTP and Appetite

◆ In a double-blind, placebo-controlled study, 28 obese individuals were randomly assigned to receive either 900 mg 5-HTP (300 mg 30 minutes before each meal) or placebo daily for 12 weeks. Subjects were prescribed a 1,200-kcal/day diet during weeks 6 through 12. Subjects were evaluated every 2 weeks for weight, feeding behavior, and energy intake (assessed by 3-day diet records). Patient compliance with 5-HTP was confirmed by urinary excretion of the 5-HTP metabolite (5-hydroxyindoleacetic acid). In the group taking 5-HTP, weight decreased significantly throughout the study (approximately 5% of body weight), but the placebo group had no significant changes in body weight. Mean total energy intake was significantly less only in the 5-HTP subjects, including a significant 50% reduction in intake of grams of carbohydrates consumed daily. Subject reports of satiety were significantly greater in the group taking 5-HTP than the group taking the placebo. Episodic nausea was reported by 80% of 5-HTP subjects during the first 6 weeks, and then reduced to 20%

of subjects for the remaining 6 weeks (rates of nausea in the placebo group were not reported) (13).

◆ In an unblinded pilot study, 14 overweight women (aged 24 to 51 years) with hyperphagia were randomly assigned to receive a placebo or 300 mg 5-HTP 30 minutes before each meal (900 mg/day total) for 12 weeks. During the first 6 weeks, subjects were not given dietary instruction. During the last 6 weeks, subjects were prescribed a 1,200-kcal diet. Every 2 weeks, body weight, diet diary, self-evaluation of appetite and satiety, and anorexia (measured by a questionnaire) were assessed. The prevalence of anorexia (related to early satiety) was higher in the 5-HTP group than in the placebo group (no statistical analysis was reported). Nausea was reported in 70% of the 5-HTP subjects and may have accounted for the loss of appetite (14).

References

1. Meyers S. Use of neurotransmitter precursors for treatment of depression. *Altern Med Rev.* 2000;5:64–71.
2. Birdsall TC. 5-hydroxytryptophan: a clinically effective serotonin precursor. *Altern Med Rev.*1998;3:271–280.
3. Michelson D, Page SW, Casey R, et al. An Eosinophilia-Myalgia Syndrome related disorder associated with exposure to L-5-Hydroxytryptophan. *J Rheumatol.* 1994;21:2261–2265.
4. Klarskov K, Johnson KL, Benson LM, et al. Eosinophilia-myalgia syndrome case-associated contaminants in commercially available 5-hydroxytryptophan. *Adv Exp Biol.* 1999;58:461–468.
5. Shaw K, Turner J, Del Mar C. Tryptophan and 5-hydroxytryptophan for depression. *Cochrane Database Syst Rev.* 2002;(1):CD003198.
6. Poldinger W, Calanchini B, Schwarz W. A functional-dimensional approach to depression: serotonin deficiency as a target syndrome in a comparison of 5-hydroxytryptophan and fluvoxamine. *Psychopathology.* 1991;24:53–81.
7. Nardini M, De Stefano R, Iannuccelli M, et al. Treatment of depression with L-5-hydroxytryptophan combined with chlorimipramine, a double-blind study. *Int J Clin Pharmacol Res.* 1983;3:239–250.
8. Ribeiro CA. L-5 Hydroxytryptophan in the prophylaxis of chronic tension-type headache: a double–blind, randomized, placebo-controlled study. For the Portuguese Head Society. *Headache.* 2000;40:451–456.
9. Maron E, Toru I, Vasar V, et al. The effect of 5-hydroxytryptophan on cholecystokinin-4-induced panic attacks in healthy volunteers. *J Psychopharmacol.* 2004;18:194–199.
10. Schruers K, van Diest R, Overbeek T, et al. Acute L-5- hydroxytryptophan administration inhibits carbon dioxide-induced panic in panic disorder patients. *Psychiatry Res.* 2002;113:237–243.
11. Bruni O, Ferri R, Milano S, et al. L-5- hydroxytryptophan treatment of sleep terrors in children. *Eur J Pediatr.* 2004;163:402–407.
12. Nicolodi M, Sicuteri F. Fibromyalgia and migraine, two faces of the same mechanism: Serotonin as the common clue for pathogenesis and therapy. *Adv Exp Med Biol.* 1996;398:373–379.

13. Cangiano C, Ceci F, Cascino A, et al. Eating behavior and adherence to dietary prescriptions in obese adult subjects treated with 5-hydroxytryptophan. *Am J Clin Nutr.* 1992;56:863–867.

14. Cangiano C, Ceci F, Cairella M, et al. Effects of 5-hydroxytryptophan on eating behavior and adherence to dietary prescriptions in obese adult subjects. *Adv Exp Med Biol.* 1991;294:591–593.

ß-Hydroxy ß-Methylbutyrate (HMB)

ß-hydroxy ß-methylbutyrate (HMB) is a metabolite of the branched-chain amino acid leucine. Approximately 5% to 10% of the leucine in the body is metabolized into HMB. HMB is believed to be converted into HMB-CoA in muscle, mammary tissue, and certain immune cells to synthesize cholesterol necessary to maintain cell function. Humans endogenously produce an estimated 0.2 to 0.4 g HMB/day in the liver and muscle depending on individual dietary leucine intake. Studies showing that HMB increases lean tissue mass and enhances the immune system in farm animals led to the addition of HMB to animal feed and prompted research on its potential for increasing lean body mass in humans (1–4).

Media and Marketing Claims	Efficacy
Increases muscle strength; reduces exercise-induced muscle damage	NR
Increases lean mass; reduces fat mass	↔
Helps resolve HIV- or cancer-related wasting	NR

Safety

- To date, there are no long-term studies (> 8 weeks) using HMB supplements (3 g/day).

- One review article summarized the safety data of 3 g/day HMB in nine human studies lasting 3 to 8 weeks' duration. HMB did not negatively affect any markers of organ or tissue function or emotional state in any of the studies. No safety issues were identified (5).

- Dosages up to 76 mg/kg (approximately 5.5 g for a person weighing 79 kg) for 8 weeks had no adverse effects on liver enzymes, lipid profiles, renal function, or the immune system in 37 untrained college men (6).

Drug/Supplement Interactions

No reported adverse interactions

Key Points

- Preliminary evidence from some studies suggests that 3 g HMB per day may increase strength and lean body mass in adults who exercise, including elderly exercisers. However, not all trials reported strength gains or improvements in body composition with HMB supplementation. New exercisers may experience more benefit than trained athletes.

- Preliminary evidence suggests that HMB may reduce markers of muscle damage caused by exercise. However, other studies showed no significant association.

- One study among patients with HIV and wasting provided promising evidence that a supplement containing HMB, glutamine, and arginine may help patients replete lean body mass, but no further research confirming these results has been published. Similar preliminary evidence with this supplement was found among cancer patients with wasting.

Food Sources

Food	HMB, mg/serving
Catfish (3 oz)	0.204–1.505
Squash (½ cup)	0.267
Avocado (1 cup)	0.165
Cauliflower (1 cup)	0.110
Asparagus (1 cup)	0.108
Cheese (1.5 oz)	0.055
Grapefruit (½)	0.026

Source: Data are from reference 7.

Most foods contain a small amount of HMB (7). Consuming food sources containing the amino acid leucine (primarily in animal products and soybeans and other legumes) enhances endogenous HMB production.

Dosage Information/Bioavailability

HMB is sold as calcium-HMB in tablets, capsules, and in some nutrition bars with suggested dosages ranging from 1 to 3 g/day. Each tablet provides 0.3 to 0.5 g, so it is often necessary to take six to nine tablets or capsules to reach the recommended dose. HMB is often sold in products containing creatine monohydrate, glutamine, carnitine, dehydroepiandrosterone, and N-acetyl cysteine.

Relevant Research

HMB and Strength, Body Composition, and Muscle Damage

- Twenty-six college football players participated in a randomized, placebo-controlled trial of 3 g HMB for 10 days. Before and after football training camp, players completed anaerobic power test, and plasma levels of testosterone, cortisol, creatine kinase, and myoglobin were measured. Although the training resulted in increased creatine kinase and decreased cortisol levels, there was no intervention effect (8). Another study focused on muscular strength effects among 35 college football players. A randomized, double-blind, crossover design with a 1-week washout was used. HMB supplementation was also 3 g/day in this study and intervention (or placebo) continued for 4 weeks. No significant improvement in muscle strength (as measured by bench press, squats, or power cleans) was demonstrated across treatments or over time, nor did body fat or weight show change (9). These studies, along with an additional study by Slater et al (in which subjects were supplemented daily with 3 g HMB standard supplement, or time-released supplement or placebo for 6 weeks, in a randomized, double-blind study) (10), suggest that HMB is not effective in improving muscle strength, athletic performance, or body composition in populations who are already trained and have favorable baseline strength and body composition.

- In a double-blind, placebo-controlled study, 37 untrained males were matched based on their body weights and assigned to one of three groups: 0 mg, 38 mg, or 76 mg HMB/kg body weight daily for 8 weeks. These dosages corresponded to approximately 0 g (placebo), 3 g, and 6 g HMB per day, respectively. Subjects performed resistance training three times per week at 80% of the maximum amount of weight they could lift at one time (one repetition maximum). The placebo group had significantly higher plasma creatine phosphokinase activity (measure of muscle damage) than both HMB groups at 48 hours after the initial training bout. No differences were noted in body fat among the three groups. However, fat-free mass increased more in the 38 mg/kg group (11).

- In a double-blind, placebo-controlled study, 31 older adults (mean age 70 years) engaging in weight training 2 days per week and walking 3 days per week were randomly assigned to receive 3 g HMB/day or a placebo for 8 weeks. Skinfold tests (SF) and computerized tomography (CT) measured fat and lean body mass. Compared with the placebo group, HMB supplementation was associated with a significant increase in percentage of body fat loss as measured by SF and CT scan. There were no significant differences between groups on upper- and lower-body strength as assessed using five different exercises and summing (one repetition) maximum for each lift (12).

- In a double-blind, placebo-controlled study, 40 experienced resistance-trained athletes were matched and randomly assigned to receive a powdered carbohydrate-protein supplement with 0 g, 3 g, or 6 g HMB for 28 days. Blood and urine samples, DEXA, and isotonic bench press and leg press 1 repetition maximum were measured at baseline and at day 28. Blood and urine HMB concentrations increased significantly with HMB supplementation. However, there were no differences between groups on general markers of body anabolic or catabolic status, muscle and liver enzyme efflux, fat-free mass, fat mass, percentage body fat, or measures of strength (13).

HMB and Wasting in HIV or Cancer

- In a mouse model of skeletal muscle loss associated with solid tumors, HMB was shown to attenuate weight loss and induce a small reduction in tumor growth rate. Protein degradation was reduced with HMB, and skeletal muscle protein synthesis increased (14). This animal study provides preliminary evidence for human studies to assess the potential for HMB to prevent muscle loss associated with cancer cachexia.

- Human studies assessing the role of HMB in cancer and AIDS wasting are restricted to the use of a supplement that combines HMB, arginine, and glutamine. One study of 68 patients with HIV and more than 5% body weight loss in the previous 3 months showed that daily intake of the HMB-containing supplement (3 g) for 8 weeks was associated with a mean weight gain of 3.0 kg, while the placebo group experienced a 0.37 kg weight gain (15). Dropout rates were high (25 of 68); therefore, results must be interpreted cautiously. A second study of cancer patients using the same regimen and weight-loss selection criteria showed that among 32 patients, the 18 randomly assigned to HMB gained a mean of 0.95 kg in 4 weeks whereas control subjects lost 0.26 kg (16). The increase in weight could be attributed to increased fat-free mass, and weight gain was sustained over the 24 weeks of intervention. Additional research using HMB alone or in combination in this highly vulnerable population is warranted.

References

1. Nissen S, Abumrad NN. Nutritional role of the leucine metabolite ß-hydroxy ß-methyl-butyrate (HMB). *J Nutr Biochem.* 1997;8:300–311.
2. Nissen S, Fuller JC, Sell J, et al. The effect of ß-hydroxy ß-methylbutyrate on growth, mortality, and carcass qualities of broiler chickens. *Poult Sci.* 1994;73:137–155.
3. Nissen S, Faidley TD, Zimmerman R, et al. Colostral milk fat percentage and pig performances are enhanced by feeding the leucine metabolite ß-hydroxy ß-methylbutyrate to sows. *J Anim Sci.* 1994;72:2332–2337.
4. Van Koeving MT, Dolezal HG, Gill DR, et al. Effects of ß-hydroxy ß-methylbutyrate on performance and carcass quality of feedlot steers. *J Anim Sci.* 1994;72:1927–1935.
5. Nissen S, Sharp RL, Panton L, et al. ß-hydroxy ß-methylbutyrate (HMB) supplementation in humans is safe and may decrease cardiovascular risk factors. *J Nutr.* 2000;130: 1937–1945.
6. Gallagher PM, Carrithers JA, Godard MP, et al. Beta-hydroxy-beta-methylbutyrate ingestion, part II: effects on hematology, hepatic and renal function. *Med Sci Sports Exerc.* 2000;32:2116–2119.

7. Zhang Z, Coates C, Rathmacher J. Occurrence of ß-hydroxy ß-methyl butyrate in foods and feeds. *FASEB J.* 8:A464.

8. Hoffman JR, Cooper J, Wendell M, et al. Effects of beta-hydroxy beta-methylbutyrate on power performance and indices of muscle damage and stress during high-intensity training. *J Strength Cond Res.* 2004;18:747–752.

9. Ransone J, Neighbors K, Lefavi R, et al. The effect of beta-hydroxy beta-methylbutyrate on muscular strength and body composition in collegiate football players. *J Strength Cond Res.* 2003;17:34–39.

10. Slater G, Jenkins D, Logan P, et al. Beta-hydroxy beta-methylbutyrate (HMB) supplementation does not affect changes in strength or body composition during resistance training in trained men. *Int J Sport Nutr Exerc Metab.* 2001;11:384–396.

11. Gallagher PM, Carrithers JA, Godard MP, et al. Beta-hydroxy-beta-methylbutyrate ingestion, part I: effects on strength and fat free mass. *Med Sci Sports Exerc.* 2000;32: 2109–2115.

12. Vukovich MD, Stubbs NB, Bohlken RM, et al. Body composition in 70-year-old adults responds to dietary ß-hydroxy ß-methylbutyrate (HMB) similarly to that of young adults. *J Nutr.* 2001;131:2049–2052.

13. Kreider RB, Ferreira M, Wilson M, et al. Effects of calcium ß-hydroxy ß-methylbutyrate (HMB) supplementation during resistance-training on markers of catabolism, body composition and strength. *Int J Sports Med.* 1999;20:503–509.

14. Smith HJ, Mukerji P, Tisdale MJ. Attenuation of proteasome-induced proteolysis in skeletal muscle by ß-hydroxy- ß-methylbutyrate in cancer-induced muscle loss. *Cancer Res.* 2005;65:277–283.

15. Clark RH, Feleke G, Din M, et al. Nutritional treatment for acquired immunodeficiency virus-associated wasting using beta-hydroxy beta-methylbutyrate, glutamine, and arginine: a randomized, double-blind, placebo-controlled study. *JPEN J Parenter Enteral Nutr.* 2000;24.133–139.

16. May PE, Barber A, D'Olimpio JT, et al. Reversal of cancer-related wasting using oral supplementation with a combination of beta-hydroxy beta-methylbutyrate, arginine and glutamine. *Am J Surg.* 2002;183:471–479.

Hydroxycitric Acid (*Garcinia cambogia*)

Hydroxycitric acid (HCA) is a compound derived from the fruit of a plant called *Garcinia cambogia* (also called Malabar tamarind) found in southeast Asia. HCA was first isolated in the late 19th century, and in the 1960s it was discovered to be a potent competitive inhibitor of the enzyme ATP-citrate-lyase. This enzyme converts citrate, a product of carbohydrate breakdown in the Krebs cycle, into acetyl coenzyme A. Acetyl coenzyme A is a substrate for fatty acid and cholesterol synthesis. Because of this biological action of HCA, some scientists theorized that HCA may inhibit fat synthesis (1,2).

Media and Marketing Claims	Efficacy
Reduces body weight	↓?
Reduces appetite/energy intake	↓?

Safety

♦ No studies have evaluated the long-term safety of HCA supplements in humans; no adverse events in humans have been reported with use up to 12 weeks duration.

♦ In overweight subjects, 12 weeks of 1,500 mg HCA daily seemed to be safe, with no reports of serious adverse effects (1,3).

♦ A review of safety/toxicity data related to HCA published in *Food Chemistry and Toxicology* indicated that up to 2,800 mg HCA per day is safe for human consumption, and that animal and limited human data do not suggest any carcinogenic/mutagenic, tolerance, or reproductive adverse events associated with its use (4).

Drug/Supplement Interactions

No reported adverse interactions

Key Points

♦ Preliminary controlled trials testing the active ingredient in *Garcinia cambogia*, hydroxycitric acid, provide only limited evidence for its efficacy in weight control.

♦ Although some research has reported beneficial effects on body composition, these trials have been criticized for poor design, and for using the herb in combination with other ingredients. Additional controlled, clinical research is needed to build on the present studies and determine the safety and efficacy of the compound.

Food Sources

Garcinia cambogia is not an ingredient or component of food in Western cultures. In India, the dried fruit and rinds of the fruit are used in cooking.

Dosage Information/Bioavailability

Garcinia cambogia extract is sold in tablets, capsules, and powders standardized to approximately 50% HCA. Manufacturers recommend taking from 250 to 1,500 mg HCA per day (500 to 3,000 mg *Garcinia cambogia*) 30 to 60 minutes before eating. Some suggest that a high-fiber diet may inhibit absorption of HCA (2,5). Excessive levels of calcium (used to stabilize HCA) and low solubility in water are also factors that may reduce bioavailability of HCA and that exist in some commercial HCA extracts (5,6).

Relevant Research

HCA and Weight Control

- In a double-blind, placebo-controlled, crossover study, 11 overweight male subjects were randomly assigned to one of three treatments for 2 weeks each, separated by 4-week washout periods. All subjects consumed three self-selected meals (with no restrictions on type or amount of food) and four isocaloric snacks daily. Additionally, one group took 500 mg HCA, another took 500 mg HCA plus 3 mg medium-chain triglycerides, and a third group took only the placebo pill. Each intervention ended with a 36-hour stay in a respiration chamber. All groups had significant weight loss, but this did not differ across groups. In addition, 24-hour energy expenditure, fat oxidation, and satiety did not differ among groups (7).

- In a double-blind, placebo-controlled study, 89 overweight female subjects (weighing 4.5 to 9 kg more than their ideal body weight) were randomly assigned to receive 400 mg HCA three times per day or a placebo for 12 weeks. Treatment was administered 30 to 60 minutes before meals for a total dosage of 1,200 mg/day. Subjects were counseled to adhere to a 1,200-kcal exchange, 30%-fat diet. Weight and body composition were assessed at baseline and every other week for the 12 weeks. Food intake and appetite variables were assessed at baseline and monthly. Both groups experienced significant loss of weight, although mean weight loss with HCA (−3.7 kg) was significantly greater than with the placebo (−2.4 kg). The reduction in fat mass was not significant. No significant effects were observed on appetite indexes (hunger ratings, mean ratings of desire to eat, fullness or sensation of thirst, stomach growling, headache, or irritability). Further, the appetite indexes were not associated with energy intake or body weight change within the active treatment subjects (3).

- In a double-blind, placebo-controlled study, 135 overweight, healthy subjects (ages 18 to 65 years) were randomly assigned to receive 1,500 mg HCA or a placebo daily for 12 weeks. HCA was administered approximately 30 minutes prior to meals. Both groups were prescribed a high-fiber, low-calorie diet plan (20% fat, 50% carbohydrate, 30% protein) and asked to maintain a stable physical activity level. Diet compliance was not quantitatively monitored during the study. Body weight was measured biweekly, and fat mass was measured at baseline and at study's end using DEXA, skinfold thickness, underwater weighing, and bioimpedance analysis). Patients in both groups lost significant amounts of weight during the trial; however, there was no difference between groups in estimated percentage of fat mass loss. Blood or tissue levels of HCA were not measured in this study (1).

- In a double-blind, placebo-controlled, crossover study, 10 sedentary male subjects (age range 22 to 38 years; BMI 22.4 to 37.6) were given, in random order, 3,000 mg HCA or a placebo for 3 days each. The objective of the study was to determine the effect of HCA on marker substrates of altered metabolism and the effect on the respiratory quotient (RQ) and energy expenditure in humans after an overnight fast and during a bout of exercise. The effects of treatment on metabolic parameters with or without moderate exercise (30 minutes at 40% maximal aerobic fitness (VO_{2max})

and 15 minutes at 60% VO_{2max}) were investigated during four laboratory visits. Energy expenditure measured by indirect calorimetry and RQ were measured for 150 minutes after an overnight fast. Blood levels of glucose, insulin, glucagon, lactate, and beta-hydroxybutyrate (marker of increased fat oxidation) were assessed. HCA treatment did not reduce RQ or affect energy expenditure during rest or during exercise compared with placebo treatment. The blood parameters measured were not significantly different between treatment groups under fasting conditions (8).

♦ A double-blind, placebo-controlled, crossover-design study randomly assigned 24 overweight subjects to 2 weeks of HCA or placebo followed by an additional 2-week intervention using the alternate treatment (HCA or placebo). Although HCA reduced energy intake significantly (15% to 30%), there was no change in reported appetite. Weight showed a trend toward reduction but did not reach statistical significance (9).

♦ Sixty overweight adults in India participated in a double-blind, placebo-controlled intervention trial using 4,667 mg HCA, 4,667 mg HCA plus niacin, or placebo for 8 weeks. All subjects consumed 2,000 kcal/day and participated in a supervised walking program. Subjects randomized to HCA or HCA with niacin demonstrated a significant increase in food left on plate after meals (as an indicator of appetite suppression). Also, those in the HCA and HCA plus niacin groups showed a significant reduction in body weight of 5% and 6.1%, respectively. The difference between these two groups was not significant. Lipid profiles also improved (10). This study was generally well-designed compared with other studies.

References

1. Heymsfield SB, Allison DB, Vasselli JR, et al. *Garcinia cambogia* (hydroxycitric acid) as a potential antiobesity agent. *JAMA*. 1998; 280:1596–1600.
2. Badmaev V, Majeed M, Conte AA, et al. *Garcinia cambogia* for weight loss [letter]. *JAMA*. 1999;282:233.
3. Mattes RD, Bormann L. Effects of (-)-hydroxycitric acid on appetitive variables. *Physiol Behav*. 2000;71:87–94.
4. Soni MG, Burdock GA, Preuss HG, et al. Safety assessment of (–)-hydroxycitric acid and Super CitriMax, a novel calcium/potassium salt. *Food Chem Toxicol*. 2004;42: 1513–1529.
5. Schaller JL. *Garcinia cambogia* for weight loss [letter]. *JAMA*. 1999; 282:234.
6. Firenzuoli F. *Garcinia cambogia* for weight loss [letter]. *JAMA*. 1999; 282:234.
7. Kovacs EM, Westerterp-Plantenga MS, Saris WH. The effects of 2-week ingestion of (-)-hydroxycitrate and (-)-hydroxycitrate combined with medium-chain triglycerides on satiety, fat oxidation, energy expenditure and body weight. *Int J Obes Relat Metab Disord*. 2001;25:1087–1094.
8. Kriketos AD, Thompson HR, Greene H, et al. (-)-Hydroxycitric acid does not affect energy expenditure and substrate oxidation in adult males in a post-absorptive state. *Int J Obes Relat Metab Disord*. 1999;23:867–873.

9. Westerterp-Plantenga MS, Kovacs EM. The effect of (-)-hydroxycitrate on energy intake and satiety in overweight humans. *Int J Obes Relat Metab Disord.* 2002;26: 870–872.

10. Preuss HG, Bagchi D, Bagchi M, et al. Effects of natural extract of (-)-hydroxycitric acid (HCA-SX) and a combination of HCA-SX plus niacin-bound chromium and *Gymnema sylvestre* extract on weight loss. *Diabetes Obes Metab.* 2004;6:171–180.

Indole-3-carbinol (I-3C)

Indole-3-carbinol (I-3C) is a compound in cruciferous vegetables such as broccoli, cabbage, cauliflower, and kale. It is also known as indole-3-methanol. I-3C stimulates cytochrome P450 detoxification enzymes in the gut and liver and is currently being studied as a cancer preventive agent. Preliminary evidence indicates that I-3C may reduce the risk of cancer in humans. However, a small number of animal studies have found the compound to have tumor-promoting effects. One biological effect of interest, in the context of estrogen-related cancers, is that I-3C seems to reduce estrogen levels (1), possibly by down-regulating estrogen receptors at select tissue sites, but the specific mechanisms have yet to be fully described. The National Cancer Institute has published a clinical development plan to test the efficacy of I-3C as a cancer chemopreventive agent (2), and a standardized supplement for trials has been developed. Research using this compound is on-going.

Media and Marketing Claims	Efficacy
Slows cancer growth	↑?

Safety

- Although no adverse events have been reported in human clinical trials, data suggest that I-3C has some tumor-promoting capabilities (3). For this reason I-3C should only be taken under the advice of a physician.

- Dietary consumption of I-3C through the consumption of cruciferous vegetables is considered safe because the dose will be significantly less than would be consumed with supplements, and there is a theoretical health-promoting synergy among active biological constituents found in cruciferous vegetables.

Drug/Supplement Interactions

I-3C induces the liver enzyme P450 and may affect the levels of medications metabolized by P450 enzymes.

Key Points

- I-3C has been developed as a chemopreventive agent for Phase I and II trials; however, data are currently limited (2). The biological mechanisms of anticancer activity have been well-described in cell-culture models, and to some extent in animal models, but additional evidence in human studies is needed, particularly those that include clinical cancer outcomes.

Food Sources

Cruciferous vegetables such as broccoli, cauliflower, kale, cabbage, and mustard greens are rich in I-3C. The specific level of I-3C found in these foods varies with cultivar, climate, cooking and processing, and no specific I-3C database is available for US-grown cruciferous vegetables. However, it is known that food sources have substantially less I-3C than commercially available supplements (100 mg/capsule; recommended intake 2 to 3 capsules/day).

Dosage Information/Bioavailability

I-3C can be purchased in tablet form. Doses between 200 to 400 mg of I-3C per day have been used to study its effects on premalignant cervical lesions and up 800 mg/day has been used in Phase I chemoprevention studies. Animal studies suggest that intraperitoneal or IV administration of I-3C does not increase urinary or plasma measures, suggesting that oral intake is important to the biological availability and actions (4). The primary metabolite measurable in human plasma after intake of I-3C is diindolylmethane (DIM). Oral administration of the NCI I-3C capsules at doses of 400 mg I-3C daily for 4 weeks followed by 800 mg daily for 4 weeks in 17 women showed a significant and sustained increase in urinary metabolites, which also resulted in a significant 66% increase in 2-hydroxyestrone to 16-alpha hydroxyestrone (5).

Relevant Research

I-3C and Cancer

- Cervical intraepithelial neoplasia (CIN) is a premalignant lesion associated with the development of cervical cancer. In an innovative study design, 27 women with CIN (confirmed pathologically) were randomly assigned in a double-blind fashion to receive placebo or 200 or 400 mg/day of I-3C orally for a period of 12 weeks. I-3C content of the supplements was confirmed using high-performance liquid chromatography (HPLC). Adherence, assessed by subject self-report and pill counts, was estimated as high throughout the study. No patients in the placebo arm showed regression of their premalignant lesions after 12 weeks (lesions were stable as measured by degree of dysplasia), whereas 50% of those receiving 200 mg I-3C and 44.4% of those receiving 400 mg demonstrated complete regression of the lesions at 12 weeks. In addition, the degree to which individual lesions regressed pathologically was dose-dependent (greatest at the higher dose of I-3C). This study suggests that short-term I-3C supplementation may have potential to reverse abnormal pathologies found on Pap smear or colposcopy; however, additional studies are needed (6).

◆ In a randomized clinical trial (unblinded) to test the hypothesis that I-3C can reduce estrogen-related cancer risk through altering estrogen metabolism, 30 healthy women (ages 26 to 45.1 years) who were assessed to be at increased risk for developing breast cancer were assigned to a fiber (cellulose) supplement, 400 mg I-3C, or placebo daily for 3 months. I-3C significantly shifted the urinary 2-OH-estrone:estriol:estrogen ratio toward increased 2-OH, a ratio associated with reduced breast cancer risk (3). Although promising, these results need to be replicated in larger sample populations in blinded studies (and perhaps in a crossover design) before clinical application can be determined.

◆ Combination therapy of I-3C and tamoxifen (estrogen-receptor modulator that reduces estrogen levels in women treated for estrogen-receptor positive tumors) has shown that they both suppress the growth of human breast cancer cells grown in culture but by different pathways, suggesting that together they may have a synergistic effect against this disease (7).

◆ To investigate the effects of I-3C on human prostate cancer cells, cultured cells were supplemented with varying concentrations of I-3C. Three cell lines were used: LNCaP (wild-type p53), DU145 (mutant p53, moderately differentiated), and PC3 (mutant p53, poorly differentiated). I-3C inhibited growth of prostate cancer cell lines by inducing cell death of the cancer cells in culture (8).

◆ In a similar experiment testing the ability of I-3C to prevent cell growth of cultured colon cancer cells (HT29), colon cancer cells were cultured in the presence of varying concentrations of I-3C. Cell proliferation was measured by ^{3}H-thymidine incorporation, the trypan blue exclusion assay, and a colorimetric assay (WST-1 kit). I-3C significantly reduced colon cancer cell proliferation in a dose-dependent manner at concentrations more than 0.1 mM (9).

◆ In another cell culture model, I-3C was tested against cultured cervical cancer cells using two separate cervical cancer cell lines, CaSki and C33A, as well as a healthy cell line (control). After adding varying concentrations of I-3C, cell viability was measured using a mitochondrial function assay, and cell death was measured using the Cell Death Detection ELISA kit from Roche Molecular Biochemicals (Indianapolis, IN) and the TUNEL assay. As with the studies mentioned previously, in this study I-3C was associated with reduced cervical cancer cell growth. In additional studies, transgenic mice known to develop cervical cancer (K14-Human Papilloma Virus16) and nontransgenic control mice were fed a diet supplemented with I-3C and then assessed for the development of cervical cancer. I-3C seemed to be protective: it was associated with reduced mutagenic changes in the cervical cells that are related to HPV16 exposure (10).

◆ To investigate the chemopreventive activity of I-3C, rats were fed AIN-76a diet supplemented with 0.02% or 0.1% I-3C for 23 days. During the feeding period, rats were exposed to the carcinogenic agent PhIP (2-amino-1-methyl-6-phenylimidazole [4,5-b] pyridine), a common carcinogen formed when meat is charred. On day 24, animals were killed for collection of blood and organs. In a second experiment, rats were fed AIN-76a and supplemented with one of six protocols: 3-methylcholanthrene (80 mg/kg) for 2 days, one of two levels of I-3C (100 or 200 mg/kg/day) for 2 days by gavage, one of two dosages of I-3C orally (0.02% or 0.1%) for 2 weeks, or a control diet for 2 weeks. After feeding periods, rats were evaluated for PhIP-DNA adducts in various tissues and white blood cells using a ^{32}P-post-labelling method. I-3C supplementation significantly reduced PhIP-DNA adducts in white blood cells and all tissues except the mammary gland in a dose-dependent manner. This study suggests that I-3C may have chemopreventive activity in PhIP-induced carcinogenesis, such as human colorectal cancers (11).

References

1. Yuan F, Chen DZ, Liu K, et al. Anti-estrogenic activities of indole-3-carbinol in cervical cells: implication for prevention of cervical cancer. *Anticancer Res.* 1999;19: 1673–1680.
2. National Cancer Institute, Division of Cancer Prevention and Control. Clinical Development Plan: Indole-3-carbinol. *J Cellular Biochem.* 1996;265:127–136.
3. Bradlow HL, Michnovicz JJ, Halper M, et al. Long-term responses of women to indole-3-carbinol or a high fiber diet. *Cancer Epidemiol Biomarkers Prev.* 1994;3:591–595.
4. Bradfield CA, Bjeldanes LF. Structure-activity relationship of dietary indoles: a proposed mechanism of action as modifiers of xenobiotic metabolism. *J Toxicol Environ Health.* 1987;21:311–323.
5. Reed GA, Peterson KS, Smith HJ, et al. A Phase I study of indole-3-carbinol in women: tolerability and effects. *Cancer Epidemiol Biomarkers Prev.* 2005;14:1953–1960.
6. Bell MC, Crowley-Nowick P, Bradlow HL, et al. Placebo-controlled trial of indole-3-carbinol in the treatment of CIN. *Gynecol Oncol.* 2000;78:123–129.
7. Cover C, Hsieh SJ, Cram EJ, et al. Indole-3-carbinol and tamoxifen cooperate to arrest the cell cycle of MCF-7 human breast cancer cells. *Cancer Res.* 1999;59:1244–1251.
8. Nachshon-Kedmi M, Yannai S, Haj A, et al. Indole-3-carbinol and 3,3'-diindoylylmethane induce apoptosis in human prostate cancer cells. *Food Chem Toxicol.* 2003;41:745–752.
9. Frydoonfar HR, McGrath DR, Spigelman AD. Inhibition of proliferation of a colon cancer cell line by indole-3-carbinol. *Colorectal Dis.* 2002;4:205–207.
10. Chen DZ, Qi M, Auborn KJ, et al. Indole-3-carbinol and diindolylmethane induce apoptosis of human cervical cancer cells and in murine HPV16-transgenic preneoplastic cervical epithelium. *J Nutr.* 2001;131:3294–3302.
11. He YH, Friesen MD, Ruch RJ, et al. Indole-3-carbinol as a chemopreventive agent in 2-amino-1-methyl-6-phenylimidazo[4,5-b]pyridine (PhIP) carcinogenesis: inhibition of PhIP-DNA adduct formation, acceleration of PhIP metabolism, and induction of cytochrome P450 in female F344 rats. *Food Chem Toxicol.* 2000;38:15–23.

Iron

Iron is one of the most plentiful trace metals on earth. It is essential for the formation of red blood cells and hemoglobin and is a constituent of myoglobin, which carries oxygen in muscle. A deficiency in iron decreases oxygen delivery to cells and can result in an iron deficiency that can lead to anemia. Initially, iron deficiency causes no symptoms, but over time symptoms develop; an untreated deficiency eventually leads to anemia. The World Health Organization identifies iron deficiency as the most common nutrition disorder in the world (1). Part of the problem is a lack of dietary iron. A study examining the nature and magnitude of iron-deficiency anemia found that as much as 80% of the world's population may be iron-deficient, and 30% of those may have iron-deficiency anemia (2). Symptoms of iron-deficiency anemia include fatigue, extreme weakness, decreased performance at work, decreased cognitive abilities, difficulty maintaining body temperature, susceptibility to infection, difficulty breathing, and glossitis (3).

There are two forms of iron: heme and non-heme. Heme-iron is the most readily absorbed and is found in meat, fish, and poultry. Non-heme iron sources are dried fruits, green-leafy vegetables, and most iron supplements. There are three types of iron supplements: ferrous sulphate, ferrous gluconate, and ferrous fumerate. Ferrous fumarate typically contains the largest amount of elemental iron. To increase absorption, dietary and supplemental sources of non-heme iron should be consumed with food and beverages rich in vitamin C. In addition, eating foods rich in oxalates or tannins or taking calcium supplements with iron-rich foods can reduce the bioavailability.

Media and Marketing Claims	Efficacy
Treats and prevents iron deficiency anemia	↑
Treats anemia of chronic disease	↔
Improves cognitive function in iron-deficient children and adolescents	↑?

Safety

- It is essential that iron supplements be stored away from children. Even at low doses, iron supplementation can result in toxicity in children. In case of suspected overdose, contact your local poison control center.

- Iron poisoning is the leading cause of poisoning death in children younger than age 6 years (4,5). Iron supplements must be in a child-safe bottle and kept in a locked cabinet.

- Iron is considered safe when taken in dosages that do not exceed the Tolerable Upper Intake Limit (UL). The UL for individuals older than 14 years is 45 mg/day; the UL for children younger than 14 is 40 mg/day (3).

- When taken in doses greater than the UL, side effects include constipation, stomach cramps, nausea, and vomiting.
- Excessive iron intake over time can lead to toxicity. Symptoms include dehydration, low blood sugar, fever, bluish colored lips and fingernails, pallor, vomiting blood, low blood pressure, fast and weak pulse, drowsiness, shock, and coma (4).
- Iron supplementation in people with normal iron stores can increase levels of oxidative DNA damage and thus contribute to increased cancer risk (6).

Drug/Supplement Interactions

- Iron taken in combination with any of the following drugs may cause serious side effects: antibiotics (quinolone, tetracycline), bisphosphonates (Fosamax), levodopa, methyldopa, penicillamine, and drugs used to treat thyroid disorders.
- Supplementation with 256 mg ferrous iron for 4 weeks in 19 Korean adults with ACE inhibitor–associated cough resulted in a significant reduction in self-reported daily mean cough score as compared with placebo (7). Further studies are needed.

Key Points

- An abundance of evidence supports the use of supplemental iron to treat iron-deficiency anemia. Several factors can contribute to iron deficiency: poor dietary intake, decreased absorption, and excessive blood loss. Individuals who may benefit the most from iron supplementation are pregnant women, preterm infants, infants and toddlers, teenage girls, women with heavy menstrual losses, people with renal failure, and people with medical conditions that affect their ability to absorb iron (8). However, even at low doses, iron supplementation can be toxic for children.
- It is a commonly held belief that many premenopausal women are iron-deficient. This belief is based on reports that menstrual bleeding is a leading cause of iron deficiency. However, an analysis of the prevalence of iron deficiency in the United States showed only 1 in 10 premenopausal women are iron-deficient (2).
- Iron supplementation in combination with red cell–promoting medications such as erythropoietin will improve red cell count and symptoms (fatigue) related to anemia of chronic disease (ie, diseases such as chronic renal failure, premature birth [9], and chemotherapy-treated cancers).
- Studies show that iron deficiency in children and adolescents is commonly associated with poor school performance and reduced cognitive function.

Food Sources

Iron is available from heme sources (found in meat, fish, and poultry) and non-heme sources (found mainly in fruit, vegetables, grains, nuts, beans, and fortified products such as cereal).

Heme Iron Sources	Iron, mg/serving
Beef, liver (3 oz)	7.5
Beef, lean ground (3 oz)	3.9
Beef, flank (3 oz)	4.3
Chicken breast, boneless (3 oz)	0.9
Chicken, liver (3 oz)	7.3
Cod, broiled (3 oz)	0.8
Flounder, baked (3 oz)	1.2
Pork, lean ham (3 oz)	1.9
Salmon, pink canned (3 oz)	0.7
Turkey, white meat (3 oz)	1.2

Source: Data are from reference 10.

Non-Heme Iron Sources	Iron, mg/serving
Baked beans, canned (½ cup)	2.0
Almonds, raw (10–12 whole)	0.7
Bagel (1 whole)	1.5
Bread, white (2 slices)	1.4
Bread, whole-wheat (2 slices)	1.7
Broccoli, raw (1 stalk)	1.1
Prune juice (½ cup)	1.5
Rice, white enriched, cooked (1 cup)	1.8
Spaghetti, enriched, cooked (1 cup)	1.6
Spinach, cooked (½ cup)	2.0

Source: Data are from reference 10.

Dosage Information/Bioavailability

Iron is available in many different forms including capsules, elixir, tablets, oral solution and suspension, chewables, and extended release tablets. Iron can also be given parenterally by injection. When choosing a supplement, read the label for elemental iron. This is the amount of iron that is available for absorption.

Daily requirements for iron in adults are 8 mg for men and 18 mg for women up until age 50, at which time the requirement is 8 mg/day for both men and women. Requirements for children are 7 mg/day for ages 1 to 3 years and 10 mg/day for ages 4 to 8 years. Menstruating girls should increase iron intake to 15 mg/day through age 19 and vegetarian adolescent girls should further increase intake to 26 mg/day (2). Iron is most efficiently absorbed when taken on an empty stomach with a high–vitamin C fruit juice, but to eliminate the possibility of upset stomach, iron supplements may be taken with food or after meals.

One of the largest influences on iron absorption is iron stores. When body stores are low, iron is more readily absorbed. When stores are high, absorption decreases to protect the body from iron toxicity (3). Several studies have shown that calcium and the tannins found in tea can decrease the absorption of non-heme iron (11). Vitamin C improves the absorption (12).

Relevant Research

Iron and Iron-deficiency Anemia

- In a double-blind, randomized, placebo-controlled trial to determine an effective dosage of daily iron to treat iron deficiency in frequent blood donors, 526 regular blood donors received either 0, 20, or 40 mg ferrous gluconate daily for 6 months. During the treatment period, men donated four units and women donated three units of whole blood. Hemoglobin levels, serum ferritin, and transferrin receptor levels were measured before each donation. Both 20 mg and 40 mg iron were effective in treating iron deficiency in frequent blood donors (13).

- To collect information on patterns of iron intake in adolescent girls and women in the United States, data from the Third National Health and Nutrition Examination Survey (NHANES III) trial were used. Daily intake of iron was determined from questions about vitamins and minerals consumed in the previous month. It was estimated that approximately 9% of nonpregnant, nonlactating adolescents, 23% of women 19 years and older, 72% of pregnant women, and 60% of lactating women consume iron supplements. Low-income and minority individuals were less likely to consume iron even though they are more likely to experience iron deficiency. Iron supplementation was associated with significant reduction in iron deficiency in women age 19 to 50 years old (14).

Iron and Anemia of Chronic Disease

- In a double-blind, placebo-controlled study conducted in cardiac surgery patients diagnosed with anemia of chronic disease, 63 patients received rhEPO (5 × 500 U/kg body weight) or placebo intravenously for 14 days before surgery. All patients also were provided 300 mg iron glycine sulfate orally each day in a single dose. rhEPO significantly increased hemoglobin, hematocrit, reticulocyte count, and red blood cell counts while decreasing transferrin saturation levels. The placebo had no effect. Interestingly, the efficacy of rhEPO was demonstrated specifically in those with anemia of chronic disease before initiation of iron supplementation and rhEPO (vs iron plus placebo) (15). Additional studies in other patient populations demonstrating anemia of chronic disease are warranted; however, in cancer patients receiving EPO, additional iron supplementation, although potentially enhancing the EPO efficacy, could also contribute to increased oxidative stress and therefore should be closely evaluated.

Iron and Cognitive Function in Iron-Deficient Children and Adolescents

- A double-blind, placebo-controlled study in 716 adolescent girls with non-anemic iron deficiency (related to menstrual blood loss) was conducted to test the hypothesis that iron supplementation improves cognitive function and, indirectly, school performance. Eighty-one girls with non-anemic iron deficiency consented to participate. Students were randomly assigned to 650 mg ferrous sulfate twice/day or placebo for 8 weeks. Ninety-six percent of the girls completed the trial. Among those receiving iron supplementation, mean serum ferritin levels increased significantly, from 12.1 to 27.3 µg/L. Both verbal test and memory testing were significantly higher in the iron-supplemented group at the end of the study, despite equivalent deficits at baseline in both groups of girls (16).

References

1. Looker AC. Prevalence of iron deficiency in the United States. *JAMA*. 1997;277: 973–976.
2. Stoltzfus RJ. Defining iron-deficiency anemia in public health terms: reexamining the nature and magnitude of the public health problem. *J Nutr*. 2001;131(2S-2):S565–S567.
3. Institute of Medicine. *Dietary Reference Intakes for Vitamin A, Vitamin K, Arsenic, Boron, Chromium, Copper, Iodine, Iron, Manganese, Molybdenum, Nickel, Silicon, Vanadium, and Zinc*. Washington, DC: National Academy Press; 2001.
4. Iron overdose. Available at: http://www.drugs.com. Accessed May 30, 2005.
5. McKevoy GK, ed. *AHFS Drug Information*. Bethesda, Md: American Society of Health- System Pharmacists; 1998.
6. Rehman A, Collis CS, Yang M, et al. The effects of iron and vitamin C co-supplementation on oxidative damage to DNA in healthy volunteers. *Biochem Biophys Res Comm*. 1998;246:293–298.
7. Lee S, Park SW, Kim DK, et al. Iron supplementation inhibits cough associated with ACE inhibitors. *Hypertension*. 2001;38:166–170.
8. Moriarty-Craige SE, Ramakrishnan U, Neufeld L, et al. Multivitamin-mineral supplementation is not as efficacious as is iron supplementation in improving hemoglobin concentrations in nonpregnant anemic women living in Mexico. *Am J Clin Nutr*. 2004;80:1308–1311.
9. Carnielli VP, Da Riol R, Montini G. Iron supplementation enhances response to high doses of recombinant human erythropoietin in preterm infants. *Arch Dis Child Fetal Neonatal Ed*. 1998;79:44–48.
10. Office of Dietary Supplements. Dietary Supplement Fact Sheet: Iron. Available at: http://ods.nih.gov/factsheets/iron.asp. Accessed March 17, 2006.
11. Samman S, Sandstrom B, Toft M, et al. Green tea or rosemary extract added to foods reduces non-heme iron absorption. *Am J Clin Nutr*. 2001;73:607–612.
12. Siegenberg D, Baynes R, Bothwell T, et al. Ascorbic acid prevents the dose-dependent inhibitory effects of polyphenols and phytates on non-heme absorption. *Am J Clin Nutr*. 1991;53:537–541.
13. Radtke H, Tegtmeier J, Rocker L, et al. Daily doses of 20 mg of elemental iron compensate for iron loss in regular blood donors: a randomized, double-blind, placebo-controlled study. *Transfusion*. 2004;44:1427–1432.

14. Cogswell ME, Kettel-Khan L, Ramakrishnan U. Iron supplement use among women in the United States: science, policy, and practice. *J Nutr.* 2003;133:S1974–S1977.
15. Sowade O, Messinger D, Franke W, et al. The estimation of efficacy of oral iron supplementation during treatment with epoetin beta (recombinant human erythropoietin) in patients undergoing cardiac surgery. *Eur J Haematol.* 1998;60:252–259.
16. Bruner AB, Joffe A, Duggan AK, et al. Randomised study of cognitive effects of iron supplementation in non-anaemic iron-deficient adolescent girls. *Lancet.* 1996;348:992–996.

Isoleucine. *See* Branched-Chain Amino Acids (BCAA).

Kava

Kava (*Piper methysticum;* also known as kava-kava) is a perennial plant native to the Pacific Islands. For centuries, kava roots have been ground into a bitter-tasting drink for ceremonial occasions in the South Pacific. The kava beverage, a psychoactive drink, is valued for its minor tranquilizing and relaxant effects. Kava pyrones (also referred to as kava lactones), the active components of the kava plant, are generally considered to be responsible for its sedative qualities. The mechanism of action on the central nervous system is not known. In vitro studies have found that certain pyrones block norepinephrine uptake. Recent studies have suggested that kava has monoamine oxidase (MAO) uptake inhibition properties. Research is conflicting regarding the capacity of kava to bind to the gamma-aminobutyric acid receptors in the brain (prescription sedatives bind to these receptors) (1,2).

Media and Marketing Claims	Efficacy
Reduces anxiety	↑?
Promotes restful sleep	NR

Safety

♦ Patients with liver disease should not use kava. The FDA released a Consumer Advisory warning in March 2002 (3) regarding the potential hepatic toxicity of kava supplements, but kava has not been removed from US markets as it has been in other nations. Kava has been banned in Switzerland, Germany, and Canada. It is not known whether the cases cited in the FDA warning were due to contamination or a particular component found in kava.

- A 50-year-old man developed acute hepatitis and required liver transplantation after taking kava extract (210 to 280 mg kava lactones/day) for 2 months. The authors of the case report noted that heavy kava intake has been associated with increased levels of gamma-glutamyltransferase, suggesting potential hepatotoxicity (4).

- Patients taking kava should have ongoing liver function tests to monitor hepatic function; abnormalities can appear within 3 weeks of use.

- The German Commission E reports that kava should be discontinued if side effects such as discoloration of skin, hair, and nails, enlargement of pupils, or disturbance of ocularmotor equilibrium develop (5).

- The Commission E report also states that kava is contraindicated in pregnancy, nursing, and endogenous depression. It should not be combined with alcohol, barbiturates, or psychopharmacological agents because of possible potentiation of sedative effects (5).

- Due to its sedative properties, kava could adversely affect motor reflexes and judgment for driving or operating heavy machinery (5).

- In Australia, heavy kava beverage consumption (300 to 400 g/week) has been associated with scaly rash, malnutrition, abnormal liver function tests, and dyskinesia (6,7).

- Cases of kava extract–associated skin lesions have been reported. Two to three weeks of kava use was associated with papules and plaques on the face, arms, back, and chest (8,9).

- A safety review for kava indicated that gastrointestinal complaints, allergic skin reactions, headaches and sensitivity to UV exposure are common and worsen at higher does of kava (10). The review also discusses the 78 cases of hepatotoxicity identified among adults using kava supplements.

- Kava should not be used for more than 3 months without medical advice.

Drug/Supplement Interactions

- Kava has potential additive, sedative effects when combined with alcohol, antianxiety medications (benzodiazepines), barbiturates, and other psychopharmacological agents.

- Kava may decrease effectiveness of drugs used in Parkinson's disease (levodopa).

- Preliminary evidence suggests that kava may interfere with medication levels of drugs metabolized through several of the P450 pathways; therefore, medication levels should be monitored with concomitant kava use.

- Concern has also been expressed about the interaction of kava with anesthetic agents (11) and/or medications metabolized through CYP 450 enzyme systems in that medication bioavailability may be altered (increased or decreased) depending on which genetic form of CYP 450 gene a person expresses (12).

- An interaction between kava and the antianxiety medication alprazolam (Xanax, a benzodiazepine) produced lethargy and disorientation in a 54-year-old man. The authors suggested that kava may have an additive sedating effect to benzodiazepines because the medication and the supplement may act on the same receptor and areas of the central nervous system (13). Additionally, if transitioning from antianxiety drugs to kava, patients must be under medical supervision to prevent potential adverse effects.

Key Points

- The FDA released a letter to health professionals seeking information on liver injury and kava products in December 2001, after approximately 25 reports of hepatic toxicity associated with the use of kava were reported in Germany and Switzerland. This was followed by an FDA Consumer Advisory in 2002 that included two cases of hepatic failure in the United States (14). To date, more than 65 cases have been reported, some leading to liver transplant or death. Whether these cases were due to contamination of the kava product has not been resolved. Safety may also be modulated by genetic predisposition to metabolize kava, although this has not been adequately tested. Numerous reports regarding the safety of kava—or lack thereof—have been published in recent years with mixed assessment of the supplement's safety profile (12,15–17). People choosing to use kava should be under medical supervision, including regular liver function testing until more is known about the potential hepatic toxicity.

- Preliminary evidence suggests kava may play a role in reducing anxiety in nonpsychotic anxiety disorders, but more research is needed before specific recommendations can be made.

- Although various books discussing kava suggest that the herb induces a deep, restful sleep and relieves insomnia and nervousness (1), controlled clinical trials are limited. One well-designed study did support efficacy for kava in reducing sleep disturbances associated with anxiety disorders. Confirmatory studies are needed.

Food Sources

Kava beverage (consumed in the South Pacific) is prepared by infusing dried kava powder in cold water for several minutes.

Dosage Information/Bioavailability

Kava is sold in liquid or powdered herbal extract preparations. Some products are standardized to contain 30% kava pyrones/lactones (equivalent to 60 to 120 mg kava pyrones). Most of the research on anxiety used a standardized kava extract, WS 1490. WS 1490 is standardized to contain 70% kava pyrones (providing approximately 210 mg kava pyrones per 300 mg daily dose). Kava can also be taken as a tea. Some products suggest taking kava on an empty stomach to maximize purported sedative effects.

Relevant Research

Kava and Anxiety

◆ The third, and most recent, Cochrane Systematic Review on the use of kava to treat anxiety was published in 2003. This review included 11 well-designed studies (645 subjects) testing the hypothesis that kava was more effective than placebo in reducing anxiety symptoms in subjects with diagnosed anxiety disorders (18). A sub–meta-analysis of six trials (345 subjects) all using the same tool to assess anxiety (the Hamilton Anxiety Scale [HAMA]) supported an intervention effect of kava above placebo. The authors call for further research in this area. Comparison studies with prescribed medications as well as placebos should be considered.

◆ One study compared kava (400 mg/day) with 10 mg buspirone plus 100 mg opipramol in the treatment of general anxiety disorder (GAD). In this study 129 outpatients received supplementation in a double-blind, randomized-design study. Multiple instruments assessed anxiety, sleep disturbance, well-being, and quality of life at baseline and again at 8 weeks. Kava-kava LI150 was shown to be as effective as buspirone plus opipramol in reducing anxiety, showing efficacy in approximately 50% of subjects (19).

◆ In a 3-month unblinded study of perimenopausal women (n = 68) who reported increased anxiety related to the transition to menopause, subjects were randomly assigned to receive 1,000 mg calcium per day alone, calcium plus 100 mg kava, or calcium plus 200 mg kava daily (20). Although anxiety symptoms decreased in the calcium-only group, the reduction was not significant. Significant reductions in anxiety were demonstrated for women taking kava supplements, and anxiety scores between calcium alone and the kava-supplemented groups were significantly different at 1 and 3 months. Depression and mood scores were not significantly different from calcium alone at the end of the study. Follow-up blinded studies assessing the efficacy of kava using a true placebo (rather than calcium) are needed. This study should also include an assessment of sleep outcomes.

◆ In a double-blind, placebo-controlled multicenter study, 101 German outpatients with anxiety disorders clinically documented by the *Diagnostic and Statistical Manual (3rd ed, revised)* were randomly assigned to receive a standardized kava extract (WS 1490) providing 210 mg kava lactones, or a placebo for 25 weeks. The total HAMA score showed a pronounced decrease in both groups; however, patients taking kava scored significantly better from week 8 until the end of the study. Kava was significantly more effective than placebo on HAMA subscores of somatic and psychic anxiety, Clinical Global Impression, Self-Report Symptom Inventory-90 Items revised, and the Adjective Mood Scale. The authors noted that WS 1490 had none of the tolerance problems typically associated with tricyclic antidepressants and benzodiazepines (21).

◆ In a double-blind, placebo-controlled study, 58 patients with anxiety disorders were randomly assigned to receive 100 mg kava extract WS 1490 three times/day or a placebo preparation for 4 weeks. In patients taking kava, anxiety as measured by HAMA, decreased significantly. The magnitude of anxiety reduction in the kava group increased during the course of the study ($P < .02$ at week 8; $P < .001$ at weeks 16 to 24) (22).

Kava and Sleep Disturbance

- Few studies have been conducted to assess the efficacy of kava for treating sleep disturbances.

- In a randomized, double-blind, placebo-controlled study in 61 patients with sleep disturbances associated with anxiety disorders, the researchers used 200 mg WS 1490 (kava) or placebo to treat sleep disturbances for a period of 4 weeks. Efficacy was assessed using the standard HAMA along with a validated sleep questionnaire and self-rating scale of well being. Kava supplementation after 4 weeks was associated with a statistically significant improvement in "quality of sleep" and "recuperative effect after sleep" scores (23). This study provides support for the clinical use of kava for sleep disturbances; however, repeat studies with larger subject populations are needed.

References

1. Singh YN. Kava: an overview. *J Ethnopharmacol*. 1992;37:13–45.
2. *Piper methysticum* (kava kava). *Altern Med Rev*. 1998;3:458–460.
3. US Food and Drug Administration, Center for Food Safety and Applied Nutrition. Kava-containing dietary supplements may be associated with severe liver injury. *FDA CFSAN Consumer Advisory*. March 25, 2002. Available at: http://www.cfsan.fda.gov/ ~dms/addskava.html. Accessed November 7, 2005.
4. Escher M, Desmeules J, Giostra E, et al. Hepatitis associated with kava, an herbal remedy for anxiety. *BMJ*. 2001;322:139.
5. Blumenthal M, ed. *The Complete German Commission E Monographs Therapeutic Guide to Herbal Medicines*. Boston, Mass: Integrative Medicine Communications; 1998.
6. Mathews JD, Riley MD, Fejo L, et al. Effects of the heavy usage of kava on physical health: summary of a pilot survey in an Aboriginal community. *Med J Aust*. 1988;148: 548–555.
7. Spillane PK, Fisher DA, Currie BJ. Neurological manifestations of kava intoxication. *Med J Aust*. 1997;167:172–173.
8. Jappe U, Franke I, Reinhold D, et al. Sebotropic drug reaction resulting from kava-kava extract therapy: a new entity? *J Am Acad Dermatol*. 1998;38:104–106.
9. Schmidt P, Boehncke WH. Delayed-type hypersensitivity reaction to kava-kava extract. *Contact Dermatitis*. 2000;42:363–364.
10. Clouatre DL. Kava kava: examining the new reports of toxicity. *Toxicology Lett*. 2004;150:85–96.
11. Raduege KM, Kleshinski JF, Ryckman JV, et al. Anesthetic considerations of the herbal, kava. *J Clin Anesth*. 2004;16:305–311.
12. Anke J, Ramzan I. Kava hepatotoxicity: are we any closer to the truth? *Planta Med*. 2004;70:193–196.

13. Almeida JC, Grimsley EW. Coma from the health food store: interaction between kava and alprazolam. *Ann Intern Med.* 1996;125:940–941.
14. Centers for Disease Control and Prevention. Hepatic toxicity possibly associated with kava-containing products—United States, Germany, and Switzerland, 1999–2002. *JAMA.* 2003;289:36–37.
15. Teschke R, Gaus W, Loew D. Kava extracts: safety and risks including rare hepatotoxicity. *Phytomedicine.* 2003;10:440–446.
16. Clouatre DL. Kava kava: examining new reports of toxicity. *Toxicol Lett.* 2004;150: 85–96.
17. Stevinson C, Huntley A, Ernst E. A systematic review of the safety of kava extract in the treatment of anxiety. *Drug Saf.* 2002;25:251–261.
18. Pittler MH, Ernst E. Kava extract for treating anxiety. *Cochrane Database Syst Rev.* 2003;(1):CD003383.
19. Boerner RJ, Sommer H, Berger W, et al. Kava-kava extract LI 150 is as effective as opipramol and buspirone in generalized anxiety disorder: an 8 week randomized, double-blind multi centre clinical trial in 129 out-patients. *Phytomedicine.* 2003;10(Suppl 4): 38–49.
20. Cagnacci A, Arangino S, Renzi A, et al. Kava-Kava administration reduces anxiety in perimenopausal women. *Maturitas.* 2003;44:103–109.
21. Volz HP, Kieser M. Kava-kava extract WS 1490 versus placebo in anxiety disorders—a randomized placebo-controlled 25-week outpatient trial. *Pharmacopsychiatry.* 1997;30: 1–5.
22. Kinzler E, Kromer J, Lehmann E. Effect of a special kava extract in patients with anxiety-tension and excitation states of nonpsychotic genesis. Double blind study with placebos over 4 weeks [in German]. *Arzneimittelforschung.* 1991;41:584–588.
23. Lehrl S. Clinical efficacy of kava extract WS 1490 in sleep disturbances associated with anxiety disorders. Results of a multicenter, randomized, placebo-controlled, double-blind clinical trial. *J Affect Disord.* 2004;78:101–110.

L-Arginine. *See* Arginine.

L-Carnitine. *See* Carnitine.

Lecithin/Choline

Lecithin, also known as phosphatidylcholine, is a phospholipid that is approximately 13% choline by weight and is found in the cell membranes and lipoproteins of plants and animals. Choline, an amine, is a precursor of the phospholipids lecithin and sphingomyelin, and the neurotransmitter acetylcholine. As part of these compounds, choline is involved in memory storage, muscle control, cell membrane signaling, and many other functions.

Because it can be synthesized in the body if excess methionine is present, choline is an essential nutrient only when demand for it exceeds the endogenous production. Although a normal diet provides sufficient choline to maintain healthy organ function, some populations are at risk for deficiency, including infants, women during pregnancy or lactation, patients with cirrhosis, and patients fed via total parenteral nutrition (TPN) (1). Several studies have reported that choline deficiency associated with long-term TPN administration results in hepatic steatosis (2–4). In healthy humans, diets deficient in choline have resulted in reduced plasma choline concentrations and the development of liver dysfunction (5). Because lecithin or choline supplementation can reverse steatosis and liver dysfunction, choline is now generally recognized as a "conditionally" essential nutrient for normal liver function (6,7).

Media and Marketing Claims	Efficacy
Improves exercise endurance	↓
Improves dementia in Alzheimer's disease	↓?
Improves memory, concentration	↓?
Improves liver health	↓?

Safety

- ◆ Choline is regarded as safe in doses less than the Tolerable Upper Intake Level (UL) of 3.5 g choline per day for adults age 19 years and older (7).

- ◆ Safety of lechithin is not well-studied. Side effects associated with high oral doses of choline (20 g) include gastrointestinal symptoms, urinary incontinence, and diarrhea.

- ◆ Excess choline (> 20 g) may cause a fishy odor because of breakdown of trimethylamine in the intestine (8).

- ◆ A depression of dopamine receptors and a disturbance of neurotransmitter balance may be a concern when taking chronically high doses of choline (8).

Drug/Supplement Interactions

No reported adverse interactions

Key Points

- ◆ Research suggests that choline is a conditionally essential nutrient. Deficiency is not a concern for most people because choline and lecithin are available in a wide variety of foods. The Institute of Medicine states that "although an AI is set for choline, there are few data to assess whether a dietary supply is needed at all stages of the life cycle and it may be that the choline requirement can be met by endogenous synthesis during some of these stages" (7).

♦ Study results are conflicting about whether choline levels decrease during exercise. However, the limited research in small numbers of subjects shows that lecithin/ choline supplements do not seem to improve exercise performance.

♦ In general, choline/lecithin supplements have not been shown to improve symptoms of Alzheimer's disease. Reduced phosphatidylcholine levels have been demonstrated in the spinal fluid of individuals with Alzheimer's disease (9), but the clinical importance of this is not fully understood.

♦ Although more controlled trials are needed to assess the claim that supplemental lecithin/choline improves memory and cognition in healthy subjects, recent evidence in women suggests lecithin is ineffective for this use.

♦ Although rare, choline deficiency has been associated with hepatic steatosis during long-term TPN administration, which is corrected by choline supplementation.

♦ A well-controlled trial assessing the efficacy of phosphatidylcholine in reducing progression of liver disease in veterans did not show clinical efficacy as compared with placebo. Human studies in this area are lacking.

Food Sources

The estimated mean intake of choline in the typical American diet is 700 to 1,000 mg/day. However, depending on food choices, it is possible to consume more than 2,000 mg/day (4). Rich sources of choline are egg yolks, spinach, organ meats, nuts, and wheat germ. Choline is available in food as lecithin and as free choline. Lecithin is used as an emulsifier in processed foods such as mayonnaise, ice cream, and salad dressings.

Food	Free Choline, mg	Lecithin, mg	Total Choline, mg
Egg (1 large)	0.2	2,009	282.3
Beef steak (3.5 oz)	0.8	466	68.8
Peanut butter (2 Tbsp)	13.0	97	26.1
Cauliflower (½ cup)	6.8	107	22.2
Coffee (6 oz)	18.6	2	19.3
Orange (1)	2.9	53	10.4
Lecithin powder (1 Tbsp/7.5 g)	—	1,725	250

Source: Data are from reference 6.

Dosage Information/Bioavailability

In 1998, the Institute of Medicine set the AI for choline as 425 mg for nonpregnant women and 550 mg for men. The AI for pregnancy is 450 mg/day. No RDA was set due to a lack of data or uncertainty in the data (7). Choline, in the form of choline chloride, choline bitartrate, or lecithin, is available as tablets, capsules, powders, and in some sport beverages. Much of the commercial lecithin sold is a mixture of phospholipids and may contain less than 50% actual lecithin (8). Some manufacturers supply 90% to 98% lecithin powder derived from soybeans. Manufacturers recommend a variety of dosages ranging from 1 to 20 g of lecithin (about 1 to 10 tablespoons of powder).

Dietary choline is absorbed in the small intestine, some of which is metabolized by gut bacteria. Lecithin is broken down by phospholipases and is absorbed into the lymph as chylomicrons via the thoracic duct, and the remaining free choline enters the portal circulation (1,7).

Relevant Research

Choline and Exercise

- ◆ Plasma choline concentrations decreased by approximately 40% in trained runners after a 26-km race. The authors hypothesized that the reductions in plasma choline associated with strenuous exercise may reduce acetylcholine release and could thereby affect endurance or performance (10).

- ◆ In a double-blind, crossover design study, 20 cyclists rode either at 150% power output or 70% output to exhaustion 1 hour after drinking a beverage with or without choline bitartrate (2.43 g). Neither group depleted serum choline during exercise with or without choline, and there were no differences in time to fatigue or work performance between groups. The authors concluded: "Trained cyclists do not deplete choline during supramaximal brief or prolonged submaximal exercise, nor do they benefit from choline supplementation to delay fatigue under these conditions" (11).

Choline and Neurological Disorders

- ◆ In the 1970s and 1980s, several small studies tested the use of choline or lecithin in individuals with Alzheimer's disease. The theory was that by increasing plasma acetylcholine levels through choline supplementation, dementia symptoms would subside. Alzheimer's disease is believed to be associated with a defect in the enzyme choline acetyl transferase, and production of the neurotransmitter acetylcholine by this enzyme is enhanced when more choline is available to the brain. Although occasionally some patients with Alzheimer's disease did respond to choline or lecithin treatment (12), the overall findings of the research did not demonstrate a benefit with choline or lecithin supplements (4,6).

- ◆ A Cochrane Database Systematic Review of lecithin supplementation for dementia included 20 studies involving 265 patients with Alzheimer's disease, 21 subjects with Parkinson's disease, and 90 individuals with self-reported memory problems. Doses of lecithin ranged from 1 to 35 g/day. The authors concluded that current evidence does not indicate that lecithin has efficacy for the treatment of patients with dementia related to Alzheimer's disease or Parkinson's disease; however, in one study of self-reported memory problems there was a statistically significant subjective improvement in memory with lechithin supplementation that warrants follow-up studies (13).

◆ A randomized, double-blind, placebo-controlled study randomly assigned 400 women (mean age 21.8 years) to lecithin (1.6 g/day), placebo, carnitine, or carnitine plus lecithin (14). Multiple measurements of cognitive function and mood were done at baseline and again at 3 days. No significant change in measures was shown. Limitations include the enrollment of healthy adults rather than those with known cognitive impairment and the short duration of intervention (3 days).

◆ A small, double-blind, placebo-controlled trial of six patients with bipolar disorder reported that 10 mg lecithin three times per day dissolved in ice cream had a therapeutic effect on symptoms of mania (hallucinations, delusions, incoherent speech) in five patients compared with the placebo phase (15). However, the dosage used was so small ($\approx$ 4 mg choline), it seems unlikely that such a quantity could ameliorate manic symptoms.

Lecithin and Liver Health

◆ Based on animal data supporting a role for phosphytidylcholine in preventing alcoholic cirrhosis, the Veteran's Administration completed a large-scale, multicenter cooperative study among 789 patients with a history of alcohol abuse (mean intake 16 drinks/day for 19 years) (16). Liver biopsy assessment of fibrotic changes was the primary outcome for this research. Four hundred twelve patients repeated a liver biopsy at 2 years. No significant difference in disease fibrotic progression was shown between the placebo and phosphytidylcholine groups. Liver function tests and bilirubin levels did show transient improvements in the choline-treated group. Although this research did not show efficacy in patients with a significant history of alcohol exposure and liver damage, earlier interventions in individuals with alcoholism who do not have substantial hepatic disease should be considered.

References

1. Zeisel SH. Choline and phosphytidylcholine. In: Shils ME, Olson JA, Shike M, et al, eds. *Modern Nutrition in Health and Disease*. 9th ed. Philadelphia, Pa: Lea & Febiger; 1999:513–523.

2. Buchman AL, Dubin M, Jenden D, et al. Lecithin increases plasma free choline and decreases hepatic steatosis in long-term total parenteral nutrition patients. *Gastroenterology.* 1992;102:1363–1370.

3. Buchman AL, Dubin MD, Moukarzel AA, et al. Choline deficiency: a cause of hepatic steatosis during parenteral nutrition that can be reversed with intravenous choline supplementation. *Hepatology.* 1995;22:1399–1403.

4. Shronts EP. Essential nature of choline with implications for total parenteral nutrition. *J Am Diet Assoc.* 1997;97:639–646, 649.

5. Zeisel SH. Choline: an important nutrient in brain development, liver function, and carcinogenesis. *J Am Coll Nutr.* 1992;11:473–481.

6. Canty DJ, Zeisel SH. Lecithin and choline in human health and disease. *Nutr Rev.* 1994;52:327–339.

7. Institute of Medicine. *Dietary Reference Intakes for Thiamin, Riboflavin, Niacin, Vitamin B-6, Folate, Vitamin B-12, Pantothenic Acid, Biotin, and Choline.* Washington, DC: National Academy Press; 1998.

8. Linder MC. Nutrition and metabolism of vitamins. In: Linder MC, ed. *Nutritional Biochemistry and Metabolism with Clinical Applications.* 2nd ed. Norwalk, Conn: Appleton & Lange; 1991:127.

9. Mulder C, Wahlund LO, Teerlink T, et al. Decreased lysophosphatidylcholine/ phosphatidylcholine ratio in cerebrospinal fluid in Alzheimer's disease. *J Neural Transm.* 2003;110:949–955.

10. Conlay LA, Saboujian LA, Wurtman RJ. Exercise and neuromodulators: choline and acetylcholine in marathon runners. *Int J Sports Med.* 1992;13:S141-S142.

11. Spector SA, Jackman MR, Sabounjian LA, et al. Effect of choline supplementation on fatigue in trained cyclists. *Med Sci Sports Exerc.* 1995;27:668–673.

12. Little A, Levy R, Chuaqui-Kidd P, et al. A double-blind, placebo-controlled trial of high dose lecithin in Alzheimer's disease. *J Neurol Neurosurg Psychiatry.* 1985;48: 736–742.

13. Higgins JP, Flicker L. Lecithin for dementia and cognitive impairment. *Cochrane Database Syst Rev.* 2003;(3):CD001015.

14. Benton D, Donohoe RT. The influence on cognition of the interactions between lecithin, carnitine and carbohydrate. *Psychopharmacology.* 2004;175:84–91.

15. Cohen BM, Lipinski JF, Altesman RI. Lecithin in the treatment of mania: double-blind, placebo-controlled trials. *Am J Psychiatry.* 1982;139:1162–1164.

16. Lieber CS, Weiss DG, Groszmann R, et al. II. Veterans Affairs Cooperative Study of polyenylphosphatidylcholine in alcoholic liver disease. *Alcohol Clin Exp Res.* 2003;27:1765–1772.

Leucine. *See* Branched-Chain Amino Acids (BCAA).

Licorice Root

Licorice *(Glycyrrhiza glabra)* is a herb that has been used in food and medicine for thousands of years. Licorice root, native to Asia, southern Europe, and the Mediterranean, is a perennial plant that grows up to 8 feet tall with an extensive root system. Also known as "sweet root," licorice contains a component that is nearly 50 times sweeter than sugar. The active constituent in licorice is glycyrrhizin, a molecule scientists believe is responsible for mimicking the action of steroid hormones such as aldosterone and estrogen. Isoflavones in licorice have also been reported to mimic estrogens in the human body (1). Used primarily to treat peptic ulcers, deglycyrrhizinated licorice is also used because of the potential side effects that occur with glycyrrhizin (2).

Media and Marketing Claims	Efficacy
Treats stomach ulcers, gastrointestinal upset such as nausea	NR
Treats eczema	NR
Prevents cancer	NR
Helps prevent heart disease	NR

Safety

+ Licorice root has Generally Recognized as Safe (GRAS) status in the United States (3).

+ Glycyrrhizic acid, a component of licorice root, can cause severe allergic reactions. The deglycyrrhizinated licorice preparation has had this component removed and is better tolerated.

+ Licorice can also cause fluid retention, hypokalemia, and metabolic alkalosis. Individuals with any type of heart disease, high blood pressure, kidney or liver disease, or problems maintaining fluid balance should not take licorice root.

+ Licorice may also decrease testosterone levels in men and estrogen levels in women, making it difficult to become pregnant.

Drug/Supplement Interaction

Licorice root taken in combination with any of the following may cause serious side effects: anticoagulant/antiplatelet drugs, aspirin, cardiac glycosides, corticosteroids, diuretics, hormone therapy, insulin, laxatives, and MAO inhibitors.

Key Points

+ Limited data suggest that licorice root may reduce dyspepsia; the one study available for review used licorice root in combination with several other herbals, including peppermint, caraway, and lemon balm. Therefore, what role, if any, licorice may play in reducing dyspepsia was not determined (4). A separate meta-analysis of a second combination herbal supplement (STW 5-II) that includes licorice (as well as bitter candytuft, peppermint, matricaria flower, caraway, and lemon balm) for the treatment of dyspepsia suggests that of the three placebo-controlled studies reviewed, there was an indication of reduced symptoms with supplementation (5).

◆ Data conflict regarding the topical use of licorice to treat eczema. A few small studies indicated an improvement, but others did not (6–8). The herbal preparation used for these studies, Zemaphyte, is no longer being manufactured.

◆ Cell culture data suggest that licorice may modulate cancer risk; no human or animal data are yet available.

◆ Preliminary evidence in one small human intervention trial supports a role for licorice in improving lipid levels.

Food Sources

Licorice root is found as a flavoring agent in a number of candies, snacks, and beverages. Licorice candy made in the United States has no or almost no active glycyrrhizin; however, European-made candies (which can be purchased in the United States) may contain varying amounts.

Dosage Information/Bioavailability

Licorice root is available in wafer, tincture, tablet, lozenge, liquid, tea, cream, and capsule formulations. To avoid potential side effects, look for licorice that has been deglycyrrhizinated (or DGL). To treat ulcers, research studies have used one to two 380-mg DGL wafers three times per day (9). Licorice should be taken intermittently to reduce dyspepsia and may lose efficacy with long term daily use.

Relevant Research

Licorice and Dyspepsia

◆ In a double-blind, randomized, placebo-controlled, multi-center study investigating the treatment of dyspepsia in 120 subjects with chronic or recurrent dyspepsia (ages 21 to 70 years), investigators found after 12 weeks of treatment with STW 5-II (herbal mix containing licorice root and other herbs as described in Key Points) that symptoms of dyspepsia improved significantly as compared with placebo (4). Although licorice root was one of the major components of STW 5-II, it also contained several other herbs. Further research is needed to determine the effect licorice root alone has on dyspepsia.

◆ A meta-analysis of three randomized, double-blind, placebo-controlled studies that included 425 patients with dyspepsia concluded that licorice in combination with other herbals (STW 5) was safe and was shown to be more effective in reducing dyspepsia than placebo (OR = 0.22; 95% CI = 0.11–0.47) (5). Additional studies in larger sample populations and with licorice as a single component are needed.

Licorice and Eczema

◆ A Cochrane Database Review assessing the efficacy of licorice and other herbal medicines in the treatment of eczema was published in 2004, and updated in 2005

(7). Four randomized, controlled trials including 159 patients were available for review. Three studies that included 159 subjects used Zemaphyte, a mixture of herbals, including licorice, and this supplement was shown to have significantly greater efficacy than placebo. None of the studies had a strong design, and sample size was low in individual studies. No further clinical trials using this product will be conducted because it is no longer being manufactured. Studies using licorice preparations for eczema are needed before efficacy can be determined.

◆ A double-blind, placebo-controlled, crossover design study of Zemaphyte (herbal blend supplement that includes licorice) was conducted in 40 Chinese patients with eczema (8). Supplement was provided for 8 weeks followed by a 4-week washout before crossing over to the alternate treatment (Zemaphyte or placebo). More than 90% of patients completed the study. Clinical symptoms improved with both Zemaphyte and placebo treatments, and no significant difference between treatments was shown. This supplement did not seem to be efficacious in the context of recalcitrant atopic dermatitis.

◆ In a study among 40 consecutive adult patients being treated for atopic dermatitis, patients were randomly assigned in a placebo-controlled, double-blind study to receive an herbal combination containing licorice root or placebo herbs for 2 months, followed by a 4-week washout and crossover to the alternate treatment group for an additional 2 months of therapy (6). The supplement contained *Ledebouriella seseloides, Potentilla chinesis, Clematis armandii, Rehmannia glutinosa, Paeonia lactiflora, Lophatherum gracile, Dictammus dascarpus, Tribulus terretris, Schizonepeta tenuifolia* and *Glycyrrhiza glabra*. The supplement resulted in a significant reduction in erythema (swelling/inflammation/redness) as compared with placebo. By self-report, patients preferred the supplement to placebo (20 vs 4 patients).

Licorice and Cancer Prevention

◆ To determine the effects of licorice root extracts on cultured breast cancer cells, MCF-7 cells were cultured in standard medium supplemented with various extracts of licorice root. Cell proliferation, apoptosis, and the expression of PARP and Bcl-2/Bax were evaluated. It was found that trichloromethane, ethyl acetate, methanol, and hexane extracts all inhibited MCF-7 cell proliferation in a time- and dose-dependent manner. Likewise, all extracts induced apoptosis in the MCF-7 cells, with a concomitant cleavage of PARP to its active, pro-apoptotic form and activation of the Bcl-2/Bax pathway (10).

◆ To assess the effects of licorice root extracts on the Bcl-2 pathway in breast and prostate cancer cells, several cell lines were cultured in the presence of various licorice root extracts and subsequently analyzed. Cell cycle arrest analysis was completed to determine whether cells had stopped growing and cells were analyzed for viability and apoptosis using the Apoalert Annexin V-EGFP method and TUNEL assay. In these studies, licorice root extracted with ethyl acetate, DMSO, and ethanol induced Bcl-2 phosphorylation and a cycle arrest (11).

Licorice and Prevention of Cardiovascular Disease

◆ In a blinded, crossover study to analyze the antiatherosclerotic effects of licorice root extracts, 12 patients with hypercholesterolemia were given either 0.1 g of licorice root extract daily for 1 month or placebo for 1 month and then immediately crossed-over to the alternate group. Fasting blood samples were drawn at baseline and after each month of supplementation. Blood samples were analyzed for paraoxonase activity, lipid peroxidation, and plasma lipids. Licorice supplementation reduced plasma LDL oxidation, aggregation, and retention as well as reduced plasma cholesterol levels and triacylglycerol levels. Total cholesterol, LDL cholesterol, and VLDL cholesterol levels were significantly reduced, the benefit of which was lost when subjects were switched to placebo. A significant reduction was also seen in mean systolic blood pressure following licorice supplementation, the benefit of which seemed to be retained while on placebo (12).

References

1. Somjen D, Knoll E, Vaya J, et al. Estrogen-like activity of licorice root constituents: glabridin and glabrene, in vascular tissues in vitro and in vivo. *J Steroid Biochem Mol Biol.* 2004;91:147–155.
2. De Smet K, Keller K, Hansell R, et al, eds. *Adverse Effects of Herbal Drugs.* Vol 3. New York, NY: Springer; 1997.
3. Food and Drug Administration. Center for Food Safety and Applied Nutrition, Office of Premarket Approval. EAFUS: a food additive database. Available at: http://vm.cfsan.fda.gov/~dms/eafus.html. Accessed March 3, 2005.
4. Madisch A, Holtmann G, Mayr G, et al. Treatment of functional dyspepsia with a herbal preparation. A double-blind, randomized, placebo-controlled multicenter trial. *Digestion.* 2004;69:45–52.
5. Melzer J, Rosch W, Reichling J, et al. Meta-analysis: phytotherapy of functional dyspepsia with the herbal drug preparation STW 5 (Iberogast). *Aliment Pharmacol Ther.* 2004;20:1279–1287.
6. Sheehan, M, Rustin MH, Atherton DJ, et al. Efficacy of traditional Chinese herbal therapy in adult atopic dermatitis. *Lancet.* 1992;340:13–17.
7. Zhang W, Leonard T, Bath-Hextall F, et al. Chinese herbal medicine for atopic eczema. *Cochrane Database Syst Rev.* 2004;(4):CD002291.
8. Fung AY, Look PC, Chong LY, et al. A controlled trial of traditional Chinese herbal medicine in Chinese patients with recalcitrant atopic dermatitis. *Int J Dermatol.* 1999;38:387–392.
9. Licorice. Available at: http://www.wholehealthmd.com. Accessed May 31, 2005.
10. Jo EH, Hong HD, Ahn NC, et al. Modulations of the Bcl-2/Bax family were involved in the chemopreventive effects of licorice root *(Glycyrrhiza uralensis Fisch)* in MCF-7 human breast cancer cell. *J Agric Food Chem.* 2004;52:1715–1719.
11. Rafi MM, Vastano BC, Zhu N, et al. Novel polyphenol molecule isolated from licorice root *(Glycrrhiza glabra)* induces apoptosis, G2/m cell cycle arrest, and Bcl-2 phosphorylation in tumor cell lines. *J Agric Food Chem.* 2002;50:677–684.

12. Fuhrman B, Volkova N, Kaplan M, et al. Antiatherosclerotic effects of licorice extract supplementation on hypercholesterolemic patients: increased resistance of LDL to atherogenic modifications, reduced plasma lipid levels, and decreased systolic blood pressure. *Nutrition.* 2002;18:268–273.

Lipoic Acid. *See* Alpha-Lipoic Acid (ALA).

Lutein

Lutein is a xanthophyll carotenoid that is a naturally occurring carotenoid pigment. Along with another carotenoid (zeaxanthin), it accumulates within the eye (1). It is thought to be important to protecting the retina in particular from oxidative damage related to UV light exposure (blue light filters) over the lifespan. Increasing intake of lutein increases not only serum levels but also macular pigment density (2). Although lutein intake has been associated with reduced incidence of age-related eye disease, the data are not unequivocal and only a small number of studies have used lutein supplementation to modulate eye health (3). Lutein is classified as a non–provitamin A carotenoid because it cannot be converted to retinol. Rich sources of lutein include spinach, cabbage, kale, and many cruciferous vegetables.

Media and Marketing Claims	Efficacy
Treats age-related macular degeneration	↑?
Treats age-related cataracts	NR
Treats retinitis pigmentosa	NR
Prevents cancer	NR

Safety

Available trials do not suggest any safety issues, even with long-term use.

Drug/Supplement Interactions

Data are not available; however, it is possible that cholesterol-lowering medications that bind to serum lipids may reduce bioavailability of lutein.

Key Points

- Investigators for the NIH Eye Disease Case-Control Study correlated macular degeneration with intake of dietary antioxidants. Higher intakes of carotenoids were associated with a reduced risk of exudative neovascular macular degeneration (4). In addition, investigators from the Third National Health and Nutrition Examination Survey reported that people between the ages of 40 and 59 years have a reduced risk of macular degeneration with high intakes of lutein and zeaxanthin (5). Studies using lutein supplementation are limited, but hold potential for a therapeutic benefit. Further, a release petition for a qualified health claim for lutein in relation to age-related macular degeneration (AMD) was denied by the FFA (Docket No. 2004Q-0180).

♦ Data from the Nurses' Health Study showed an inverse relationship between the need for cataract surgery and increasing intakes of lutein and zeaxanthin (6). Again, lutein supplementation trials for the prevention of cataracts have not been conducted.

♦ One study has tested the hypothesis that lutein supplementation reduces retinitis pigmentosa in humans, but this study was poorly designed. Further research is needed.

♦ Although some epidemiological evidence suggests a role for dietary lutein in cancer prevention, lutein supplementation trials in humans have not be conducted. Cell-culture studies using select tumor types suggest lutein can induce cell death in cancerous cells.

Food Sources

Food	Lutein, mg/serving
Spinach, cooked (1 cup)	13.3
Savoy cabbage, raw (1 cup)	10.2
Greens, cooked (1 cup)	8.4
Broccoli, cooked (1 cup)	3.4
Peas, cooked (1 cup)	3.2
Spinach, raw (1 cup)	1.8
Green pepper, sliced (1 cup)	0.9

Source: Data are from reference 7.

Dosage Information/Bioavailability

Lutein can be obtained through dietary sources such as spinach, broccoli, and eggs. Lutein supplements include tablets, capsules, and softgels. The most common dosage is 6 mg/day, but some studies used as much as 40 mg/day. One study, using multiple dosage levels of lutein (2.4 to 30 mg) suggests that there is a plateau point at which supplementation translates to improved optical density, and this point is achieved more rapidly and was slightly higher with larger doses of lutein (8). Another study assessed the effect of 9 mg lutein per day on serum levels in young adults vs elderly and showed no age-dependent effects (9). An in vivo model of lutein absorption using human intestinal cells demonstrated that uptake of lutein from oil-based supplementation was greater than for spinach and exceeded beta carotene uptake (10). A 6-week study of lutein supplement pharmacokinetics conducted among 19 healthy volunteers assigned varying doses (0 mg, 4.1 mg, 20.5 mg) indicated that 18 days of supplementation was required to reach steady-state concentration (11). There was no indication in this study that lutein supplementation altered levels of other carotenoids as measured in the serum. Bioavailability of lutein may be reduced in obesity; for this reason, it has been hypothesized that incidence of AMD may increase as incidence of obesity increases in the American population (12).

Relevant Research

Lutein and Age-Related Macular Degeneration

- A double-blind, randomized, placebo-controlled trial assessed whether lutein or lutein plus other supplements improved visual function in 90 male veterans with atrophic AMD. The subjects with AMD received lutein (10 mg/day), lutein plus antioxidants (10 mg lutein plus a high-antioxidant multivitamin-mineral supplement [OcuPower, Nutraceutical Sciences Institute, Boynton Beach, FL] that contained 15,000 IU beta-carotene, 1,500 mg vitamin C, 500 IU d-alpha tocopherol, B vitamins, and 400 IU vitamin D-3), or placebo. Visual function, macular pigment optical density, and contrast sensitivity were tested at the beginning of the study and after 12 months. Lutein alone or in combination with the antioxidant multivitamin-mineral supplement improved visual function in AMD as assessed by eye macular pigment optical density, visual acuity, contrast sensitivity and self-reported glare recovery (13).

- To determine the effects of lutein supplementation on patients with choroideremia (hereditary primary choroid degeneration), 13 patients with choroideremia and 40 control subjects received 20 mg lutein/day. Researchers assessed changes in eye exams, serum carotenoids, and macular pigment and absolute sensitivity of the fovea with a 650 nm target. Oral supplementation with lutein increased macular pigment levels but did not affect absolute foveal sensitivity in all patients or control subjects. (14).

- In a small pilot study, which was nonrandomized but controlled, 30 patients with AMD and eight age-matched control subjects were assigned (50% to one group and 50% to the other) either no treatment or an antioxidant supplement containing 15 mg lutein, 20 mg vitamin E, and 18 mg nicotinamide daily for 6 months (15). Focal electroretinogram amplitudes improved with antioxidant supplementation for both those with AMD and healthy control subjects. Whether lutein will arrest of the degenerative process is unknown, and improved study design is warranted before appropriate conclusions can be drawn from these results.

Lutein and Age-related Cataracts

- In a double-blind, randomized, placebo-controlled trial to evaluate the effects of lutein and alpha-tocopherol on serum carotenoid and tocopherol levels and visual performance in patients with cataracts subjects received lutein (15 mg/day), alpha-tocopherol

(100 mg/day), or placebo three times per week for up to 24 months. A total of 17 patients were enrolled in this study; 15 completed the study. Visual performance was assessed by best corrected distance and glare sensitivity estimates. Serum carotenoid and tocopherol levels were determined by high-performance liquid chromatography (HPLC). Among those supplemented with lutein, serum lutein levels showed a steady increase between baseline and 12 months as well as a significant increase above baseline even at 24 months. Visual acuity and glare sensitivity as well as biochemical and hematologic values were assessed every 3 months. A trend toward loss of visual function was noted in the alpha-tocopherol and placebo groups but a statistically significant improvement in visual acuity was found in the lutein-supplemented group (16).

Lutein and Retinitis Pigmentosa

- Only one study in humans was identified which evaluated the role of lutein supplementation on visual acuity in patients with retinitis pigmentosa (a group of usually inherited diseases marked by progressive loss of retinal response and contraction of the field of vision). In this small pilot study, 16 subjects were supplemented with 40 mg/day lutein for 9 weeks followed by 20 mg/day for 15 additional weeks (17). Ten of the 16 subjects also took a combination of self-prescribed supplements that included dehydroepiandrosterone (DHEA), B-complex vitamins, and digestive enzymes. Visual acuity was tested using a self-administered computer-based test. At 2- to 4-weeks after supplementation, subjects began to report improved visual acuity. Subjects with blue eyes seemed to have the most improvement. This study has several flaws, including no control or placebo groups, no randomization to a treatment, no blinding, self-administered testing, and use of concurrent dietary supplements.

Lutein and Cancer Prevention

- To determine the effective dose of beta carotene and lutein in the chemoprevention of azoxymethane-induced colon carcinogenesis, male F344 rats were maintained on AIN-76a diets with or without beta carotene or lutein supplementation. The tolerated dose of each supplement was determined by analysis of body weights, signs of toxicity, or microscopic analysis of the colon, small intestine, stomach, liver, and kidney. The effect of supplementation on aberrant crypt foci formation (ACF) induced by azoxymethane (AOM) was determined by histologic examination following diet supplementation after AOM exposure. In these studies, beta carotene at 100 or 200 ppm exhibited chemopreventive activity for AOM-induced ACF formation. Lutein also exhibited chemopreventive activity, but only at the 200 ppm dose. High doses of 1,000 or 2,000 ppm lutein increased colonic ACF formation, suggesting a carcinogenic potential (18).

References

1. Stahl W. Macular carotenoids: lutein and zeaxanthin. *Dev Ophthalmol.* 2005;38:70–88.
2. Alves-Rodrigues A, Shao A. The science behind lutein. *Toxicol Lett.* 2004;150:57–83.

3. Mozaffarieh M, Sacu S, Wedrich A. The role of the caortenoids, lutein and zeaxanthin in protecting against age-related macular degeneration: a review based on controversial evidence. *Nutr J.* 2003;2:1–8.

4. Seddon JM, Ajani UA, Sperduto RD, et al. Dietary carotenoids, vitamins A, C, and E, and advanced age-related macular degeneration. *JAMA.* 1994;272:1413–1420.

5. Brown L, Rimm EB, Seddon JM, et al. A prospective study of carotenoid and risk of cataract extraction in US men. *Am J Clin Nutr.* 1999;70:517–524.

6. Chasen-Taber L, Willett WC, Seddon JM, et al. A prospective study of carotenoid and vitamin A intakes and risk of cataract extraction in US women. *Am J Clin Nutr.* 1999;70: 509–516.

7. United States Department of Agriculture Agricultural Research Service Nutrient database laboratory, National Nutrient Standard Reference, Release 16, 2004. Available at: http://www.ars.usda.gov. Accessed March 17, 2006.

8. Bone RA, Landrum JT, Guerra LH, et al. Lutein and zeaxanthin dietary supplements raise macular pigment density and serum concentrations of these carotenoids in humans. *J Nutr.* 2003;133:992–998.

9. Cardinault N, Gorrand JM, Tyssandier V, et al. Short-term supplementation with lutein affects biomarkers of lutein status similarly in young and elderly subjects. *Exp Gerontol.* 2004;38:573–582.

10. Chitchumroonchokchai C, Schwartz SJ, Failla ML. Assessment of lutein bioavailability from meals and a supplement using simulated digestion and caco-2 human intestinal cells. *J Nutr.* 2004;134:2280–2286.

11. Thurmann PA, Schalch W, Aebischer JC, et al. Plasma kinetics of lutein, zeaxanthin and 3-dehydro-lutein after multiple oral doses of a lutein supplement. *Am J Clin Nutr.* 2005;82:88–97.

12. Johnson EJ. Obesity, lutein metabolism and age-related macular degeneration: a web of connections. *Nutr Rev.* 2005;63:9–15.

13. Richer S, Stiles W, Stakute L, et al. Double-masked, placebo-controlled, randomized trial of lutein and antioxidant supplementation in the intervention of atrophic age-related macular degeneration: the Veterans LAST study (Lutein Antioxidant Supplementation Trial). *Optometry.* 2004;75:216–230.

14. Duncan JL, Aleman TS, Gardner LM, et al. Macular pigment and lutein supplementation in choroideremia. *Exp Eye Res.* 2002;74:371–381.

15. Falsini B, Piccardi M, Iarossi G, et al. Influence of short-term antioxidant supplementation on macular function in age-related maculopathy: a pilot study including electrophysiologic assessment. *Ophthalmology.* 2003;110:51–60.

16. Olmedilla B, Granado F, Blanco I, et al. Lutein, but not alpha-tocopherol, supplementation improves visual function in patients with age-related cataracts: a 2-y double-blind, placebo-controlled pilot study. *Nutrition.* 2003;19:21–24.

17. Dagnelie G, Zorge IS, McDonald TM. Lutein improves visual function in some patients with retinal degeneration: a pilot study via the Internet. *Optometry.* 2000;71: 147–164.

18. Raju J, Swamy MV, Cooma I, et al. Low doses of beta-carotene and lutein inhibit AOM-induced rat colonic ACF formation but high doses augment ACF incidence. *Int J Cancer.* 2005;113:798–802.

Lycopene

Lycopene is a naturally occurring carotenoid pigment that is classified as a non–provitamin A carotenoid. Lycopene is an open-chain unsaturated carotenoid that imparts red color to tomatoes, guava, watermelon, and pink grapefruit. Although not as potent as beta carotene, lycopene acts as an antioxidant and affects cell growth and communication. The antioxidant capacity of lycopene is of interest to investigators studying the potential of lycopene to prevent cancer by decreasing oxidative DNA damage and to prevent cardiovascular disease by reducing lipid peroxidation. Most research addressing the association between lycopene and disease risk reduction has been based on reported dietary intake rather than lycopene supplementation. Here we review studies using supplemental lycopene.

Media and Marketing Claims	Efficacy
Decreases risk of prostate cancer	↔
Prevents other cancers	NR
Reduces symptoms of exercise-induced asthma	NR
Prevents atherosclerosis	NR

Safety

There have been no scientific studies specifically evaluating the safety of lycopene supplementation. However, supplementation trials indicate that lycopene supplementation is safe. Supplementation is usually at or below 30 mg/day, and no adverse effects have been reported over several weeks of use.

Drug/Supplement Interactions

None

Key Points

- The data suggesting a role for lycopene in prostate cancer prevention are largely based on dietary lycopene exposure in the context of case-control and cohort studies (1) as well as in vitro cell culture studies (2). Few lycopene supplementation trials exist; however, cell culture and a few animal studies support a protective role.

- As with prostate cancer, current evidence for a protective role of lycopene in breast, lung, colorectal, and oral cancer are predominantly based on dietary exposure or serum lycopene measures in cases vs controls; lycopene supplementation studies are lacking.

- In a small clinical trial, 30 mg lycopene daily for 1 week showed a protective effect against exercise-induced asthma in some patients (3).

- The potential role of lycopene supplementation in reducing the risk for atherosclerosis or modulating cardiac events stems from its antioxidant activity, which has been associated with reduced lipid peroxidation. However, prospective lycopene supplementation trials in humans have not been done.

Food Sources

Food	Lycopene, mg/serving
Tomato sauce (½ cup)	21.9
Tomato puree (½ cup)	20.8
Marinara sauce (½ cup)	20.0
Tomato paste (2 Tbsp)	18.2
Tomato juice (½ cup)	13.2
Vegetable cocktail juice (V-8) (½ cup)	11.7
Tomato, raw (½ cup)	8.3
Pink grapefruit (1 medium)	8.0

Source: Data are from reference 4.

Dosage Information/Bioavailability

Data suggest that 10 servings of tomato products per week reduce the risk of prostate cancer by as much as 35% (5); this is approximately equivalent to 15 to 20 mg/day. In an animal model, human dosage equivalents of 15 mg/day were effective in significantly increasing plasma lycopene levels. Small human intervention studies report dosages between 4 and 30 mg/day. One study assessed the effect of lycopene vs tomato juice in increasing buccal cell lycopene levels (which could be important to oral cancer prevention studies) and showed lycopene beadlet supplements increased buccal cell lycopene levels to significant levels within 1 week, whereas tomato juice response was evident after 2 weeks of supplementation. Interestingly, after 3 weeks both showed similar effects on buccal cell lycopene concentrations (5). Supplements are available in capsule and softgel (beadlet). Lycopene in the *cis*-isomer form is more bioavailable; however, lycopene supplement manufacturers generally do not clarify the isomer form. Other factors that affect bioavailability include: concurrent dietary fat intake, which enhances absorption; high BMI, which is associated with reduced absorption; and concurrent beta carotene supplementation, which has been shown to increase lycopene absorption in males (6).

Relevant Research

Lycopene and Prostate Cancer

- In a prospective study to evaluate the efficacy of lycopene for the treatment of patients with metastatic prostate cancer unresponsive to hormone therapy, 20 consecutive patients were given 10 mg of lycopene daily for 3 months. Serum PSA levels, Eastern Cooperative Oncology Group performance status (ECOG PS), bone pain, records of lower urinary tract symptoms (LUTS), and uroflowmetry were evaluated. One patient experienced a normalization of PSA levels, 30% experienced a partial response, 50% remained stable, and 15% had progression of cancer. ECOG PS improved in the lycopene group as well. Finally, lycopene was helpful for reduction of bone pain and LUTS (7).

◆ In a pilot study, 26 subjects with active prostate cancer (early stage) were randomly assigned to no supplementation vs tomato oleosresin (a new supplement containing 15 mg lycopene) supplementation twice daily (8). Patients receiving the lycopene supplement for 3 weeks prior to their scheduled prostatectomy showed significantly reduced tumor volume and grade when tumors were analyzed postoperatively. Supplementation also resulted in an 18% reduction in PSA levels prior to surgery, whereas the control group showed a 14% increase in PSA; however, this was not significantly different. The findings of this pilot study encourage additional intervention studies in a statistically relevant number of subjects.

Lycopene and the Prevention of Other Cancers

◆ In a randomized, placebo-controlled study of lycopene supplementation at a dosage of 4 vs 8 mg/day conducted among patients with oral leukoplakia (precursor lesion for oral cancer), a dose-response effect was demonstrated (9). Twenty patients entered into each lycopene supplement arm, and 18 were randomly assigned to the placebo. After 3 months of supplementation, the 8 mg/day dosage resulted in an 80% reduction in lesion size while the 4 mg/day dose reduced the lesions by a mean of 66.5%. A 12% reduction was shown in the placebo group, as might be expected because precancerous lesions have been shown in many tissue types to spontaneously regress. This study provides preliminary evidence of a therapeutic benefit in the reversal of early lesions that have the potential to develop into oral cancer.

◆ In a lung cancer model study of lycopene supplementation conducted among ferrets who were exposed to tobacco smoke, 1.1 mg/kg/day (15 mg human dose) or 4.3 mg/kg/day (60 mg human dose) or no lycopene was administered daily for 9 weeks (10). Lycopene supplementation was associated with a significant increase in insulin-like growth factor binding protein 3 levels and a lower insulin-like growth factor 1:binding protein ratio, suggesting a reduced risk for cancer. In addition, supplementation at either dosage (as compared with placebo) resulted in inhibition of smoke-related tissue abnormalities as well as a significant reduction in proliferation markers associated with increased cancer risk.

Lycopene and Exercise-induced Asthma

◆ The only available research assessing the effect of lycopene supplementation on exercise-induced asthma (EIA) was a double-blind, randomized, crossover design study conducted among 20 patients (13 males, 7 females) with EIA (3). Patients were randomly assigned to receive LYC-O-MATO (providing 30 mg lycopene per day) or placebo for a period of 7 days, followed by a 4-week washout and then assignment to the alternate treatment group (lycopene or placebo). This study used a standardized exercise protocol that included a 7-minute run at 80% submaximal effort workload on a motorized treadmill followed by an 8-minute rest. Lung function tests using a spirograph were completed at baseline and after each supplementation period and included measures of lung function before and after the standard exercise as well as after the 8-minute rest period. Eleven patients (55%) demonstrated a significant improvement in postexercise pulmonary function with lycopene supplementation. Forced expiratory volume (FEV) decreased by 14.7% after exercise during lycopene supplementation; in comparison, the mean decrease in FEV was 26.5% after exercise during placebo supplementation. This effect was thought to be related to in vivo antioxidant effects. This study, while well designed, had a small sample size, and further research is needed in this area.

Lycopene and Atherosclerosis Prevention

◆ In a prospective, nested case-control study, 499 men with cardiovascular disease were matched with an equal number of men without cardiovascular disease to determine whether plasma lycopene levels were associated with cardiovascular disease in men. Baseline and follow-up blood samples were analyzed for total lycopene, other carotenoids, and retinol by HPLC; plasma lipids and C-reactive protein were also evaluated. Researchers were blinded to these assessments. No association was found between plasma lycopene levels and relative risk of cardiovascular disease in this cohort of men (11).

◆ Conversely, plasma lycopene data from the prospective Kuopio Ischemic Heart Disease Risk Factor trial (n = 725 men) showed that men in the lowest quartile of serum lycopene had a 3.3-fold increased risk for an acute coronary event or stroke (12). Similar findings were seen in the Rotterdam Study where a case-control analysis of serum lycopene levels from 108 patients with aortic stenosis and 108 healthy controls showed that adults with the highest levels of serum lycopene were at the lowest risk for atherosclerosis; however the protective effect was significant only among current and former smokers (OR = 0.35; 95% CI = 0.13–0.94) (13). Although an increase in plasma lycopene levels would be expected after lycopene supplementation, no lycopene supplements were used in these trials and thus the efficacy of lycopene supplementation cannot be directly derived from these findings.

References

1. Etminan M, Takkouche B, Caamano-Isorna F. The role of tomato products and lycopene in the prevention of prostate cancer: a meta-analysis of observational studies. *Cancer Epidemiol Biomarkers Prev.* 2004;13:340–345.
2. Obermuller-Jevic UC, Olano-Martin E, Corbacho AM, et al. Lycopene inhibits the growth of normal human prostate epithelial cells in vitro. *J Nutr.* 2003;133:3356–3360.
3. Neuman I, Nahum H, Ben-Amotz A. Reduction of exercise-induced asthma oxidative stress by lycopene, a natural antioxidant. *Allergy.* 2000;55:1184–1189.

4. United States Department of Agriculture Agricultural Research Service Nutrient database laboratory, National Nutrient Standard Reference, Release 16, 2004. Available at: http://www.ars.usda.gov. Accessed March 17, 2006.

5. Paetau I, Khachik F, Brown ED, et al. Chronic ingestion of lycopene-rich tomato juice or lycopene supplements significantly increases plasma concentrations of lycopene and related tomato carotenoids in humans. *Am J Clin Nutr.* 1998;68:1187–1195.

6. Johnson EJ, Qin J, Krinsky NI, Russell RM. Ingestion by men of a combined dose of beta-carotene and lycopene does not affect the absorption of beta-carotene but improves that of lycopene. *J Nutr.* 1997;127:1833–1837.

7. Ansari MS, Gupta NP. Lycopene: a novel drug therapy in hormone refractory metastatic prostate cancer. *Urol Oncol.* 2004;22:415–420.

8. Kucuk O, Sarkar FH, Sakr W, et al. Phase II randomized clinical trial of lycopene supplementation before radical prostatectomy. *Cancer Epidemiol Biomarkers Prev.* 2001;10:861–868.

9. Singh M, Krishanappa R, Bagewadi A, et al. Efficacy of oral lycopene in the treatment of oral leukoplakia. *Oral Oncol.* 224;40:591–596.

10. Liu C, Lian F, Smith DE, et al. Lycopene supplementation inhibits lung squamous metaplasia and induces apoptosis via up-regulating insulin-like growth factor-binding protein 3 in cigarette smoke-exposed ferrets. *Cancer Res.* 2003;63;3138–3144.

11. Sesso HD, Buring JE, Norkus EP, et al. Plasma lycopene, other carotenoids, and retinol and the risk of cardiovascular disease in men. *Am J Clin Nutr.* 2005;81:990–997.

12. Rissanen T, Voutilainen S, Nyyssonen K, et al. Lycopene, atherosclerosis, and coronary heart disease. *Exp Biol Med.* 2002;227:900–907.

13. Klipstein-Grobusch K, Launer LJ, Geleijnse JM, et al. Serum carotenoids and atherosclerosis. The Rotterdam Study. *Atherosclerosis.* 2000;148:49–56.

Lysine

Lysine is an essential amino acid involved in the synthesis of cross-linking proteins (collagen and elastin) and is a precursor of carnitine. Low-lysine diets produce lower growth rates and nitrogen retention in animals and humans than diets in which the lysine/tryptophan ratio is 5 or more. (Proteins are considered to have a high biological value if they have approximately 5 to 8 times as much lysine as tryptophan by weight.) Of all the essential amino acids, lysine is one of the most strongly conserved by the body. Lysine is usually the limiting amino acid in diets based on grains (1).

Media and Marketing Claims	Efficacy
Stops growth of herpes virus and canker sores	↔
Enhances calcium absorption	NR

Safety

- Three g/day for as long as 1 year seems to be safe (1).

- Lysine and arginine are antagonistic because they share a common transport system in the blood. Excess lysine intake may interfere with arginine metabolism (1).

- Diets high in lysine or with a high lysine-to-arginine ratio were reported to have a hypercholesterolemic effect in animal studies (2–4).

- To date, there have been no reported cases of acute toxicity with lysine supplementation (1).

Drug/Supplement Interactions

- Lysine competes with the amino acid arginine for absorption.

- Lysine may increase supplemental calcium absorption.

Key Points

- Research is conflicting on the role of lysine in treating herpes simplex infection. Dietary protein intake and lysine-to-arginine ratios were not controlled in any of the studies, although subjects were instructed to avoid arginine-rich foods. The amount supplemented in these studies was comparable to an amount that can be obtained from the diet (see Food Sources, later in this entry). Although more research is needed on the potential role of lysine against herpes infection, these patients can be encouraged to increase consumption of lysine-rich foods within the context of an overall healthful diet.

- Preliminary animal studies and one human trial suggest that lysine enhances calcium absorption and retention. Controlled clinical trials are needed to more clearly determine the potential role of supplemental lysine in the treatment or prevention of osteoporosis.

Food Sources

Lysine is found in animal proteins and in potatoes and legumes (lentils, soybeans, lima beans). Wheat flour, maize, rice, oats, and peanuts are low in lysine. Lysine is easily damaged during the processing of foods and animal feeds (5). Dietary lysine intakes are highly variable and can be as low as 2 g/day if protein intake is 50 g/day, and as high as 8 to 9 g/day on a diet high in energy and animal protein (1). The estimated dietary lysine requirement for adults is 12 mg/kg/day (6).

Food	Lysine, mg/serving
Beef, ground (3.5 oz)	1,892
Salmon, Atlantic (3 oz)	1,727
Tofu, firm (½ cup)	1,309
Beans, black (1 cup)	1,064
Milk, nonfat (1 cup)	818
Peanuts (½ cup)	621
Cheese, mozzarella (1 oz)	559
Egg (1)	452
Spinach, boiled (½ cup)	164
Corn, boiled (½ cup)	116
Bread, whole-wheat (1 slice)	85

Source: Data are from reference 7.

Dosage Information/Bioavailability

Lysine is sold as free form L-lysine hydrochloride, usually in 500-mg tablets or capsules. It is also sold in combination with other amino acid supplements. Studies have shown that free lysine hydrochloride added to food or in supplements is absorbed at a similar rate as amino acids from dietary proteins (1).

Relevant Research

Lysine and Herpes Simplex Virus

♦ Researchers have hypothesized that lysine may treat the herpes simplex virus because growth of the virus seems to be inhibited by high intracellular concentrations of lysine and low levels of arginine (8,9).

♦ In a double-blind, placebo-controlled, multicenter study, 52 subjects with genital and oral-facial herpes simplex infection were randomly assigned to receive 1,000 mg of lysine as lysine monohydrochloride divided into three doses or a placebo daily for 6 months. Subjects were instructed to avoid foods containing large amounts of arginine, but this was not monitored. With lysine supplementation, there was a significant decrease in the mean number of infections, symptoms, and severity and healing time. Specifically, subjects treated with lysine had 2.4 fewer herpes outbreaks and 2.3 fewer days of infection compared with the placebo group (10).

♦ In a double-blind, placebo-controlled, crossover study, 26 subjects with a history of recurring genital herpes lesions received, in random order, 1,000 mg lysine or a placebo daily for 6 months each. For 1 year before the study, subjects recorded the frequency of herpetic lesions. All subjects were instructed to avoid foods high in arginine, but this was not monitored. At the end of the first 6-month period, the frequency of lesions in those subjects given lysine did not differ significantly from those given the placebo (39 lesions in the lysine group vs 44 lesions in the placebo group). In contrast, subjects who began taking lysine during the second 6-month test period reported significantly fewer lesions than those who had reverted to placebo (12 lesions in the lysine group vs 31 in the placebo group). The authors speculated that a placebo effect may have occurred during the first 6-month period. Low serum lysine concentrations were associated with a significant increase in lesion frequency, and high concentrations were associated with a significant decrease in lesion frequency. The serum lysine-to-arginine ratio showed no correlation with lesion occurrence. The authors concluded: "Prophylactic lysine may be useful in managing selected cases of recurrent herpes simplex labialis *if* serum lysine levels can be maintained at adequate concentrations" (11).

◆ In a double-blind, placebo-controlled study, 21 patients with a history of severe frequently occurring herpes simplex infection were randomly assigned to receive 1,200 mg lysine as lysine hydrochloride divided into three doses or a placebo for 4 to 5 months. Patients were evaluated at baseline, at 3 months, and at the end of the study. Subjects were instructed to avoid arginine-rich foods and to keep a diary of symptoms. There were no changes in episode frequency, duration, or severity of episodes between groups (12).

◆ In a double-blind, placebo-controlled, crossover study, 41 patients with recurrent herpes simplex infections were randomly assigned to receive one of four treatments for 48 weeks: (*a*) 1,248 mg lysine as lysine monohydrochloride for 24 weeks, followed by a placebo for 24 weeks; (*b*) placebo for 24 weeks followed by 1,248 mg lysine as lysine monohydrochloride for 24 weeks (*c*) 624 mg lysine for 24 weeks followed by a placebo; or (*d*) placebo for 24 weeks followed by 624 mg lysine for 24 weeks. Subjects were instructed to avoid arginine-rich foods and increase lysine foods, but this was not monitored. Patients were assessed at the baseline, 12, 24, 36, and 48 weeks. In the high-dose lysine group, there was a significant decrease in herpes outbreaks compared with the placebo phase. There were no significant changes in the lower dose lysine group. There were also no differences in self-reported healing times among groups (13).

Lysine and Calcium Metabolism/Bone Health

◆ In a comparative study, 30 women age 33 to 65 years (15 healthy, 15 with osteoporosis) were given an acute oral load of calcium chloride (3 g elemental calcium) administered either with or without 400 mg lysine. Both the lysine and control groups experienced an increase in plasma total calcium. A progressive increase in urinary calcium excretion was observed after calcium alone but not in the healthy subjects taking calcium plus lysine. In a second study, 45 postmenopausal women with osteoporosis were randomly assigned to receive one of three treatments: (*a*) 800 mg lysine, (*b*) 800 mg valine, or (*c*) 800 mg tryptophan. Lysine, but not valine or tryptophan, significantly increased intestinal absorption of calcium as measured by fractional absorption of calcium by stable isotope administration. The authors concluded: "Our results suggest that L-lysine can both enhance intestinal calcium absorption and improve the renal conservation of the absorbed calcium. The combined effects may contribute to a positive calcium balance, thus suggesting a potential usefulness of L-lysine supplements for both preventative and therapeutic interventions in osteoporosis" (14).

◆ Lysine supplementation in animals has been shown to increase calcium absorption (14).

References

1. Flodin NW. The metabolic roles, pharmacology, and toxicology of lysine. *J Am Coll Nutr.* 1997;16:7–21.
2. Kurowska EM, Carroll KK. Hypercholesterolemic responses in rabbits to selected groups of dietary essential amino acids. *J Nutr.* 1994;124:364–370.
3. Sanchez A, Rubano DA, Shavlik GW, et al. Cholesterolemic effects of the lysine/arginine ratio in rabbits after initial early growth. *Arch Latinoam Nutr.* 1988;38:229–238.
4. Leszcynski DE, Kummerow FA. Excess dietary lysine induces hypercholesterolemia in chickens. *Experientia.* 1982;38:266–267.
5. Ostrowski HT. Analysis for availability of amino acid supplements in foods and feeds: biochemical and nutritional implications. *Adv Exp Med Biol.* 1978;105:497–547.
6. Matthews DE. Proteins and amino acids. In: Shils ME, Olson JA, Shike M, et al, eds. *Modern Nutrition in Health and Disease.* 9th ed. Philadelphia, Pa: Lea & Febiger; 1999:11–48.
7. Pennington JAT. *Bowes and Church's Food Values of Portions Commonly Used.* 17th ed. Philadelphia, Pa: Lippincott-Raven Publishers; 1998.
8. Tankersley RW Jr. Amino acid requirements of herpes simplex virus in human cells. *J Bacteriol.* 1964;87:609–613.
9. Griffith RD, DeLong DC, Nelson JD. Relation of arginine-lysine to herpes simplex growth in tissue culture. *Chemotherapy.* 1981;27:209–213.
10. Griffith RS, Walsh DE, Myrmel KH, et al. Success of L-lysine therapy in frequently recurrent herpes simplex infection. Treatment and prophylaxis. *Dermatologica.* 1987;175:183–190.
11. Thein DJ, Hurt WC. Lysine as a prophylactic agent in the treatment of recurrent herpes simplex labialis. *Oral Surg Oral Med Oral Pathol.* 1984;58:659–666.
12. DiGiovanna JJ, Blank H. Failure of lysine in frequently recurrent herpes simplex infection. Treatment and prophylaxis. *Arch Dermatol.* 1984;120:48–51.
13. McCune MA, Perry HO, Muller SA, et al. Treatment of recurrent herpes simplex infections with L-lysine monohydrochloride. *Cutis.* 1984;34:366–373.
14. Civitelli R, Villareal DT, Agnusdei D, et al. Dietary L-lysine and calcium metabolism in humans. *Nutrition.* 1992;8:400–405.

Magnesium

The second most abundant intracellular cation in the body, magnesium is involved in more than 300 enzymatic reactions. It interacts with other electrolytes (eg, calcium, potassium); plays a role in neuromuscular activity, excitation, and contraction; and is involved in bone function. Magnesium also stabilizes the structure of adenosine triphosphate (ATP) in ATP-dependent enzyme reactions. The body contains a total of 20 to 28 g magnesium, with 60% in bone, 27% in muscle, 1% in extracellular fluid, and the remainder in soft tissue and other fluids. Hypomagnesemia may result from renal dysfunction, endocrine disorders, malabsorption syndromes, use of loop diuretics or digitalis, chronic alcoholism, diabetes mellitus, and excessive diarrhea. A deficiency is associated with cardiac and neuromuscular changes, including muscle weakness, spasms, tetany, convulsions, hypokalemia, hypocalcemia, and arrhythmias (1).

The numerous clinical applications for intravenous administration of magnesium are not discussed here because IV magnesium is not considered a dietary supplement. IV applications are used for such conditions as pre-eclampsia, acute myocardial infarction, arrhythmia, asthma, cancer-associated neuropathic pain, exacerbation of chronic obstructive pulmonary disease, and torsade de pointes.

Media and Marketing Claims	Efficacy
Supports heart health	↔
Reduces blood pressure	↔
Improves blood glucose control in diabetes	↔
Reduces pain associated with migraine headaches	↔
Reduces symptoms of PMS	↔
Enhances exercise performance	↓?
Relieves constipation	↑

Safety

◆ For males and females age 9 years or older, the Tolerable Upper Intake Level (UL) for magnesium from supplements/pharmacological agents is 350 mg/day; the UL does not include magnesium intake from food and water (2).

◆ Magnesium supplements are considered relatively nontoxic for healthy individuals because excess amounts are eliminated by the kidney. However, soft stools and osmotic diarrhea have been reported by some subjects who took more than 500 mg elemental magnesium via supplements daily, which could result in dehydration and neurological symptoms (1).

Drug/Supplement Interactions

- In patients with renal insufficiency, chronic use of magnesium-containing drugs (antacids or cathartics) may cause hypermagnesemia. The effects of elevated serum magnesium include hypotension, nausea, decreased mental status, alterations in cardiac function, paralysis, central nervous system disorders, and death (1).

- Taking magnesium supplements in addition to magnesium-containing drugs (antacids, cathartics) may exceed the UL and may be associated with diarrhea, dehydration, and electrolyte imbalances.

- Use of magnesium supplements with aminoglycoside antibiotics, such as amikacin, gentamicin, kanamycin, streptomycin, and tobramycin, can cause neuromuscular weakness or paralysis.

- Magnesium supplementation should be taken at least 2 hours before or after biphosphonates such as alendronate sodium (Fosamax) and risedronate sodium (Actonel) because magnesium will decrease absorption of these medications.

- Magnesium also decreases absorption of certain quinine antibiotics, such as ciprofloxacin, levofloxacin, and ofloxacin, as well as tetracycline.

- Potassium-sparing diuretics also spare magnesium. Therefore, magnesium levels should be monitored in individuals taking these medications and magnesium.

Key Points

- Magnesium is necessary for the proper functioning of muscle, including the heart muscle. A magnesium deficiency (rare in healthy individuals) results in negative effects on cardiac and neuromuscular functions. Preliminary evidence suggests that magnesium supplements may benefit individuals with mitral valve prolapse. Larger controlled clinical trials are needed to substantiate the potential role of magnesium supplements in various heart conditions. If dietary intake is inadequate, patients with cardiovascular disease should be encouraged to consume magnesium-rich foods and take a magnesium supplement (providing no more than the UL).

- The role of magnesium supplements in reducing blood pressure has not been confirmed. Epidemiological studies have suggested an inverse relationship between dietary magnesium and blood pressure. The data from clinical trials are conflicting, and the reduction in blood pressure, if any, is small. Loop and thiazide diuretics, used in the treatment of hypertension, can induce magnesium depletion that can be corrected by increasing intake of magnesium-rich foods or by taking a magnesium supplement providing no more than the UL, provided that renal function is normal.

- Individuals with diabetes are at risk for poor magnesium status. However, magnesium supplements generally have not improved glycemic control in people with type 1 or type 2 diabetes. This may be because researchers were not able to fully restore subjects' intracellular magnesium status. More research is needed. This population should be encouraged to increase dietary magnesium or take a supplement only if there is no sign of renal insufficiency. A physician should be consulted to make recommendations regarding magnesium supplementation in individuals at risk for renal insufficiency.

◆ The research on the efficacy of magnesium in migraine headaches is conflicting and requires further study.

◆ Preliminary research suggests that magnesium supplements may reduce mild premenstrual symptoms. In some studies, only symptoms of fluid retention were affected, whereas in other studies, only symptoms related to mood were improved. More research is needed.

◆ Athletes in sports in which competition is organized by weight-range classifications may not be meeting the RDA for magnesium, but research from well-controlled studies generally does not support an ergogenic benefit of magnesium supplements.

◆ Magnesium, usually as a component of over-the-counter medications to treat constipation, but also as a dietary supplement, can promote bowel movements by helping pull fluid from the body into the digestive tract.

Food Sources

Good sources of magnesium are whole grains, dark-green leafy vegetables, nuts, legumes, and fish.

Food	Magnesium, mg/serving
Spinach, (½ cup)	78
Beans, black (½ cup)	60
Potato, baked, with skin	55
Peanuts (1 oz)	50
Sea bass (3 oz)	45
Rice, brown (½ cup)	42
Squash, butternut (½ cup)	30
Milk, nonfat (1 cup)	28
Chicken breast, skinless (½)	25

Source: Data are from reference 3.

Dosage Information/Bioavailability

The RDA for magnesium is 400 mg for men age 19 to 30 years, 310 mg for women age 19 to 30 years, 420 mg for men age 31 years or older, and 320 mg for women age 31 years or older (3). Magnesium is sold in single preparations, in combination with calcium, or in multivitamin-mineral supplements providing 10 to 500 mg in the form of magnesium citrate, aspartate, acetate, glycinate, hydroxide, lactate, carbonate, chloride, pidolate, or oxide. In one study, magnesium citrate was found to be more soluble and bioavailable than magnesium oxide (4). Because magnesium oxide and hydroxide are not soluble, they are often used as an osmotic laxative (1). Absorption of dietary magnesium varies from 14% to 70%, depending on the dosage (fractional absorption is inversely related to intake). The kidneys regulate magnesium excretion and conserve the mineral when intake is low (1). Diets high in saturated fats, sugar, caffeine, and alcohol may increase magnesium needs (5).

Relevant Research

Magnesium Status and Intake

♦ According to 24-hour recall data from the Third National Health and Nutrition Examination Survey (1999–2000), median magnesium intake is 326 mg/day in non-Hispanic white men, 237 mg/day in non-Hispanic white women, 237 mg/day among African-American men and 177 mg/day among African-American women. Mexican American men reported intakes of 297 mg/day whereas Mexican American women reported intakes of 221 mg/day. Thus, total magnesium intake was reported to be higher among men and whites. Intake was also shown to decrease with age (6).

♦ Magnesium status is difficult to assess because plasma levels represent only 1% of total body magnesium and are not reflective of intracellular stores. A variety of diagnostic tests assess magnesium nutriture, but none are flawless. Blood mononuclear cell magnesium concentrations are thought to be more reliable than serum levels. Likewise, ionized magnesium (IMg^{2+}) is considered a better indicator of magnesium status than total serum concentrations. Urinary levels of magnesium increase with supplementation but do not provide a quantitative measure of magnesium status (1).

♦ Magnesium depletion is common among patients in intensive care (1). In one study, approximately 50% of critically ill patients presented with magnesium depletion, which was related to a higher morbidity and mortality compared with patients with adequate magnesium status (7).

♦ Risk factors associated with poor magnesium status include uncontrolled diabetes, cardiovascular disease, alcohol ingestion, severe diarrhea, and steatorrhea, and the use of renal magnesium-wasting drugs (eg, loop diuretics such as furosemide) (1).

Magnesium and Cardiovascular Disease

♦ Much of the research of magnesium in cardiovascular disease has been done with individuals with type 2 diabetes and is described under diabetes and magnesium later in this section.

♦ In a prospective, observational study (Atherosclerosis Risk in Communities [ARIC]), 13,922 subjects (from four US communities) without coronary heart disease (CHD) were followed up for 4 to 7 years. After adjusting for sociodemographic variables, waist-to-hip ratio, smoking, alcohol intake, exercise, diuretic use, fibrinogen levels, cholesterol levels, and hormone replacement therapy, the relative risk of development of CHD was statistically significantly correlated to low serum magnesium levels in women, but not in men. (The relative risk from the highest to lowest quartile of serum magnesium in women was 1.00, 0.92, 0.48, and 0.44). However, the adjusted relative risk of development of CHD was not statistically correlated with dietary magnesium intake in women or men (8). Results from the same ARIC population were reported in an earlier analysis of 15,248 subjects. Mean serum magnesium was significantly less in subjects with prevalent cardiovascular disease, hypertension, and diabetes. Dietary magnesium was inversely associated with serum insulin, HDL cholesterol, and systolic and diastolic blood pressure (9). Whether low magnesium contributed to the development of disease or was a consequence thereof is difficult to determine in these at-risk populations.

- Serum magnesium levels were compared in 141 subjects (age 16 to 57 years) with mitral valve prolapse syndrome (MVP) and 40 healthy control subjects (age 19 to 49 years) living in the same area. The incidence of low magnesium levels differed significantly between subjects with MVP and control subjects (60% vs 5%, respectively). Subjects with MVP with low serum magnesium (n = 70) were entered into a double-blind, crossover study and were given magnesium supplements (in random order) or a placebo daily for 5 weeks each (week 1 = 497 mg [21 mmol] magnesium as magnesium carbonate; weeks 2 to 5 = 330 mg [14 mmol] magnesium). Serum magnesium increased significantly with magnesium supplementation (0.63 ± 0.11 mmol/L to 0.73 ± 0.08 mmol/L), but not with the placebo. Weakness, chest pain, dyspnea, palpitations, and anxiety decreased significantly after magnesium supplementation and compared with placebo. Mean daily excretion of catecholamines (norepinephrine and epinephrine) decreased significantly with magnesium but not with placebo. The authors hypothesized that the reduction in symptoms could have been caused by an antiadrenergic effect of magnesium (10).

Magnesium and Blood Pressure

- A comprehensive review of the role of magnesium in blood pressure control provides insight into the molecular and physiological aspects of this association (11). Although the exact pathophysiology of hypertension is not known, magnesium appears to improve heart muscle contractibility as well as to improve the tonal quality of vascular tissue.

- The Canadian Hypertension Education Program Evidence-Based Recommendations Task Force states that one should "maintain an adequate intake of potassium, magnesium, and calcium" to improve blood pressure control (12).

- A meta-analysis of magnesium supplementation for blood pressure control included 20 trials, 14 with hypertensive subjects and 6 with normotensive subjects (total n = 1,220). Magnesium supplementation resulted in a small overall reduction in blood pressure, estimated at –0.6 mm Hg for systolic blood pressure and –0.8 mm Hg for diastolic blood pressure. A dose-dependent effect was also demonstrated, indicating a 4.3 mm Hg reduction in systolic blood pressure per 10 mmol/day (237 mg/day) increase in magnesium supplementation (13). Prospective dose-related, placebo-controlled trials are needed.

♦ In a double-blind, placebo-controlled, randomized study, 300 normotensive women from the Nurses' Health Study II whose reported intake of magnesium, potassium, and calcium were between the 10th and 15th percentile, received daily supplements of (*a*) 336 mg (14 mmol) magnesium as magnesium lactate, (*b*) 1,200 mg (30 mmol) calcium, (*c*) 40 mEq (40 mmol) potassium, (*d*) all three supplements together, or (*e*) a placebo for 16 weeks. The mean reductions in systolic and diastolic blood pressures between treatment and placebo groups were statistically significant for the potassium-supplemented group (−2.0 mm Hg systolic, −1.7 mm Hg diastolic), but not for the calcium- or magnesium-supplemented groups. The combination supplement did not enhance the blood pressure-reducing effect of potassium supplements alone (14).

♦ In a double-blind, placebo-controlled trial, 698 healthy subjects with high-normal diastolic blood pressure (80 to 89 mm Hg) were randomly assigned to receive one of three treatments daily for 6 months: (*a*) 360 mg magnesium as magnesium diglycine, (*b*) 1,000 mg calcium, or (*c*) placebo. There was no significant change in blood pressure at 3 or 6 months. Analyses stratified by baseline intakes of calcium, magnesium, sodium, or initial blood pressures also found no effect of supplementation on blood pressure (15).

Magnesium and Diabetes

♦ Hypomagnesemia occurs in an estimated 30% of individuals with type 2 diabetes, especially those not under good metabolic control (1,16–18).

♦ In an epidemiological study comparing baseline intake of magnesium in 42,782 men and 85,060 women (of which 1,333 men and 4,085 women prospectively developed type 2 diabetes), there was a significant 33% to 34% reduction in risk for diabetes in adults within the highest quintile of dietary magnesium intake (19).

♦ A randomized, double-blind, placebo-controlled trial of 63 individuals with type 2 diabetes with demonstrated reduced serum magnesium levels was conducted using 50 mL magnesium chloride solution (containing 50 g magnesium chloride per 1,000 mL solution) or placebo daily for 16 weeks. Magnesium supplementation increased serum magnesium levels and reduced insulin resistance (HOMA-IR index) as well as fasting blood glucose and A1C as compared with placebo (20).

♦ In a study in India, 20 subjects with type 2 diabetes and 54 age- and gender-matched control subjects took a daily supplement of 600 mg magnesium for 12 weeks. Magnesium supplementation was associated with a significant improvement in lipid profile but did not modulate serum glucose over time (21). Of interest, mean serum magnesium level was significantly less in the diabetes group as compared with the control group at the initiation of the study.

Magnesium and Migraine Headaches

♦ In a study of 118 children ages 3 to 17 years with a history of at least weekly migraine-type headaches, children were randomly assigned in a double-blind design to receive

9 mg magnesium oxide per kilogram of body weight or placebo divided into three daily doses for a 16-week period. Although 192 children were contacted for participation, only 40% enrolled in the study and completion rate was 73%. Intent-to-treat analysis demonstrated a significant reduction in headache frequency and severity in the magnesium-treated group that was not shown in the placebo group. However, there was no statistically significant difference between the two groups at the end of study, indicating that although the placebo group did report improvements in migraine status over time, it was not enough to reach statistical significance. This study provides preliminary data to pursue this hypothesis in a larger number of children (22).

♦ According to one review, 50% of individuals have reduced levels of ionized magnesium during an acute migraine attack. The authors further discussed the potential role of magnesium in the pathogenesis of migraines, noting that magnesium concentration affects serotonin receptors, nitric oxide synthesis and release, and other migraine-related receptors and neurotransmitters (23).

♦ An oral magnesium–loading study (3,000 mg) was conducted in individuals with migraines and control subjects to determine whether those suffering from migraines have a systemic deficiency of magnesium. Magnesium lactate was administered over a 24-hour period to 20 patients with migraines and 20 healthy control subjects. At the start of the study, there were no significant differences in serum or urinary magnesium levels between groups. Compared with the control group, subjects with migraine had significantly lower urinary magnesium excretion after magnesium supplementation. This supports the hypothesis that people with migraines demonstrate magnesium retention when supplemented due to a systemic deficiency that promotes increased magnesium retention with supplementation (24).

♦ In a double-blind, placebo-controlled, prospective multicenter study, 69 patients experiencing two to six migraine attacks without aura per month, and a history of migraine for at least 2 years, were randomly assigned to receive 480 mg (20 mmol) magnesium or a placebo divided into two doses daily for 12 weeks. There were no differences between groups in the number of migraine days or migraine attacks at the end of 4 weeks. Final assessments of efficacy by doctor and patients showed no benefit of magnesium supplementation. The trial was discontinued because interim analysis revealed a lack of response to treatment. Forty-five percent of patients receiving magnesium experienced mild adverse effects (soft stool, diarrhea) compared with 23% in the placebo group (25).

♦ In a double-blind, placebo-controlled, multicenter study, 81 subjects with a mean migraine attack frequency of 3.6 per month were randomly assigned to receive 576 mg (24 mmol) magnesium (as trimagnesium dicitrate) daily or a placebo for 12 weeks. All patients were assessed at baseline and for 4 weeks prior to treatment. At weeks 9 to 12, self-reported migraine frequency had decreased significantly (by 41.6%) in the magnesium group compared with a 15.8% reduction in the placebo group. The number of days with migraine and medication consumption for symptomatic treatment per patient also decreased significantly in the magnesium group.

Intensity of attacks and drug consumption per attack tended to decrease with magnesium, but was not statistically significant. Diarrhea and gastric irritation occurred in 4% to 18% of the treatment group (26).

Magnesium and Premenstrual Syndrome

◆ Blood magnesium levels were measured at different times in the menstrual cycle in 26 women with confirmed PMS and 19 female control subjects of the same age. At each sampling time, magnesium concentrations (in erythrocyte and mononuclear blood cells but not plasma) were statistically lower in subjects with PMS than in controls. However, the lower magnesium concentrations were not confined to the luteal phase, when PMS symptoms typically occur. Additionally, magnesium measures did not correlate with severity of mood symptoms (27).

◆ Another study of 105 women with PMS reported that erythrocyte magnesium concentration, but not plasma magnesium, was significantly lower than that of a normal population (28).

◆ In a double-blind, placebo-controlled, crossover study, 38 women were randomly assigned to receive 200 mg magnesium as magnesium oxide or a placebo daily for two menstrual cycles each. Subjects kept a daily record of symptoms grouped into six categories (anxiety, craving, depression, hydration, other, and total overall symptoms). In the first menstrual cycle, there was no difference among treatment results. In the second month there was a significant reduction of symptoms of "hydration" (weight gain, swelling of upper extremities, breast tenderness, abdominal bloating) with magnesium supplementation compared with placebo (29).

◆ In a double-blind, placebo-controlled, crossover study, 44 women (mean age 32 years) were given, in random order, one of four treatments for one menstrual cycle: (*a*) 200 mg magnesium (oxide); (*b*) 50 mg vitamin B-6; (*c*) 200 mg magnesium plus 50 mg vitamin B-6; or (*d*) a placebo. During the study, each subject recorded daily symptoms on a 5-point scale in a menstrual diary of 30 symptoms that were grouped into categories (anxiety, craving, depression, hydration, other). Urinary magnesium output was not affected by treatment, suggesting poor absorption of the magnesium. There were no overall differences in symptoms among treatments, but a modest significant reduction in premenstrual anxiety-related symptoms was associated with the magnesium plus vitamin B-6 combination (30).

Magnesium and Exercise Performance

◆ Several studies have reported that athletes in weight-controlled sports often do not consume adequate dietary magnesium because of food-restriction practices (31). A review of current research suggest that studies evaluating the relationship between magnesium status and exercise performance are limited by poor study design and lack of effective measurement of magnesium status (32).

◆ In a magnesium depletion-repletion study, postmenopausal women ages 45 to 71 years (mean age 59.7 years) ate a diet containing 112 mg magnesium/day plus 200 mg supplemental magnesium/day for 35 days, followed by a diet with 112 mg diet for 93 days, followed by 112 mg diet plus 200 mg supplemental magnesium per day for an additional 49 days. Twelve subjects began the study, and 10 completed it. Subjects exercised to submaximal workload (80% of age-related peak heart rate). Magnesium depletion was verified with measures of red blood cell and skeletal muscle magnesium levels. Functional response was measured by duration, and submaximal ergocycle exercise was maintained from baseline through the magnesium depletion (low-magnesium) phase of the study. Peak and cumulative oxygen uptake and peak heart rate increased during magnesium depletion period as compared with the magnesium repletion period, indicating less efficient work economy when magnesium levels are low (33).

♦ In a randomized, placebo-controlled, crossover study of 121 physically active women screened for study participation, 36% (44 subjects) had baseline hypomagnesiumemia (34). Twenty women at the low end of the distribution for plasma magnesium levels and 20 at the high end of plasma magnesium were randomly assigned to the intervention study. Thirty two of the subjects completed extensive exercise testing followed by a 4-week magnesium intervention of 212 mg/day or placebo and repeat exercise testing, a 6-week washout, and then a crossover to magnesium or placebo for an additional 4 weeks. Of the women who dropped out of the study, 7 were in the magnesium-first group and one was in the placebo-first group; these subjects were not included in the data analysis. Outcomes included resting blood pressure, treadmill testing for anaerobic threshold, maximal workload, submaximal running efficiency, heart rate, maximum oxygen consumption (VO_{2max}), and plasma magnesium levels. In this study, no significant difference in performance (anaerobic treadmill, incremental treadmill) or recovery was shown between the magnesium-supplemented group and the placebo group. However, with a 20% dropout rate, the study was likely not statistically powered to detect significant differences in such a small number of subjects.

♦ In a meta-analysis, researchers who examined 12 studies of exercise and magnesium supplementation reported that most evidence does not suggest a benefit from supplementation on performance (strength, anaerobic, aerobic). When only peak treadmill speed during a VO_{2max} test was examined, the evidence was equivocal. The authors noted several limitations in the studies that hinder assessment, including use of different exercise modes and intensities; variable training status and age of subjects; subject-selection favoring males; varying dosages of supplementation (116 to 500 mg/day); lack of magnesium status assessment; and lack of control for dietary magnesium intake (35).

♦ In a double-blind, placebo-controlled study, 20 athletes with low-normal serum magnesium levels were randomly assigned to receive 500 mg magnesium as magnesium oxide or a placebo daily for 3 weeks. Supplementation did not increase the magnesium concentration in serum or any cellular compartment studied. There was no effect of magnesium on exercise performance by submaximal and maximal ergometer measurements, neuromuscular activity, or muscle-related symptoms. The authors concluded: "Magnesium supplementation in athletes with low-normal serum magnesium did not improve performance and failed to increase the body's magnesium stores" (36).

♦ In a small, double-blind, placebo-controlled study, 20 marathon runners were assigned to receive 365 mg magnesium daily or a placebo for 4 weeks before and 6 weeks after a marathon race. Subjects were pair-matched by performance on a treadmill test. Magnesium supplementation did not increase muscle or serum magnesium concentrations. There were no differences between groups in the extent of muscle damage or the rate of recovery of muscle function. The authors concluded that runners who have adequate magnesium status would not experience a benefit from supplementation (37).

Magnesium and Bowel Function

♦ Magnesium citrate, sulfate, and hydroxide salts are typically used when preparing for bowel surgery or diagnostic procedures on the colon. Magnesium can be beneficial as a laxative. The most potent form of magnesium as a laxative is magnesium sulfate salt (38).

References

1. Shils ME. Magnesium. In: Shils ME, Olson JA, Shike M, Ross AC, eds. *Modern Nutrition in Health and Disease.* 9th ed. Philadelphia, Pa: Lea & Febiger; 1999:169–192.
2. Institute of Medicine. *Dietary Reference Intakes for Calcium, Phosphorus, Magnesium, Vitamin D, and Fluoride.* Washington, DC: National Academy Press; 1997.
3. Pennington JA. *Bowes and Church's Food Values of Portions Commonly Used.* 17th ed. Philadelphia, Pa: Lippincott-Raven Publishers; 1998.
4. Lindberg JS, Zobitz MM, Poindexter JR, et al. Magnesium bioavailability from magnesium citrate and magnesium oxide. *J Am Coll Nutr.* 1990;9:48–55.
5. Schaafsma G. Bioavailability of calcium and magnesium. *Eur J Clin Nutr.* 1997;51(Suppl 1):S13-S16.
6. Ford ES, Mokdad AH. Dietary magnesium intake in a national sample of US adults. *J Nutr.* 2003;133:2879–2882.
7. Olerich MA, Rude RK. Should we supplement magnesium in critically ill patients? *New Horiz.* 1994;2:186–192.
8. Liao F, Folsom AR, Brancati FL. Is low magnesium concentration a risk factor for coronary heart disease? The Atherosclerosis Risk in Communities (ARIC) Study. *Am Heart J.* 1998;136:480–490.
9. Ma J, Folsom AR, Melnick SL, et al. Associations of serum and dietary magnesium with cardiovascular disease, hypertension, diabetes, insulin, and carotid arterial wall thickness: the ARIC study. Atherosclerosis Risk in Communities Study. *J Clin Epidemiol.* 1995;48:927–940.
10. Lichodziejewska B, Klos J, Rezler J, et al. Clinical symptoms of mitral valve prolapse are related to hypomagnesemia and attenuated by magnesium supplementation. *Am J Cardiol.* 1997;15:768–772.

11. Touyz RM. Role of magnesium in the pathogenesis of hypertension. *Mol Aspects Med.* 2003;24:107–136.

12. Touyz RM, Campbell N, Logan A, et al; Canadian Hypertension Education Program. The 2004 Canadian recommendations for the management of hypertension: Part III— Lifestyle modifications to prevent and control hypertension. *Can J Cardiol.* 2004;20: 55–59.

13. Jee SH, Miller ER, Guallar E, et al. The effect of magnesium supplementation on blood pressure: a meta-analysis of randomized clinical trials. *Am J Hypertens.* 2002;15:691–696.

14. Sacks FM, Willet WC, Smith A, et al. Effect on blood pressure of potassium, calcium, and magnesium in women with low habitual intake. *Hypertension.* 1998;31:131–138.

15. Yamamoto ME, Applegate WB, Klag MJ, et al. Lack of blood pressure effect with calcium and magnesium supplementation in adults with high-normal blood pressure. Reports from phase I of the Trials of Hypertension Prevention (TOHP). Trials of Hypertension Prevention (TOHP) Collaborative Research Group. *Ann Epidemiol.* 1995;5:96–107.

16. Resnick L, Altura BT, Gupta R, et al. Intracellular and extracellular magnesium depletion in type 2 (non-insulin-dependent) diabetes mellitus. *Diabetologia.* 1993;36: 767–770.

17. Crook M, Couchman S, Tutt P, et al. Erythrocyte, plasma total, ultrafiltrable and platelet magnesium in type 2 (non-insulin-dependent) diabetes mellitus. *Diabetes Res.* 1994;27:73–79.

18. Vanroelen L, Gaal L, Van Rooy P, et al. Serum and erythrocyte magnesium level in type I and type II diabetes. *Acta Diabetol.* 1985;22:185–190.

19. Lopez-Ridaura R, Willett WC, Rimm EB, et al. Magnesium intake and risk of type 2 diabetes in men and women. *Diabetes Care.* 2004;27:134–140.

20. Rodriguez-Moran M, Guerrero-Romero F. Oral magnesium supplementation improves insulin sensitivity and metabolic control in type 2 diabetic subjects: a randomized double-blind controlled trial. *Diabetes Care.* 2003;26:1147–1152.

21. Lal J, Vasudev K, Kela AK, et al. Effect of oral magnesium supplementation on the lipid profile and blood glucose of patients with type 2 diabetes mellitus. *J Assoc Phys India.* 2003;51:37–42.

22. Wang F, Van Den Eeden SK, Ackerson LM, et al. Oral magnesium oxide prophylaxis of frequent migrainous headache in children: a randomized, double-blind, placebo-controlled trial. *Headache.* 2003;43:601–610.

23. Mauskop A, Altura BM. Role of magnesium in the pathogenesis and treatment of migraines. *Clin Neurosci.* 1998;5:24–27.

24. Trauninger A, Pfund Z, Koszegi T, et al. Oral magnesium load test in patients with migraine. *Headache.* 2002;42:114–119.

25. Pfaffenrath V, Wessely P, Meyer C, et al. Magnesium in the prophylaxis of migraine— a double-blind placebo-controlled study. *Cephalalgia.* 1996;16:436–440.

26. Peikert A, Wilimzig C, Kohne-Volland R. Prophylaxis of migraine with oral magnesium: results from a prospective, multi-center, placebo-controlled and double-blind randomized study. *Cephalalgia.* 1996;16:257–263.

27. Rosenstein DL, Elin RJ, Hosseini JM, et al. Magnesium measures across the menstrual cycle in premenstrual syndrome. *Biol Psychiatry.* 1994;35:557–561.

28. Sherwood RA, Rocks BF, Stewart A, et al. Magnesium and the premenstrual syndrome. *Ann Clin Biochem.* 1986;23:667–670.

29. Walker AF, De Souza MC, Vickers MF, et al. Magnesium supplementation alleviates premenstrual symptoms of fluid retention. *J Womens Health.* 1998;7:1157–1165.

30. De Souza MC, Walker AF, Robinson PA, et al. A synergistic effect of a daily supplement for one month of 200 mg magnesium plus 50 mg vitamin B6 for the relief of anxiety-related premenstrual symptoms: a randomized, double-blind, crossover study. *J Womens Health Gend Based Med.* 2000;9:131–139.

31. Haymes EM, Clarkson PM. Minerals and trace minerals. In: Berning JR, Nelson S, eds. *Nutrition for Sport and Exercise.* 2nd ed. Gaithersburg, Md: Aspen Publishers; 1998: 91–92.

32. Bohl CH, Volpe SL. Magnesium and exercise. *Crit Rev Food Sci Nutr.* 2002;42:533–563.

33. Lukaski HC, Nielsen FH. Dietary magnesium depletion affects metabolic responses during submaximal exercise in postmenopausal women. *J Nutr.* 2002;132:930–935.

34. Finstad EW, Newhouse IJ, Lukaski HC, et al. The effects of magnesium supplementation on exercise performance. *Med Sci Sports Exerc.* 2001;33:493–498.

35. Newhouse IJ, Finstad EW. The effects of magnesium supplementation on exercise performance. *Clin J Sport Med.* 2000;10:195–200.

36. Weller E, Bachert P, Meinck HM, et al. Lack of effect of oral Mg-supplementation on Mg in serum, blood cells, and calf muscle. *Med Sci Sports Exerc.* 1998;30:1584–1591.

37. Terblanche S, Noakes TD, Dennis SC, et al. Failure of magnesium supplementation to influence marathon running performance or recovery in magnesium-replete subjects. *Int J Sport Nutr.* 1992;2:154–164.

38. Anderson PO, Knoben JE. *Handbook of Clinical Drug Data.* 8th ed. Stamford, Conn: Appleton and Lange, 1997.

Ma Huang *(Ephedra sinica)*

Ma huang, the dried stem of the three ephedra species *(Ephedra sinica, Ephedra equisetina, Ephedra intermedia),* has been a part of Chinese medicine for 5,000 years. The herb has traditionally been used for a number of conditions, including colds, flu, fever, chills, headache, edema, asthma, wheezing, and lack of perspiration. The alkaloids of ma huang, ephedrine and pseudoephedrine, are found in many over-the-counter cold and asthma medications (synthetic form) and dietary supplements (botanical form). Ephedra alkaloids are powerful central nervous system (CNS) stimulants. Ephedrine, a sympathomimetic agent, causes vasoconstriction and cardiac stimulation. Pseudoephedrine enhances bronchodilation and decreases symptoms of nasal congestion.

Because dietary supplements containing ephedrine alkaloids can pose serious health risks, the FDA published a final rule banning ephedra and ephedra-containing products from the US market in 2002 (1). This rule was based on thousands of adverse event reports submitted voluntarily by the industry, health care providers, and individuals. This ruling is currently under legal challenge by a dietary supplement manufacturer, and there is concern the ruling could be overturned despite the wealth of reports indicating the health risks associated with ephedra use. Contact the FDA for up-to-date information on regulations.

Media and Marketing Claims	Efficacy
Increases metabolism for weight loss	Do *not* use due to safety issues; products with ephedra have been banned by the FDA.

Safety

♦ The FDA banned ephedra and ephedra-containing products from the US market in 2002 after compiling numerous reports of adverse events for ma huang, including heart attack, stroke, tremors, insomnia, and death in individuals otherwise in good health after using ma huang/ephedrine products (1). Legal challenges to this ban continue.

♦ Most of the adverse events were related to cardiovascular symptoms, with hypertension as the single most frequent negative event, followed by palpitations, tachycardia, or both, stroke, and seizures (2).

♦ However, another study did not find adverse events. In a randomized, double blind trial testing the acute cardiac response to ephedra, 27 overweight adults took Xenadrine (335 mg ephedra, 910 mg guarana, 200 mg caffeine) or placebo twice a day for 7 days, increasing to two tablets twice a day for an additional 7 days. There were no significant changes in blood pressure, heart rate, echocardiogram, serum glucose, or sleep quality over time or between treatment groups (3). The Xenadrine study was funded by Cytodyne Technologies, the manufacturer of the supplement under study.

♦ A randomized, controlled, crossover study conducted in 15 overweight, otherwise healthy volunteers (mean age 27 years) showed that a single dose of a dietary supplement (MetaboLife) containing ephedra plus caffeine, along with 17 other ingredients, was associated with a prolonged QTc interval and higher systolic blood pressure (4).

♦ A blinded, randomized, crossover study assessed acute changes (during a 3-hour period) in resting energy expenditure, heart rate, and blood pressure in response to ephedra (20 mg ephedra alkaloids) combined with caffeine vs placebo in four healthy men and four healthy women (5). In this controlled study, ephedra-caffeine supplement use was associated with a significant increase in heart rate and, systolic blood pressure compared with baseline, and resting energy expenditure was significantly higher during the last 30 minutes of measurement in the ephedra-caffeine group as compared with placebo ($P = .05$).

- Case reports of ischemic and hemorrhagic stroke have been associated with ephedrine use (6). A case-control report refutes this association (7); however, dose may be an important risk factor.

- Case reports of psychosis related to use of ephedra-containing supplements have also been published (8).

- Ephedrine-induced nephrolithiasis has been reported with use of ma huang extract (9).

- Individuals with hypertension, cardiovascular disease, thyroid disease, diabetes, neurological disorders, and men experiencing difficulty urinating because of an enlarged prostate should take special precautions to avoid ma huang/ephedra because it acts as a heart and central nervous system (CNS) stimulant (1).

- To prevent potential excessive CNS and cardiovascular stimulation, ma huang/ephedrine supplements should not be combined with monoamine oxidase inhibitors (MAOIs), medications containing pseudoephedrine or ephedrine, or other caffeine-containing weight-loss remedies (1).

Drug/Supplement Interactions

- Excessive CNS and cardiovascular stimulation may occur when ma huang is combined with MAOIs, medications containing pseudoephedrine or ephedrine, or large sources of caffeine, such as weight-loss remedies or caffeine-containing analgesics.

- Ma huang/ephedra should not be combined with any medications used to treat heart disease, hypertension, depression, Parkinson's disease, asthma, or diabetes.

- Ma huang/ephedra may cause excessive CNS stimulation when combined with other stimulant herbs such as kola nut and guarana.

Key Points

- Ma huang/ephedra is a "natural" product with drug-like actions. Because the alkaloid content of ma huang is variable, self-medicating is dangerous, especially if products contain high amounts of ephedrine or if they are taken in excess. The FDA has banned ephedra from the US dietary supplement market.

- Studies have found that ephedrine plus caffeine increases weight loss and reduces body fat in healthy, obese subjects. However, in clinical trials, herbal preparations of ephedra with kola nut or guarana have been associated with palpitations, increased heart rate, transient increases in blood pressure, insomnia, irritability, and chest pain. Many experts contend that the risks associated with self-supplementing with ephedra products far outweigh the weight-loss benefits.

- Ephedrine is similar in chemical structure to the illegal drug methamphetamine, which produces a feeling of increased energy and euphoria. Some manufacturers have used this fact to falsely claim that ma huang produces the same effects "naturally." Although ma huang may seem to increase energy because of its stimulatory effect on the CNS, there is no evidence that it produces a "high" similar to that from amphetamines. In March 2000, FDA stated that "street drugs" containing ephedra and marketed as dietary supplements are not legal because they are considered unapproved and misbranded drugs.

Food Sources

None

Dosage Information/Bioavailability

Ma huang (*E sinica*) contains up to 3.3% ephedra alkaloids. Ma huang is sold (illegally) in tablets, capsules, tinctures, and teas in doses ranging from 5 to 75 mg ephedrine alkaloids. (In comparison, asthma medications contain 24 mg ephedrine hydrochloride and cold medications contain 60 mg to 120 mg pseudoephedrine hydrochloride.) Supplements are prepared from the powdered stems and aerial portions of the herb or from dried herbal extracts. The powdered stems and aerial portions typically contain lower levels of ephedra alkaloids than the dried extracts, which contain much higher alkaloid concentrations (10).

When ephedra was still marketed legally, an analysis of nine commercial ma huang products showed varying levels of alkaloids ranging from 0.3 to 56 mg, with one product having no detectable ephedrine-type alkaloids (11). A separate analysis of 20 ephedra products reported variability in ephedra alkaloid contents (ephedrine content ranged from 1.1 to 15.3 mg per dose) (12). In addition, there were significant lot-to-lot variations in alkaloid content in four samples, and half of the products had discrepancies between label claims for ephedra alkaloid content and actual content (in excess of 20%). Ma huang supplements formulated as extracts (found in most dietary supplements) are more rapidly absorbed than those formulated from the ground stem and aerial portions. The mean values of the rate of absorption and maximum plasma levels were 0.49 to 3.9 hours for the powdered herb and 1.36 to 2.8 hours for the extract formulations (10,12,13).

Relevant Research

Ephedra (Ma Huang) vs Ephedrine

- ♦ A randomized, crossover study of 10 subjects investigated the pharmacokinetics of ephedrine from three commercially available ma huang products compared with a 25-mg ephedrine hydrochloride capsule. Pharmacokinetic parameters for botanical ephedrine were similar to the synthetic form. The authors concluded: "The increased incidence of ma huang toxicity does not stem from differences in the absorption of botanical ephedrine compared with synthetic ephedrine; rather, it results from accidental overdose often prompted by exaggerated off-label claims and a belief that 'natural' medicinal agents are inherently safe" (14).

Ephedrine (Synthetic) and Weight Loss

♦ A meta-analysis of weight-loss studies involving ephedra and ephedrine reviewed 530 articles, 22 of which were considered for inclusion in terms of placebo-control (15). Results were generally nonsignificant for supplements containing ephedrine, ephedra, ephedrine plus caffeine, or ephedra plus herbs. Only one well-designed study evaluated the efficacy of ephedra alone (Metabolite) in weight loss. During a 3-month intervention, weight loss with ephedra was 0.8 kg/month greater than with placebo, but this difference did not reach statistical significance. Other supplements that contained ephedrine also lacked efficacy. No studies lasted more than 6 months. The minimal clinical relevance of this short-term weight loss intervention would limit any recommendation for its use, regardless of the FDA ban.

♦ A 12-week, double-blind, placebo-controlled study of a multiconstituent, ephedra-containing supplement was conducted in 102 overweight/obese adults. The study demonstrated a significantly greater loss of body weight (and decrease in BMI) and waist circumference in those randomly assigned to the ephedra-containing supplement (16). Body composition did not change in either group. Blood pressure did not increase with the ephedra-based product. Of importance, independent analysis of supplement ingredients indicated that the actual ephedra content of the supplement was 50% less than what was stated on the product label.

♦ A 6-month randomized, double-blind study was conducted at Columbia University to evaluate the weight-loss efficacy of ephedra plus kola nut (90 mg ma huang) vs placebo in 167 overweight and obese adults (17). Outcomes included changes in blood pressure, body weight, and cardiac function. Compared with placebo, the dietary supplement was associated with significantly more weight loss, greater reduction in body fat, greater decrease in LDL, and greater increase in HDL. The statistical analysis employed was based on intent-to-treat; therefore, the last available anthropometric measurements were used for subjects who dropped after the initial 4-week phase of the intervention to fill in missing data points throughout the remainder of the study. Blood pressure and heart rate increased significantly, but there were no reports of stroke or myocardial infarction. The carried-forward analysis is of some concern because those who do not lose weight are more likely to discontinue study visits.

♦ In a double-blind, placebo-controlled study, 67 overweight but otherwise healthy men and women (ages 25 to 55 years) were randomly assigned to receive ma huang and guarana (72 mg ephedrine alkaloids plus 240 mg caffeine/Metabolife 356) or a placebo daily for 8 weeks. Subjects were encouraged to limit dietary fat to 30% of energy intake and to exercise moderately. Baseline evaluation included medical and nutrition history, exam, blood and urine studies, electrocardiogram (ECG), and body composition measurements. Twenty-four subjects in each group completed the study. Compared with the placebo, the ma huang/guarana group lost significantly more weight and body fat, and waist and hip circumferences and triglyceride levels decreased significantly. Mean systolic blood pressure was significantly more at week 6 in the ephedra/guarana group. Heart rate (beats/minute) was significantly higher with the ephedra/guarana combination throughout the study. No abnormalities were observed with ECG in either group at baseline or week 8. Eight of the subjects in the ma huang/guarana group (23%) and zero from the placebo group withdrew from the study because of adverse side effects, including elevated blood pressure, palpitations, extreme irritability, and chest pain. The authors concluded that critical questions regarding the risks and benefits of the supplement must be answered (18).

References

1. FDA final rule. Available at: http://www.fda.gov/oc/initiatives/ephedra. Accessed May 25, 2005.
2. Haller CA, Benowitz NL. Adverse cardiovascular and central nervous system events associated with dietary supplements containing ephedra alkaloids. *N Engl J Med.* 2000;343:1833–1888.
3. Kalman D, Incledon T, Gaunaurd I, et al. An acute clinical trial evaluating the cardiovascular effects of an herbal ephedra-caffeine weight loss product in healthy overweight adults. *Int J Obes Relat Metab Disord.* 2002;26:1363–1366.
4. McBride BF, Karapanos AK, Krudysz A, et al. Electrocardiographic and hemodynamic effects of a multicomponent dietary supplement containing ephedra and caffeine: a randomized controlled trial. *JAMA.* 2004;291:216–221.
5. Vukovich MD, Schoorman R, Heilman C, et al. Caffeine-herbal ephedra combination increases resting energy expenditure, heart rate and blood pressure. *Clin Exp Pharmacol Physiol.* 2005;32:47–53.
6. Bruno A, Nolte KB, Chapin J. Stroke associated with ephedrine use. *Neurology.* 1993;43:1313–1316.
7. Morgenstern LB, Viscoli CM, Kernan WN, et al. Use of ephedra-containing products and risk for hemorrhagic stroke. *Neurology.* 2003;60:132–135.
8. Walton R, Manos GH. Psychosis related to ephedra-containing herbal supplement use. *South Med J.* 2003;96:718–720.
9. Powell T, Hsu FF, Turk J, et al. Ma huang strikes again: ephedrine nephrolithiasis. *Am J Kidney Dis.* 1998;32:153–159.
10. Gurley BJ, Gardner SF, Hubbard MA. Content versus label claims in ephedra-containing dietary supplements. *Am J Health-Syst Pharm.* 2000;57:963–969.
11. Betz JM, Gay ML, Mossoba MM, et al. Chiral gas chromatographic determination of ephedrine-type alkaloids in dietary supplements containing ma huang. *J AOAC Int.* 1997;80:303–315.
12. Gurley B. Extract versus herb: effect of formulation on the absorption on rate of botanical ephedrine from dietary supplements containing ephedra (ma huang). *Ther Drug Monit.* 2000;22:497.
13. White LM, Gardner SF, Gurley BJ, et al. Pharmacokinetics and cardiovascular effects of ma-huang (*Ephedra sinica*) in normotensive adults. *J Clin Pharmacol.* 1997;37:116–122.
14. Gurley BJ, Gardner SF, White LM, et al. Ephedrine pharmacokinetics after ingestion of nutritional supplements containing *Ephedra sinica* (ma huang). *Ther Drug Monit.* 1998;20:439–445.

15. Shekelle PG, Hardy ML, Morton SC, et al. Efficacy and safety of ephedra and ephedrine for weight loss and athletic performance: a meta-analysis. *JAMA*. 2003;289: 1537–1545.

16. Coffey CS, Steiner D, Baker BA, et al. A randomized double-blind placebo-controlled clinical trial of a product containing ephedrine, caffeine, and other ingredients from herbal sources for treatment of overweight and obesity in the absence of lifestyle treatment. *Int J Obes Relat Metab Disord*. 2004;28:1411–1419.

17. Boozer CN, Daly PA, Homel P, et al. Herbal ephedra/caffeine for weight loss: a 6-month randomized safety and efficacy trial. *Int J Obes Relat Metab Disord*. 2002;26: 593–604.

18. Boozer CN, Nasser JA, Heymsfield SB, et al. An herbal supplement containing ma huang-guarana for weight loss: a randomized, double-blind, trial. *Int J Obes Relat Metab Disord*. 2001;25:316–324.

Melatonin

Synthesized from tryptophan, melatonin is the major hormone produced by the pineal gland, located in the brain. Studies have shown that melatonin plays a role in regulating circadian rhythm and reducing core body temperature. Reduced melatonin secretions have been associated with aging, Alzheimer's disease, diabetes, cancer, and cardiovascular disease; however, its role in the etiology and pathophysiology of these conditions is unknown. Additionally, melatonin has been studied as a potential anticancer agent based on evidence from in vitro and animal research suggesting that the hormone has antiproliferative, antioxidative, and immunostimulatory mechanisms of action. Melatonin became available in 1993 as a dietary supplement marketed as a sleep-aid for insomnia and jet lag (1–4).

Media and Marketing Claims	Efficacy
Regulates sleep-awake cycles	↔
Reduces jet lag	↑?
Reduces cancer risk; eases side effects of cancer treatment	NR
Prevents and treats migraines	NR
Enhances sex drive	NR

Safety

- To date, short-term human studies in small numbers of subjects have not reported any harmful effects of melatonin supplementation (3).

- The toxicity of 10 mg melatonin per day for 28 days was assessed in 40 volunteers randomly assigned to melatonin (n = 30) or placebo (n = 10) in a double-blind fashion. Melatonin had no effect on complete blood count; urinalysis; sodium, potassium, or calcium levels; total protein levels; albumin; blood glucose; triglycerides; total cholesterol, HDL, LDL, or VLDL cholesterol; urea; creatinine; uric acid; liver enzymes; thyroid hormones (T3, T4, TSH); ratio of leutinizing hormone to follicle stimulating hormone; cortisol; or serum melatonin (5).

♦ The long-term effects and the safety of melatonin supplementation have not been studied. Melatonin supplements could theoretically suppress endogenous melatonin production, which could further aggravate sleep disorders (6).

♦ A double-blind, placebo-controlled study of nine healthy men in a sleep laboratory reported that morning administration of melatonin impaired psychomotor function for 6 hours. Morning supplementation with melatonin may affect alertness and reflexes (7).

♦ Individuals should not drive automobiles or machinery for several hours after taking melatonin.

♦ Melatonin from animal pineal gland should be avoided due to potential contamination from toxins.

Drug/Supplement Interactions

♦ Melatonin production is increased with administration of fluvoxetine (antidepressant); the additive effect of melatonin supplementation is unknown.

♦ Endogenous melatonin production may be reduced by beta blockers, valproic acid, corticosteroids, or fluvoxetine.

♦ Oral contraceptives increase endogenous melatonin levels.

♦ Melatonin may interfere with or reduce efficacy of immune suppressive medications.

♦ Individuals taking other sleep medications should not take melatonin.

♦ The decision to supplement with melatonin while undergoing chemotherapy for cancer should be made under the supervision of an oncologist.

Key Points

♦ Some research suggests that melatonin hastens sleep onset, although this has not been consistent across all studies. The FDA has awarded orphan drug status for this application of melatonin in health (8). One review article attributes contradictory results to study design differences with varying times of melatonin administration, dosage levels, types of subjects (normal vs insomniacs), and subjective vs objective measures of improvement. The authors concluded: "There is not yet a convincing body of evidence using generally accepted measures that melatonin administration improves sleep in insomniacs with noncircadian sleep disturbance" (9). Although the research is not discussed here, melatonin may also improve sleep in the blind and children with autism.

- Data for the use of melatonin to reduce jet lag suggest that supplementation may be effective. Individuals with sleep disorders or jet lag should consider maximizing nighttime endogenous melatonin production by: avoiding alcohol and caffeine, which reduce melatonin levels; increasing exposure to light during the day; avoiding sleeping late or taking naps longer than 30 minutes; and sleeping in a cool, dark environment. However, supplemental melatonin may also ease symptoms of jet lag.

- Preliminary controlled studies suggest that high doses of melatonin administered in addition to chemotherapy may reduce some, but not all, chemotherapy-induced side effects. More definitive research is needed before any recommendations can be made regarding melatonin administration and cancer. The decision to supplement with melatonin should be made under the supervision of an oncologist.

- Preliminary evidence suggests that regular, low-dose melatonin supplementation may reduce the intensity or frequency of migraines. Larger, well-designed studies are needed (10).

- Although the pineal gland secretes higher levels of melatonin during sexual maturation than during adulthood (11), there is currently no evidence from controlled clinical trials that melatonin supplements enhance sexual function or drive. There is some concern that increasing melatonin levels in children could offset gonadal development, but this is theoretical at this time.

- In a study of longitudinal secretion of melatonin with age, investigators noted a significant decrease in 24-hour melatonin secretion in women, but not men, associated with aging. This warrants further study and may explain inconsistencies in efficacy of melatonin in select studies (12).

Food Sources

A minimal amount of melatonin is found in food, although more extensive studies are needed to define the levels of melatonin in a wider variety of food products (13). Melatonin is produced by plants, with the highest known amounts found in rice, barley, sweet corn, and oats (14). According to one report, ingesting 3 mg melatonin, would require eating 120 bananas or 30 bowls of rice (15). Currently, the unknown impact of variables such as absorption from the gut and processing by the liver make it difficult to calculate how much a melatonin-containing food would have to be consumed to affect mood/sleep (13).

Dosage Information/Bioavailability

Melatonin is sold as capsules and tablets. Manufacturers recommend dosages ranging from 3 to 5 mg (studies have used dosages ranging from 0.1 to 2,000 mg). Some researchers have expressed concern about the safety, purity, and potency of melatonin sold in health food stores and pharmacies (2). Melatonin is absorbed rapidly and has a half-life in plasma of approximately 45 minutes (3). Labels suggest taking melatonin supplements a few hours before sleep time. Although the research is not conclusive, timing of administration varies depending on whether melatonin is used to advance the body clock (as in eastward travel), to treat delayed–sleep phase syndrome, or to treat insomnia. Sach et al describe melatonin administration as developed by the Sleep and Mood Disorders Laboratory at Oregon Health Sciences University (3).

Relevant Research

Melatonin and Sleep

◆ In a study of 517 adults (older than age 55 years) with insomnia, nocturnal melatonin secretion was measured. A subsample of 372 patients completed an intervention that included 2 weeks of placebo and 3 weeks of 2 mg melatonin (controlled-release) to determine the effect on sleep, evaluated with the Leeds Sleep Evaluation Questionnaire (16). Patients with insomnia demonstrated significantly lower melatonin secretion in a cross-sectional analysis as compared with age-matched healthy volunteers and younger healthy volunteers. "Low excretors" of melatonin also demonstrated the greatest response to the nightly melatonin supplement. Thus, the investigators suggest that correction of depleted melatonin levels may improve sleep; individuals with normal melatonin levels are unlikely to find benefit.

◆ In a study of 157 individuals with Alzheimer's disease who had less than 7 hours of restful sleep per night (as assessed by monitored sleep using wrist actigraphy in Alzheimer's disease research centers) and who had at least two episodes of awakening at night during a 1-week period, subjects were randomly assigned to placebo, 2.5 mg slow-release melatonin, or 10 mg melatonin daily for 2 months. The results showed no significant differences in measures of sleep (total sleep time, awakening at night, wake-time after sleep onset, and day-to-night sleep ratio) across groups, although there was a trend toward increased total sleep time with a dose of 10 mg/day (17).

◆ Numerous studies have focused on the role of melatonin in enhancing sleep patterns in children with neurodevelopmental disabilities. Many of these studies have limitations in design. Several studies suggest that these children have depleted melatonin levels. A systematic review of randomized, placebo-controlled clinical trials yielded only three studies, with a total of 35 child subjects, that were thought to be of sufficient scientific integrity. The results showed that time to sleep was reduced in two studies, but total sleep time and awakenings were not modulated by melatonin supplementation (18).

◆ In a double-blind, placebo controlled study conducted among mentally retarded children with or without epilepsy, 25 children were randomly assigned to sustained-release melatonin with an initial dose of 3 mg, increasing as tolerated to 9 mg if the lower dose was ineffective (thus raising questions about how blinding could be maintained). This study, published after the systemic review, also supported a role for melatonin in enhancing sleep onset in mentally retarded persons (19).

◆ Melatonin may also enhance sleep in children with insomnia of unknown origin. In a study of 62 children randomly assigned to 5 mg melatonin or placebo at 7 PM nightly, melatonin supplementation after 4 weeks resulted in significantly improved

Functional Status scores and a 57-minute reduction in time to sleep, but total sleep time did not change (20).

◆ In a double-blind, placebo-controlled study, 34 elderly subjects with insomnia who were taking benzodiazepines to induce sleep were randomly assigned to receive 2 mg controlled-release melatonin or a placebo nightly for 6 weeks. Subjects were encouraged to reduce their benzodiazepine dosage by 50% during week 2 and by 75% during weeks 3 and 4, and to eliminate it by weeks 5 and 6. In a second single-blind phase of the study, melatonin was administered for 6 weeks to all subjects, who were encouraged to discontinue benzodiazepine therapy. Drug intake and subjective sleep quality scores were reported daily. By the end of the first phase, 14 of 18 subjects taking melatonin but only 4 of 16 placebo subjects were able to discontinue benzodiazepine therapy, and the difference between groups was significant. In addition, sleep quality scores were significantly higher in the melatonin group. Six additional subjects in the placebo group eliminated benzodiazepine therapy during the open phase. Follow-up 6 months later revealed that of the 24 subjects in the melatonin group who discontinued benzodiazepine, 19 maintained good quality sleep (21).

Melatonin for Jet Lag and Night Shift Work

◆ A Cochrane Systematic Review of melatonin for jet lag including 10 trials that meet evidence-based criteria for review states that "melatonin is remarkably effective in preventing or reducing jet lag and occasional, short-term use appears to be safe. It should be recommended to all traveler's flying across five or more time zones, particularly in the easterly direction, and especially if they have experienced jet lag on previous journeys" (22).

◆ In double-blind, placebo-controlled study, 257 Norwegian physicians who had visited New York for 5 days were randomly assigned to receive one of four regimens: (*a*) a placebo; (*b*) 5.0 mg melatonin at bedtime; (*c*) 0.5 mg melatonin at bedtime; or (*d*) 0.5 mg melatonin taken on a shifting schedule. Jet lag ratings were made on the day of travel from New York back to Oslo (6 hours eastward) and for the next 6 days in Norway. Main outcome measures were scores on the Columbia Jet Lag Scale (identifies prominent daytime symptoms of jet lag). In all groups, there was a marked increase in total jet lag score on the first day home, followed by improvement during the next 5 days. However, there were no differences in jet lag, sleep onset, time of awakening, hours slept, or hours napping among any of the groups (23).

◆ In a double-blind, placebo-controlled study, 137 subjects flying from Switzerland to the United States and back (six to nine time zones) received randomly one of four treatments on the eastbound flight back to Switzerland and at bedtime on 4 consecutive nights after the flight: (*a*) 5 mg melatonin; (*b*) 10 mg zolpidem (hypnotic); (*c*) a combination of the two; or (*d*) a placebo. Alleviation of jet lag was assessed by daily sleep logs, symptoms questionnaires, and the Profile of Mood States. On the last day of treatment, all subjects completed Visual Analog Scales on overall jet lag ratings and treatment effectiveness. At baseline and during the days after the flight, motor activity was measured by wrist-worn ambulatory monitors in a subgroup of subjects (n = 49). Seventy-nine percent of the subjects took the medication between 5 pm and 9 pm as instructed; 21% ingested the treatment later. All active treatments were associated with a significant reduction in jet lag severity, with zolpidem rated as the most effective. Zolpidem significantly improved subjective sleep quality on night flights, reduced overall jet lag feelings, and alleviated sleep disturbances and confusion associated with jet lag. However, zolpidem and the combination of melatonin and zolpidem were not tolerated as well as melatonin alone. Confusion associated with jet lag, morning sleepiness, and nausea were highest in the combination group, and this was confirmed by actigraphy, which showed significantly reduced motor activity in the first hour after waking only in the combination group. The authors suggested that future research evaluate using one dose of zolpidem for sleep while on the aircraft, and melatonin for the following days after the intercontinental flight (24).

◆ In a double-blind, placebo-controlled trial, 52 flight crew employees were randomly assigned to three groups: (*a*) early melatonin (5 mg melatonin for 3 days before arrival continuing for 5 days after returning home); (*b*) late melatonin (placebo for 3 days followed by 5 mg melatonin for 5 days); or (*c*) a placebo. All subjects began taking capsules at 7 AM to 8 AM Los Angeles time 2 days before their departure from home to New Zealand (corresponding to 2 AM to 3 AM New Zealand time). Subjects then took one capsule on the return flight at 12 PM New Zealand time and continued taking one capsule between 10 PM to 12 PM for 5 days after arrival in New Zealand. (Researchers did not indicate why the large window of time from 10 PM to 12 PM was chosen.) For 6 days after arrival home, subjects completed daily questionnaires measuring subjective impressions of fatigue, jet lag, activity, and sleepiness. Subjects in the late melatonin group reported less jet lag and sleep disturbance than did the placebo group. However, subjects in the early melatonin group reported a worse recovery of energy and alertness than did the placebo group. The authors concluded that timing of the melatonin dose seemed to affect the subjective effects of jet lag (25).

◆ In a double-blind, placebo-controlled, crossover study, 18 emergency physicians working between two and five consecutive night shifts were given 10 mg sublingual melatonin or a placebo each morning after night shifts. Although there were trends toward improvement, melatonin intake did not have a significant effect on self-reported day sleep and night alertness (26).

◆ In a similar double-blind, placebo-controlled, crossover study, 19 emergency medicine residents who worked at least two night shifts per week received in random order 1 mg melatonin or a placebo 30 to 60 minutes prior to their daytime sleep session, for 3 consecutive days after each night shift. Subjects switched to the other treatment during their subsequent night shifts the following week. Quality of daytime sleep was assessed by wrist actigraphs—a device that measures sleep motion and correlates with sleep efficiency, total sleep time, time in bed, and sleep latency. The Profile of Mood States and the Stanford Sleepiness Scale evaluated mood and sleepiness. There were no differences in any of the parameters measured between either treatment (27).

Melatonin and Cancer

♦ In a controlled trial, 80 subjects with metastatic solid tumors (lung, breast, and gastrointestinal cancers) and in poor clinical condition were randomly assigned to receive chemotherapy alone or chemotherapy plus melatonin (20 mg/day). Melatonin resulted in a significant reduction in frequency of thrombocytopenia, malaise, and asthenia compared with controls. There was an insignificant trend toward less stomatitis and neuropathy with melatonin, but it had no affect on alopecia or vomiting. The authors concluded: "This pilot study seems to suggest that concomitant administration of the pineal hormone melatonin during chemotherapy may prevent some chemotherapy-induced side effects, particularly myelosuppression and neuropathy" (28).

♦ In a controlled study, 50 subjects with brain metastases caused by solid neoplasms were randomly assigned to receive supportive care alone (steroids plus anticonvulsant drugs) or supportive care plus melatonin (20 mg/day). The survival at 1 year rate, free-from-brain-progression period, and mean survival time were significantly higher in subjects treated with melatonin. The control subjects had a significant increase in metabolic and infective complications compared with melatonin-treated subjects (29).

♦ Another randomized controlled study providing melatonin intravenously plus chemotherapy to individuals with advanced non–small-cell lung cancer reported a significant increase in percentage of subjects living at 1 year after treatment compared with chemotherapy alone (15 of 34 melatonin subjects vs 7 of 36 control subjects) (30).

♦ In a randomized study of 250 individuals with metastatic solid tumors (lung, breast, gastrointestinal, or head and neck cancers), 20 mg melatonin daily plus chemotherapy reduced the frequency of thrombocytopenia, neurotoxicity, cardiotoxicity, stomatitis, and asthenia compared with chemotherapy alone (31).

♦ A prospective study that analyzed 24-hour urinary 6-sulfaoxymelatonin levels in 127 women diagnosed with breast cancer and 353 control subjects showed no significant association between melatonin levels and future breast cancer risk (32).

♦ A review of mechanistic studies evaluating the potential role of melatonin in modulating cancer risk found strong evidence that melatonin reduces oxidative damage and DNA damage, which may promote cancer (33).

♦ In addition, some researchers now speculate that exposure to light at night reduces melatonin levels and contributes to cancer risk; however, this is only observational data (34).

Melatonin and Migraines

♦ In an open-label study, 34 subjects with recurrent migraines were given 3 mg melatonin just before bedtime for 3 months following a 1-month run-in. Individuals with sleep disturbances were excluded, and subjects had to demonstrate recurrent but not chronic daily headaches during the run-in phase to participate. Thirty two of the 34 who successfully completed run-in completed the study. No subjects reported an increase in headaches, and 78% reported a greater than 50% reduction in headaches; complete response was shown in 8 of the 32 subjects. In addition to decreasing headache frequency, melatonin also significantly reduced headache intensity and duration (10). Although promising, this study is limited by the lack of a control group and blinding.

References

1. Defrance R, Quera-Salva MA. Therapeutic applications of melatonin and related compounds. *Horm Res.* 1998;49:142–146.
2. Cupp MJ. Melatonin. *Am Fam Physician.* 1997;56:1421–1425.
3. Sack RL, Lewy AJ, Hughes RJ. Use of melatonin for sleep and circadian rhythm disorders. *Ann Med.* 1998;30:115–121.
4. Panzer A, Viljoen M. The validity of melatonin as an oncostatic agent. *J Pineal Res.* 1997;22:184–202.
5. de Lourdes M, Seabra V, Bignotto M, et al. Randomized, double-blind clinical trial, controlled with placebo, of the toxicology of chronic melatonin treatment. *J Pineal Res.* 2000;29:193–200.
6. Guardiola-Lemaitre B. Toxicology of melatonin. *J Biol Rhythms.* 1997;12:697–706.
7. Graw P, Werth E, Krauchi K, et al. Early morning melatonin administration impairs psychomotor vigilance. *Behav Brain Res.* 2001;121:167–172.
8. FDA. Office of Orphan Products Development. List of orphan designations and approvals. Available at: www.fda.gov/orphan/designat/list.htm. Accessed March 31, 2005.
9. Mendelson WB. Efficacy of melatonin as a hypnotic agent. *J Biol Rhythms.* 1997;12:651–656.
10. Peres MFP, Zukerman E, da Cunha Tanuri F, et al. Melatonin, 3 mg, is effective for migraine prevention. *Neurology.* 2004;63:757.
11. Cavallo A, Ritschel WA. Pharmacokinetics of melatonin in human sexual maturation. *J Clin Endocrinol Metab.* 1996;81:1882–1886.
12. Kin NM, Nair NP, Schwartz G, et al. Secretion of melatonin in healthy elder subjects: a longitudinal study. *Ann N Y Acad Sci.* 2004;1019:326–329.
13. Reiter RJ, Tan DX, Burkhardt S, et al. Melatonin in plants. *Nutr Rev.* 2001;59:286–290.
14. Hattori A, Migitaka H, Iigo M, et al. Identification of melatonin in plants and its effects on plasma melatonin levels and binding to melatonin receptors in vertebrates. *Biochem Mol Biol Int.* 1995;35:627–634.
15. Lamberg L. Melatonin potentially useful but safety, efficacy remain uncertain. *JAMA.* 1996;276:1011–1014.
16. Leger D, Laudon M, Zisapel N. Nocturnal 6-sulfatoxymelatonin excretion in insomnia and its relation to the response to melatonin replacement therapy. *Am J Med.* 2004;116:91–95.

17. Singer C, Tractenberg RE, Kaye J, et al; Alzheimer's Disease Cooperative Study. A multicenter, placebo-controlled trial of melatonin for sleep disturbance in Alzheimer's disease. *Sleep.* 2003;26:893–901.

18. Phillips L, Appleton RE. Systematic review of melatonin treatment in children with neurodevelopmental disabilities and sleep impairment. *Dev Med Child Neurol.* 2004;46:723.

19. Coppola G, Iervolino G, Mastrosimone M, et al. Melatonin in wake-sleep disorders in children, adolescents and young adults with mental retardation with or without epilepsy: a double-blind, cross-over, placebo-controlled trial. *Brain Dev.* 2004;26:373–376.

20. Smits MG, van Stel HF, van der Heijden K, et al. Melatonin improves health status and sleep in children with idiopathic chronic sleep-onset insomnia: a randomized placebo-controlled trial. *J Am Acad Child Adolesc Psychiatry.* 2003;42:1286–1293.

21. Garfinkel D, Zisapel N, Wainstein J, et al. Facilitation of benzodiazepine discontinuation by melatonin: a new clinical approach. *Arch Intern Med.* 1999;159:2456–2460.

22. Herxheimer A, Petrie KJ. Melatonin for the prevention and treatment of jet lag. *Cochrane Database Syst Rev.* 2002;2:CD001520.

23. Spitzer RL, Terman M, Williams JB, et al. Jet lag: clinical features, validation of a new syndrome-specific scale, and lack of response to melatonin in a randomized, double-blind trial. *Am J Psychiatry.* 1999;156:1392–1396.

24. Suhner A, Schlagenhauf P, Hofer I, et al. Effectiveness and tolerability of melatonin and zolpidem for the alleviation of jet lag. *Aviat Space Environ Med.* 2001;72:638–646.

25. Petrie K, Dawson AG, Thompson L, et al. A double-blind trial of melatonin as a treatment for jet lag in international cabin crew. *Biol Psychiatry.* 1993;33:526–530.

26. Jorgensen KM, Witting MD. Does exogenous melatonin improve day sleep or night alertness in emergency physicians working night shifts? *Ann Emerg Med.* 1998;31: 699–704.

27. Jockovich M, Cosentino D, Cosentino L, et al. Effect of exogenous melatonin on mood and sleep efficiency in emergency medicine residents working night shifts. *Acad Emerg Med.* 2000;7:955–958.

28. Lissoni P, Tancini G, Barni S, et al. Treatment of cancer chemotherapy-induced toxicity with the pineal hormone melatonin. *Support Care Cancer.* 1997;5:126–129.

29. Lissoni P, Barni S, Ardizzoia A, et al. A randomized study with the pineal hormone melatonin versus supportive care alone in patients with brain metastases due to solid neoplasms. *Cancer.* 1994;73:699–701.

30. Lissoni P, Paolorossi F, Ardizzoia A, et al. A randomized study of chemotherapy with cisplatin plus etoposide versus chemoendocrine therapy with cisplatin, etoposide and the pineal hormone melatonin as a first-line treatment of advanced nonsmall cell lung cancer patients in a poor clinical state. *J Pineal Res.* 1997;23:15–19.

31. Lissoni P, Barni S, Mandala M, et al. Decreased toxicity and increased efficacy of cancer chemotherapy using the pineal hormone melatonin in metastatic solid tumour patients with poor clinical status. *Eur J Cancer.* 1999;35:1688–1692.

32. Travis RC, Allen DS, Fentiman IS, et al. Melatonin and breast cancer: a prospective study. *J Natl Cancer Inst.* 2004;96:475–482.

33. Reiter RJ, Tan DX, Gitto E, et al. Pharmacological utility of melatonin in reducing oxidative cellular and molecular damage. *Pol J Pharmacol.* 2004;56:159–170.

34. Schernhammer ES, Schulmeister K. Melatonin and cancer risk: does light at night compromise physiologic cancer protection by lowering serum melatonin levels? *Br J Cancer.* 2004;90:941–943.

Methylsulfonylmethane (MSM)

Methylsulfonylmethane (MSM) is a naturally occurring sulfur-containing compound found in the body. It is an odorless, water-soluble derivative of dimethylsulfoxide (DMSO). DMSO was first used as an industrial solvent in paint thinners and antifreeze. Later, it was used in veterinary medicine and approved for human use for arthritis. DMSO is currently available in health food stores as a topical ointment for arthritis and as a prescription drug for intravesicular instillation for interstitial cystitis. Clinical trials in the 1960s and 1970s reported that topical DMSO has an analgesic effect in patients with osteoarthritis, rheumatoid arthritis, gout, and soft tissue conditions, although not all studies demonstrate benefits. In addition, some uncomfortable side-effects such as odor and garlic taste in the mouth are associated with DMSO. Because MSM is a metabolic product of DMSO and is odorless, it has been hypothesized that it might have the same beneficial effects on arthritis and other inflammatory diseases. Despite the numerous Web sites, *The Miracle MSM* book, and anecdotal data that support use of MSM, there is a lack of research to substantiate these claims (1).

Media and Marketing Claims	Efficacy
Relieves arthritis pain	NR
Decreases allergy symptoms	NR
Reduces heartburn	NR
Reduces muscular pain	NR
Reduces symptoms of asthma	NR

Safety

- There are some anecdotal reports that MSM may cause mild gastrointestinal discomfort.
- Intake of 2,600 mg MSM per day for 30 days has been well-tolerated.

Drug/Supplement Interactions

No adverse interactions have been reported.

Key Points

- Few well-designed human studies have assessed the efficacy of MSM in reducing symptoms of arthritis.

- Only one open-label clinical trial has evaluated the effect of MSM on allergies (2). Clearly, much more well-controlled research is needed.
- MSM is marketed as a treatment for heartburn, muscular pain, and asthma; however, there are no scientific data to support these uses.

Food Sources

Small amounts of MSM are found in milk, fish, grains, and fruits and vegetables (1).

Dosage Information/Bioavailability

MSM is sold in capsules or tablets (often with glucosamine), with some manufacturers recommending dosages ranging from 500 to 8,000 mg/day. MSM is also available in topical creams. MSM is produced synthetically from DMSO.

Relevant Research

MSM and Arthritis

- In a randomized, blinded, placebo-controlled study conducted in 118 adults with osteoarthritis, subjects were randomly assigned to receive (*a*) glucosamine (500 mg), (*b*) MSM (500 mg), (*c*) a combination, or (*d*) placebo three times daily for 12 weeks (3). Several outcomes scales were included to assess response, including visual analogue scale pain intensity, 15-meter walking time, swelling index, and patient use of supplemental medications for pain control. All three treatments resulted in a significant improvement in pain index and swelling scores over time as compared with placebo. Concurrent use of other medications makes interpretation more difficult. This study may support further research using this supplement.

MSM and Allergic Rhinitis

- Only one study has evaluated the efficacy of MSM in the treatment of seasonal allergies. In this open-label study, 55 subjects with seasonal allergies consumed 2,600 mg MSM daily for 30 days. Outcome assessment included Seasonal Allergy Symptom Questionnaire, IgE, C-reactive protein, and plasma histamine. Self-report data suggested an improvement in upper respiratory airway symptoms at 7 days, which was maintained throughout the 30 days; however, IgE and plasma histamine levels were not modulated. This suggests a strong placebo effect that will need to be tested in a randomized, blinded, and placebo-controlled study (2).

References

1. John H, Laudahn G. Clinical experiences with the topical application of DMSO in orthopedic diseases: evaluation of 4180 cases. *Ann N Y Acad Sci.* 1967;141:506–516.
2. Barrager E, Veltmann JR, Schauss AG, et al. A multicentered, open-label trial on the safety and efficacy of methylsulfonylmethane in the treatment of seasonal allergic rhinitis. *J Altern Complement Med.* 2002;8:167–173.

3. Lawrence RM. Methylsulfonylmethane: a double-blind study of its use in degenerative arthritis. *Int J Anti Aging Med*. 1998;1:50.

Milk Thistle *(Silybum marianum)*

Milk thistle *(Silybum marianum)* has been used in the United States since the late 19th century, when physicians began to use the seeds to treat ailments of the kidney, liver, and spleen. In 1986, milk thistle was approved in Germany for the treatment of liver disease. The four active components, isosilybinin, sillbinin, silychristin, and silydianin, of milk thistle are collectively known as "silymarin." Silymarin, a plant flavonoid, displaces toxins from the liver, allowing for liver cell regeneration (1). This function has led researchers to investigate the protective mechanisms of milk thistle against poisonous mushrooms, toluene, and acetaminophen (2). Mechanisms of action include antioxidant activity, membrane permeability effects, as well as possibly anti-inflammatory or immune-enhancing effects.

Media and Marketing Claims	Efficacy
Reduces liver damage in patients with alcohol-induced liver damage (cirrhosis)	↔
Treats viral hepatitis	↓?
Improves general liver health	NR
Prevents cancer	NR

Safety

◆ Standardized milk thistle extracts seem to be safe with minimal occurrence of side effects. The more commonly reported side effects include gastrointestinal upset and allergic skin rash.

◆ Adverse events reported in published studies include nausea, diarrhea, dyspepsia, and headache, but these same symptoms were frequently reported in the placebo groups as well.

Drug/Supplement Interactions

◆ Milk thistle may alter the bioavailability of medications that are metabolized by cytochrome P450 (3).

◆ Some early reports raised concern that milk thistle might interfere with the bioavailability of indinavir, an antiretroviral medication (in the protease inhibitor class) used to treat HIV. However, a more recent, well-designed study using a three-period, randomized, controlled trial design found that milk thistle did not seem to alter the pharmacokinetics of indinavir (4).

- Silymarin/milk thistle may increase clearance of glucuronidated drugs, such as select statin medications, acetaminophen, diazepam, digoxin and/or morphine.
- Silymarin may chelate iron and may slow calcium metabolism (5). Additional research is needed.

Key Points

- In 2005, the Agency for Healthcare research and Quality published a review of the evidence regarding the use of milk thistle for hepatic diseases (6). Sixteen prospective intervention studies were included in the analysis, 14 of which were randomized, blinded, and placebo-controlled. The review concluded that "clinical efficacy of milk thistle is not clearly established. Interpretation of evidence is hampered by poor study methods and/or poor quality reporting in publications."
- In a review of the clinical efficacy and safety of milk thistle for treatment of liver diseases, investigators concluded that milk thistle may play a role in treatment of alcoholic liver cirrhosis (7).
- Studies of the role of milk thistle in improving liver health in individuals with hepatitis remain inconclusive, but to date the research does not generally support a benefit. A few small trials suggest liver function tests can improve, but changes are generally the same for placebo. Long-term clinical outcome studies are lacking.
- Milk thistle may improve liver function tests in individuals showing abnormalities related to liver toxicity due to hepatotoxic exposures (7,8).
- Despite frequent reported use of milk thistle by people with cancer to enhance liver function after chemotherapy, there is no clinical trial evidence to support this use.
- Cell culture data suggest that milk thistle may reduce the risk of cancer, particularly skin and prostate cancer, because milk thistle has been shown to induce cancer cell death, reduce prostate-specific antigen (PSA) levels, and prevent cancer cells from forming a blood supply that would lead to metastasis.

Food Sources

None

Dosage Information/Bioavailability

Milk thistle is available as a tincture, tablet, softgel, liquid, and capsule. To ensure effectiveness, the supplement should contain no less than 70% to 80% silymarin. Hepatic conditions have been treated with 240 to 420 mg/day.

Relevant Research

Milk Thistle and Cirrhosis of the Liver

- A review of the use of silymarin/milk thistle in liver disease identified five well-designed clinical trials that assessed the efficacy of this supplement as a treatment for liver cirrhosis (total n = 602). For these five trials, supplement use was associated with a nonsignificant 4.2% reduction in death (7). Encephalopathy incidence was significantly reduced in one trial, but the other trials did not report on this outcome.

◆ One of the first studies to investigate the role of milk thistle in cirrhosis of the liver (alcohol- and non-alcohol-related) was a double-blind, placebo-controlled, randomized study published in 1989 (9). Subjects received either 140 mg silymarin (n = 87) or placebo (n = 83) three times/day for 41 months. Fourteen subjects in the treatment group and 10 in the placebo group dropped out of the study, and mortality accounted for the loss of 24 patients in the treatment group and 37 in the placebo group. Thus, the overall survival rate was significantly less in the placebo group at 4 years ($P = .036$). Efficacy of treatment was greatest in those diagnosed with alcohol-related cirrhosis of the liver.

◆ A multicenter, randomized, double-blind, placebo-controlled study was conducted by Pares et al in Spain using silymarin at a dosage of 150 mg three times/day (10). The study enrolled 200 subjects with a history of alcoholic cirrhosis. One hundred twenty-five subjects remained in the study at 2 years. Fifteen were lost to follow-up after the initial enrollment visit, and 42 patients dropped out of the study (27 from the silymarin group vs 12 from the placebo group). Eighteen patients died during the course of the study, and the mortality rates were similar for the silymarin and placebo groups. These results suggest that silymarin is ineffective in changing survival rates in individuals with alcoholic cirrhosis; however, the differential and substantial dropout rates reported, as well as the number of subjects who stopped drinking alcohol (54 in the silymarin group and 59 in the placebo group), may have limited the potential for silymarin to show a therapeutic effect.

◆ A double-blind, placebo-controlled, randomized 4-week intervention study was conducted in 1982 in 106 consecutive patients diagnosed with alcohol-induced cirrhosis. Completion rate was 92% (97 patients: 14 women, 83 men). The mean age of participants was 35.2 years in the treated group and 38.8 in the control group. Compared with the control group, daily treatment with 420 mg silymarin (n = 47) was associated with a significant decrease in SGOT and SGPT levels after 4 weeks, as well as decreased (though nonsignificant) bilirubin levels. Further, histological review of liver biopsy tissues before and after treatment also showed that silymarin was associated with a reduction in fatty liver in a significant number of subjects as compared with placebo (11).

Milk Thistle and Hepatitis

◆ Pares et al's multicenter study (10) (described in the previous section) included a secondary analysis of 75 subjects with anti–hepatitis C antibodies. Twenty-nine of these subjects (13 on supplement and 16 on placebo) had anti-hepatitis antibodies on sera analysis. Four subjects, all of whom had been randomly assigned to placebo, died over the 24-month study period, indicating a potential survival benefit for milk thistle supplementation ($P = .056$). The study was underpowered in terms of numbers to test the hypothesis that silymarin treatment is effective for hepatitis C, but it does provide preliminary evidence to support more studies.

- A retrospective analysis was conducted in Germany to compare silymarin dosages of 420, 840 or 1,260 mg/day in 40 subjects with hepatitis C. This study focused on changes in liver function tests over time. Subjects were enrolled if they showed persistent elevation in alanine aminotransferase. Patients had to restrict alcohol intake to less than 30 g/day. The average treatment duration was slightly more than 4 months. The results indicated no change in liver function or bilirubin levels over time or between groups; however, the retrospective nature of the study and small sample size limit interpretation (12).

- A study of 177 patients with hepatitis C residing in Egypt was conducted using a prospective, randomized, controlled design (13). Subjects were randomly assigned either to silymarin (Legalon, a brand manufactured in Germany), with a mean dosage of 124.5 mg three times daily, or a standard multivitamin for a period of 12 months. Silymarin had no significant effect on hepatitis C viral load, serum liver function tests, or ultrasound examination of liver fibrosis over time or compared with the multivitamin group.

- A Cochrane review of several herbal therapies for the treatment of hepatitis C virus concluded that there is "no firm evidence supporting medicinal herbs for HCV infection, and further randomized studies are justified" (14). This report included only one study with milk thistle supplementation; that study showed improved liver function tests.

Milk Thistle and General Liver Health

- The primary medical literature databases (MEDLINE, EMBASE, CINAHL, dissertation abstracts, Micromedex, and BIOSIS and alternative medicine registries including AMED, MAPRALERT, CISCOM) were reviewed to assess the safety and efficacy of milk thistle in the treatment of liver disease (15). A total of 1,726 studies were identified in research published before 1999. In 14 trials (total n = 1,209) that were included in a meta-analysis using random effects modeling, milk thistle seemed safe and may have been effective. In terms of mortality, the overall odds ratio was 0.8 (95% CI = 0.5–1.5). Evaluation of histological parameters found no difference between milk thistle and placebo in liver tissues. Likewise, there was no statistical difference in biochemical markers of liver damage, such as elevated liver enzymes.

- A pilot study was conducted among workers exposed to hepatotoxic chemicals (toluebe and/or xylene), 25% of whom demonstrated abnormal liver function after 5 to 20 years of exposure. Thirty workers took 140 mg silymarin three times daily for 30 days whereas 19 were given no treatment (workers decided for themselves whether or not to take the supplement) (8). Compared with baseline values, liver function tests improved significantly in the treated group but not the untreated group. Interpretation of these results is limited because this study was not blinded, placebo-controlled, or randomized, and the study sample population consisted of only 49 subjects.

Milk Thistle and Cancer

- To assess the growth inhibitory effects of silybinin, the main active component of milk thistle, against human prostate cancer, DU145 prostate carcinoma cells were implanted subcutaneously into nude mice that were then fed AIN-93m purified diet supplemented with 0%, 0.05%, or 0.1% silybinin for 60 days. In a second experiment the nude mice were fed the diet for 3 weeks prior to implantation of DU145 cells and maintained on their respective diets for an additional 6 weeks. Tumor growth was monitored twice a week and at the study's termination. Also at study termination, the level of IGFBP-3 secretion by tumor cells was determined using the Quantikine human IGFBP-3 immunoassay kit from R&D Systems. It was found that silybinin inhibited xenograft tumor growth in a dose-dependent manner. The effect was even more pronounced when nude mice had silybinin-supplemented diets prior to tumor implantation. Mice supplemented with silybinin demonstrated increased secretion of IGFBP-3 (16).

◆ Using isomers of silybinin A and B, investigators cultured three different prostate cancer cell lines to determine the anticancer effects (17). In this study, silybinin suppressed prostate cancer growth as well as PSA excretion.

◆ A review of experimental data on the role of silybinin as chemopreventive against prostate cancer has been published (18). A separate review focused on the anticarcinogenic effects silybinin in the context of skin cancer and found that this compound has anti-inflammatory and antioxidant properties (19).

References

1. Schulz V, Hansel R, Tyler VE. *Rational Phytotherapy: A Physician's Guide to Herbal Medicine.* 3rd ed. Berlin, Germany: Springer-Verlag; 1998:215,218.
2. Muriel P, Garciapina T, Perez-Alvarez V, et al. Silymarin protects against paracetamol-induced lipid peroxidation and liver damage. *J Appl Toxicol.* 1992;12:439–442.
3. Gurley BJ, Gardner SF, Hubbard MA, et al. In vivo assessment of botanical supplementation on human cytochrome P450 phenotypes: *Citrus aurantium, Echinacea purpurea,* milk thistle, and saw palmetto. *Clin Pharmacol Ther.* 2004;76:428–440.
4. Mills E, Wilson K, Clarke M, et al. Milk thistle and indinavir: a randomized controlled pharmacokinetics study and meta-analysis. *Eur J Clin Pharmacol.* 2005;61:1–7.
5. Flora K, Hahn M, Rosen H, et al. Milk thistle (Silybum marianum) for the therapy of liver disease. *Am J Gastroenterol.* 1998;93:139–143.
6. Agency for Healthcare Research and Quality. Milk thistle: Effects on liver disease and cirrhosis and clinical adverse effects. Summary. Evidence Report/Technology Assessment: Number 21 (2005). Available at: http://www.ahrq.gov/clinic/epcsums/milktsum.htm. Accessed August 11, 2005.
7. Saller R, Meier R, Brignoli R. The use of silymarin in the treatment of liver diseases. *Drugs.* 2001;61:2035–2063.
8. Szilard S, Szentgyorgyi D, Demeter I. Protective effect of Legalon in workers exposed to organic solvents. *Acta Med Hung.* 1988;45:249–256.
9. Ferenci P, Dragosics B, Dittrich H, et al. Randomized controlled trial of silymarin treatment in patients with cirrhosis of the liver. *J Hepatol.* 1989;9:105–113.
10. Pares A, Planas R, Torres M, et al. Effects of silymarin in alcoholic patients with cirrhosis of the liver: results of a controlled, double-blind, randomized and multicenter trial. *J Hepatol.* 1998;28:615–621.

11. Salmi HA, Sarna S. Effect of silymarin on chemical, functional, and morphological alterations of the liver. A double-blind, controlled study. *Scand J Gastroenterol*. 1982;17: 517–521.
12. Huber R, Futter I, Ludtke R. Oral silymarin for chronic hepatitis C: a retrospective analysis comparing three dose regimens. *Eur J Med Res*. 2005;10:68–70.
13. Tanamly MD, Tadros F, Labeeb S, et al Randomised double-blinded trial evaluating silymarin for chronic hepatitis C in an Egyptian village: study description and 12-month results. *Dig Liver Dis*. 2004;36:752–759.
14. Liu J, Manheimer E, Tsutani K, et al. Medicinal herbs for hepatitis C virus infection: a Cochrane hepatobiliary systematic review of randomized trials. *Am J Gastroenterol*. 2003;98:538–544.
15. Jacobs BP, Dennehy C, Ramirez G, et al. Milk thistle for the treatment of liver disease: a systematic review and meta-analysis. *Am J Med*. 2002;113:506–515.
16. Singh RP, Dhanalakshmi S, Tyagi AK, et al. Dietary feeding of silibinin inhibits advance human prostate carcinoma growth in athymic nude mice and increases plasma insulin-like growth factor-binding protein-3 levels. *Cancer Res*. 2002;62:3063–3069.
17. Singh RP, Agarwal R. A cancer chemopreventive agent, silibinin, targets mitogenic and survival signaling in prostate cancer. *Mutat Res*. 2004;555:21–32.
18. Davis-Searles PR, Nakanishi Y, Kim NC, et al, Milk thistle and prostate cancer: effects of pure flavonolignans from Silybum marianum on antiproliferative endpoints in human prostate cells. *Cancer Res*. 2005;65:4448–4457.
19. Katiyar SK. Silymarin and skin cancer prevention: anti-inflammatory, antioxidant and immunomodulatory effects (review). *Int J Oncol*. 2005;26:169–176.

Minerals. *See* Boron; Calcium; Chromium; Magnesium; Potassium; Selenium; Vanadium; Zinc.

N-Acetylcysteine (NAC)

N-acetylcysteine (NAC) is derivative of the sulfur-containing amino acid cysteine. First introduced as a mucolytic drug in the 1960s, NAC has also been used successfully as an antidote for acetaminophen toxicity (1). In the body, NAC is a precursor of reduced glutathione (GSH), an endogenous antioxidant. Because NAC has demonstrated antioxidant activity in vitro and can be converted into the antioxidant GSH, it has been proposed to be beneficial in treating conditions such as acute and chronic bronchitis, acute respiratory distress syndrome, HIV infection, cancer, and some cardiovascular diseases (2–5). There is a fine line between medical use of NAC for diagnoses (such as acetaminophen poisoning or select use as an adjuvant agent in cancer therapy or for acute viral hepatitis) and supplemental over-the-counter use. This needs to be considered when reviewing evidence for NAC and when making recommendations regarding its use.

Media and Marketing Claims	Efficacy
Prevents and treats influenza and respiratory illnesses	NR
Improves markers of immune function in HIV patients	↑?
Prevents free-radical damage associated with exercise	NR
Enhances fertility	NR

Safety

♦ NAC has been used for 3 decades with few side effects (mild side effects include nausea and rash). No adverse effects were reported in people with HIV supplemented with 6,000 to 8,000 mg NAC per day for 1 year.

♦ NAC seems to have antiplatelet effects; this suggests that it should not be used in patients before elective surgery (6).

♦ Intravenous NAC is an FDA-approved prescription medication used for the treatment of acetaminophen toxicity.

Drug/Supplement Interactions

♦ NAC reduces acetaminophen absorption by charcoal in the clinical setting of acetaminophen overdose.

♦ Intravenous NAC along with nitroglycerin has been associated with hypotension in cardiac patients.

Key Points

♦ NAC has been used in Europe to treat bronchitis, acute respiratory distress disease, and other lung diseases (4). Recent preliminary evidence suggests that NAC may reduce respiratory symptoms related to the influenza virus in elderly subjects. Additional studies are needed to confirm this use.

♦ Studies in patients with HIV suggest that NAC can increase glutathione levels and improve parameters of immune function. In one open trial, NAC was associated with increased length of survival. Controlled clinical trials are needed in this population to further determine its effects on survival.

♦ There is a lack of well-controlled clinical trials demonstrating that oral NAC supplementation in humans has a favorable effect on exercise performance by reducing oxidative damage or enhancing immunity.

♦ Although still limited, evidence suggests that NAC may be useful in increasing ovulatory cycles and pregnancy rates in women with polycystic ovary syndrome. This may be related to either improved insulin sensitivity and/or antioxidant properties that may reduce the cystic characteristics of the ovum (7).

♦ Individuals undergoing coronary procedures or contrast-dye imaging studies are sometimes at risk for renal damage. Reports suggest NAC may be efficacious in reducing these events (8,9), but evidence is conflicting (10). This application for NAC is a medical intervention that must be under the guidance of a physician.

Food Sources

NAC is a form of cysteine found in animal proteins (eggs, dairy, meat, poultry, fish) and some vegetable proteins (eg, soybeans) (11).

Food	Cysteine, mg/serving
Chicken, roasted, skinless and boneless (½ breast)	318.2
Soybeans, green (1 cup)	203.4
Beef, lean (3 oz)	190.4
Egg (1 large)	144.5
Peanut butter (2 Tbsp)	116.8
Milk, whole (1 cup)	73.2
Cheese, cheddar (1½ oz)	53.2

Source: Data are from reference 12.

Dosage Information/Bioavailability

There is no RDA for NAC. NAC is sold in tablets providing doses of 200 to 600 mg. Most manufacturers suggest taking 1,200 to 2,400 mg/day with food.

Relevant Research

NAC and Influenza Virus and Respiratory Illness

- Several European studies since 1980 have reported that prophylactic treatment with NAC (600 mg/day) may reduce the duration—and in some trials, the incidence—of chronic bronchitis (13–18).

- A meta-analysis of NAC used in bronchopulmonary disease was conducted in studies from 1980 through 1995. Of 21 trials reviewed, eight double-blind, placebo-controlled studies lasting from 2 to 6 months were selected for analysis. NAC dosages varied: 400 mg (one study), 600 mg (five studies), 1,200 mg (one study), and 600 mg three times per week (one study). The primary endpoint was the incidence of acute exacerbations of disease in seven of eight trials and clinical assessment in the other. The results showed that NAC therapy had a significant effect compared with a placebo. The authors concluded that oral NAC may prevent acute exacerbations of chronic bronchitis and thus may decrease morbidity and health care costs (19).

- In a randomized, double-blind multicenter study in Italy, 262 subjects (most older than 65 years, 62% with nonrespiratory chronic degenerative diseases such as cardiovascular disease, arthritis, and diabetes) were randomly assigned to receive effervescent tablets of 1,200 mg NAC divided into two doses or a placebo daily for 6 months. Subjects' self-reported signs and symptoms of influenza-like episodes were reviewed at monthly intervals by clinicians in addition to a complete medical examination. The subjects taking NAC supplements experienced a statistically significant decrease in influenza-like episodes, severity of condition, and length of time confined to bed as compared with the placebo group. Although NAC supplementation did not prevent subclinical influenza infection as assessed by antibody response to the A/H_1N_1 Singapore 6/86 virus, only 25% of those who contracted the virus in the NAC group developed a symptomatic form vs 79% in the placebo group; the difference between treatments was significant (4).

NAC and HIV

◆ Because individuals with AIDS typically have decreased levels of glutathione in their lymphocytes and plasma, some researchers have suggested that NAC may benefit people with AIDS by increasing intracellular levels of glutathione, thereby potentially suppressing HIV replication (20). Although clinical studies have shown that low GSH levels are associated with poor survival in subjects with HIV (20), the effectiveness of NAC supplementation has not been confirmed.

◆ Daily NAC supplementation (3,200 to 8,000 mg) during an 8-week randomized, double-blind, placebo-controlled trial restored blood GSH levels in subjects with CD4 counts less than 200 compared with a placebo. After this phase, the majority of subjects in both arms of the study were offered NAC for a 6-month open-label phase. Survival was evaluated 2 years after initiation of NAC. During the 2-year period, NAC-supplemented subjects (n = 25) with a CD4 count less than 200 survived significantly longer than a comparable group of non-NAC supplemented subjects (n = 19). Despite this finding, the authors emphasized that "no conclusion can be drawn until NAC is administered in a properly controlled prospective clinical trial with survival as a primary endpoint" (20).

◆ In a double blind, placebo-controlled trial, 81 individuals with HIV (low GSH, CD4 < 500, and no opportunistic infections) were randomly assigned to receive 8,000 mg NAC in effervescent tablets dissolved in water each day for 8 weeks. The trial was followed by an optional open-label drug for up to 24 weeks. Blood GSH levels and CD4 GSH levels significantly increased in NAC-supplemented subjects to normal levels. Baseline GSH levels in the placebo group did not change during the study. NAC was well tolerated during the 8-month study. The authors suggested that because NAC appeared to increase protection against oxidative stress and enhanced the immune system, NAC therapy could be valuable in other conditions of GSH deficiency or oxidative stress such as rheumatoid arthritis, Parkinson's disease, hepatitis, liver cirrhosis, septic shock, and diabetes. In addition, they advised individuals with HIV to avoid drugs and activities that further deplete GSH levels, such as ultraviolet light, alcohol, and acetaminophen (21).

◆ In a double-blind, placebo-controlled trial, 40 individuals with HIV on antiretroviral therapy and 29 individuals with HIV not on antiretroviral drugs were randomly assigned to receive NAC (dose individually adjusted dependent on plasma glutamine levels) or a placebo daily for 7 months. Immunological parameters (natural killer cell, CD4 functions and the viral load) were the main outcome measures.

NAC-supplemented subjects had a significant increase in immunological functions and plasma albumin concentrations. NAC had an inconsistent effect on the viral load, which, the authors noted, requires further study. The authors hypothesized that the impairment of immune function in subjects with HIV results at least partly from cysteine deficiency, which can be replenished by NAC supplementation (22).

♦ In a double-blind, placebo-controlled trial, 45 individuals with HIV not on retroviral drugs were randomly assigned to receive 400 mg NAC twice daily or a placebo for 4 months. Before the study, subjects had low plasma cysteine levels, high free-radical activity in neutrophils, and increased tumor necrosis factor-α (TNF-α) levels. After treatment, plasma cysteine levels increased to normal and the decline of the CD4+ lymphocyte count apparent prior to the study was less severe after NAC supplementation compared with placebo. TNF-α levels also decreased significantly in the NAC group. NAC had no effect on free-radical production by neutrophils (23).

♦ In a double-blind, controlled study, 238 subjects with HIV were randomly assigned to receive 3 g NAC or no treatment 1 hour before each dose of the antibiotic trimethoprim-sulfamethoxazole (TMP-SMX) twice daily. TMP-SMX was initiated as primary *Pneumocystis carinii* pneumonia prophylaxis. It was hypothesized that adverse reactions to TMP-SMX observed in individuals with HIV may be due to systemic glutathione deficiency that may be ameliorated by NAC supplementation. Within 2 months, 45 subjects had to discontinue TMP-SMX because of fever, rash, or pruritis. NAC had no effect on hypersensitivity reaction to the antibiotic (24).

NAC and Exercise

♦ In a double-blind, placebo-controlled study, 14 oarsmen were randomly assigned to receive 6 g NAC or a placebo daily for 3 days before a 6-minute "all-out" ergometer rowing trial. NAC did not attenuate the reduction in lymphocyte proliferation and natural killer cell activity associated with intense exercise, nor did it affect levels of lymphocyte subsets (CD4+, CD8+, CD16+, or CD19+ cells) as compared with the placebo (25).

♦ Other research has reported that NAC may reduce oxidative stress and muscle fatigue. However, one study was uncontrolled (26) and the other study was not applicable to supplementation because NAC was administered intravenously during exercise (27).

NAC and Polycystic Ovary Syndrome

♦ Use of NAC to enhance pregnancy rates and increase ovulatory cycles in women with polycystic ovary syndrome (PCOS) is gaining attention (28).

♦ In a placebo-controlled, double-blind study, 150 women with PCOS were randomly assigned to receive clomophene citrate plus adjuvant NAC (1,200 mg) or placebo daily for 5 days starting on day 3 of the ovulatory cycle. A marked 48% increase in ovulation rate and a 21.3% increase in pregnancy were demonstrated with NAC as compared with placebo (7). This study suggests strong clinical efficacy, but the findings need to be replicated before clinical recommendations can be made.

References

1. Smilkstein MJ, Gary MD, Knapp MS, et al. Efficacy of oral N-acetylcysteine in the treatment of acetaminophen over-dose. *J Med.* 1988;24:1557–1562.
2. Moldeus P, Cotgreave IA, Berggren M. Lung protection by thiol-containing antioxidant: N-acetylcysteine. *Respiration.* 1986;50(Suppl 1):S31-S42.
3. Droge W, Gross A, Hack V, et al. Role of cysteine and glutathione in HIV infection and cancer cachexia: therapeutic intervention with N-acetylcysteine. *Adv Pharmacol.* 1997;38:581–600.
4. De Flora S, Grassi C, Carati L. Attenuation of influenza-like symptomatology and improvement of cell-mediated immunity with long-term N-acetylcysteine treatment. *Eur Respir J.* 1997;10:1535–1541.
5. Flanagan RJ, Meredith TJ. Use of N-acetylcysteine in clinical toxicology. *Am J Med.* 1991;91(3C):S131-S139.
6. Anfossi G, Russo I, Massucco P, et al. N-acetyl-L-cysteine exerts direct anti-aggregating effect on human platelets. *Eur J Clin Invest.* 2001;31:452–461.
7. Rizk AY, Bedaiwy MA, Al-Inany HG. N-acetyl-cysteine is a novel adjuvant to clomiphene citrate in clomiphene citrate-resistant patients with polycystic ovary syndrome. *Fertil Steril.* 2005;83:367–370.
8. Tepel M, van der Giet M, Statz M, et al. The antioxidant acetylcysteine reduces cardiovascular events in patients with end-stage renal failure: a randomized, controlled trial. *Circulation.* 2003;107:992–995.
9. Shyu KG, Cheng JJ, Kuan P. Acetylcysteine protects against acute renal damage in patients with abnormal renal function undergoing a coronary procedure. *J Am Coll Cardiol.* 2002;40:1383–1388.
10. Oldemeyer JB, Biddle WP, Wurdeman RL, et al. Acetylcysteine in the prevention of contrast-induced nephropathy after coronary angiography. *Am Heart J.* 2003;146:E23
11. Linder MC, ed. *Nutritional Biochemistry and Metabolism.* 2nd ed. Norwalk, Conn: Appleton & Lange; 1991.
12. Stipanuk MH. Homocysteine, cysteine, and taurine. In: Shils ME, Olson JA, Shike M, Ross AC, eds. *Modern Nutrition in Health and Disease.* 9th ed. Philadelphia, Pa: Lea & Febiger; 1999:543–559.
13. Multicenter Study Group. Long-term acetylcysteine in chronic bronchitis: a double-blind, controlled study. *Eur J Respir Dis.* 1980;61:93–108.
14. Boman G, Backer U, Larsson S, et al. Oral acetylcysteine reduces exacerbation rate in chronic bronchitis: a report of a trial organized by the Swedish Society for Pulmonary Diseases. *Eur J Respir Dis.* 1983;64:405–415.
15. Rasmussen JB, Glennow G. Reduction in days of illness after long-term treatment with N-acetylcysteine controlled release tablets in patients with chronic bronchitis. *Eur J Respir Dis.* 1988;1:351–355.
16. British Thoracic Society Research Committee. Oral N-acetylcysteine and exacerbation rate in patients with chronic bronchitis and severe airways obstruction. *Thorax.* 1985;40:832–835.
17. Parr DG, Huitson A. Oral N-acetylcysteine in chronic bronchitis. *Br J Dis Chest.* 1987;81:341–348.

18. Riise BT, Larsson S, Larsson P, et al. The intrabronchial microbial flora in chronic bronchitis patients: a target for N-acetylcysteine therapy? *Eur Respir J*. 1994;7:94–101.
19. Grandjean EM, Berthet P, Ruffman R, et al. Efficacy of oral long-term N-acetylcysteine in chronic bronchopulmonary disease: a meta-analysis of published double-blind, placebo-controlled clinical trials. *Clin Ther*. 2000;22:209–221.
20. Herzenberg LA, De Rosa SC, Dubs JG, et al. Glutathione deficiency is associated with impaired survival in HIV disease. *Proc Natl Acad Sci USA*. 1997;94:1967–1972.
21. De Rosa SC, Zaretsky MD, Dubs JG, et al. N-acetylcysteine replenishes glutathione in HIV infection. *Eur J Clin Invest*. 2000;30:915–929.
22. Breitkreutz R, Pittack N, Nebe CT, et al. Improvement of immune functions in HIV infection by sulfur supplementation: two randomized trials. *J Mol Med*. 2000;78:55–62.
23. Akerlund B, Jarstrand C, Lindeke B, et al. Effect of N-acetylcysteine (NAC) treatment on HIV-1 infection: a double-blind placebo-controlled trial. *Eur J Clin Pharmacol*. 1996;50:457–461.
24. Walmsley SL, Khorasheh S, Singer J, et al. A randomized trial of N-acetylcysteine for prevention of trimethorprim-sulfamethoaxazole hypersensitivity reactions in *Pneumocystis carinii* pneumonia prophylaxis (CTN 057). Canadian HIV Trials Network 057 Study Group. *J Acquir Immune Defic Syndr Hum Retrovirol*. 1998;19:498–505.
25. Nielsen HB, Secher NH, Kappel M, et al. N-acetylcysteine does not affect the lymphocyte proliferation and natural killer cell activity responses to exercise. *Am J Physiol*. 1998;275:R1227-R1231.
26. Sen CK, Rankinen T, Vaisanen S, et al. Oxidative stress after human exercise: effect of N-acetylcysteine supplementation. *J Appl Physiol*. 1994;76:2570–2577.
27. Reid MB, Stokic DS, Koch SM, et al. N-acetylcysteine inhibits muscle fatigue in humans. *J Clin Invest*. 1994;94:2468–2474.
28. Kilic-Okman T, Kucuk M. N-acetyl-cysteine treatment for polycystic ovary syndrome. *Int J Gyn Obest*. 2004;85:296–297.

Niacin. *See* Vitamin B-3 (Niacin).

Noni Juice

Noni juice is a liquid supplement made from the fruit of the noni plant *(Morinda citrifolia)* found in Polynesia, China, and India. The juice is available through local noni distributors who are part of a multilevel marketing firm. Noni juice advertisements and marketing literature feature endorsements by physicians and testimonials that the juice can heal a variety of health conditions. Noni is a relatively new supplement, only available in the United States since 1996.

Media and Marketing Claims	Efficacy
Prevents cancer	NR
Improves immunity	NR
Reduces blood pressure	NR
Improves cholesterol levels	NR
Acts as a natural pain reliever	NR

Safety

◆ Noni juice contains approximately the same amount of potassium as orange juice. There is one report of a man with renal insufficiency who presented with hyperkalemia after self-medicating with noni juice (1).

◆ Noni juice may reduce the clinical efficacy of warfarin (2).

◆ The high potassium content of noni juice could cause hyperkalemia in individuals with kidney disease.

Drug/Supplement Interactions

No reported adverse interactions

Key Points

◆ Experimental and animal studies suggest that differential compounds found in the noni fruit may exert some anticancer activity. For example, noni fruit has been shown to reduce angiogenesis in a breast cancer cell line model (3) and to arrest cancer cell growth in a mouse model of lung tumorogenesis. However, there is no research in humans at this time to substantiate these results, with the exception of published case reports (4).

◆ There are currently no published clinical trials available to support the use of noni juice to treat or prevent any health condition.

Food Sources

The noni fruit is the only source of noni juice.

Dosage Information/Bioavailability

Noni juice is sold in bottles prepared from ripened Tahitian noni fruit. The juice is extracted from the mashed fruit and bottled for use. A typical serving is 8 ounces. Not all noni juices are pasteurized. There are no scientific data on the purported active ingredients; thus, bioavailability is not known.

Relevant Research

♦ A review of the traditional use of *Morinda citrifolia* (noni) provides anecdotal evidence of the potential health benefits of noni from natural medicinal experience, including its role in immunity, cancer, blood pressure control, and pain control (5).

♦ In an animal study, a polysaccharide isolated from noni juice was found to enhance the survival of mice having Lewis lung cancer. Noni juice extract stimulated the release of tumor necrosis factor-alpha, interleukin-1beta (IL-1beta), IL-10, IL-12 p70, interferon-gamma (IFN-gamma), and nitric oxide, but had no effect on IL-2 and suppressed IL-4 release. The polysaccharide also improved survival time when combined with suboptimal doses of standard chemotherapeutic drugs (6).

References

1. Mueller BA, Scott MK, Sowinski KM, et al. Noni juice (*Morinda citrifolia*): a hidden potential for hyperkalemia? *Am J Kidney Dis.* 2000;35:330–332.
2. Carr ME, Klotz J, Bergeron M. Coumadin resistance and the vitamin supplement "noni." *Am J Hematol.* 2004;77:103.
3. Hornick CA, Myers A, Sadowska-Krowicka H, et al. Inhibition of angiogenic initiation and disruption of newly established human vascular networks by juice from Morinda citrifolia (noni). *Angiogenesis.* 2003;6:143–149.
4. Wong DK. Are immune responses pivotal to cancer patient's long term survival? Two clinical case-study reports on the effects of Morinda citrifolia (noni). *Hawaii Med J.* 2004;63:182–184.
5. Wang MY, West BJ, Jensen CJ, et al. Morinda citrifolia (noni): a literature review and recent advances in noni research. *Acta Pharmacol Sin.* 2002;23:1127–1141.
6. Hirazumi A, Furusawa E. An immunomodulatory polysaccharide-rich substance from the fruit juice of Morinda citrifolia (noni) with antitumor activity. *Phytother Res.* 1999;13:380–387.

Pancreatin

The pancreas secretes enzymes (pancreatin) into the gastrointestinal tract to aid digestion. Pancreatin contains three classes of enzymes: (*a*) amylases, which hydrolyze starch molecules into sugars; (*b*) lipases, which hydrolyze fat molecules (insufficient lipase causes steatorrhea); and (*c*) proteases (chymotrypsin, trypsin, and carboxypeptidase), which digest protein into amino acids. Oral supplementation of pancreatin is an established medical treatment for such diseases as chronic pancreatitis, cystic fibrosis, and pancreatic cancer.

Less frequently, pancreatic enzymes have been prescribed for celiac disease, inflammatory bowel disease, primary biliary cirrhosis, total gastrectomy, and dyspepsia (1).

Media and Marketing Claims	Efficacy
Helps improve digestion in pancreatic enzyme deficiency*	↑
Helps improve digestion in people with normal enzyme activity	NR
Enhances immunity	NR
Helps reduce the risk of pancreatic cancer	NR
Medical use for cystic fibrosis, pancreatitis.	

Safety

- The effects of long-term use of exogenous enzymes by healthy subjects is unknown, but some theorize that this may permanently reduce the ability of the digestive system to secrete endogenous enzymes. In one study, pancreatic enzymes acutely administered to healthy subjects reduced postprandial endogenous pancreatic enzyme secretion; however, there were no reported acute adverse effects on bile acid secretion, gastroduodenal motility, or gastrointestinal hormone release (2).

- People with diabetes are at risk of hypoglycemia when using pancreatin and a case of diabetic ketoacidosis has been reported (3).

- Individuals with hypersensitivity to pork may react unfavorably to pancreatic extracts of porcine origin (4).

- Pancreatic extracts form insoluble complexes with folic acid, which may impair folate absorption (4).

- Dietary fiber may interfere with the activity of enzymes in vitro and in vivo (5).

- Some products have reportedly been contaminated with *Salmonella*.

- Use of pancreatic enzymes for a medical diagnosis such as cystic fibrosis or pancreatitis should be medically supervised. Guidelines for therapeutic uses are available (6,7).

Drug/Supplement Interactions

- May decrease effectiveness of the diabetes medication acarbose (Precose).
- Can decrease absorption of folic acid supplements.

Key Points

- Pancreatic enzymes are effective in the treatment of documented gastrointestinal disorders if there is clinical evidence of pancreatic insufficiency (chronic pancreatitis).

- Pancreatic function may be impaired in nonpancreatic digestive disorders including inflammatory bowel disease, celiac disease, malabsorption conditions, hepatobiliary disease, gastrectomy, and dyspepsia. The few studies on enzyme treatment for "nonpancreatic" disorders suggest that short-term pancreatin administration does not seem to benefit subjects with dyspepsia but may have some application in young children with celiac disease. Further, controlled trials are needed to elucidate the effects and determine dosage of supplemental enzymes in subjects with these intestinal disorders.

- At the current time, the possibility that the digestion process is enhanced by exogenous enzyme supplementation in healthy subjects has not been studied. Controlled clinical research is needed to determine whether supplemental enzymes enhance digestion in healthy individuals and whether their long-term use is safe.

- There is little research available to evaluate the marketing claim that exogenous pancreatic enzymes improve immunity.

- Preliminary evidence from in vitro studies showed that pancreatin in combination with other proteolytic enzymes is cytotoxic to tumor cells and in mouse models of pancreatic cancer; however, no controlled clinical trials have tested this in humans. (*See also* Bromelain.)

Food Sources

None. Pancreatic enzymes from meat products are destroyed by cooking. Pancreatic enzymes are produced endogenously.

Dosage Information/Bioavailability

Pancreatic enzymes derived from the bovine and porcine pancreas are available in tablets and capsules. The United States Pharmacopoeia (USP) has set standards for the level of activity of pancreatin. Each milligram must have a minimum of 25 USP units of amylase, 2 USP units of lipase, and 25 USP units of protease activity. One USP standard is referred to as pancreatin 1 × (500 mg), which provides 12,500 USP units amylase activity, 1,000 USP units of lipase activity, and 12,500 USP units of protease activity. Many commercial products are sold as four times USP standard, or pancreatin 4 × USP (50,000 USP units amylase activity, 4,000 USP units lipase activity, and 50,000 USP units protease) equivalent to 2,000 mg. Pancreatin is also available as 10 × USP or 5,000 mg.

To prevent inactivation of enzymes by gastric acid, many preparations are enteric-coated. The activity of individual preparations depends on a variety of factors, including pH of gastrointestinal secretions, the intestinal location where the enteric-coated enzyme disintegrates (gastric acid destroys enzymes), and whether the enzyme is consumed with food (4,8). In patients with pancreatic insufficiency, pancreatin is taken with meals to enhance effectiveness, but should not be taken with acidic foods that reduce the pH and reduce bioavailability.

There is some concern that among healthy adults, supplementation with pancreatic enzymes (proteases, lipases, and amylases) can suppress endogenous production in a dose-dependent manner due to the feedback mechanism for exocrine pancreatic secretion (9).

Relevant Research

Pancreatin and Gastrointestinal Disorders

◆ In a single-blind, placebo-controlled, crossover design study, 37 individuals with non-ulcer dyspepsia took a placebo or 30,000 mg pancreatin (units not specified) divided into three doses daily for 24 days each. Before the study, all subjects underwent endoscopy, which revealed no significant clinical differences between groups. Subjects recorded their global dyspeptic complaints on a visual analogue scale each day of the trial. There were no differences in gastrointestinal symptoms (abdominal pain, nausea, heartburn, stool abnormalities, early satiety) between treatments (10).

◆ In a double-blind, placebo-controlled study, 40 children (mean age 14.5 months) diagnosed with celiac disease were randomly assigned to receive the contents of two capsules of pancreatic enzymes with every meal (1 capsule = 5,000 IU lipase, 2,900 IU amylase, 330 IU protease) or a placebo for 60 days. On the day of diagnosis, day 30, and day 60 after beginning isocaloric gluten-free diets, a series of anthropometric measurements were taken. After 30 days, subjects in the pancreatin group had significantly greater weight gain and weight-for-age increase. Increases in weight-for-height, height Z score ([observed height – mean height for sex and age]/standard deviation for sex and age), arm circumference, and subscapular and triceps skinfold measurements were greater in the pancreatin group than the placebo group, but the differences were not significant. After 60 days, there were no differences between groups. The authors concluded that pancreatic enzyme therapy seemed to improve anthropometric measurements in young children with celiac disease in the first 30 days after diagnosis, with apparent attenuation of the benefits thereafter (11).

Pancreatin and Immunity

◆ A review article hypothesized the potential beneficial role of pancreatic enzymes in immune complex diseases (AIDS, rheumatoid arthritis, multiple sclerosis, Crohn's disease, ulcerative colitis). The authors suggested that enzyme supplementation removes tissue-bound immune complexes, thereby enhancing immune function (increased macrophage and natural killer cell activity), which may be beneficial to individuals with HIV (12). However, no controlled clinical trials have adequately tested this hypothesis.

◆ In a descriptive study of IgE levels (proinflammatory cytokine) in 86 individuals with chronic pancreatitis (73 men and 13 women) vs 52 healthy control subjects, serum IgE was significantly higher in subjects with chronic pancreatitis and particularly in those with high alcohol intake (> 25 g/day). Alcohol abstinence and pancreatic enzymes were associated with lower IgE levels, indicating a role in reducing the inflammatory process in this population (13).

♦ *See* Bromelain for additional studies of combination enzyme supplements that include pancreatin.

Pancreatin and Pancreatic Cancer

♦ In a study of mice induced with pancreatic cancer, mice were fed standard diet or standard diet plus pancreatic enzymes in drinking water. Mice receiving pancreatic enzymes showed prolonged survival as well as reduced tumor size. The mechanism for enhanced survival was thought to be delayed malnutrition because the pancreatic enzyme intake was also associated with reduced steatorrhea, improved biliary function, and improved glucose control, whereas markers of tumor-specific effects such as apoptosis and growth factors were not different across treatment groups (14).

♦ A double-blind study of the effect of pancreatic enzymes on body weight in individuals with unresectable pancreatic cancer (n = 21) randomly assigned subjects to receive either high-dose pancreatic enzymes or placebo daily for 8 weeks. Pancreatic enzyme replacement was associated with improved body weight (gain of 1.2% vs loss of 3.7% for placebo), which could be attributed to increased energy intake as reported on subject food records (15). In addition, energy intake seemed to be modulated by fat tolerance, with subjects receiving enteric-coated pancreatic enzymes demonstrating improved fat absorption (based on questionnaire of bowel function/symptoms). Studies in larger numbers of subjects and for longer duration are warranted.

References

1. Gullo L. Indication for pancreatic enzyme treatment in non-pancreatic digestive diseases. *Digestion.* 1993;54(Suppl 2):43–47.
2. Dominguez-Munoz JE, Birckelbach U, Glasbrenner B, et al. Effect of oral pancreatic enzyme administration on digestive function in healthy subjects: comparison between two enzyme preparations. *Ailment Pharmacol Ther.* 1997;11:403–408.
3. O'Keefe SJ, Cariem AK, Levy M. The exacerbation of pancreatic endocrine dysfunction by potent pancreatic exocrine supplements in patients with chronic pancreatitis. *J Clin Gastroenterol.* 2001;32:319–323.
4. Lankisch PG. Enzyme treatment of exocrine pancreatic insufficiency in chronic pancreatitis. *Digestion.* 1993;54(Suppl 2):21–29.
5. Leng-Peschlow E. Interference of dietary fibres with gastrointestinal enzymes in vitro. *Digestion.* 1989;44:200–210.
6. Schibli S, Durie PR, Tullis ED. Proper usage of pancreatic enzymes. *Curr Opin Pulm Med.* 2002;8:542–546.
7. Layer P, Keller J. Lipase supplementation therapy: standards, alternatives, and perspectives. *Pancreas.* 2003;26:1–7.
8. Guarner L, Rodriguez R, Guarner F, et al. Fate of oral enzymes in pancreatic insufficiency. *Gut.* 1993;34:708–709.
9. Walkowiak J, Witmanowski H, Strzykala K, et al. Inhibitions of endogenous pancreatic enzyme secretion by oral pancreatic enzyme treatment. *Eur J Clin Invest.* 2003;33:65–69.

10. Kleveland PM, Johannessen T, Kristensen P, et al. Effect of pancreatic enzymes in non-ulcer dyspepsia. A pilot study. *Scand J Gastroenterol*. 1990;25:298–301.
11. Carroccio A, Iacono G, Montalto G, et al. Pancreatic enzyme therapy in childhood celiac disease. *Dig Dis Sci*. 1995;40:2555–2560.
12. Stauder G, Ransberger K, Steichhan P, et al. The use of hydrolytic enzymes as adjuvant therapy in AIDS/ARC/LAS patients. *Biomed Pharmacother*. 1988;42:31–34.
13. Raithel M, Dormann H, Harsch IA, et al. Immunoglobulin E production in chronic pancreatitis. *Eur J Gastroenterol Hepatol*. 2003;15:801–807.
14. Saruck M, Standop S, Standop J, et al. Pancreatic enzyme extract improves survival in murine pancreatic cancer. *Pancreas*. 2004;28:401–412.
15. Bruno MJ, Haverkort EB, Tijssen GP, et al. Placebo controlled trial of enteric coated pancreatin microsphere treatment in patients with unresectable cancer of the pancreatic head region. *Gut*. 1998;42:92–96.

Pantothenic Acid

Pantothenic acid (pantethine) is an essential water-soluble B vitamin (B-5). It is physiologically active as part of two coenzymes: acetyl coenzyme A (CoA) and acyl carrier protein. Pantothenic acid functions in the oxidation of fatty acids and carbohydrates for energy production and the synthesis of fatty acids, ketones, cholesterol, phospholipids, steroid hormones, and amino acids. Because pantothenic acid is widely distributed in foods, deficiency is extremely rare. Depletion studies have shown that deficiency is associated with fatigue and depression in humans and dysfunction in adrenal cortex, nervous system, and respiratory function in animals (1).

Media and Marketing Claims*	Efficacy
Reduces cholesterol	NR
Improves exercise performance	NR
Reduces pain and other symptoms of arthritis	NR
Reduces stress	NR

Dozens of other marketing claims have been made for pantothenic acid; there is no evidence to support most of these claims.

Safety

- High doses of calcium pantothenate are relatively nontoxic in rats, dogs, rabbits, and humans. The lethal dose (LD_{50}) for mice was 10 g/kg body weight, which led to death from respiratory failure (1).
- No reported serious adverse effects.
- A Tolerable Upper Intake Level (UL) has not been defined; dosages up to 10 g/day seem to be safe.

Drug/Supplement Interactions

No reported adverse interactions

Key Points

* There is a lack of well-controlled studies testing the effects of pantothenic acid in cholesterol reduction. More research is needed to verify the cholesterol-lowering claims, which are based on poorly controlled studies.

* The limited research on pantothenic acid/pantethine has not found an ergogenic benefit from supplementation during exercise.

* Much more research is needed to determine the potential role of pantothenic acid supplements in treating rheumatoid or osteoarthritis.

* Although pantothenic acid has been referred to as the "anti-stress" vitamin by some supplement marketers because of its central role in adrenal cortex function and cellular metabolism, there is currently no evidence from controlled studies to suggest that pantothenic acid reduces feelings of stress or anxiety.

Food Sources

Pantothenic is found in most plant and animal foods. Good sources are liver, egg yolk, fresh vegetables, legumes, yeast, and whole grains. The average American diet provides approximately 5.8 mg pantothenic acid daily. Pantothenic acid is stable at a neutral pH. It has been estimated that 15% to 20% of pantothenic acid in raw meat is destroyed by cooking and that 37% to 78% of the vitamin is lost in vegetables during processing (1).

Food	Pantothenic Acid, mg/serving
Mushrooms, cooked (½ cup)	1.68
Potato, baked with skin	1.12
Chicken breast (3.5 oz)	0.92
Egg (1)	0.70
Catfish (3 oz)	0.65
Lentils (½ cup)	0.63
Beef, broiled, lean ground (3.5 oz)	0.38
Rice, brown (½ cup)	0.28

Source: Data are from reference 2.

Dosage Information/Bioavailability

There is no RDA for pantothenic acid; however, the adequate intake (AI) is set at 5 mg/day for adults (3). Pantothenic acid is available in multivitamin supplements and single preparations in doses ranging from 5 to 500 mg in the form of calcium pantothenate, calcium panthenol, sodium pantothenate, or sodium panthenol. Pantethine, a metabolite of pan-tothenic acid used in several studies, is also available in supplements. Information on pan-tothenic acid bioavailability in humans is limited (4). However, in one controlled study, the bioavailability of dietary pantothenate (5.8 mg/day) ranged from 40% to 61% in healthy men (5).

Relevant Research

Pantothenic Acid/Pantethine and Cholesterol

♦ In a double-blind, placebo-controlled crossover study, 29 subjects (11 with type IIB hyperlipidemia, 15 with type IV hyperlipidemia, and 3 with isolated low HDL cholesterol levels) were randomly assigned to receive 900 mg pantethine or a placebo daily for 8 weeks each. In subjects with type IIB hyperlipidemia, pantethine signifi-cantly reduced plasma total and LDL cholesterol. In subjects with type IV hyperlipi-demia, pantethine had a variable effect on LDL levels. In subjects with type IIB or type IV hyperlipidemia, plasma triglyceride levels decreased when pantethine was given as the first treatment, but the reduction was less when the regimen was pre-ceded by the placebo. There was no change in HDL cholesterol in subjects with type IV hyperlipidemia or low HDL cholesterol (6).

Pantothenic Acid/Pantethine and Exercise Performance

♦ In a double-blind, placebo-controlled study, six highly trained cyclists were ran-domly assigned to receive 1.8 g of a pantethine/pantothenic acid compound plus 1 g allithiamin (an efficiently absorbed thiamin derivative) or a placebo for 7 days before a 50-km ride on a cycle ergometer that was followed by a 2,000-meter time trial. This protocol was completed on two separate occasions. There were no significant differ-ences in measures of heart rate, respiratory gas exchange, ratings of perceived exer-tion, or blood lactate, glucose, and free fatty acids between groups. There were also no differences in time to complete the 2,000-meter trial. The authors concluded that supplementation with allithiamin and pantethine did not alter exercise metabolism or exercise performance (7).

♦ In a double-blind, placebo-controlled study, 18 highly trained distance runners were given 1 g pantothenic acid or a placebo daily for 2 weeks. Subjects were instructed not to change their diets or training schedules. At the start and end of the study, each subject completed two treadmill runs to exhaustion separated by 2 weeks. There were no significant differences between groups in run time, pulse rate, or blood cor-tisol or blood glucose levels (8).

Pantothenic Acid and Arthritis

♦ In a double-blind, placebo-controlled trial, 94 individuals with arthritis (27 with rheumatoid arthritis) were randomly assigned to receive increasing doses of calcium pantothenate (500 mg for 2 days, 1,000 mg for the next 3 days, 1,500 mg for the next

4 days, and 2,000 mg for the remaining days in the study) or a placebo daily for 2 months. Subjects were permitted to take only paracetamol for pain. There were no significant reductions in either group in the duration of morning stiffness or disability. Both groups experienced significant relief of pain, although neither resulted in any reduction of paracetamol. Physician assessment did not differ between treatment groups. When subjects with rheumatoid arthritis were analyzed separately, the group receiving pantothenate showed significant reductions in morning stiffness, disability, and pain, but not paracetamol use. The placebo group had no changes. The authors did not speculate why pantothenate seemed to benefit patients with rheumatoid arthritis but not subjects with osteoarthritis (9).

References

1. Plesofsky-Vig N. Pantothenic acid. In: Shils ME, Olson JA, Shike M, et al, eds. *Modern Nutrition in Health and Disease.* 9th ed. Philadelphia, Pa: Lea & Febiger; 1999:423–432.
2. Pennington JA. *Bowes and Church's Food Values of Portions Commonly Used.* 17th ed. Philadelphia, Pa: Lippincott; 1998.
3. Institute of Medicine. *Dietary Reference Intakes for Thiamin, Riboflavin, Niacin, Vitamin B-6, Folate, Vitamin B-12, Pantothenic Acid, Biotin, and Choline.* Washington, DC: National Academy Press; 1998.
4. van den Berg H. Bioavailability of pantothenic acid. *Eur J Clin Nutr.* 1997;51(Suppl 2): S62-S63.
5. Tarr JB, Tamura T, Stokstad EL. Availability of vitamin B6 and pantothenate in an average American diet in man. *Am J Clin Nutr.* 1981;34:1328–1337.
6. Gaddi A, Descovich GC, Noseda G, et al. Controlled evaluation of pantethine, a natural hypolipemic compound, in patients with different forms of hyperlipidemia. *Atherosclerosis.* 1984;50:73–83.
7. Webster MJ. Physiological and performance responses to supplementation with thiamin and pantothenic acid derivatives. *Eur J Appl Physiol.* 1998;77:486–491.
8. Nice C, Reeves AG, Brinck-Johnsen T, et al. The effects of pantothenic acid on human exercise capacity. *J Sports Med Phys Fitness.* 1984;24:26–29.
9. General Practitioner Research Group. Calcium pantothenate in arthritic conditions. A report from the General Practitioner Research Group. *Practitioner.* 1980;224:208–211.

Pau d'arco

Pau d'arco is an herb that comes from the inner bark of the *Tabebuia avellanedae* tree. Native to Brazil but also grown in other South American and Central American countries, the tree is an evergreen that can grow up to 125 feet tall. Because of the increasing demand for pau d'arco, the trees are at risk of becoming extinct. Pau d'arco is commonly used in South American countries and by South American tribes to treat cancer, diabetes, infections, and asthma. However, there are no scientific data to support the effectiveness of pau d'arco.

Media and Marketing Claims	Efficacy
Kills cancer cells	NR
Treat diabetes	NR
Improves immunity	NR
Reduce asthmatic symptoms	NR

Safety

* There have been no studies conducted on the safety and efficacy of pau d'arco at standard doses (between 1 and 4 g pau d'arco per day).

* Serious side effects, including severe nausea, vomiting, dizziness, anemia, and bleeding, have been shown to occur with high doses of pau d'arco (estimated at 1.5 lapachol, the primary constituent in pau d'arco) (1). Long-term use (> 7 days) has also been associated with the onset of these side effects as well.

Drug/Supplement Interaction

Pau d'arco prolongs blood clotting time. Taking it with anticoagulant/antiplatelet drugs may increase risk of bleeding.

Key Points

* Pau d'arco is sold in many health-food stores as a "cure" for cancer. There are no scientific data to support this claim.

* NIH tested pau d'arco in the early 1970s for its effectiveness in treating cancer. Investigators found that at very high (1.5 g lapachol) doses pau d'arco could kill cancer cells in vitro, but the side effects were too severe to continue with further studies (1).

* No data are available to assess the use of pau d'arco in diabetes, immunity, or asthma.

Food Sources

None

Dosage Information/Bioavailability

Pau d'arco is available as a tincture, softgel, ointment, powder, tablet, liquid, tea, or capsule. Typical usage is 1,000 mg three times per day. Pau d'arco can also be consumed as a tea using 1 teaspoon dried herb per 1 cup boiling water steeped for 5 to 15 minutes (2).

Relevant Research

Due to extreme side effects associated with pau d'arco in clinical trials conducted more than 30 years ago, very little notable research is being done on this supplement (1). In fact, a search of common medical literature databases suggests that no studies exist. However, in vitro research using lapachol has suggested that this compound may have antimetastatic activity in vitro (3).

References

1. Block JB, Serpick AA, Miller W, et al. Early clinical studies with lapachol (NSC-11905). *Cancer Chemother Rep 2*. 1974;4:27–28.
2. Pau d'arco. Available at: www.healthandage.com. Accessed May 31, 2005.
3. Balassiano IT, De Paulo SA, Henriques SN, et al. Demonstration of the lapachol as a potential drug for reducing cancer metastasis. *Oncol Rep*. 2005;13:329–333.

Phosphatidylserine

Phosphatidylserine (PS) is a naturally occurring phospholipid in the brain cortex. PS is involved in neuronal membrane function and may influence membrane-mediated biological activities and receptor functions. Research suggests that PS causes biochemical brain changes by acting on neurotransmitter systems (acetylcholine, norepinephrine, serotonin, dopamine) (1,2). Because PS plays a role in brain cell function, some proponents have proposed administering oral PS to prevent or reverse age-related neurochemical deficits. Additionally, PS may also be involved in blunting adrenocorticotropin hormone (ACTH) and cortisol production associated with physical stress. Because elevated cortisol levels have a protein catabolic effect on skeletal muscle and have been associated with overtraining (3), proponents of PS supplementation have extrapolated applications for body builders.

Media and Marketing Claims	Efficacy
Reduces age-related memory loss, including that which is related to Alzheimer's disease	↑?
Increases intelligence	NR
Reduces muscle breakdown	NR
Decreases physical stress	NR

Safety

- Bovine-derived PS supplements are taken from the bovine cortex. Although there have been no adverse reports in studies using bovine cortex–derived phosphatidylserine

(BC-PS), some researchers warned that, "in terms of safety, the brain cortex is not a suitable material for food use, because some encephalopathies such as mad cow disease (bovine spongiform encephalopathy) or Kuru disease in humans are orally infectious through prion contaminated brain" (4). This concern led to the development of soybean-lecithin and cabbage-derived PS (SL-PS) supplements. To date, however, BC-PS has been shown in numerous studies to be well-tolerated for as long as 6 months with no serious side effects.

♦ Dosages of 600 mg per day have been associated with insomnia.

Drug/Supplement Interactions

No reported adverse interactions

Key Points

♦ Several studies suggest that BC-PS may improve learning and memory (recall of misplaced objects and numbers, face recognition) in older individuals with cognitive disorders. A few studies in patients with less severe symptoms of Alzheimer's disease suggest some efficacy in the short-term (16 weeks).

♦ Controlled trials have not tested the hypothesis that PS increases intelligence quotient or improves recall of frequently misplaced objects and memory of numbers in healthy individuals with normal cognitive function.

♦ Limited research exists regarding the ability of BC-PS to blunt the physical stress response to exercise. More research is needed to determine whether PS is beneficial to athletes.

♦ A blunted stress-response has been shown among young adults taking daily PS (5). More research is needed with larger sample size and improved study design before PS should be considered for improving mood and adaptation to increased stress.

Food Sources

Common foods have trace amounts of PS, although the total estimated daily intake is 80 mg (4).

Dosage Information/Bioavailability

PS is sold in 100- to 400-mg tablets, capsules, powders, and chewing gum; these products are synthetically derived from soybean lecithin (SL-PS). Note that most studies have used PS derived from bovine cortex (BC-PS). Labels recommend taking dosages ranging from 100 to 800 mg/day. Some products combine SL-PS with other phospholipids, including lecithin and cephalin.

Relevant Research

PS and Cognitive Function in the Aging Population

◆ In a double-blind, placebo-controlled, multicenter study in Italy, 494 elderly subjects with moderate to severe cognitive impairment as determined by the Mini Mental State Examination and the Reisberg Global Deterioration scale were randomly assigned to receive 300 mg BC-PS or a placebo daily for 6 months. Changes in behavior and cognitive performance were measured using the Plutchik Geriatric Rating Scale and the Buschke Selective Reminding Test at baseline, and at 3 and 6 months. Of the 494 subjects enrolled, 425 (215 PS- and 210 placebo-treated subjects) completed the 6-month trial. After 3 and 6 months, cognitive and behavioral parameters improved significantly in the PS group compared with the placebo group. Clinical evaluation and laboratory tests demonstrated that PS was well-tolerated (2).

◆ In a double-blind, placebo-controlled study, 149 subjects with age-associated memory impairment were randomly assigned to receive 200 mg BC-PS or a placebo daily for 12 weeks. Fourteen subjects did not complete the study, and these subjects were equally divided between treatments. The PS subjects improved significantly on performance tests related to learning and memory tasks of daily life such as face, name, object, and telephone number recognition and recall. Within subjects in the PS supplement group, those who had scored at a relatively low level before treatment were more likely to benefit from PS (6).

◆ In a double-blind, placebo-controlled study, 51 individuals (mean age 71 years) in the early stages of Alzheimer's disease were randomly assigned to receive 300 mg BC-PS or a placebo daily for 12 weeks. Efficacy measures included a 12-item, clinical global improvement scale (CGI), a 25-item psychiatric rating scale (completed by a study psychiatrist based on an extended interview with each patient), and the Memory Assessment Clinics Family Rating Scale. After 12 weeks, the PS group improved significantly on three of the 12 CGI variables (ability to maintain concentration and two overall global items on the scale). On the psychiatric rating scale, subjects in the PS supplement group improved significantly on 5 of 25 parameters related to memory impairment and ability to recall names and events compared with the placebo subjects. The authors emphasized that PS seemed to exert a mild therapeutic effect, which may not be effective for individuals with middle- or late-stage Alzheimer's disease (7).

◆ Additional double-blind, placebo-controlled studies have shown that 300 mg of BC-PS improved cognitive function in subjects with senile dementia, Alzheimer's disease, or and Parkinson's disease (8–10).

PS and Physical Stress

◆ A double-blind, placebo-controlled, crossover design study was conducted using oral BC-PS. Nine healthy men underwent three experiments with a bicycle ergometer. Just prior to exercise, within 10 minutes, each subject received either a placebo,

200 mg BC-PS, or 400 mg BC-PS twice per day. BC-PS at 400 mg twice daily attenuated the exercise-induced ACTH and cortisol responses. The authors concluded that "chronic administration of PS may counteract stress-induced activation of the hypothalamo-pituitary-adrenal axis in man" (11).

PS and Acute Stress Response/Mood Enhancement

♦ In a randomized, double-blind, placebo-controlled study designed to test the effects of PS supplementation on the subjects' responsiveness to stress, healthy participants were assigned to one of four groups (10 men and 10 women per group): 400 mg PS per day, 600 mg PS per day, 800 mg PS per day, or placebo for 3 weeks followed by exposure to the Trier Social Stress Test. Mean age of subjects ranged from 25.3 to 30.1 years across treatment groups. Stress outcomes included ATCH and cortisol levels as well as MDBF (Mehrdimensionaler Befindlichkeitsfragebogen) psychological well-being questionnaire. PS supplementation was associated with significantly reduced serum ACTH and cortisol response to the mental and emotional stressor, but only at the 400-mg dose (5). No differences in MDBF scores from baseline or across supplementation groups were demonstrated. Additional research is needed to more fully elucidate the reason for the dose-specific response and to verify efficacy in larger sample populations.

References

1. Calderini G, Bellini F, Bonetti AC, et al. Pharmacological properties of phosphatidylserine in the aging brain. *Clin Trials J.* 1987;24:9–17.
2. Cenacchi T, Bertoldin T, Farina C, et al. Cognitive decline in the elderly: a double-blind, placebo controlled, multicenter study on efficacy of phosphatidylserine administration. *Aging (Milano).* 1993;5:123–133.
3. Urhausen A, Gabriel H, Kindermann W. Blood hormones as markers of training stress and overtraining. *Sports Med.* 1995;20:251–276.
4. Sakai M, Yamatoya H, Kudo S. Pharmacological effects of phosphatidylserine enzymatically synthesized from soybean lecithin on brain functions in rodents. *J Nutr Sci Vitaminol (Tokyo).* 1996;42:47–54.
5. Hellhammer J, Fries E, Buss C, et al. Effects of soy lecithin phosphatidic acid and phosphatidylserine complex (PAS) on the endocrine and psychological responses to mental stress. *Stress.* 2004;7:119–126.
6. Crook TH, Tinkleberg J, Yesavage J, et al. Effects of phosphatidylserine in age-associated memory impairment. *Neurology.* 1991;41:644–649.
7. Crook T, Petrie W, Wells C, et al. Effects of phosphatidylserine in Alzheimer's disease. *Psychopharmacol Bull.* 1992;28:61–66.
8. Funfgeld EW, Baggen M, Nedwidek P, et al. Double-blind study with phosphatidylserine (PS) in Parkinsonian patients with senile dementia of Alzheimer's type (SDAT). *Prog Clin Biol Res.* 1989;317:1235–1246.
9. Amaducci L. Phosphatidylserine in the treatment of Alzheimer's disease: results of a multicenter study. *Psychopharmacol Bull.* 1988;24:130–134.

10. Delwaide PJ, Gyselnynck-Mambourg AM, Hurlet A, et al. Double-blind randomized controlled study of phosphatidylserine in senile demented patients. *Acta Neurol Scand.* 1986;73:136–140.
11. Monteleone P, Maj M, Beinat L, et al. Blunting by chronic phosphatidylserine administration of the stress-induced activation of the hypothalamo-pituitary-adrenal axis in healthy men. *Eur J Clin Pharmacol.* 1992;41:385–388.

Phytosterols

Plant sterols and plant stanols are present in fruit, vegetables, nuts, seeds, legumes, and many other plant sources. Collectively known as *phytosterols,* both are fundamental components of plant-cell membranes. Phytosterols have chemical structures similar to that of cholesterol, but they do not have an ethyl or methyl group on their side chain as cholesterol does. Because phytosterols do not have an ethyl or methyl group on their side chains, the body absorbs little or no phytosterols; thus, they do not cause some of the adverse events associated with dietary cholesterol. The most abundant plant sterol is beta-sitosterol, comprising almost 80% of all phytosterols. Others include campesterol, stigmasterol, and trace amounts of stanols such as sitostanol.

As early as the 1950s, phytosterols were recognized for their potential to treat hypercholesterolemia. Currently, there is substantial evidence supporting the efficacy of phytosterols in the treatment of high cholesterol, but most research is related to the development of plant sterol–enriched food products rather than dietary supplements per se (1–3).

Media and Marketing Claims	Efficacy
Treats hypercholesterolemia	↑
Eases symptoms of an enlarged prostate	↔

Safety

- Phytosterols have been well-tolerated and effectively used in many clinical trials (1–4). The most commonly reported side effects have been gastrointestinal disturbances, including bloating, diarrhea, and nausea.

Drug/Supplement Interactions

Although plant sterols may reduce carotenoid and vitamin E bioavailability, substantial decreases in carotenoid levels and/or tocopherol levels will not occur with standard functional food doses of plant sterols (5,6).

Key Points

◆ In September 2000, the FDA authorized the use of health claims about the role of plant sterol or plant stanol esters in reducing the risk for coronary heart disease on food labels for foods containing these substances (7). This authorization was based on the FDA's conclusion that plant sterol and plant stanol esters reduce the risk of coronary heart disease by blocking absorption of dietary cholesterol, which reduces serum cholesterol levels.

◆ Both plant sterols and stanols have been effective at reducing total and LDL cholesterol but have had little effect on HDL (8). These findings include one study among 7 familial hypercholesterolemic prepubertal children (9).

◆ The enrichment of foods with plant sterol or plant stanol esters is a recent development in functional foods; enrichment aims to enhance the ability of certain foods to reduce serum cholesterol.

◆ Beta-sitosterol has shown some efficacy in reducing symptoms of an enlarged prostate, particularly with regard to improving urinary flow. However, studies are limited and not consistent in this finding.

◆ *See also* Gamma-oryzanol.

Food Sources

Phytosterols are nonnutritive components of many foods. Therefore, eating a variety of fruits and vegetables will ensure a good intake. Seafood, peas, nuts, seeds, and whole-grains are good sources.

Dosage Information/Bioavailability

Phytosterol supplements are available in capsule, tablet, softgel, and liquid forms. A therapeutic dosage to reduce serum cholesterol is 3.4 to 5.1 g/day (10). To treat benign prostatic hyperplasia, a standard dosage is 60 to 130 mg two to three times per day (4). Phytosterols can also be found in some commercially prepared margarines. Manufacturer claims suggest that 3 teaspoons per day may help reduce cholesterol levels.

In a double-blind, randomized, placebo-controlled study to determine whether plant sterols affect the bioavailability of beta carotene and alpha tocopherol, and to investigate the effects of plant sterols on cholesterol absorption, 26 men with normal serum cholesterol levels consumed a low-fat, milk-based beverage or the same beverage supplemented with either free sterols or sterol esters for 1 week each (5). Cholesterol absorption and bioavailability of beta carotene and alpha tocopherol were assessed. In this study, milk enriched with either free sterols or sterol esters reduced cholesterol absorption in these men (5). Both free sterols and sterol esters also reduced the bioavailability of beta carotene and alpha tocopherol, with plant sterol esters having the most substantial reduction in beta carotene bioavailability.

A recent report from the Olestra Post-Marketing Surveillance Study of 2,535 adults (ages 30 to 60 years) and their offspring (n = 272; ages 12 to 17 years) showed that mean reported daily consumption of Olestra was 78 mg in the adults and 74 mg in the adolescents (6). Among adult subjects at the highest levels of intake (> 1.3 g/week), there was a significant reduction in alpha-carotene (22%) and beta-carotene (10%) as well as beta-cryptoxanthin (6.5%) and lycopene (12%). Carotenoid levels were also reduced in adolescents. However, these reductions were not statistically significant. Other fat soluble nutrients (retinol, 25[OH]vitamin D3, and alpha-tocopherol) were not significantly changed with Olestra intake in the adolescents. Of these nutrients, only alpha-tocopherol was reduced (by 3.2%) in adults.

Relevant Research

Plant Sterols and Stanols and Hyperlipidemia

- To determine the efficacy of plant sterols/stanols in the treatment of hyperlipidemia, 25 subjects with hyperlipidemia were randomly assigned to one of two groups: 14 subjects incorporated plant sterol–enriched margarine (25 g/day) into their diets vs 11 who ate their usual diet. Serum lipids were evaluated at baseline and 12 weeks later, at the study's end. Serum cholesterol decreased in 5 of the subjects who incorporated margarine into their diet, whereas no change was seen in the control subjects (11).

- A single-blind, randomized, placebo-controlled, repeated-measure study compared the effect on serum lipids of intake of meat products enriched with plant sterols and calcium, magnesium, and potassium vs control meat products. Twenty-one normo-cholesterolemic subjects (15 men, 6 women) were recruited, and all 21 completed the study. Subjects consumed enriched meat products for 3 weeks, followed by 3 weeks' consumption of control meat, and then consumed enriched meats for an additional 3 weeks. Serum lipids were analyzed at baseline and during the first and third weeks of each 3-week study phase. Total cholesterol and LDL levels decreased significantly after the second enriched–meat product consumption phase. No other significant changes were identified (12).

- A randomized, single-blind, placebo-controlled, parallel arm study evaluated the effects of plant sterols and/or endurance training on plasma lipids and lipoprotein cholesterol levels. Subjects were selected for participation if they demonstrated elevated serum cholesterol and BMI between 18 to 40, were between the ages of 40 to 70 years, and reported a previously sedentary lifestyle. Eighty-four subjects met selection criteria, and 74 (20 men and 54 women) completed the study. Subjects were randomly assigned after stratification for age and serum cholesterol levels to one of four interventions (sterol-enriched spread alone, exercise with placebo margarine spread, sterol spread and exercise, or control) for 8 weeks. Fasting blood samples were taken on days 0, 53, 54, and 55 for analysis of plasma lipid profiles. Sterol spread with or without exercise, was associated with significantly reduced total cholesterol as compared with pretreatment levels. Exercise alone did not reduce total cholesterol significantly. However, it significantly increased HDL and decreased triacylglycerol levels as well as total body fat as compared with baseline. The combined sterols and exercise program provided the most total benefit on lipid profiles (13).

Plant Sterols and Stanols and Benign Prostatic Hypertrophy

- In a randomized, double-blind, placebo-controlled study, 200 subjects with benign prostatic hypertrophy/hyperplasia took 20 mg beta-sitosterol or placebo three times daily for a period of 6 months (4). Responsiveness was assessed using standardized scales, including the International Prostate Symptom Score, urine flow, and prostate gland volume. Both groups showed some clinical response; however, only the beta-sitosterol group reached significance, with a mean symptom score decrease of 7.4 points. Both peak urine flow and residual urine volume also responded significantly to supplementation. However, prostate volume did not respond to either treatment.

♦ In a randomized, double-blind, placebo-controlled trial using Azuprostat (a beta-sitosterol supplement) at a dosage of 130 mg/day for 6 months, 177 subjects with benign prostatic hyperplasia also showed clinical responsiveness to beta-sitosterol supplementation (14). In this study, symptom scores as measured by the International Prostate Symptom Score (IPSS) were reduced by a mean of 5.4 points, but peak urine volume and urinary residual volume did not show a significant change with beta-sitosterol or placebo.

References

1. Hallikainen MA, Usitupa MI. Effects of 2 low-fat stanol ester-containing margarines on serum cholesterol concentrations as part of a low-fat diet in hypercholesterolemic subjects. *Am J Clin Nutr.* 1999;69:403–410.
2. Jones PJ, Ntanios FY, Raeini-Sarjaz M, et al. Cholesterol-lowering efficacy of a sitostanol-containing phytosterol mixture with a prudent diet in hyperlipidemic men. *Am J Clin Nutr.* 1999;69:1144–1150.
3. Miettinen TA, Puska P, Gylling H, et al. Reduction of serum cholesterol with sitostanol-ester margarine in a mildly hypercholesterolemic population. *N Engl J Med.* 1995;333:1308–1312.
4. Berges RR, Windeler J, Trampisch HJ, et al. Randomised, placebo-controlled, double-blind clinical trial of beta-sitosterol in patients with benign prostatic hyperplasia. Beta-sitosterol Study Group. *Lancet.* 1995;345:1529–1532.
5. Richelle M, Enslen M, Hager C, et al. Both free and esterified plant sterols reduce cholesterol absorption and the bioavailability of beta-carotene and alpha-tocopherol in normocholesterolemic humans. *Am J Clin Nutr.* 2004;80:171–177.
6. Neuhouser ML, Rock CL, Kristal AR, et al. Olestra is associated with slight reductions in serum carotenoids but does not markedly influence serum fat-soluble vitamin concentrations. *Am J Clin Nutr.* 2006;83:624–631.
7. FDA authorizes new coronary heart disease health claim for plant sterol and plant stanol esters. 2000. Available at: http://www.fda.gov/bbs/topics/ANSWERS/ANS01033.html. Accessed May 5, 2006.
8. Weststrate JA, Meijer GW. Plant sterol-enriched margarines and reduction of plasma total- and LDL-cholesterol concentrations in normocholesterolaemic and mildly hypercholesterolaemic subjects. *Eur J Clin Nutr.* 1998;52:334–343.
9. Becker M, Staab D, Von Bergman K. Long-term treatment of severe familial hypercholesterolemia in children: effect of sitosterol and bezafibrate. *Pediatrics.* 1992;89:138–142.

10. Blair S, Capuzzi D, Gottlieb S, et al. Incremental reduction of serum total cholesterol and low density lipoprotein cholesterol with the addition of plant sterol ester-containing spread to statin therapy. *Am J Cardiol.* 2000;86:46–52.

11. Patch CS, Tapsell LC, Williams PG. Plant sterol/stanol prescription is an effective treatment strategy for managing hypercholesterolemia in outpatient clinical practice. *J Am Diet Assoc.* 2005;105:46–52.

12. Tapola NS, Lyyra ML, Karvonen HM, et al. The effect of meat products enriched with plant sterols and minerals on serum lipids and blood pressure. *Int J Food Sci Nutr.* 2004;55:389–397.

13. Varady KA, Ebine N, Vanstone CA, et al. Plant sterols and endurance training combine to favorably alter plasma lipid profiles in previously sedentary hypercholesterolemic adults after 8 wk. *Am J Clin Nutr.* 2004;80:1159–1166.

14. Klippel KF, Hiltl DM, Schipp B. A multicentric, placebo-controlled, double-blind clinical trial of beta-sitosterol (phytosterol) for the treatment of benign prostatic hyperplasia. German BPH-Phyto Study group. *Br J Urol.* 1997;80:427–432.

Policosanol

Policosanol is derived from sugar cane wax, beeswax, or wheat germ. The supplement derived from sugar cane wax and has been referred to as a "natural statin" that is used to treat hypercholesterolemia (1). This supplement is approved for treatment of high cholesterol in more than 20 countries (2). Policosanol has also been found in a few studies to be effective for treating intermittent claudication (3).

Policosanol supplements manufactured from beeswax may not be as effective as policosanol derived from sugar cane wax in reducing cholesterol levels. (Wheat germ policosanol, which is available in the Netherlands, has not been shown to significantly reduce blood lipid levels.)

Policosanol seems to reduce lipid levels and treat intermittent claudication through several biological mechanisms, including reduced platelet aggregation, increased antioxidant activity, increased bile acid secretion, inhibition of hepatic cholesterol synthesis, and down-regulation of HMG-CoA reductase. Studies comparing the efficacy of policosanol with standard medications for lipid control suggest a comparative response in some patient populations.

It is important to note that most of the published research for policosanol comes from one research team. Reviews of the evidence for policosanol in the reduction of lipid levels and intermittent claudication are available from both *American Journal of Health-System Pharmacy* (4) and *Alternative Medicine Reviews* (5).

Media and Marketing Claims	Efficacy
Treats hypercholesterolemia*	↔
Improves intermittent claudication	NR

Studies generally limited to one research group.

Safety

◆ Policosanol is generally well-tolerated. Side effects are rare and generally limited to weight loss (6).

◆ To investigate the tolerability of policosanol in an elderly population, 5, 10, or 20 mg/day policosanol was provided to 2,252 individuals eligible for cholesterol-lowering and/or antiplatelet medications. The dosage was determined by atherosclerotic risk profile. Subjects were evaluated every 6 months for follow-up. All subjects had substantial vascular disease as well as other risk factors such as hypercholesterolemia, hypertension, or diabetes mellitus. Treatment duration varied; however, half were still enrolled after 2 years and 18% at 3 years. Adverse events were recorded on case-report forms. In this study, 31 subjects (approximately 1.5%) experienced serious adverse events, including 18 deaths, mostly from vascular events such as myocardial infarction or ventricular arrhythmia. Overall, the authors concluded, "long-term tolerability of policosanol in elderly patients at high vascular risk was very good, as assessed under conditions of routine clinical practice" (7).

◆ In a study assessing the concomitant effects of policosanol and beta-blockers on blood pressure, elderly subjects (n = 205) were randomly assigned to add policosanol (5 mg/day) or placebo to their daily beta-blocker treatment for a period of 3 years (8). Mild to moderate adverse events were reported in approximately 18% of subjects vs 28% in the placebo group. Severe adverse event reports were 3.1% in the policosanol group and 14.0% in the placebo group and were characterized as "vascular.

Drug/Supplement Interactions

Individuals may experience increased bleeding and bruising when taking policosanol with other medications that alter bleeding time or platelet aggregation. A dosage of 20 mg policosanol per day is similar to 100 mg/day of aspirin in terms of reducing platelet aggregation, but policosanol does not affect coagulation time (9).

Key Points

◆ Although several studies from a single research team suggest that policosanol may be as effective as statins in reducing serum cholesterol levels in individuals with hypercholesterolemia, a 2006 double-blind, placebo-controlled study showed that policosanol was no more effective than placebo in lowering LDL cholesterol.

◆ In a double-blind, placebo-controlled study of the effects of policosanol in individuals with intermittent claudication, investigators found that subjects in the treatment group were able to improve their walking distance as compared with the placebo group (3). More research is needed to support these findings.

Food Sources

None

Dosage Information/Bioavailability

Pharmacokinetic studies of policosanol bioavailability in humans are lacking. Policosanol is available in capsule, softgel, and tablet forms. Doses of 5 to 10 mg taken twice/day have been used in studies on hypercholesterolemia and intermittent claudication (1,3).

Relevant Research

Policosanol and Hypercholesterolemia

◆ In a randomized, double-blind, placebo-controlled, parallel-group study conducted in Germany among 143 patients (61% women, 39% men) who presented with LDL cholesterol levels equal or greater than 150 mg/dL, policosanol was no more effective than placebo in lowering LDL cholesterol levels (10). During the initial 6 weeks, subjects received dietary counseling (Step I National Cholesterol Education Program guidelines) for hyperlipidemia and took a placebo. Patients were then randomly assigned, in five equal groups, to 10, 20, 40, or 80 mg policosanol (Dalmer Labs, La Habana, Cuba) or placebo daily for a period of 12 weeks. After run-in, participant dropout rates were minimal and equivalent across groups; intent-to-treat analysis considered all subjects in the final determination of treatment effect. Mean age was 53.8 to 58.7 years across treatment groups and mean BMI was elevated (26.8–27.7). LDL cholesterol levels decreased by an average of 15 mg/dL in the placebo group from baseline to 12 weeks, likely in response to dietary change. Changes in LDL for policosanol groups were 17 mg/dL (10-mg dose); 10 mg/dL (20-mg dose); 5 mg/dL (40-mg dose); and 13 mg/dL (80-mg dose), suggesting no significant difference as compared with placebo and no clear dose-response.

◆ A meta-analysis of herbal therapies for the treatment of hyperlipidemia reviewed data from 52 trials including 4,596 subjects. The authors reported that policosanol supplementation was associated with a significantly reduced LDL cholesterol by an average of 23.7% (n = 29 studies), whereas plant sterols and stanol esters were associated with an 11% decrease (n = 23 studies), and placebo reduced LDL cholesterol by 2.3% (11).

◆ In a double-blind study, 129 obese individuals with type II hypercholesterolemia were randomly assigned in a to receive 5 mg policosanol or placebo daily for 3 years (12). Both groups were instructed on the Step I American Heart Association diet for 5 weeks prior to randomization. At the 12-month assessment point, policosanol treatment was associated with significant reductions in LDL and total cholesterol (24.3% and 15.8%, respectively). By the 3-year timepoint, the mean LDL cholesterol decrease was 31.8% in the policosanol group, whereas the placebo group showed no significant change. Tolerance was also reportedly high, with only 30 patients dropping out of the study. However, nine subjects in the placebo group and three in the policosanol group reported serious adverse events and almost 30% of subjects in each group reported mild to moderate side effects. In a follow-up of a larger cohort of 239 overweight adults with type 2 diabetes (13), intent-to-treat analysis showed a similar therapeutic response, with LDL levels reduced by 21.2% at 12 months, total cholesterol reduced by 17.5%, and HDL cholesterol increased by a mean of slightly more than 10% with policosanol. Although these findings are promising, double-blind studies are needed.

- In a randomized, double-blind, parallel-group study of elderly women being treated for hypercholesterolemia, 10 mg/day of policosanol was found to be just as effective as 10 mg/day of fluvastatin (Lescol) for reducing cholesterol (14). In this study, all subjects first discontinued all lipid-lowering medications and were counseled to follow a Step I diet for 4 weeks prior to supplement therapy. The mean total cholesterol levels at baseline were 6.5 and 6.7 mmol/L for the policosanol and fluvastatin groups, respectively. After 4 weeks, total cholesterol decreased approximately 10%in both groups to a mean of 5.84 and 6.02 mmol/L, respectively. This trend continued over time. At 8 weeks, total cholesterol levels were 5.24 mmol/L and 5.57 mmol/L for policosanol and fluvastatin, respectively. In addition, both groups demonstrated a significant drop in LDL cholesterol and triglycerides and a significant increase in HDL cholesterol levels during the same time period.

- The same investigative team tested the efficacy of policosanol in comparative studies with acipimox and lovastatin and found policosanol to be associated with significantly greater improvements in blood lipids than these prescription medications (15,16). However, it is not clearly stated whether investigators were blinded to medication assignment.

- A double-blind, randomized, placebo-controlled trial investigated whether policosanol interacts with beta-blocker medications when they are taken together by older adults. Two hundred five hypercholesterolemic subjects older than 60 years taking beta-blockers were given 5 mg policosanol or placebo daily for 3 years. After 1 year of treatment, the policosanol group had significantly reduced total cholesterol, LDL, and triglyceride levels. Their HDL levels increased significantly. These effects continued through the end of the study. The placebo group reported more adverse events (n = 30) than the policosanol group (n = 18), with vascular events being the most common (8).

- In a double-blind, randomized, placebo-controlled study to compare the effects of two doses of policosanol on platelet aggregation in healthy individuals (n = 47) and those with hypercholesterolemia (n = 47), subjects received 20 or 40 mg of policosanol or placebo daily for 30 days. Platelet aggregation was assessed at baseline and following the supplementation period. In healthy and hypercholesterolemic subjects, both doses of policosanol significantly reduced platelet aggregation induced by arachidonic acid, collagen, and adenosine diphosphate (ADP) when compared with placebo and with baseline measures of platelet aggregation. Both doses of policosanol significantly reduced LDL and total cholesterol levels while increasing HDL (17).

- In a double-blind, randomized, placebo-controlled study to investigate the effects of policosanol on LDL lipid peroxidation in vitro, healthy volunteers received 5 or 10 mg policosanol or placebo for 8 weeks. LDL cholesterol was tested for susceptibility to lipid peroxidation at baseline and at the end of the supplementation period.

Policosanol significantly and dose-dependently reduced lipid peroxidation as determined by conjugated diene generation, macrophage-mediated oxidation, and malondialdehyde generation studies. Policosanol also significantly reduced LDL and total cholesterol levels while significantly increasing levels of HDL cholesterol as compared with baseline and placebo (18).

♦ A double-blinded study of individuals with mildly elevated cholesterol levels in the Netherlands showed that among the 58 subjects randomly assigned to receive wheat germ policosanol or placebo, a 4 week intervention produced no significant change in serum lipid profiles (19). There was no significant change in lipids over time and nor was there a significance difference between treatment and placebo groups. This was one of the few studies of policosanol conducted outside of Cuba and by different researchers than the team that conducted most of the studies cited in this entry. The sample size of the Netherlands study was smaller than the Cuban studies, and the potential to modulate lipids may have been less likely in this study because of the mild elevations in lipids shown at baseline and the unique form of policosanol (wheat germ).

Policosanol and Intermittent Claudication

♦ A double-blind, randomized trial comparing policosanol (10 mg) to lovastatin (20 mg) for the treatment of moderately severe intermittent claudication was conducted with 28 subjects for 20 weeks (20). Treatment response was evaluated by using a treadmill to measure walking distance until claudication. At 20 weeks, policosanol treatment was associated with a significant increase in initial and total claudication distance over baseline measures and as compared with lovastatin, which showed no significant effect. Sample size for this study was small and a placebo group was not included, but this study provides preliminary support for efficacy of policosanol in the clinical setting of intermittent claudication.

♦ An earlier study by the same lead investigator enrolled 62 subjects with intermittent claudication (3). In this trial, 31 subjects were randomly assigned to placebo and 31 to 10 mg policosanol twice each day for 6 months. Initial claudication distance increased significantly by 73.2 meters after treatment with policosanol but did not change with placebo. Absolute claudication distance (maximum distance tolerance) also increased significantly with policosanol treatment, from 229.5 to 365.4 meters. Arm/ankle pressure ratios did not change in either group.

References

1. Pons P, Mas R, Illnait J, et al Efficacy and safety of policosanol in patients with primary hypercholesterolemia. *Curr Ther Res.* 1992;52:507–513.
2. Gouni-Berthold I, Berthold HK. Policosanol: clinical pharmacology and therapeutic significance of a new lipid-lowering agent. *Am Heart J.* 2002;143:356–365.

3. Castano G, Mas R, Roca J, et al. A double-blind, placebo-controlled study of the effects of policosanol in patients with intermittent claudication. *Angiology.* 1999;50:123–130.

4. Pepping J. Policosanol. *Am J Health Syst Pharm.* 2003;60:1112–1115.

5. Monograph. Policosanol. *Altern Med Rev.* 2004;9:312–317.

6. Fernandez L, Mas R, Illnait J, et al. Policosanol: results of a postmarketing surveillance control on 27,879 patients. *Curr Ther Res.* 1998;59:717,722.

7. Fernandez S, Mas R, Gamez R, et al. A pharmacological surveillance study of the tolerability of policosanol in the elderly population. *Am J Geriatr Pharmacother.* 2004;2: 219–229.

8. Castano G, Mas R, Gamez R, et al. Concomitant use of policosanol and beta-blockers in older patients. *Int J Clin Pharmacol Res.* 2004;24:65–77.

9. Arruzzabala ML, Valdes S, Mas R, et al. Effect of policosanol successive dose increases on platelet aggregation in healthy volunteers. *Pharmacol Res.* 1996;43:181–185.

10. Berthold HK, Unverdorben S, Degenhardt R, Bulitta M, Gouni-Berthold I. Effect of policosanol on lipid levels among patients with hypercholesterolemia or combined hyperlipidemia: a randomized controlled trial. *JAMA.* 2006;295:2262–2269.

11. Chen JT, Wesley R, Shamburek RD, et al. Meta-analysis of natural therapies for hyperlipidemia: plant sterols and stanols versus policosanol. *Pharmacotherapy.* 2005;25: 171–183.

12. Mas R, Castano G, Fernandez J, et al. Long-term effects of policosanol on obese patients with type II hypercholesterolemia. *Asia Pac J Clin Nutr.* 2004;12(Suppl):S102.

13. Mas R, Castano G, Fernandez J, et al. Long-term effects of policosanol on older patients with type 2 diabetes. *Asia Pac J Clin Nutr.* 2004;13(Suppl):S101.

14. Fernandez JC, Mas R, Castano G, et al. Comparison of the efficacy, safety and tolerability of policosanol versus fluvastatin in elderly hypercholesterolaemic women. *Clin Drug Invest.* 2001;21:103–113.

15. Crespo N, Illnait J, Mas R, et al. Comparative study of the efficacy and tolerability of policosanol and lovastatin in patients with hypercholesterolemia and noninsulin dependent diabetes mellitus. *Int J Clin Pharmacol Res.* 1999;19:117–127.

16. Alcocer L, Fernandez L, Campos E, et al. A comparative study of policosanol versus acipimox in patients with type II hypercholesterolemia. *Int J Tissue React.* 1999;21: 85–92.

17. Arruzazabala ML, Molina V, Mas R, et al. Antiplatelet effects of policosanol (20 and 40 mg/day) in healthy volunteers and dyslipidaemic patients. *Clin Exp Pharmacol Physiol.* 2002;29:891–897.

18. Menéndez R, Mas R, Amor AM, et al. Effects of policosanol treatment on the susceptibility of low density lipoprotein (LDL) isolated from healthy volunteers to oxidative modification in vitro. *Br J Clin Pharmacol.* 2000;50:255–262.

19. Lin Y, Rudrum M, van der Wielden RP, et al. Wheat germ policosanol failed to lower plasma cholesterol in subjects with normal to mildly elevated cholesterol concentrations. *Metabolism.* 2004;53:1309–1314.

20. Castrano G, Mas R, Fernandez L, et al. Effects of policosanol and lovastatin in patients with intermittent claudication: a double-blind comparative pilot study. *Angiology.* 2003;54:25–38.

Potassium

Potassium, the most abundant intracellular cation, is one of the major minerals responsible for maintaining osmotic pressure in the intra- and extracellular environments. The steep potassium gradient from inside to outside cells, sustained by the sodium pump, creates the membrane potential and membrane charge found in every cell. Potassium is involved in the regulation of neuromuscular excitability and contraction, glycogen formation, protein synthesis, and correction of imbalances in acid-base metabolism. Excessive extracellular potassium levels (hyperkalemia) interfere with normal heart and nerve function and may be caused by acidosis and tissue damage (myocardial infarction or renal failure). Hypokalemia, although rare, may result from poor dietary intake, gastrointestinal losses due to diarrhea or laxative use, bulimia, advanced liver disease, or excessive renal losses due to diuretic therapy. Nondiuretic medications such as steroids, carbenoxolone, and digoxin, and excess natural licorice, also negatively affect potassium status (1,2).

The role of potassium as it relates to blood pressure and high-sodium diets has been investigated. Epidemiological studies have reported an inverse relationship between potassium intake and blood pressure in patients with hypertension (3).

Media and Marketing Claims	Efficacy
Controls blood pressure; prevents strokes	↑?
Decreases risk of muscle cramping with exercise	NR

Safety

♦ Because of the risk for serious adverse effects (including sudden death), potassium supplements should only be taken when prescribed by a physician. Excess consumption of electrolyte replacements, including potassium supplements, can be harmful if serum potassium levels increase beyond normal values.

♦ People with renal disease are at high risk for hyperkalemia and should not take potassium supplements. Similarly, individuals with diabetes should not take potassium.

♦ High-dose potassium chloride prescriptions (6,000 to 12,000 mg/day) have been associated with gastrointestinal lesions, hemorrhage, and obstruction, primarily in individuals with delayed intestinal transit time (4).

♦ When combined with angiotensin-converting enzyme (ACE) inhibitors, potassium supplements may cause hyperkalemia. People on ACE inhibitors should not take potassium supplements (5).

♦ People taking potassium-sparing diuretics should not take potassium supplements.

♦ Liberal use of potassium-containing salt substitutes has caused hyperkalemia in individuals with compromised cardiovascular or renal function (2).

- Healthy adults with normal renal function will tolerate 2,400 mg/day without developing hyperkalemia.

Drug/Supplement Interactions

- A hyperkalemic reaction may occur when potassium supplements are taken in combination with ACE inhibitors (captopril, enalapril). Therefore, people taking ACE inhibitors should not take potassium supplements.

- Do not use potassium supplements if taking potassium-sparing diuretics (amiloride, spironolactone, triamterene).

- Potassium levels may become dangerously elevated when potassium supplements or salt substitutes containing potassium are combined with potassium-sparing diuretics. Individuals should discuss with their physician before using.

- Many medications can contribute to low serum levels of potassium (eg, loop and thiazide diuretics, beta-2-agonists, diflucan, glucocorticoids, amphotericin, tetracyclines).

Key Points

- Potassium supplements should be taken only when prescribed by a physician (*see* Safety).

- Evidence suggests that potassium supplements cause small but significant reductions in blood pressure, particularly in individuals with hypertension or those consuming diets low in potassium. However, evidence from the Dietary Approaches to Stop Hypertension (DASH) study suggests that a diet rich in fruits, vegetables, and low-fat dairy foods, with reduced saturated and total fat (dietary potassium intake = 4,415 mg/day) is associated with significant reductions in systolic and diastolic blood pressure, particularly isolated systolic hypertension.

- Diets high in sodium and processed foods and low in fruits, vegetables, dairy, and whole-grains may not provide enough potassium to meet minimum requirements. Some diuretic medications also cause potassium losses. Adjusting the diet to include more potassium-rich whole foods is preferable to over-the-counter potassium supplements. In addition, it is possible to achieve potassium intakes comparable to amounts used in the blood pressure studies by increasing consumption of fruits, vegetables, low-fat dairy, and legumes (*see* Food Sources). Many potassium-rich foods are also excellent sources of many other beneficial nutrients such as fiber, phytochemicals, vitamins, and minerals that play a role in disease prevention.

- Low-level potassium replacement may be indicated for individuals who exercise intensively, but potassium supplements likely play no role in preventing muscle cramping. Sodium replacement reduces risk of cramping.

- Many people believe that sustained exercise with loss of body fluids and electrolytes can result in hypokalemia and muscle cramping. However, muscle cramping associated with exercise is actually associated with sodium status. Although prolonged exercise should be accompanied by some level of potassium replacement through food selections or consumption of sport beverages, cramping is best avoided by ensuring adequate sodium intake before, during, and after exercise.

Food Sources

Food*	Potassium, mg/serving	Sodium, mg/serving
Figs (10)	1,331	21
Beans, kidney (1 cup)	713	4
Avocado (½ medium)	530	53
Molasses, blackstrap (1 Tbsp)	498	11
Orange juice (1 cup)	473	2
Banana (1 medium)	451	1
Milk, nonfat (1 cup)	406	126
Salmon (3 oz)	327	52
Sweet potato (½ cup)	302	21
Mushrooms (½ cup)	278	2
Chicken breast (½)	240	70
Sunflower seeds (1 oz)	139	1
Bread, whole-wheat (1 slice)	71	148
Cheese, mozzarella (1 oz)	19	106

Many processed foods are relatively high in sodium and low in potassium.
Source: Data are from reference 6.

Dosage Information/Bioavailability

Over-the-counter potassium supplements are available in liquids, tablets, or capsules in the form of potassium gluconate, aspartate, citrate, or hydrochloride. Each dose provides no more than 99 mg per serving, as mandated by the FDA because of potential dangers associated with self-dosing (*see* Safety). Potassium is also available in higher amounts by prescription. Commercial salt substitutes also contain considerable amounts of potassium (195 to 2,340 mg/teaspoon) (3). The Adequate Intake for healthy adults is 4,700 mg/day (7). The average US dietary intake of potassium is approximately 2,500 mg/day (3).

Relevant Research

Potassium and Blood Pressure

◆ In a meta-regression analysis study assessing risk factors for hypertension in adults from the United States, Netherlands, Finland, Italy, and the United Kingdom, low potassium intake was associated with a 4% to 17% increased risk for developing hypertension (8).

◆ A meta-analysis report summarized the results of 33 randomized clinical trials (a total of 2,609 subjects) examining potassium supplementation for hypertension. All trials included adult subjects ranging from ages 18 to 79 years. Twenty trials included subjects with hypertension and 12 trials included subjects with normal blood pressure. Three of the studies were single-blind, and seven had no placebo control. The results from each study were pooled after weighting the results for individual studies by the inverse of its variance for blood pressure change. Potassium supplements were associated with a significant reduction in mean systolic and diastolic blood pressure (–4.44 mm Hg, –2.45 mm Hg, respectively). After exclusion of a trial with extreme results, potassium supplementation was still associated with significant reductions in systolic and diastolic blood pressure (–3.11 mm Hg, –1.97 mm Hg, respectively). These effects seemed to be the greatest in studies in which subjects had higher intakes of sodium (9).

◆ In a double-blind, placebo-controlled study, 300 women with normal blood pressure (mean age 39 years) from the Nurses' Health Study II whose reported intakes of potassium, calcium, and magnesium were between the 10th and 15th percentiles were randomly assigned to receive one of five supplements for 16 weeks: (*a*) 1,564 mg (40 mmol) potassium; (*b*) 1,200 mg calcium; (*c*) 336 mg magnesium; (*d*) all three minerals together; or (*e*) a placebo. The mean differences among the treatment and placebo groups were significant for potassium supplements (–2.0 mm Hg systolic, –1.7 mm Hg diastolic) (10).

◆ In a double-blind, placebo-controlled trial, 87 healthy African Americans (systolic blood pressure, 100 to 159 mm Hg; diastolic blood pressure, 70 to 94 mm Hg) were randomly assigned to receive 3,127 mg (80 mmol) potassium or a placebo while following a low-potassium diet (1,251 to 1,368 mg/day [32 to 35 mmol/day]) for 21 days. Nine blood pressure readings were taken during three visits during the trial. There were no differences in blood pressure between groups at the baseline. The potassium-supplemented group had significantly lower systolic (–6.9 mm Hg) and diastolic (–2.5 mm Hg) blood pressure compared with the placebo group (11).

◆ In a double-blind, placebo-controlled trial, 125 subjects with untreated mild or borderline hypertension were randomly assigned to one of four treatments for 6 months: (*a*) 2,345 mg (60 mmol) potassium plus 1,000 mg calcium; (*b*) 2,345 mg potassium plus 360 mg magnesium; (*c*) calcium plus magnesium; or (*d*) a placebo. Blood pressure measurements were taken at the baseline, and at 3 and 6 months of treatment. There were no significant differences in dietary intakes of potassium, calcium, or magnesium among groups during the study. The mean differences in changes in blood pressure between treatment and placebo groups were not significant. The authors concluded that "this trial provides little evidence of an important role of combinations of cation supplements in the treatment of mild or borderline hypertension" (12).

◆ In a randomized, multicenter trial (DASH), 459 subjects with systolic blood pressure less than 160 mm Hg and diastolic blood pressures between 80 and 95 mm Hg were randomly assigned to one of three controlled diets for 8 weeks: (*a*) control diet—low in fruits and vegetables and low-fat dairy, and a 37% fat diet typical of the average diet in the United States (mean dietary potassium intake = 1,752 mg/day); (*b*) diet rich in fruits and vegetables (total dietary fat = 37%; mean potassium intake = 4,101 mg/day); or (*c*) combination diet rich in fruits and vegetables and low-fat dairy products and with reduced saturated fat and total fat (total dietary fat = 25%; mean potassium intake = 4,415 mg). Prior to the study, all subjects were fed control diets for 3 weeks. Sodium intake and body weight were maintained at constant levels. The combination diet resulted in a significant reduction in systolic (–5.0 mm Hg) and diastolic (–3.0 mm Hg) blood pressure compared with subjects on the control diet. The fruit and vegetable–rich diet resulted in a statistically significant reduction of systolic (–2.8 mm Hg) and diastolic (–1.1 mm Hg) blood pressure compared with the control diet, an association that was attributed to increased dietary potassium exposure. Among the 133 subjects with hypertension, the combination diet significantly reduced systolic and diastolic pressure by 11.4 and 5.5 mm Hg more, respectively, than the control diet. Subjects without hypertension also experienced significant reductions of systolic and diastolic blood pressure by 3.5 mm Hg and 2.1 mm Hg (13).

Potassium and Exercise-Associated Muscle Cramping

- ◆ In a study, 72 runners who had participated in an ultradistance road race were divided into those with postexercise cramping and those without (control). Post-race cramping was associated with depleted serum sodium levels and elevated serum magnesium levels. No significant association between cramping and potassium status was found (14).

- ◆ Research on whether shifts in extracellular and intermuscular potassium during exercise are associated with increased fatigue or reduced performance is somewhat controversial; investigators suggest only low-level replacement is needed (15,16).

References

1. Oh MS. Water, electrolyte, and acid-base balance. In: Shils ME, Olson JA, Shike M, et al, eds. *Modern Nutrition in Health and Disease.* 9th ed. Philadelphia, Pa: Lea & Febiger; 1999:105–139.
2. Riccardella D, Dwyer J. Salt substitutes and medicinal potassium sources: risks and benefits. *J Am Diet Assoc.* 1985;85:471–474.
3. Tobian L. Dietary sodium chloride and potassium have effects on the pathophysiology of hypertension in humans and animals. *Am J Clin Nutr.* 1997;65(2 Suppl):S606–S611.
4. McMahon FG, Akdamar K, Ryan JR, et al. Upper gastrointestinal lesions after potassium chloride supplements: a controlled clinical trial. *Lancet.* 1982;2:1059–1061.
5. Burnakis TG, Mioduch HJ. Combined therapy with captopril and potassium supplementation. A potential for hyperkalemia. *Arch Intern Med.* 1984;144:2371–2372.
6. Pennington JA. *Bowes and Church's Food Values of Portions Commonly Used.* 17th ed. Philadelphia, Pa: Lippincott-Raven Publishers; 1998.
7. Institute of Medicine. *Dietary Reference Intakes for Water, Potassium, Sodium, Chloride, and Sulfate.* Washington, DC: National Academy Press; 2004.

8. Geleijnse JM, Kok FJ, Grobbee DE. Impact of dietary and lifestyle factors on the prevalence of hypertension in Western populations. *Eur J Public Health.* 2004;14:235–239.

9. Whelton PK, He J. Potassium in preventing and treating high blood pressure. *Semin Nephrol.* 1999;19:494–499.

10. Sacks FM, Willett WC, Smith A, et al. Effect on blood pressure of potassium, calcium, and magnesium in women with low habitual intake. *Hypertension.* 1998;31:131–138.

11. Brancati FL, Appel LJ, Seidler AJ, et al. Effect of potassium supplementation on blood pressure in African Americans on a low-potassium diet. A randomized, double-blind, placebo-controlled trial. *Arch Intern Med.* 1996;156:61–67.

12. Sacks FM, Brown LE, Appel L, et al. Combinations of potassium, calcium, and magnesium supplements in hypertension. *Hypertension.* 1995;26:950–956.

13. Appel LJ, Moore TJ, Obarzanek E, et al. A clinical trial of the effects of dietary patterns on blood pressure. *N Engl J Med.* 1997;16:1117–1124.

14. Schwellnus MP, Nicol J, Laubscher R, et al. Serum electrolyte concentrations and hydration status are not associated with exercise associated muscle cramping (EAMC) in distance runners. *Br J Sports Med.* 2004;38:488–492.

15. Mohr M, Nordsborg N, Nielsen JJ, et al. Potassium kinetics in human muscle interstitium during repeated intense exercise in relation to fatigue. *Pflugers Arch.* 2004;448:452–456.

16. Nielson JJ, Mohr M, Klarskov C, et al. Effects of high-intensity intermittent training on potassium kinetics and performances in human skeletal muscle. *J Physiol.* 2004; 554:857–870.

Pygeum

Pygeum is made from the bark of the African plum tree *(Pygeum africanum),* an evergreen tree native to higher elevations in central and southern Africa. It been used in many parts of the world to treat benign prostatic hyperplasia (BPH), a common condition in men older than 50 years. Pygeum has antiproliferative effects on prostatic fibroblasts and epithelial cells in rat models (1).

Media and Marketing Claims	Efficacy
Reduces symptoms of benign prostatic hyperplasia	↑?

Safety

- ◆ Pygeum has been well-tolerated in clinical trials. Reported side effects include mild gastrointestinal upset, including diarrhea and constipation (2). A study using a dosage of 100 mg/day for 12 months resulted in minimal adverse events (3).

Drug/Supplement Interactions

None

Key Points

- ◆ Pygeum may be effective in the treatment of BPH, but human studies are limited. Urinary symptoms improved and urinary discomfort decreased in individuals taking pygeum (4). In a review of clinical data published during the last 25 years, investigators concluded that pygeum is an effective and well-tolerated treatment for mild to moderate symptomatic BPH (5).

Food Sources

None

Dosage Information/Bioavailability

Pygeum is available in liquid, tablet, capsule, and softgel forms. To treat BPH, dosages of 50 mg twice/day or 100 mg once/day are equally effective (2). Some studies have used as much as 200 mg/day with no adverse effects (5).

Relevant Research

Pygeum and Benign Prostatic Hyperplasia

- ◆ According to a review of evidence related to the clinical use of *Pygeum africanum,* this dietary supplement has been used to treat mild to moderate symptomatic BPH for more than 35 years. This article describes the biological mechanisms of action, including anti-inflammatory, bladder contractility, inhibition of fibroblast proliferation, and enhanced adrenal androgen activity (5). Open-label studies that did not include a control group (n = 31 studies with 1,310 patients with BPH) generally support a therapeutic benefit of pygeum in short-term use (21 days to 4 months) at doses ranging from 75 to 200 mg/day. Most of these studies had fewer than 50 subjects. The review separately describes the evidence from double-blind, placebo-controlled studies (n = 12; 358 subjects using pygeum and 359 placebo subjects). The authors conclude, "taken as whole the results show a statistically significant benefit for *P Africanum* extract over placebo."

- ◆ The largest trial was published by Barlet et al in 1990. In this 60-day, double-blind, placebo controlled study of 263 men with BPH (255 completed the trial), daily supplementation with 100 mg pygeum significantly increased maximum urinary flow rate and voided volume, as compared with placebo. The pygeum group also had significant reductions in residual volume, nocturia, daytime urinary frequency, and overall self-reported improvement in prostate health (6).

- In a double-blind, randomized, placebo-controlled study to determine the efficacy of pygeum and stinging nettle extracts in the treatment of BPH, subjects ranging in age from 52 to 86 years (half with high blood pressure and 25% with diabetes) were given a combination of *Pygeum africanum* and *Urtica dioica* extracts (n = 27) or placebo (n = 22) for 6 months and then evaluated for improvement. There was no difference between the two groups in terms of International Prostate Symptoms Score, Quality of Life Scores, or maximum urinary flow rate at study end. However, the dosage used (25 mg/day) was much lower than what was used in studies that report efficacy (100 mg/day) (7).

- In a meta-analysis of 18 randomized, placebo-controlled trials (1,562 men) in which supplementation lasted at least 30 days, the safety and efficacy of pygeum in the treatment of BPH was evaluated. In only six studies did pygeum provide significant symptomatic urinary flow improvement as compared with placebo. The supplement was well-tolerated (2). Long term efficacy should be assessed because current studies have not determined the efficacy over prolonged periods of time (greater than 6 months).

- In a double-blind, randomized, two-phase study to compare the safety and efficacy of pygeum in the treatment of BPH, 223 subjects with BPH (ages 58 to 72 years) were initially randomly assigned to a 2-month intervention with 100 mg pygeum every evening or 50 mg pygeum twice per day (morning and evening). Next, the remaining subjects (n = 174) met inclusion criteria for randomization to continue with phase 2 of the study, which was open-label. This phase prescribed 100 mg pygeum once/day for 10 months. Symptom improvement, quality of life, and urinary flow were evaluated, including the International Prostate Symptom Scale (IPSS). Results showed that during 2-month phase (phase 1) the mean IPSS was reduced equally in both groups (35% to 38% across groups) as did nocturia and quality of life. During phase 2 (10 months of intervention), the IPSS scores were further reduced, with a total 46% reduction in symptoms from baseline (3).

- In an open-label, three-center study initiated to determine the efficacy of tadenan (*Pygeum africanum* extract) in the treatment of BPH, 85 men in general good health between the ages of 50 and 75 years were given 50 mg of the extract twice per day for 2 months followed by a third month in which no treatment was provided. Subjects were evaluated for symptomatic complaints, quality of life, nocturia, and urodynamics. Statistically significant improvements were found in symptoms and quality of life as well as reduced nocturia frequency and urodynamic parameters. However, the findings should be viewed with caution because the study was not blinded nor placebo-controlled (8).

References

1. Yablonsky F, Nicolas V, Riffaud JP, et al. Antiproliferative effect of *Pygeum africanum* extract on rat prostatic fibroblasts. *J Urol.* 1997;157:2881–2887.
2. Ishani A, MacDonald R, Nelson D, et al. *Pygeum africanum* for the treatment of patients with benign prostatic hyperplasia: a systematic review and quantitative meta-analysis. *Am J Med.* 2000;109:654–664.

3. Chatelain C, Autet W, Brackman F. Comparison of once and twice daily dosage forms of *Pygeum africanum* extract in patients with benign prostatic hyperplasia: a randomized, double-blind, study, with long-term open label extension. *Urology.* 1999;54:473–478.

4. Wilt T, Ishani A, MacDonald R, et al. Pygeum africanum for benign prostatic hyperplasia. *Cochrane Database Syst Rev.* 2002;CD001044.

5. Andro MC, Riffaud JP. *Pygeum africanum* extract for the treatment of patients with benign prostatic hyperplasia. A review of 25 years of published experience. *Curr Ther Res.* 1995;56:796–817.

6. Baret A, Albrecht J, Aubert A, et al. Efficacy of *Pygeum africanum* extract in the treatment of micturitional disorders due to benign prostatic hyperplasia. Evaluation of objective and subjective parameters. *Wien Klin Wochenschr.* 1990;102:667–673.

7. Melo EA, Bertero EB, Rios LA, et al. Evaluating the efficiency of a combination of *Pygeum africanum* and stinging nettle (*Urtica dioica*) extracts in treating benign prostatic hyperplasia (BPH): double-blind, randomized, placebo controlled trial. *Int Braz J Urol.* 2002;28:418–425.

8. Breza J, Dzurny O, Borowka A, et al. Efficacy and acceptability of tadenan (*Pygeum africanum* extract) in the treatment of benign prostatic hyperplasia (BPH): a multicentre trial in central Europe. *Curr Med Res Opin.* 1998;14:127–139.

Pyridoxine. *See* Vitamin B-6 (Pyridoxine).

Pyruvate

Pyruvate, a 3-carbon molecule, is produced endogenously from phosphoenolpyruvate in the end stages of glycolysis. It can be reduced to lactate in the cytosol or decarboxylated to acetyl coenzyme A in the mitochondria. Some researchers have hypothesized that pyruvate supplementation may spare oxidation of glucose, thus improving sports endurance by sparing glycogen. Preliminary investigations found that pyruvate prevented the development of hepatic steatosis in rats receiving chronic ethanol feedings. These findings led to additional research testing pyruvate supplementation on fat metabolism in animals and humans (1,2).

Media and Marketing Claims	Efficacy
Weight loss aid	↔
Improves exercise endurance	↔
Reduces cholesterol	↔

Safety

- There are no studies testing the safety of pyruvate supplementation for more than 6 weeks.
- Flatus, diarrhea, and borborygmus were reported in most subjects ingesting pyruvate and dihydroxyacetone.

Drug/Supplement Interactions

No reported adverse interactions

Key Points

- In preliminary studies in small numbers of obese subjects, mainly on very-low-calorie diets, pyruvate enhanced weight loss and fat loss. These studies have been criticized for reliance on bioelectrical impedance, which is not generally regarded as an effective measure of body fat in obese subjects. Other studies have reported enhanced weight loss in overweight subjects who took pyruvate supplements.
- In two preliminary laboratory studies, 7 days of supplementation with pyruvate and dihydroxyacetone improved exercise endurance in untrained subjects. However, pyruvate had no ergogenic effect on exercise in two studies of trained athletes. Much more research is needed before the claim that pyruvate enhances exercise endurance can be supported. In addition, athletes should be cautioned that pyruvate supplementation has been associated with gastrointestinal distress, which could interfere with sport performance.
- One preliminary study showed that pyruvate had no effect on blood lipids in hyperlipidemic subjects on low-fat diets, but another study reported that pyruvate prevented lipids from increasing in subjects on high-fat diets. More research is needed to clarify these findings and to explore the possible mechanisms involved. It is not prudent to suggest that individuals take pyruvate supplements with the notion that it allows them to eat a high-fat diet without consequences.
- Commercially available pyruvate supplements do not contain dihydroxyacetone and are not available in the high doses used in many of the research studies.

Food Sources

Pyruvate is found in animal products; however, food sources have not been quantified.

Dosage Information/Bioavailability

Pyruvate is sold in the form of sodium or calcium pyruvate in capsules or tablets supplying 0.5 to 1 g pyruvate per serving. This dose is considerably less than those used in research, which typically provided 25 to 50 g pyruvate in addition to dihydroxyacetone (another three-carbon metabolite of carbohydrate metabolism).

Relevant Research

Pyruvate and Weight Loss

- A review of dietary supplements used for weight loss published in the *American Journal of Clinical Nutrition* suggests that pyruvate may improve body composition; however, pyruvate supplementation was no better than placebo in modulating body weight (3). Only two studies using pyruvate were included in the systematic review, and both enrolled obese adults (n = 52 and n = 104). Subjects were randomized to 6 g pyruvate per day or placebo in a double-blind design.

- In a double-blind, placebo-controlled study, 26 healthy overweight men and women (BMI > 27) were randomly assigned to receive 6 g pyruvate or a placebo daily for 6 weeks. All subjects participated in an exercise program consisting of a 45- to 60-minute aerobic/anaerobic routine three times weekly. Body composition was determined by bioelectrical impedance. (Researchers stated that they used a newer technology of bioelectrical impedance that is more accurate than previous versions used in the Stanko et al studies, described later.) All subjects were instructed by a dietitian to follow a 2,000-kcal diet. There were no significant differences in dietary intake as assessed by food records between groups. After 6 weeks, there was a significant decrease in body weight (–1.2 kg), body fat (–2.5 kg), and percentage body fat (23% pretrial vs 20.3% 6 weeks posttrial) in the pyruvate group. Profile of Mood States (POMS) fatigue and vigor scores were significantly improved for the pyruvate group at week 6 (vigor) and weeks 4 and 6 (fatigue). There was no significant change in total lean body mass in the pyruvate group. The placebo group demonstrated significant improvements for POMS vigor at weeks 2 and 4, but no changes in body weight, body fat, or percentage body fat (4).

- In a double-blind, placebo-controlled study, 53 overweight subjects (BMI > 25) were randomly assigned to one of three groups for 6 weeks: (*a*) 6 g pyruvate (total of 10 capsules, also containing zinc, vitamin B-6, chromium, cranberry powder, dehydroacetone, and corn silk); (*b*) a placebo; and (*c*) control. The first two groups received dietary counseling, and all three groups engaged in supervised circuit training exercise three times per week. At study's end, subjects taking the pyruvate supplement experienced significant decreases in fat mass, percentage body fat, and increases in lean body mass as measured by bioelectrical impedance. Despite the exercise regimen, the placebo and control groups had no significant changes in body composition. In addition, the pyruvate group was the only group in which POMS fatigue and vigor ratings scores improved (5).

- In a randomized, placebo-controlled study, 13 obese women (mean BMI 38.9) confined to a metabolic ward were given 16 g pyruvate and 12 g dihydroxyacetone or a placebo of 26 g polyglucose; both served as isocaloric substitutions for a portion of the carbohydrate content of the diet for 21 days. Subjects were instructed to control energy expenditure and to closely monitor dietary compliance. All subjects were fed 500-kcal hypocaloric, liquid diets (60% carbohydrate, 40% protein) for 21 days. Body composition as determined by bioelectrical impedance, energy deficit (calculated from metabolic rates measured by using a metabolic cart and compared with weight and fat loss), and nitrogen metabolism (assessed by analyzing all urine and stool samples for 21 days and estimating insensible nitrogen losses) were measured. Subjects receiving pyruvate and dihydroxyacetone had significantly greater weight loss (6.5 kg vs 5.6 kg) and fat loss (4.3 kg vs 3.5 kg) than the placebo group subjects. There were no differences between groups in resting metabolic rate, nitrogen balance, and hematology indexes. The authors acknowledged that, "with the small differences in body composition changes observed in the present study, the sensitivity of any technique available for measurement of body composition is in question. Therefore, our results must be considered preliminary" (6).

- In a similar randomized, placebo-controlled study by the same investigators, 14 obese women confined to bed in a metabolic ward were given 30 g pyruvate or 22 g polyglucose as placebo as part of a 1,000-kcal hypocaloric, liquid diet (68% carbohydrate, 22% protein) for 21 days. Body composition, energy deficit, and nitrogen metabolism were measured using the same methods as the previously cited study. Subjects fed pyruvate had significantly greater weight loss (5.9 vs 4.3 kg) and fat loss (4.0 vs 2.7 kg) than the placebo group (7).

Pyruvate and Exercise Endurance

- In a double-blind, placebo-controlled, crossover study, seven trained cyclists received in random order 7 g pyruvate (calcium pyruvate) or a placebo daily for 1 week each, with a 2-week washout period. Subjects cycled at 74% to 80% of their maximum oxygen consumption until exhaustion. There were no differences in performance times between the two trials. Measured blood indexes (insulin, peptide C, glucose, lactate, glycerol, free fatty acids) were not affected. In a separate study reported in the same article, a range of pyruvate doses were administered to nine recreational athletes to determine what dose might increase blood pyruvate concentration. The 7-, 15-, and 25-g doses of pyruvate did not significantly affect blood levels of pyruvate, glucose, lactate, glycerol, or free fatty acids during a 4-hour period after ingestion (8).

- In a double-blind, placebo-controlled study, 42 college football players were randomly assigned to one of four treatments daily for 5 weeks: (*a*) creatine monohydrate; (*b*) calcium pyruvate; (*c*) combination (60% pyruvate plus 40% creatine); or (*d*) a placebo. Creatine alone and pyruvate alone were administered in three doses providing 0.22 g/kg/day (mean dose for a 100-kg subject = 22 g). The combination product provided 0.13 and 0.09 g/kg/day for pyruvate and creatine, respectively. Exercise tests were performed before and after the supplementation period while subjects continued their normal training schedules. Body composition was assessed using hydrostatic weighing and measuring seven skinfold sites. Food diaries recorded at weeks 1 and 5 revealed no significant differences in total energy intake or macronutrients across time or among groups. Compared with placebo and pyruvate alone, subjects receiving creatine and creatine plus pyruvate had significantly greater increases in body mass, lean body mass, one repetition maximum (RM) bench press, combined one RM squat and bench press, and static vertical jump power output. Percentage body fat, fat mass, and cycle peak power, total work performed, blood lactate concentration, and ratings of perceived exertion during cycle ergometry did not differ among groups. In the pyruvate group, 6 of 11 subjects reported mild headaches that subsided after 2 weeks. The authors concluded that creatine supplementation seems to have beneficial effects on body composition and anaerobic exercise, but that pyruvate supplementation does not offer any additional advantages (9).

◆ In a double-blind, placebo-controlled, crossover design study, 10 untrained, free-living males on controlled diets (55% carbohydrate, 15% protein, 30% fat, 35 kcal/kg) took, in random order, 25 g sodium pyruvate plus 75 g dihydroxyacetone added to pudding or 100 g polyglucose added to pudding (placebo) for 7 days each, with a 7- to 14-day washout period. Diets were administered at the research site. (Details of diet administration were not provided). Subjects performed submaximal exercise on an arm ergometer to exhaustion at the end of each 7-day diet. Muscle biopsies were taken before and immediately after exercise to assess muscle glycogen. Subjects taking pyruvate plus dihydroxyacetone (PD) supplements exercised significantly longer than placebo subjects (160 vs 133 minutes). Resting triceps muscle glycogen was significantly greater than during placebo administration but did not differ between trials at the point of exhaustion. Arterial and venous glucose difference (glucose extraction) was significantly greater before exercise and after 60 minutes of exercise, but not at exhaustion during PD supplementation compared with the placebo. Whole-arm fractional glucose extraction was significantly greater before exercise, after 60 minutes of exercise, and at exhaustion with PD supplementation compared with placebo. There were no differences in respiratory exchange ratios, plasma free fatty acids, ß-hydroxybutyrate, glycerol, catecholamines, and insulin between groups. The authors hypothesized that pyruvate increased endurance by augmenting sources of carbohydrate for fuel used during exercise (10).

◆ In a similar double-blind, placebo-controlled, crossover study by the same research team, eight untrained, free-living male subjects on controlled high-carbohydrate diets (70% carbohydrate, 18% protein, 12% fat, 35 kcal/kg) were supplemented in random order with 25 g sodium pyruvate plus 75 g dihydroxyacetone or 100 g polyglucose for 7 days each, with a 7- to 14-day washout period. All meals were given to the subjects at the research site, but were consumed on an outpatient basis. After each diet, subjects exercised to exhaustion on the cycle ergometer at 70% of maximum oxygen consumption. Blood samples and muscle biopsies were taken. Endurance capacity was significantly improved after pyruvate plus dihydroxyacetone (PD) supplementation compared with placebo (79 vs 66 minutes). Whole-leg arterial and venous glucose difference (glucose extraction) was significantly greater at rest and after 30 minutes of exercise, but not at exhaustion during PD supplementation compared with placebo. There were no differences between treatments on muscle glycogen content or other blood parameters. The authors concluded that a 20% increase in leg endurance following PD supplementation may have been caused by increased glucose availability for oxidation by exercising muscle (11).

Pyruvate and Blood Lipids

- In a randomized, placebo-controlled study, 34 free-living subjects with hyperlipidemia consumed a low-fat, low-cholesterol diet for 4 weeks, followed by 6 more weeks of the same diet supplemented with 22 to 44 g pyruvate (7% of the diet) or 18 to 35 g polyglucose. There were no significant differences between groups in dietary intake (assessed by 3-day food records at weeks 0 and 6). Pyruvate supplementation had no effect on plasma total, LDL, and HDL cholesterol levels or triglycerides. However, subjects taking pyruvate experienced a mild but significant reduction in weight (–0.6 kg) and fat mass (–0.4 kg) compared with subjects in the placebo group (12).

- In a randomized, placebo-controlled study, 40 subjects with hyperlipidemia consumed a high-fat (45% to 74% of energy from fat, 18% to 20% of energy from saturated fat), high-cholesterol (560 to 620 mg per day), anabolic diet (0.11 MJ to 0.12 MJ/kg body weight) for 4 weeks, followed by 6 more weeks of supplementation of the same diet with 36 to 53 g pyruvate or 21 to 37 g polyglucose (placebo) as a portion of carbohydrate energy. Pyruvate supplementation resulted in a significant reductions in plasma total cholesterol (4% decrease from baseline) and LDL cholesterol (5% decrease), compared with no change in placebo subjects. There were no differences between groups in triglyceride and HDL cholesterol changes. Pyruvate supplementation significantly reduced resting heart rate and blood pressure, leading the authors to speculate that pyruvate may have a positive inotropic effect on cardiac muscle (13).

References

1. Sukula WR. Pyruvate: beyond the marketing hype. *Int J Sport Nutr.* 1998;8:241–249.
2. Ivy JL. Effect of pyruvate and dihydroxyacetone on metabolism and aerobic capacity. *Med Sci Sports Exerc.* 1998;30:837–843.
3. Pittler MH, Ernst E. Dietary supplements for body-weight reduction: a systematic review. *Am J Clin Nutr.* 2004;79:529–536.
4. Kalman D, Colker CM, Wilets I, et al. The effects of pyruvate supplementation on body composition in overweight individuals. *Nutrition.* 1999;15:337–340.
5. Kalman D, Colker CM, Stark R, et al. Effect of pyruvate supplementation on body composition and mood. *Curr Ther Res.* 1998;59:793–802.
6. Stanko RT, Tietze DL, Arch JE. Body composition, energy utilization, and nitrogen metabolism with a severely restricted diet supplemented with dihydroxyacetone and pyruvate. *Am J Clin Nutr.* 1992;55:771–776.
7. Stanko RT, Tietze DL, Arch JE. Body composition, energy utilization, and nitrogen metabolism with a 4.25 MJ/day low-energy diet supplemented with pyruvate. *Am J Clin Nutr.* 1992;56:630–635.

8. Morrison MA, Spriet LL, Dyck DJ. Pyruvate ingestion for seven days does not improve aerobic performance in well-trained individuals. *J Appl Physiol.* 2000;89:549–556.

9. Stone MH, Sanborn K, Smith LL, et al. Effects of in-season (5 weeks) creatine and pyruvate supplementation on anaerobic performance and body composition in American football players. *Int J Sport Nutr.* 1999;9:146–165.

10. Stanko RT, Robertson RJ, Spina RJ, et al. Enhancement of arm exercise endurance capacity with dihydroxyacetone and pyruvate. *J Appl Physiol.* 1990;68:119–124.

11. Stanko RT, Robertson RJ, Galbreath RW, et al. Enhanced leg exercise endurance with a high-carbohydrate diet and dihydroxyacetone and pyruvate. *J Appl Physiol.* 1990;69: 1651–1656.

12. Stanko RT, Reynolds HR, Hoyson R, et al. Pyruvate supplementation of low-cholesterol, low-fat diet: effects on plasma lipid concentrations and body composition in hyperlipidemic patients. *Am J Clin Nutr.* 1994;59:423–427.

13. Stanko RT, Reynolds HR, Lonchar KD, et al. Plasma lipid concentrations in hyper-lipidemic patients consuming a high-fat diet supplemented with pyruvate for 6 wk. *Am J Clin Nutr.* 1992;56:950–954.

Red Clover

Red clover, a perennial herb that grows wild in Asia, Europe, and some parts of the United States, has been used medicinally to treat several ailments. Although red clover is purported to relieve chest congestion, prevent heart disease, and relieve menopausal symptoms, there is no scientific data to support any of these claims. Red clover is thought to be one of the richest herbal sources of isoflavones, including biochanin, daizein, formononetin, and genistein.

Media and Marketing Claims	Efficacy
Relieves breast tenderness	NR
Relieves symptoms of menopause	NR
Prevents osteoporosis	NR

Safety

Red clover has Generally Recognized as Safe (GRAS) status in the United States (1).

Drug/Supplement Interactions

- Red clover may inhibit drugs that metabolized by cytochrome P450 enzymes.
- Red clover may interfere with anticoagulant/antiplatelet drugs and estrogen therapy.
- Red clover may decrease the effectiveness of tamoxifen.

Key Points

+ Preliminary data suggests that taking red clover may relieve breast pain and tenderness, but the number of good quality, human intervention trials conducted is insufficient to substantiate this claim (2).

+ There are conflicting data regarding the use of red clover in menopause. The large, multicenter Isoflavone Clover Extract (ICE) Study found red clover to be ineffective in reducing hot flashes (3), whereas a smaller study, funded by the supplement manufacturer, found it to be more effective than placebo in reducing hot flashes (4).

+ Preliminary studies are conflicting on the role of red clover in osteoporosis prevention. More scientific data are needed to support or refute the use of red clover for this purpose.

Food Sources

None

Dosage Information/Bioavailability

Red clover is available as a tea, tincture, capsule, or tablet. Traditionally taken as a tea, 2 to 3 teaspoons dried herb are added to 1 cup boiling water and steeped for 10 to 15 minutes. As much as 3 cups can be consumed per day. A standard dosage of red clover extract generally provides 40 to 160 mg isoflavones per day (2).

Relevant Research

Red Clover and Breast Tenderness

+ In a double-blind, randomized, placebo-controlled study to determine the efficacy isoflavones in the treatment of cyclical mastalgia, 83 healthy premenopausal with regular menses and complaints of moderate breast pain were enrolled, but only 18 received 40 or 80 mg of isoflavones extracted from red clover or a placebo for three menstrual cycles (65 women dropped out of the study prior to starting the study intervention). Subjects completed a daily breast pain and menstrual diary card during the study period and received a clinical breast exam at baseline and at the study's end. The isoflavones extracted from red clover had a positive effect on breast pain compared with placebo, but only the group taking the 40-mg dose demonstrated statistically significant improvement from baseline. Improvement was not dose-related, perhaps because of the small number of patients who completed the trial (2).

+ The efficacy of red clover isoflavone supplementation in reducing breast mammographic density was tested in a randomized, placebo-controlled, double-blind study among 205 women between 49 and 65 years of age (3). The women recruited to the trial demonstrated significant breast density as scored using the Wolfe categorization system. In this trial, subjects received a red clover–derived isoflavone supplement (1 mg genistein, 0.5 diadzein, 26 mg biochanin A, 16 mg formononetin) or placebo for 12 months to assess changes in mammographic breast density (associated with breast pain/tenderness), serum estradiol, follicle stimulating hormone (FSH), luteinizing hormone (LH), and lymphocyte tyrosine kinase activity. Among the 177 women who completed the trial, there were no significant differences between the groups in terms of mammographic breast density, serum hormone levels, or lymphocyte kinase activity. This suggests that the supplementation was not clinically efficacious for this use. However, both groups demonstrated a nonsignificant reduction in breast mammographic density over time.

Red Clover and Menopause

- The Isoflavone Clover Extract (ICE) Study was a randomized, controlled clinical trial testing the hypothesis that red clover supplements would be more effective than placebo in reducing hot flashes and improving menopausal quality of life among 169 postmenopausal women with hot flashes (4). Women received Promensil (41 mg total isoflavones) or Rimostil (28.6 mg total isoflavones) or placebo in 1:1:1 ratio. All study supplements were provided by Novogen Ltd (Sydney, Australia). Supplements were taken twice/day for 12 weeks, and 98% of subjects completed the intervention. Subjects in all groups reported a significant reduction in hot flashes, with the Promensil group having the most immediate and greatest response—a 41% reduction in symptoms. Greene Climacteric Symptom Scale was used to quantify distress related to vasomotor symptoms. All three groups showed improvement over time (week 12 compared with baseline), but no statistically significant difference across groups at any time point was shown.

- In a single-blind, randomized, placebo-controlled trial to investigate the safety and efficacy of red clover isoflavones in the treatment of postmenopausal hot flashes, 30 women between the ages of 49 and 65 years, received either the red clover extract Promensil (Novogen Ltd, Sydney, Australia) or placebo for 12 weeks after a 4-week period in which all subjects received the placebo. Eligible subjects had to have a minimum of five hot flashes per day at baseline and were evaluated for change in the number of flashes and menopausal symptoms as assessed using the Greene Climacteric Scale Score. Urinary isoflavone levels were assessed to determine adherence/compliance to the intervention. Hot flashes decreased from a mean of 6 per day to a mean of 5 per day during the run-in period. During active intervention, the number of hot flashes decreased on average over time by 44% in the supplementation group compared with the placebo group. This difference was considered statistically significant by week 8. The Greene Score also showed some improvement in menopausal symptoms with treatment and worsening of symptoms in the placebo group, but statistical significance across groups was not shown. This study was funded by the supplement manufacturer. That fact and the single-blind design suggest cautious interpretation of the data is warranted (5).

Red Clover and Osteoporosis

♦ A double-blind, randomized, placebo-controlled trial assessed the effects of red clover–derived isoflavones on spine and hip bone density, and markers of bone turnover including bone ALP, PINP, total pyridinoline and total deoxypyridinoline. In the study, 205 women between the ages of 49 and 65 years, 68% of whom were postmenopausal and all of whom demonstrated dense mammographic breast tissue patterns (Wolfe P2 or DY) were given a supplement (1 mg genistein, 0.5 mg daidzein, 26 mg biochanin A, and 16 mg formononectin) or a placebo for 1 year. Subjects were evaluated at baseline and after 1 year for changes in bone density using dual x-ray absorptiometry (DEXA) as well as blood biomarkers of bone health. A significant protection against loss of bone mineral density in the lumbar spine was shown with supplementation over time and as compared with placebo, but efficacy was not demonstrated for bone density at the hip (6). There was also a significant increase in markers of bone formation (bone ALP and PINP) in the treatment group.

♦ In a double-blind, randomized, placebo-controlled trial to compare the effects of red clover isoflavones on lipids and bone turnover markers, 252 women received Promensil (82 mg total isoflavones), Rimostil (57.2 mg total isoflavones), or placebo for 12 weeks. (Promensil and Rimostil are both manufactured by Novogen Ltd, Sydney, Australia.) Subjects were evaluated at baseline and at study's end for changes in serum osteocalcin, and urinary N-telopeptide, as well as total and HDL cholesterol, LDL cholesterol, and triglycerides. There were no significant changes in markers of bone turnover in this study. Likewise, no statistically significant changes detected with isoflavone supplementation in total cholesterol, LDL, or HDL levels. However, a significant decrease in serum triglycerides, especially in women with elevated triglycerides at baseline, was demonstrated (7).

References

1. Food and Drug Administration, Center for Food Safety and Applied Nutrition, Office of Premarket Approval. EAFUS: a food additive database. Available at: http://vm.cfsan.fda.gov/~dms/eafus.html. Accessed March 30, 2005.

2. Ingram DM, Hickling C, West L, et al. A double-blind randomized controlled trial of isoflavones in the treatment of cyclical mastalgia. *Breast.* 2002;11:170–174.

3. Atkinson C, Warren RM, Sala E, et al. Red-clover-derived isoflavones and mammographic breast density: a double-blind, placebo-controlled trial. *Breast Cancer Res.* 2004;6:R170-R179.

4. Tice JA, Ettinger B, Ensrud K, et al. Phytoestrogen supplements for the treatment of hot flashes: the isoflavone clover extract (ICE) study: a randomized controlled trial. *JAMA.* 2003;290:207–214.

5. van de Weijer PHM, Barentsen R. Isoflavones from red clover (Promensil) significantly reduce menopausal hot flush symptoms compared with placebo. *Maturitas.* 2002;42:187–193.

6. Atkinson, C, Compston JE, Day NE, et al. The effects of phytoestrogen isoflavones on bone density in women: a double-blind, randomized, placebo-controlled trial. *Am J Clin Nutr.* 2004;79:326–333.

7. Schult TM, Ensrud KE, Blackwell T, et al. Effect of isoflavones on lipids and bone turnover markers in menopausal women. *Maturitas.* 2004;48:209–218.

Red Yeast Rice

Red yeast rice is a dietary staple in China, Japan, and Asian communities in the United States. Produced by fermenting the yeast *Monascus purpureus* with red rice, it has been used for centuries in China as a preservative, spice, and food colorant. Red yeast rice has also been used in China for thousands of years as a drug to improve circulation, relieve gastrointestinal distress, and prevent diarrhea. Currently, scientists are investigating the efficacy of red yeast rice to reduce serum cholesterol.

Red yeast rice was previously available in the United States as a supplement marketed under the name Cholestin (Pharmanex, Provo, Utah), and some of the research cited in this entry used this particular product. However, in 2001, a US district court ruled that because Cholestin contained the drug lovastatin, it could not be sold without a prescription. (Cholestin is still sold in the United States, but the lovastatin has been replaced with policosanol.) Other products, such as Choleser-Reg (HongQu) have also been cited by FDA to contain HMG-COA reductase inhibitors and as such have also been restricted for sale. However, it is likely that other similar products containing cholesterol-lowering medications are also on the market, but as yet have not been identified by FDA for legal action.

Media and Marketing Claims	Efficacy
Treats hypercholesterolemia	↑
Treats dyslipidemia related to HIV	NR

Safety

◆ Red yeast rice is generally well-tolerated when taken within dosage guidelines; reported side effects are mild gastritis, heartburn, flatulence, dizziness, and nausea (1).

◆ One case of anaphylaxis from the inhalation of red yeast rice has been reported (2).

Drug/Supplement Interactions

Because of the constituent lovastatin in red yeast rice products, patients taking this supplement to reduce cholesterol should notify their physician. The combined medications could lead to excess lowering of cholesterol levels. Also, because statins can affect liver function, the combined treatment may result in an exacerbation of the elevated liver enzyme levels.

Key Points

- ◆ Lovastatin, a popular cholesterol-lowering prescription drug, was isolated in Cholestin. According to the manufacturer, the product has been reformulated to respond to the FDA concern that it contains lovastatin. Several studies have shown red yeast rice to have lipid-lowering effects. However, HDL levels either remained the same or were elevated with use of Cholestin (when it contained red yeast rice).

- ◆ A pilot study indicated that red yeast rice was effective in treating individuals with dyslipidemia related to HIV. More studies are needed before a final recommendation can be made.

Food Sources

The only natural food source is red yeast rice itself.

Dosage Information/Bioavailability

Red yeast rice is available over the counter in capsule or tablet form. For treatment of hypercholesterolemia, research suggests a dosage of 1,200 mg twice a day (3). It is suspected that most of the red yeast rice supplements that have been shown to reduce cholesterol in the scientific literature have shown efficacy due to the statin content. The presence of statin in red yeast rice has been determined to be illegal under current FDA ruling; however, for most over-the-counter products there is no information as to the presence or absence of statins in each specific supplement. In addition, it is unknown whether other active constituents in red yeast rice are efficacious in lowering cholesterol independent of the statin content.

Relevant Research

Red Yeast Rice and Hypercholesterolemia

- ◆ To determine the effects of xuezhikang (an extract of red yeast rice) on high-fat meal postprandial triglyceride levels, 50 Chinese subjects with coronary heart disease were randomly assigned to receive 600 mg xuezhikang two times/day (300 mg Cholestin and 10 mg natural lovastatin per capsule) or no intervention (control group) for 6 weeks. Thirty-three men and 17 women (mean age 58.1 years) were enrolled in the study. All subjects received 4 weeks of dietary counseling prior to randomization as well as aspirin, metoprolol, and fosinopril. Fasting lipid profiles were evaluated at baseline and at the end of 6 weeks of intervention. Subjects also completed an oral high-fat tolerance test, in which 50 g of fat was consumed as part of an 800-kcal meal consumed over 15 minutes; blood samples were analyzed before the meal and 2, 4, and 6 hours after the meal. In the xuezhikang group, fasting serum lipids (total cholesterol, LDL, triglycerides, and Apo A1 and Apo B) decreased significantly from baseline levels whereas HDL levels increased significantly. At baseline, postprandial triglyceride levels were significantly elevated in response to the high-fat test meal; however, with the repeat meal challenge after 6 weeks of xuezhikang, serum triglyceride levels were significantly lower at all time points measured as compared with both baseline time-specific measures and as compared with the control group (4).

◆ In a double-blind, randomized, placebo-controlled trial to investigate the effects of Cholestin in the treatment of hyperlipidemia, 83 subjects with elevated fasting lipids received either 2.4 g red rice yeast or a control rice powder daily for 12 weeks. Subjects completed food frequency questionnaires at baseline and at weeks 8 and 12. Liver and kidney function were also analyzed at baseline and at week 12. Fasting lipids were measured at baseline and weeks 8, 9, 11, and 12. Total cholesterol, LDL cholesterol, and triglyceride levels all decreased significantly in the red yeast rice supplementation group compared with the placebo group. It is noteworthy that the treatment group consumed statistically significant less total fat, saturated fat, monounsaturated fat, and polyunsaturated fat at week 12 compared with baseline. Therefore, it is not possible to determine the effect of the supplement vs the effect of the reduced-fat diet. Subjects in the treatment group also consumed significantly less total fat and polyunsaturated fat than subjects in the control group (3).

Red Yeast Rice and Dyslipidemia Associated with HIV

◆ In a double-blind, randomized, placebo-controlled pilot study to investigate the safety and efficacy of Cholestin in the treatment of dyslipidemia associated with HIV, 12 subjects (6 per group) received either 1.2 g Cholestin or placebo for 8 weeks. Fasting serum lipid profiles, liver function tests, HIV-1 RNA, and CD4 cell counts were evaluated at baseline, and at weeks 2 and 8 of treatment. Both total cholesterol and LDL levels decreased significantly in the Cholestin group compared with the placebo group, whereas HDL and triglyceride levels did not change. No adverse events were associated with Cholestin (5).

References

1. Wang J, Lu A, Chi J. Multicenter clinical trial of the serum lipid-lowering effects of a *Monascus purpureus* (red yeast) rice preparation from traditional Chinese medicine. *Curr Ther Res.* 1997;58:964–978.
2. Wigger-Alberti W, Bauer A, Hipler UC, et al. Anaphylaxis due to Monascus purpureus-fermented rice (red yeast rice). *Allergy.* 1999;54:1330–1331.
3. Heber D, Yip I, Ashley JM, et al. Cholesterol-lowering effects of a proprietary Chinese red-yeast-rice dietary supplement. *Am J Clin Nutr.* 1999;69:231–236.
4. Zhao SP, Liu L, Cheng YC, et al. Effect of xuezhikang, a Cholestin extract, on reflecting postprandial triglyceridemia after a high-fat meal in patients with coronary heart disease. *Atherosclerosis.* 2003;168:375–380.
5. Keithley JK, Swanson B, Sha BE, et al. A pilot study of the safety and efficacy of Cholestin in treating HIV-related dyslipidemia. *Nutrition.* 2002;18:201–204.

Resveratrol

Resveratrol (3,5,4'-trihydroxy-*trans*-stilbene) is a natural constituent of several edible plant products, including grapes, eucalyptus, and peanuts. Because resveratrol is found in the skins of grapes, it is also a component of red wine. (Grape skins are not used in the production of white wine, so white wine has much less resveratrol than red wine does.) It was not until the early 1990s that researchers became interested in resveratrol as the agent responsible for "the French paradox"—the notion that in France, the intake of saturated fat is higher than in other European countries, but mortality from coronary heart disease is low. Although this notion has not been confirmed, animal studies have shown that resveratrol is effective at reducing inflammation and has some antitumor properties (1).

Media and Marketing Claims	Efficacy
Provides cardiovascular protection in humans	NR
Prevents cancer	NR

Safety

 ♦ No adverse reactions have been reported; however, little is known about the bioavailability of resveratrol in humans.

Drug/Supplement Interactions

Resveratrol inhibits platelet aggregation and may increase the risk of bleeding when taken in combination with anticoagulant/antiplatelet drugs.

Key Points

 ♦ Currently, all the studies with resveratrol have been completed using cell lines or animal models. Although no clinical trials have tested the efficacy of resveratrol treatment in humans, some epidemiological data suggest that resveratrol may play an important role in cardioprotection.
 ♦ The anti-inflammatory properties of resveratrol are thought to potentially reduce mortality from heart disease and cancer (2,3).
 ♦ In vitro data suggest that resveratrol may decrease cancer risk at several sites, including colon, lung, and basal cell carcinoma. In vivo data is currently lacking, and more studies are needed to determine the efficacy of resveratrol consumption for disease prevention.

Food Sources

Food	Resveratrol, mg/serving
Peanuts, boiled (1 cup)	0.32–1.28
Red wine (5 oz)	0.30–1.07
Red grapes (1 cup)	0.24–1.25
Red grape juice (5 oz)	0.17–1.30
Peanuts, raw (1 cup)	0.01–0.26
White wine (5 oz)	0.01–0.27

Source: Data are from reference 4.

Dosage Information/Bioavailability

Resveratrol supplements are available in capsule and tablet form in 10 to 200 mg doses. Due to a lack of human clinical trials, a therapeutic dosage has yet to be established.

Relevant Research

Resveratrol and Coronary Heart Disease

♦ Several epidemiological studies have indicated that moderate alcohol consumption has a cardioprotective effect (5,6). This protective effect has been shown to be conferred specifically from flavonoid-containing red wine (7). To this end, investigators have studied individual flavonoids in red wine to determine their cardioprotective roles. Both animal and cellular studies have shown resveratrol to have cardioprotective effects (8–10). Future efforts should focus on well-designed clinical trials to establish the usefulness of resveratrol as a cardioprotective agent.

Resveratrol and Cancer

♦ To characterize the chemopreventive activity of resveratrol, several in vitro experiments were done (11). Using the carrageenan-induced paw edema model, investigators demonstrated that resveratrol has anti-inflammatory properties. Resveratrol also inhibited free-radical formation in human promyelocytic leukemia (HL-60) cells treated with 12–0-tetradecanoylphorbol-13-acetate (TPA). In addition, resveratrol inhibited the mutagenic response in *Salmonella* TM677 cells treated with 7,12-dimethylbenz(a)anthracene (DMBA). In vivo studies in mice also demonstrated chemopreventive activity. In mice with tumor initiation by DMBA and promotion by TPA, resveratrol reduced the number of tumors formed in a dose-dependent manner. Resveratrol was shown to inhibit tumor initiation, tumor promotion, and tumor progression.

♦ Resveratrol has been shown to induce apoptosis and inhibit tumor growth in gastric and pancreatic cancer cell lines (12,13). In these cells, it acts in both a dose- and time-dependent manner. Resveratrol did not induce apoptosis in colon cancer cells, but it did inhibit tumor growth (14).

References

1. Hwang D, Fischer NH, Jang BC, et al. Inhibition of the expression of inducible cyclooxygenase and proinflammatory cytokines by sesquiterpene lactones in macrophages correlates with the inhibition of MAP kinases. *Biochem Biophys Res Commun.* 1996;226:810–818.
2. Chen Y, Tseng SH, Lai HS, et al. Resveratrol-induced cellular apoptosis and cell cycle arrest in neuroblastoma cells and antitumor effects on neuroblastoma in mice. *Surgery.* 2004;136:57–66.
3. Holmes-McNary M, Baldwin AS Jr. Chemopreventive properties of trans-resveratrol are associated with inhibition of activation of the IkappaB kinase. *Cancer Res.* 2000;60:3477–3483.
4. Linus Pauling Institute at Oregon State University. Micronutrient Information Center. Resveratrol. 2005. Available at: http://lpi.oregonstate.edu/infocenter/phytochemicals/resveratrol. *Accessed April* 30, 2006.
5. Rimm EB, Giovannucci EL, Willet WC, et al. Prospective study of alcohol consumption and risk of coronary disease in men. *Lancet.* 1991;338:464–468.
6. Klatsky AL. Epidemiology of coronary heart disease-influence of alcohol. *Alcohol Clin Exp Res.* 1994;18:88–96.
7. Seigneur M. Bonnet J, Dorian B, et al. Effect of consumption of alcohol, white wine, and red wine on platelet function and serum lipids. *J Appl Cardiol.* 1990;5:215–222.
8. Hung LM, Chen JK, Huang SS, et al. Cardioprotective effect of resveratrol, a natural antioxidant derived from grapes. *Cardiovasc Res.* 2000;47:549–555.
9. Pace-Asciak CR, Hahn S, Diamandis EP, et al. The red wine phenolics *trans*-resveratrol and quercetin block human platelet aggregation and eicosanoid synthesis: implications for protection against coronary heart disease. *Clin Chim Acta.* 1995;235:207–219.
10. Wu JM, Wang ZR, Hsieh TC, et al. Mechanism of cardioprotection by resveratrol, a phenolic antioxidant present in red wine. *Int J Mol Med.* 2001;1:8–17.
11. Jang M, Cai L, Udeani GO, et al. Cancer chemopreventive activity of resveratrol, a natural product derived from grapes. *Science.* 1997;275:218–220.
12. Zhou HB, Chen JJ, Wang WX, et al. Anticancer activity of resveratrol on implanted human primary gastric carcinoma cells in nude mice. *World J Gastroenterol.* 2005;11:280–284.
13. Ding XZ, Adrian TE. Resveratrol inhibits proliferation and induces apoptosis in human pancreatic cancer cells. *Pancreas.* 2002;25:e71–e76.
14. Schneider Y, Vincent F, Duranton B, et al. Anti-proliferative effect of resveratrol, a natural component of grapes and wine, on human colonic cancer cells. *Cancer Lett.* 2000;158:85–91.

Riboflavin. *See* Vitamin B-2 (Riboflavin).

Royal Jelly

Royal jelly is a milky substance secreted from the pharyngeal glands of young worker honeybees *(Apis mellifera)*. During the early stages of growth, female bee larvae feed on royal jelly, but only the queen bee continues to consume royal jelly while the other larvae become sexually immature worker bees. Because royal jelly causes the queen bee to become fertile, grow large, and live several years (compared with the lifespan of a few weeks for worker bees), some have extrapolated that royal jelly will have beneficial effects in humans.

Chemical analysis has shown that half of the dry weight of royal jelly is protein, with the remainder made up of free amino acids, fatty acids, sugars, and vitamins and minerals (specific quantities not reported). Royalisin, a protein, and 10-hydroxy-2-decenoic acid, a fatty acid, have been identified in royal jelly as potential antibiotic agents (1–3).

Media and Marketing Claims	Efficacy
Improves immunity	NR
Contributes to a healthy heart	NR
Reduces blood pressure	NR
Improves stamina; reduces fatigue	NR
Prevents cancer	NR
Reduces premenstrual symptoms	NR
Improves mental health, cognition	NR

Safety

- In a study using Femal (Natumin Pharma, Huskvarna, Sweden) (royal jelly supplement), subjects took 120 mg/day for 2 months without evidence of adverse events (4).
- There have been several reports of asthma attacks and anaphylaxis following ingestion of royal jelly (5–7). Testing of patients with these symptoms revealed that they were true IgE-mediated hypersensitivity reactions (8).
- According to a study of 461 subjects in Hong Kong who were reported royal jelly users, nine subjects (7%) reported 14 adverse reactions, such as eczema, rhinitis, acute asthma, urticaria. Subjects reporting adverse reactions also had a history of clinical allergies (9).
- Royal jelly is contraindicated in individuals with asthma or atopy. Specific allergic symptoms include rhinitis, acute asthma, eczema, conjunctivitis, pruritis, urticaria, and in some cases angioedema. Most symptoms occur within 2 hours of ingestion (7).
- Orally, short-term royal jelly is well-tolerated at a dosage of 12 mg/day.

Drug/Supplement Interactions

No reported adverse interactions

Key Points

- ◆ Although certain components of royal jelly may have antibacterial properties, much more research needs is needed to substantiate claims that royal jelly fights infection. It is also worthy to note that royal jelly was bactericidal to *Lactobacillus* and *Bifidobacteria,* which are considered to be beneficial to intestinal health. (*See* Acidophilus/*Lactobacillus Acidophilus* [LA].)

- ◆ Several poorly controlled trials (reported in journals that could not be accessed) are used to support claims that royal jelly benefits the cardiovascular system. However, there is no evidence from well-controlled clinical trials that royal jelly improves cardiovascular disease risk factors.

- ◆ A few animal studies have been published in recent years supporting a role for royal jelly in immunity, blood pressure control, and fatigue. These limited studies do not warrant use of royal jelly for these conditions, but instead offer preliminary data for future research.

- ◆ Preliminary data from a screening of the constituents in royal jelly to elicit the biological activities suggested that royal jelly has cytotoxic and antiproliferative activity against select cancer cell lines (10).

- ◆ One randomized, placebo-controlled study of royal jelly in premenstrual syndrome suggests efficacy; further research is warranted (4).

- ◆ There is no research testing the effectiveness of royal jelly on mental health and cognition.

- ◆ Given the number of asthmatic and anaphylactic reactions reported, royal jelly is contraindicated in individuals with a history of asthma or allergic reactions.

Dosage Information/Bioavailability

Royal jelly is often combined with ginseng, raw honey, bee pollen, and B vitamins in the form of a capsule or tablet. Royal jelly is usually sold in 1-g tablets containing approximately 30 to 150 mg royal jelly. In addition, royal jelly is a popular ingredient added to blended fruit beverages.

Relevant Research

Royal Jelly and Immunity and Antibacterial Properties

- ◆ Royal jelly contains an antibacterial protein recently identified as royalisin (0.3 mg/g of royal jelly). In an in vitro study, royalisin isolated from royal jelly was reported to have potent antibacterial activity against gram-positive bacteria (including *Clostridium, Corynebacterium, Leuconostoc, Staphylococcus, Lactobacillus, Bifidobacterium,* and *Streptococcus*) comparable with the effective concentrations of various antibiotics. (*Lactobacillus* and *Bifidobacterium* are considered beneficial bacteria in the colon.) Royalisin had no effect on gram-negative bacteria. The authors propose using royalisin as an antibacterial compound to preserve food (1).

- In a cell culture model, royal jelly was added to mouse macrophages previously stimulated with interferon-gamma, resulting in inhibition of several proinflammatory cytokines, including tumor necrosis factor-alpha, interleukin-6, and interleukin-1 (11).

- A study in mice found that royal jelly (1 g/kg) significantly decreased serum levels of antigen-specific IgE and inhibited histamine release from mast cells, resulting in suppression of immediate hypersensitivity reactions of ear skin (12).

Royal Jelly and Cardiovascular Disease

- A systematic review and meta-analysis were conducted examining the effect of royal jelly on atherosclerosis in 17 animal studies and nine human trials (5 placebo-controlled) in European and Asian journals. In the animal studies, royal jelly significantly decreased serum and liver total lipids and cholesterol levels in rats and rabbits and also retarded the formation of atheromas in rabbits fed a high-fat diet. Meta-analysis of the controlled human trials reported that royal jelly (in dosages ranging from 30 to 100 mg/day for 3 to 6 weeks) resulted in a significant reduction in total cholesterol levels and normalization of HDL and LDL in subjects with hyperlipidemia. The authors hypothesized that royal jelly may decrease reabsorption of cholesterol in the gastrointestinal tract and increase its excretion in the bile. However, the studies evaluated did not control subjects' dietary intake, weight, or use of medications, which would have skewed the overall results (13). (Note: None of the studies included in this analysis are available in English, so they were not directly evaluated for this book.)

Royal Jelly and Blood Pressure

- In a rat model of hypertension (spontaneously hypertensive rats), rats were given specific peptides isolated from protease-treated royal jelly "Protease N Amano" (Amano Enzyme Inc, Aichi, Japan) in an escalated dose approach. With a single dose of MIX and IY+VY+IVY peptides, systolic blood pressure decreased in a statistically significant, dose-dependent manner, and this decrease in blood pressure was sustained for a mean of 8 hours (14). Prematurely, the author concluded, "it is considered that intake of peptides, as a functional food would be beneficial for improving blood pressure in people with hypertension." This conclusion was made despite *any* human data of safety or efficacy for royal jelly in individuals with hypertension.

Royal Jelly and Fatigue

- In an experimental model of mouse fatigue, mice previously trained to swim were randomly assigned to receive royal jelly, royal jelly that had been stored under refrigeration for 7 days, or a control supplement just before a swim challenge. Mice were placed in water for a 15-minute swim, rested, and then swam again until they reached fatigue. The group receiving fresh royal jelly showed delayed fatigue onset as well as reduced lactic acid levels in muscle after exercise; this effect was not apparent with previously stored royal jelly (15). Because this is the only study of this type and no human studies have been published to date, further research is needed before recommendations for humans can be made.

Royal Jelly and Premenstrual Syndrome

◆ In a randomized, placebo-controlled, double-blind, crossover study of Femal (Natumin Pharma, Huskvarna, Sweden), a royal jelly–based supplement, 32 women with premenstrual symptoms were randomly assigned to Femal or placebo for two menstrual cycles, and then switched to the alternate treatment for two additional cycles. Several scales for quantifying premenstrual symptoms were applied. The royal jelly supplement resulted in significant improvements in several symptom inventories, including Premenstrual Tension Syndrome Observer score, irritability, edema, and overall well-being (4). In addition, women on Femal had less weight gain with menstrual cycling. Although this was a generally well-designed study, it was limited by the lack of a washout period between treatments and should be replicated with an added washout period of sufficient duration to ensure no carryover effects. In addition, more objective measures of premenstrual syndrome should be included.

References

1. Fujiwara S, Imai J, Fujiwara M, et al. A potent antibacterial protein in royal jelly. *J Biol Chem.* 1990;265:11333–11337.
2. Vittek J. Effect of royal jelly on serum lipids in experimental animals and humans with atherosclerosis. *Experientia.* 1995;51:927–935.
3. Palma MS. Composition of freshly harvested Brazilian royal jelly: identification of carbohydrates from the sugar fraction. *J Agricultural Res.* 1992;31:42–44.
4. Winther K, Hedman C. Assessment of the effects of the herbal remedy Femal on the symptoms of premenstrual syndrome: a randomized, double-blind, placebo-controlled study. *Curr Ther Res.* 2002;63:344–353.
5. Peacock S, Murray V, Turton C. Respiratory distress and royal jelly. *BMJ.* 1995;311: 1472.
6. Larporte JR, Ibaanez L, Vendrell L, et al. Bronchospasm induced by royal jelly. *Allergy.* 1996;51:440.
7. Harwood M, Harding S, Beasley R, et al. Asthma following royal jelly. *NZ Med J.* 1996;109:325.
8. Thien FC, Leung R, Baldo BA, et al. Asthma and anaphylaxis induced by royal jelly. *Clin Exp Allergy.* 1996;26:216–222.
9. Leung R, Ho A, Chan J, et al. Royal jelly consumption and hypersensitivity in the community. *Clin Exp Allergy.* 1997;27:333–336.
10. Salazar-Olivo LA, Paz-Gonzalez V. Screening of biological activities present in honeybee (*Apis mellifera*) royal jelly. *Toxicol In Vitro.* 2005;19:645–651.
11. Kohno K, Okamoto I, Sano O, et al. Royal jelly inhibits the production of proinflammatory cytokines by activated macrophages. *Biosci Biotechnol Biochem.* 2004;68:138–145.
12. Oka H, Emori Y, Kobayashi N, et al. Suppression of allergic reactions by royal jelly in association with the restoration of macrophage function and the improvement of Th1/Th2 cell responses. *Int Immunopharmacol.* 2001;1:521–532.

13. Leung R, Thien FC, Baldo B, et al. Royal jelly-induced asthma and anaphylaxis: clinical characteristics and immunologic correlations. *J Allergy Clin Immunol*. 1995;96: 1004–1007.

14. Tokunaga KH, Yoshida C, Suzuki KM, et al. Antihypertensive effect of peptides from royal jelly in spontaneously hypertensive rats. *Biol Pharm Bull*. 2004;27:189–192.

15. Kamakura M, Mitani N, Fukuda T, et al. Antifatigue effect of fresh royal jelly in mice. *J Nutr Sci Vitaminol (Tokyo)*. 2001;47:394–401.

S-adenosylmethionine (SAM-e)

S-adenosylmethionine (SAM-e) was first discovered in the 1950s, and approximately 20 years later was stabilized into a salt, which has been used in clinical investigations. SAM-e is synthesized in all living cells from methionine and adenine triphosphate (ATP) and is involved in a wide variety of metabolic reactions. The production of SAM-e is tied closely to folate and vitamin B-12 metabolism. SAM-e functions primarily in the transferring of methyl groups to substrates such as nucleic acids, proteins, polysaccharides, fatty acids, and phospholipids. After donating its methyl group, SAM-e is converted into S-adenosyl-homocysteine, which is hydrolyzed into adenosine and homocysteine. The homocysteine can be further converted into cysteine and indirectly into glutathione, both of which are intracellular antioxidants (1–4).

In Europe, where SAM-e is available as a drug, it has been investigated for its possible role in the management of osteoarthritis and depression. The mechanism of action behind the potential anti-inflammatory and antidepressant effects of SAM-e are not fully understood. It has been hypothesized that SAM-e stimulates the production of proteoglycans in cartilage that may cushion joints. There are numerous theories about how SAM-e may affect depression, including increased synthesis of the neurotransmitters serotonin, dopamine, and norepinephrine. SAM-e became available in the United States in March 1999 (1–4).

Media and Marketing Claims	Efficacy
Reduces arthritis symptoms	↑?
Reduces symptoms of fibromyalgia	NR
Reduces symptoms of depression	↑?
Improves liver health	↑?
Promotes a healthy gallbladder	NR

Safety

♦ In a controlled trial of SAM-e (1,600 mg/day for 19 days), a 65-year-old man with depression experienced a manic episode. The subject had no prior history of mania (5). A similar event occurred in an woman taking SAM-e at a dosage of 1,600 mg for

4 weeks (6). The authors of that study report that SAM-e was well-tolerated among other recipients and that the mania reversed with discontinuation of SAM-e.

◆ Mild gastrointestinal distress may occur at the beginning of treatment (4).

◆ Safety is well-demonstrated for use as long as 2 years.

Drug/Supplement Interactions

◆ Intravenous SAM-e taken with the antidepressant clomipramine (Anafranil) can result in serotonin syndrome.

◆ SAM-e taken with other antidepressants may speed onset of antidepressant action. Meperidine (Demerol), monamine oxidase inhibitors (MAOIs), pentazocine (Talwin), and tramdol (Ultram) may have additive sedative effects if taken with SAM-e.

◆ SAM-e may interact with levodopa (7).

Key Points

◆ Several controlled trials suggest that SAM-e may relieve symptoms of osteoarthritis, at least as effectively as traditional nonsteroidal anti-inflammatory drugs (NSAIDs). Further, SAM-e seems to be better tolerated, without the serious adverse effects on the gastrointestinal tract and cartilage that are associated with NSAID use. The Agency for Healthcare Research and Quality published a 2002 evidence report on SAM-e (8) that states that SAM-e seems to be effective for reducing arthritis pain. More clinical data are needed to determine whether SAM-e actually supports cartilage regeneration.

◆ Some evidence from a few trials suggests that SAM-e may relieve pain in individuals with fibromyalgia, although not all research agrees. More controlled research with larger numbers of subjects is needed before supplementation can be recommended to this population.

◆ Several studies of IV and oral supplementation demonstrate that SAM-e exerts antidepressant activity, at least as effectively as some tricyclic medications. However, SAM-e has not been tested against selective serotonin reuptake inhibitors such as fluoxetine (Prozac). Severely depressed individuals should be under the care of a health professional and should not self-medicate with SAM-e.

◆ Laboratory research and some clinical trials suggest that IV or oral SAM-e may protect against liver damage. In addition, individuals with advanced liver disease, especially alcoholic liver cirrhosis, who received a pharmaceutical preparation of SAM-e (AldoMet) had improved survival or delay of liver transplantation (9). Because more data are needed, individuals with liver disease should discuss SAM-e supplementation with their health care provider.

◆ Currently there is no research testing the effectiveness of SAM-e on gallbladder function.

♦ A review of the molecular, biological, and clinical aspects of SAM-e was published in the *American Journal of Clinical Nutrition* in 2002 (10).

Food Sources

None

Dosage Information/Bioavailability

SAM-e is sold in several forms wherein an additional compound (tosylate, disulfate tosylate, disulfate ditosylate, 1,4 butanedisulfate) is added for stability. Manufacturers typically recommend taking 400 to 1,200 mg per day. In most studies researchers have used enteric-coated tablets to promote maximum absorption. In an analysis of 13 brands of SAM-e by ConsumerLab.com, six brands did not contain the amount of SAM-e they purported to contain on their labels (11).

In animal experiments and human studies with small numbers of subjects, enteric-coated tablets of SAM-e increased plasma and synovial fluid levels of SAM-e (1). In one study, eight healthy men and women were given 400 mg SAM-e (in two enteric-coated tablets) after an overnight fast. Blood samples were collected before taking SAM-e, and 3, 6, and 9 hours afterwards. In women, SAM-e concentrations were 6- and 3.5-fold higher than baseline values after 3 and 6 hours, respectively. In men, peak levels occurred after 6 hours (3.7- fold higher than baseline) (1,12).

Relevant Research

SAM-e and Osteoarthritis

♦ In a randomized, double-blind, crossover study of SAM-e was compared with celecoxib (Celebrex) for the treatment of knee osteoarthritic pain. Sixty-one subjects were assigned to either (*a*) 600 mg SAM-e supplement twice daily for 8 weeks followed by 100 mg celecoxib for 8 weeks (*b*) celecoxib for 8 weeks followed by SAM-e for 8 weeks. Fifty-six subjects completed the study. After 4 weeks, celecoxib was associated with a greater reduction in pain than SAM-e, but by 8 weeks both agents demonstrated equal efficacy for reducing pain of osteoarthritis and both also showed significant reduction in pain from baseline (13). Given recent concerns with the long-term safety of Cox-2 inhibitors such as celecoxib, SAM-e may prove useful for treatment of knee osteoarthritis pain in some individuals.

♦ A meta-analysis of clinical trials assessing the efficacy of SAM-e for osteoarthritis was published in 2002. The analysis included 11 qualified studies published in MEDLINE, EMBASE, CAMPAIN, Scientific citation index, International Pharmaceutical Abstracts, the Cochrane Complementary Medicine Field Registry, NIH Office of Dietary Supplements Database, and/or Microindex. A total of 1,442 subjects (70% female) with a mean age of 60.3 years and reported history of osteoarthritis for a mean of 5.7 years were included in the analysis. The authors reported that SAM-e supplementation was associated with a 31% improvement in functional measures, and comparable to NSAIDs for reducing pain (14). The authors noted that the number of well-designed studies is limited.

♦ The Agency for Healthcare Research and Quality report supports a role for SAM-e in reducing pain in a manner generally equivalent to anti-inflammatory medications. Again, studies are limited in number (15).

♦ In a double-blind, placebo-controlled study, 81 individuals (ages 40 to 85 years) with knee osteoarthritis were randomly assigned to receive daily IV bolus of 400 mg SAM-e for 5 days followed by either (*a*) an oral enteric-coated SAM-e tablets (200 mg × 3) for 23 days or (*b*) an IV placebo for 5 days followed by oral placebo for 23 days. All subjects participated in a 7-day washout period before the study. Acetaminophen use was permitted and recorded throughout the study, but no other analgesic or antiarthritic medications were allowed. Six times during the study (enrollment, after washout, after second and fourth IV injections, and after 9 days and 23 days of oral therapy), subjects completed the Stanford Health Assessment Questionnaire disability and pain scales and visual analogue scales for rest and walking pain. Physicians assessed swelling, tenderness, and range of motion. Subjects were assigned to one of two groups for statistical analysis: Group A, subjects with mild arthritis (n = 48), and Group B, subjects with more severe global arthritis (n = 33). In Group A, the SAM-e-treated group had a significantly greater reduction in overall pain and rest pain, but no other differences in other parameters when compared with the placebo group. In Group B, the response to treatment did not differ between groups. However, the authors noted that baseline characteristics of the two subgroups of subjects in Group B differed significantly and thus may have flawed the results. Four patients treated with SAM-e and one treated with placebo withdrew from the study due to adverse events (neurological symptoms and chest pain) during the IV treatment. There were no significant differences in laboratory studies (complete blood count, white cell differential count, urinalysis, stool hemoccult) between groups (16).

♦ In a double-blind, comparative, multicenter study, 734 subjects with clinically diagnosed hip or knee osteoarthritis were randomly assigned to receive 1,200 mg SAM-e, 750 mg naproxen (NSAID), or a placebo daily for 30 days. Subjects were instructed not to use any pain medications during the study. All subjects underwent clinical exams at the beginning, after 2 weeks, and at the end of treatment. The following parameters were assessed: (*a*) night pain and day pain, and (*b*) degree of difficulty doing specific activities, such as standing up from a chair, going upstairs, and walking on an even floor. At the end of the study, physicians and subjects each evaluated the efficacy and tolerability of treatments. Forty subjects withdrew from the study because of side-effects (10 withdrew from the SAM-e group, 17 from the naproxen group, and 13 from the placebo group). SAM-e and naproxen exerted the same analgesic activity, and both were significantly more effective than the placebo. The efficacy of SAM-e and naproxen were rated the same by subjects and physicians; ratings for both were statistically superior to the placebo. The tolerability of SAM-e was significantly better than for naproxen and did not differ from the placebo, according to both subject and physician evaluations. Side effects (gastrointestinal, headache, dizziness, hypersomnia, insomnia) occurred in 28% of the SAM-e group, 47% of the naproxen group, and 25% of the placebo group (17).

◆ In a double-blind, comparative trial, 48 subjects (mean age = 65 years) with diagnosed knee osteoarthritis were randomly assigned to receive enteric-coated tablets of SAM-e (1,200 mg) or piroxicam (20 mg) (an NSAID) for 84 days. A 7-day single-blind initial washout period preceded the trial to exclude subjects demonstrating a placebo-effect. Pain, active and passive motility, morning stiffness, and distance covered before the onset of pain were assessed at the beginning, at the end, and every 28 days of the study. The residual therapeutic activity of SAM-e and piroxicam was assessed for 56 days posttreatment. During this time, all subjects were given placebos and clinical parameters were reevaluated every 14 days. Forty-five subjects completed the study. Both SAM-e and piroxicam demonstrated significant improvement in the total pain score after 28 days of treatment. The other clinical parameters (morning stiffness, distance walked before the onset of pain, active and passive motility) improved significantly in both groups after approximately day 56. There were no significant differences in efficacy or tolerability between groups. Clinical improvement was maintained significantly longer in subjects treated with SAM-e than in patients taking piroxicam. The authors noted that the clinical effect of SAM-e seems to be delayed compared with piroxicam, but that its effect lasts longer after discontinuation of therapy (18).

◆ In a double-blind, comparative, multicenter study, 150 subjects (ages 45 to 75 years) with hip and knee osteoarthritis were randomly assigned to receive 1,200 mg SAM-e or 1,200 mg ibuprofen (NSAID) daily for 30 days. There was an initial washout period of 5 days for all subjects. Subjective parameters of pain (rest pain, night pain, loading pain, active movement pain, passive movement pain, and muscle spasm) were recorded at baseline and at days 16 and 31. At the end of the trial, physicians and subjects rated efficacy and tolerability. Both groups reported improvement in subjective pain symptoms. Likewise, physician and subject evaluation of treatments were favorable for both SAM-e and ibuprofen. There were no differences in laboratory tests between groups. Minor side effects were reported in five subjects treated with SAM-e and in 16 subjects taking ibuprofen (19).

SAM-e and Fibromyalgia

◆ In a double-blind, placebo-controlled study in Denmark, 44 subjects with primary fibromyalgia were randomly assigned to receive 800 mg SAM-e or a placebo daily for 6 weeks. Subjects were discouraged from using analgesic or anti-inflammatory drugs. They were permitted to use acetaminophen if needed. Use of drugs was documented. There was no washout period. Tender point score, isokinetic muscle strength, disease activity, subjective symptoms (visual analog scale), mood parameters, and side effects were evaluated. There were significant improvements in disease activity, pain experienced during the last week, fatigue, morning stiffness, and mood (as evaluated by the Face Scale) in the subjects taking SAM-e compared with those taking the placebo. There were no differences between groups in the tender point score, isokinetic muscle strength, mood evaluated by the Beck Depression Inventory, and side effects (20).

◆ In a double-blind, placebo-controlled, crossover study, 34 subjects with primary fibromyalgia received intravenously 600 mg SAM-e or a placebo daily for 10 days. There were no significant differences in improvement in the primary outcome (tender point change between the two treatment groups). There was a trend toward improvement of subjective pain at rest, pain on movement, and overall well-being in the SAM-e group, but this was not significant. There was no effect on isokinetic muscle strength, Zerrsen self-assessment questionnaire, or mood evaluated by the Face Scale (21).

◆ In a double-blind, placebo-controlled, crossover study, 25 subjects (ages 33 to 55 years) with primary fibromyalgia were randomly assigned to receive intravenously 200 mg SAM-e or placebo daily for 21 days, followed by a 2-week washout period before switching to the other treatment. Pain (counting the number of subjective painful areas and the number of muscle and tendon tender points) and depression (using the Hamilton Depression Rating Scale and an Italian questionnaire for the self-evaluation of depression [SAD]) were assessed at entry, at days 21 and 35, and at study's end. Six patients withdrew from the study for unexplained reasons; two other subjects withdrew after abscesses developed at their injection sites. SAM-e treatment resulted in a significant decrease in pain, evaluated as the number of trigger points plus painful sites. Placebo treatment had no effect on these parameters. Scores on both the Hamilton and SAD scales decreased significantly after SAM-e treatment, but not with the placebo (22).

SAM-e and Depression

◆ The results of two double-blind, placebo-controlled, multicenter studies testing the use of SAM-e for depression have been reported together in one article (23). Subjects with previously diagnosed depression were randomly assigned to either SAM-e (1,600 mg by mouth in one study, 400 mg intramuscular (IM) in the other in the other) or 150 mg imipramine per day. All subjects also received placebo daily throughout the study. In the study comparing oral SAM-e with oral imipramine, 281 patients were randomly assigned to one of the two treatments, and treatment was continued for a period of 6 weeks. In the IM SAM-e vs oral imipramine study, 295 patients received study treatment for a period of 4 weeks (subjects were given placebo daily as well keep IM vs oral administration routes blinded). Outcome was based on the Hamilton Rating Depression Scale. In both studies, SAM-e was as effective as imipramine in reducing depressive symptoms from baseline ($P < .001$), but did not differ significantly across treatment groups. The number and severity of adverse events favored SAM-e use; subjects receiving imipramine were more likely to report dry mouth, constipation, and tachycardia than those in the SAM-e group.

◆ In a study of subjects with major depression disorder unresponsive or partially responsive to serotonin uptake inhibitors or venlafaxine, SAM-e was provided open-label at a dosage of 800 to 1,600 mg/day for 6 weeks as adjuvant therapy with the medication. Thirty individuals were enrolled in the study. Addition of SAM-e was associated with improved clinical response in 50% of subjects (24). Although promising, this research will need to be replicated before use is recommended in this clinical context.

♦ A meta-analysis of double-blind, randomized trials conducted between 1972 and 1992 on the impact on depression from parenteral or oral SAM-e compared with placebo or tricyclic antidepressants (TCAs) yielded six studies (n = 200 subjects) of SAM-e vs placebo, three of which used oral SAM-e tablets. Four trials were selected for meta-analysis of SAM-e compared with TCAs (n = 201 subjects), with two trials using oral SAM-e tablets. Results demonstrated a greater response rate with SAM-e compared with the placebo, with a global effect size ranging between 17% and 38%, depending on the definition of response. SAM-e had an antidepressant effect comparable to standard TCAs. The authors noted that the heterogeneity of the placebo-controlled trials made data interpretation difficult (25).

♦ A double-blind, placebo-controlled study included 80 women (ages 45 to 59 years) between 6 and 36 months after either natural menopause or hysterectomy and clinically diagnosed with major depressive disorder or dysthmia per *Diagnostic and Statistical Manual of Mental Disorders*-III-R criteria. Subjects were randomly assigned to receive 1,600 mg SAM-e or placebo daily for 30 days. All subjects were given placebos in an initial washout period of 1 week. Treatment efficacy was evaluated using the Hamilton Depression Rating Scale (HAM-D) and the Rome Depression Inventory (RDI) at baseline and at days 10 and 30. Additionally, patients completed the Minnesota Multiphasic Personality Inventory (MMPI), at baseline and day 30. At the end of the study, clinicians evaluated improvement using the Clinician Global Impression Improvement Scale (CGI-I). Ten patients in each treatment group dropped out for reduced compliance (60 completed the study). There were no significant differences at baseline in HAM-D scores between groups. From day 10 of the study, depressive symptoms improved significantly as measured by the HAM-D, RDI, MMPI, and CGI-I in subjects treated with SAM-e compared with subjects taking the placebo (26).

SAM-e and Liver Function

♦ The role of SAM-e in hepatic function has been described (27), and it has been suggested that SAM-e deficiency related to reduced synthesis is central to the pathogenesis of liver injury (28).

♦ In a study of individuals with cancer receiving chemotherapy, 50 patients with newly diagnosed chemotherapy-induced liver dysfunction were provided 1,600 mg SAM-e daily for the duration of their chemotherapy (duration varied among patients). SAM-e was associated with a significant improvement in liver function tests (including AST, ALT, and LDH) within one week of supplementation and remained significantly reduced through the remainder of the chemotherapy despite multiple courses of chemotherapy (29). This study is limited because supplementation was not placebo-controlled, nor was there a control group identified. Further studies in this area are needed.

♦ In a double-blind, placebo-controlled, multicenter trial in Spain, 123 adults (106 men, 17 women, mean age 51 years) with alcoholic liver cirrhosis were randomly assigned to receive 1,200 mg SAM-e or a placebo daily for 2 years. Seventy-five patients were in Child-Turcotte grading class A, 40 in class B, and 8 in class C. (Class A indicates least severe liver disease, and class C indicates more advanced liver disease.) There were no significant differences between the treatment and placebo groups with regard to age, sex, previous episodes of major cirrhosis complications, Child-Turcotte classification, or liver function tests. The overall mortality and liver transplantation rates were not significantly different between the placebo group and the SAM-e group. However, when subjects in Child-Turcotte class C (more advanced liver disease) were excluded from analysis, the overall mortality and transplantation rates were significantly reduced in the subjects taking SAM-e compared with the placebo group. In addition, the differences between the groups in the 2-year survival curves (time to death or liver transplantation) also significantly favored SAM-e (9).

♦ Two review articles discuss animal and human studies that reported parenteral SAM-e prevents or reverses hepatotoxicity due to drugs and chemicals such as alcohol, acetaminophen, steroids, or lead (30,31). Researchers in one review discussed data indicating that individuals with cirrhosis may have an acquired metabolic block in hepatic conversion of methionine to SAM-e, and they proposed that exogenous SAM-e may be an essential nutrient in these patients to normalize overall hepatic transmethylation and transsulfuration activity (31).

♦ In one study in baboons, IV SAM-e attenuated alcohol-induced liver injury (32).

References

1. Stramentinoli G. Pharmacologic aspects of S-adenosylmethionine. *Am J Med.* 1987;83(Suppl 5A):S35-S42.
2. Baldessarini RJ. Neuropharmacology of S-adenosyl-L-methionine. *Am J Med.* 1987;83(Suppl 5A):S95-S103.
3. Bottiglieri T, Hyland K, Reynolds EH. The clinical potential of ademetionine (S-adeosylmethionine) in neurological disorders. *Drugs.* 1994;48:137–152.
4. Chavez M. SAMe: S-adenosylmethionine. *Am J Health Syst Pharm.* 2000;57:119–123.
5. Kagan BL, Sultzer DL, Rosenlicht N, et al. Oral S-adenosylmethionine in depression: a randomized, double-blind, placebo-controlled trial. *Am J Psychiatry.* 1990;147:591–595.
6. Goren JL, Stoll AL, Damico KE, et al. Bioavailability and lack of toxicity of S-adenosyl-L-methionine (SAMe) in humans. *Pharmacotherapy.* 2004;24:1501–1507.
7. Charlton CG, Crowell B. Parkinson's disease like effects of S-adenosyl-L-methionine: effects of L-dopa. *Pharmacol Biochem Behav.* 1992;43:423–431.
8. Hardy M, Coulter I, Morton SC, et al. S-*Adenosyl-L-Methionine for Treatment of Depression, Osteoarthritis, and Liver Disease. Summary, Evidence Report/ Technology Assessment*:

Number 64. Rockville, Md: Agency for Healthcare Research and Quality; 2002. AHRQ Publication No. 02-E033. Available at: http://www.ahrq.gov/clinic/epcsums/samesum. htm. Accessed March 17, 2006.

9. Mato JM, Camara J, Fernandez de Paz J, et al. S-adenosylmethionine in alcoholic liver cirrhosis: a randomized, placebo-controlled double-blind, multicenter trial. *J Hepatol.* 1999;30:1081–1089.

10. Lieber CS, Packer L. S-Adenosylmethionine: molecular, biological, and clinical aspects—an introduction. *Am J Clin Nutr.* 2002;76(suppl):S1148-S1150.

11. ConsumerLab.com. Product Review: SAMe. Available at: http://www.consumerlab. com/results/same.asp. Accessed July 7, 2002.

12. Giulidori P, Stamentinoli G. A radioenzymatic method for S-adenosyl-L-methionine determination in biological fluids. *Anal Biochem.* 1984;137:217–220.

13. Najm WI, Reinsch S, Hoehler F, et al. S-adenosyl methionine (SAMe) versus celecoxib for the treatment of osteoarthritis symptoms: a double-blind crossover trial. *BMC Musculoskelet Disord.* 2004;5:6.

14. Soeken KL, Lee WL, Bausell RB, et al. Safety and efficacy of S-adenosylmethionine (SAMe) for osteoarthritis. *J Fam Pract.* 2002;51:425–430.

15. Agency for Healthcare Research and Quality. S-Adenosyl-L-Methionine (SAMe) for Depression, Osteoarthritis, and Liver Disease. 2002. AHRQ publication 02-E033. Available at: http://www.ahrq.gov/clinic/tp/sametp.htm. Accessed October 28, 2005.

16. Bradley JD, Flusser D, Katz BP, et al. A randomized, double-blind, placebo-controlled trial of intravenous loading with S-adenosylmethionine (SAM) followed by oral SAM therapy in patients with knee osteoarthritis. *J Rheumatol.* 1994;21:905–911.

17. Caruso I, Pietrogrande V. Italian double-blind multicenter study comparing S-Adenosylmethionine, naproxen, and placebo in the treatment of degenerative joint disease. *Am J Med.* 1987;83(Suppl 5A):66–71.

18. Maccagno A, Di Giorgio EE, Caston OL, et al. Double-blind controlled clinical trial of oral S-adenosylmethionine versus piroxicam in knee osteoarthritis. *Am J Med.* 1987;83(Suppl 5A):72–77.

19. Marcolongo R, Girodano N, Colombo B, et al. Double-blind, multicenter study of the activity of S-adenosylmethionine in hip and knee osteoarthritis. *Curr Ther Res.* 1985;37:82–94.

20. Jacobsen S, Danneskiold-Samsoe B, Andersen RB. Oral S-adensoylmethionine in primary fibromyalgia. Double-blind clinical evaluation. *Scand J Rheumatol.* 1991;20:294–302.

21. Volkman H, Norregaard J, Jacobsen S, et al. Double-blind, placebo-controlled crossover study of intravenous S-adenosyl-L-methionine in patients with fibromyalgia. *Scand J Rheumatol.* 1997;26:206–211.

22. Tavoni A, Vitali C, Bombardieri S, et al. Evaluation of S-adenosylmethionine in primary fibromyalgia. A double-blind crossover study. *Am J Med.* 1987;83(Suppl 5A): 107–110.

23. Delle Chiaie R, Pancheri P, Scapicchio P. Efficacy and tolerability of oral and intramuscular S-adenosyl-Lmethionine 1,4-butanedisulfonate (SAMe) in the treatment of

major depression: comparison with imipramine in multicenter studies. *Am J Clin Nutr.* 2002;76(Suppl):S1172-S1176.

24. Alpert JE, Papakostas G, Mischoulon D, et al. S-adenosyl-L-methionine (SAMe) as an adjunct for resistant major depressive disorder: an open trial following partial or non response to selective serotonin reuptake inhibitors or venlafaxine. *J Clin Psychopharmacol.* 2004;24:661–664.

25. Bressa GM. S-adenosyl-l-methionine (SAMe) as antidepressant: meta-analysis of clinical studies. *Acta Neurol Scand.* 1994;154:7–14.

26. Salmaggi P, Bressa GM, Nicchia G, et al. Double-blind, placebo-controlled study of S-adenosyl-L-methionine in depressed postmenopausal women. *Psychother Psychosom.* 1993;59:34–40.

27. Lieber CS. S-Adenosyl-L-methionine: its role in the treatment of liver disorders. *Am J Clin Nutr.* 2002;76(Suppl):S1183–S1187.

28. Martinez-Chantar ML, Garcia-Trevijano ER, Latasa MU, et al. Importance of a deficiency in S-adenosyl-L-methionine synthesis in the pathogenesis of liver injury. *Am J Clin Nutr.* 2002;76(Suppl):S1117–S1182.

29. Santini D, Vincenzi B, Massacesi C, et al. S-adenosylmethionine (AdoMet) supplementation for treatment of chemotherapy-induced liver injury. *Anticancer Res.* 2003;23:5173–5179.

30. Friedel HA, Goa KL, Benfield P. S-adenosyl-l-methionine. A review of its pharmacological properties and therapeutic potential in liver dysfunction and affective disorders in relation to its physiological role in cell metabolism. *Drugs.* 1989;38:389–416.

31. Chawla RK, Bonkovsky HL, Galambos JT. Biochemistry and pharmacology of S-adenosyl-l-methionine and rationale for its use in liver disease. *Drugs.* 1990;40:98–110.

32. Lieber CS, Casini A, DeCarli LM, et al. S-adenosyl-l-methionine attenuates alcohol liver injury in the baboon. *Hepatology.* 1990;11:165–172.

St John's Wort *(Hypericum perforatum)*

St John's wort (SJW; *Hypericum perforatum*), a yellow-flowering plant, has been used in traditional folk medicine for hundreds of years to treat a variety of disorders. Recently, the herb has gained popularity as a remedy for mild to moderate depression. The mechanism by which SJW might affect depression is unknown. One theory is that the herb may increase serotonin levels similar to serotonin reuptake inhibitors. It may also inhibit reuptake of monoamines, dopamine noradrenaline, and neurotransmitters GABA and glutamate (1). Another theory suggests that SJW may reduce cortisol levels.

SJW contains many compounds, including naphthodianthrones (hypericin and pseudohypericin), flavonoids (quercetin, quercitrin, hyperin), phloroglucinols (hyperforin and adhyperforin), essential oil, and xanthones (2). Although the active components have not been identified, some researchers believe its effects may be caused by hypericin, pseudohypericin, or hyperforin.

Media and Marketing Claims	Efficacy
Alleviates depression	↑?
Promotes emotional well-being	NR

Safety

♦ Studies indicate daily use of 900 mg supplementation for as long as 8 weeks is safe.

♦ Reported side effects with SJW include gastrointestinal symptoms, dizziness, headache, allergic reactions, and fatigue (3). Rash, insomnia, and hypoglycemia have also been reported with regular use. A review of adverse events identified in the context of randomized trials suggests that adverse events are comparable to placebo, with dropout rates associated with adverse events ranging from 0% to 5.7% (4).

♦ SJW may cause photosensitivity, especially in fair-skinned individuals, at dosages more than 2 g/day.

♦ Individuals with Alzheimer's disease should not use SJW because it may cause psychosis or increase dementia.

♦ Case reports of SJW-associated generalized anxiety disorder have been reported and may be associated with acute discontinuation of the supplement (5).

♦ Discontinuation of SJW has also been associated with insomnia, weight loss, and headache.

♦ SJW may interact adversely with anesthesia (hypotension); discontinue use of SJW prior to surgery.

Drug/Supplement Interactions

♦ Do not combine SJW with antidepressant medications (tricyclics, serotonin reuptake inhibitors, monoamine oxidase inhibitors; selective serotonin reuptake inhibitors [sertraline/paroxetine], nefazodone) to prevent possible dangerous additive effects.

♦ SJW seems to decrease the effectiveness of several prescription drugs, including oral contraceptives, protease inhibitor indinavir (used in HIV treatment), theophylline (bronchodilator), digoxin, and numerous other drugs for epilepsy, heart disease, depression, immunosuppression, psychosis (amitriptylene, alprazolam, clopidogrel, simvastatin, theophylline, warfarin, etc). The negative drug interactions are believed to be due to SJW's inhibition of human cytochrome P450 enzymes (6–9).

♦ There have been several reports of organ rejection after transplant when SJW is combined with the immunosuppressant drug cyclosporin A (10–14). In addition, SJW may decrease levels of digoxin and indinavir (protease inhibitor used to treat HIV) (15,16).

♦ In addition to possibly reducing the efficacy of oral contraceptives, SJW may contribute to midcycle breakthrough bleeding (17).

- Following the release of reports of drug interactions, the FDA warned health professionals of potential adverse effects of using SJW with other drugs that are metabolized via the P450 enzyme pathway, including oral contraceptives, antiepileptics, anti-inflammatories, antidepressants, antivirals, some antiretrovirals, benzodiazepines, beta-blockers, and several other drugs for cardiovascular diseases.

- The effects of taking SJW in addition to standard antidepressant medications have not been studied. It has been suggested that this combination could result in "serotonin syndrome," a condition characterized by flushing, lethargy, confusion, agitation, tremors, and sweating. A washout period of 2 weeks has been recommended to prevent the possible dangerous additive effects of psychoactive drugs and SJW (18).

- Cytochrome P450 (CYP450) activity in the elderly may be decreased, making them more susceptible to herb-mediated changes in CYP450 activity and adversely affecting drug efficacy and/or toxicity, especially with SJW use. Twelve healthy individuals ages 60 to 76 years were randomly assigned using an open-label random sequence design to receive four botanical supplements, SJW, garlic oil, *Panax* ginseng, and ginkgo biloba, for a period of 28 days each followed by a 30-day washout period, to test the effects of each supplement on CYP450 enzyme activity. A significant induction of CYP34A (approximately 140%) and CYP2E1 activity (approximately 28%) were observed when pre- and post-SJW phenotypic ratios were compared (19).

- Increased risk for photosensitivity when combined with aminolevulinic acid.

Key Points

- Clinical trials in Europe have suggested that, compared with placebo, SJW may improve symptoms of mild to moderate depression. SJW also may have similar benefits and fewer side effects compared with antidepressants. Some have criticized that the dosages, preparations, and the inclusion criteria have not been consistent in clinical research of SJW.

- Studies in patients with major depression are contradictory. Much more evidence is needed before SJW can be recommended as an alternative to antidepressants for severe depression. Individuals with severe depression should be under the care of a mental health professional.

- There is no evidence that SJW elevates mood or improves emotional well-being in individuals without clinical depression.

- SJW negatively interacts with several prescription drugs. Patients and physicians need to be aware of these interactions to prevent possible adverse effects.

Food Sources

None

Dosage Information/Bioavailability

SJW dried extract is available in tablets, capsules, teas, powders, and tinctures. It is also commonly added to products that contain valerian root, kava, or black cohosh. Labels suggest protecting the herb from heat or light to preserve its active components. Most clinical studies used 300 mg SJW extract as tablets (standardized to 0.3% hypericin) taken three times per day (900 mg extract total). In one study, ingestion of 300 to 900 mg SJW extract increased plasma levels of hypericin and pseudohypericin in 2.0 to 2.6 hours and 0.3 to 1.1 hours, respectively. Plasma levels reached a steady state after 4 days of supplementation (20).

Relevant Research

St John's Wort and Mild to Moderate Depression

◆ A meta-analysis conducted in 2005 included 37 double-blind and randomized studies using SJW to treat depression (21). Large studies among patients with major depression generally showed limited effect, whereas smaller studies among patients with mild to moderate depression support efficacy. The authors conclude that inconsistencies and confusion remain and that there is some concern about report bias toward negative trials in recent years as the reports about interactions between SJW and numerous medications gain attention.

◆ A comparison of two meta-analyses assessing the efficacy of SJW for the treatment of depression was conducted in the United Kingdom. Authors first reproduced an earlier meta-analysis (n = 15 studies, 7 with nonsignificant results) and then expanded the meta-analysis to include three more recent studies of the topic (n = 18 studies, 10 with nonsignificant results) (22). All studies were conducted between 1979 and 2003, and were conducted in a randomized, placebo-controlled, double-blind fashion and included an intent-to-treat analytical approach. Both meta-analyses resulted in small but significant overall differences in depression as measured using Hamilton Rating Scale for Depression (HAMD) as compared with placebo. However, the statistical analysis also showed that with larger study populations and an increased number of trials included in the meta-analysis, the efficacy of SJW for depression was less pronounced.

◆ In a double-blind study of 140 individuals with moderate depression, subjects were randomly assigned to either 900 mg SJW or placebo for 6 weeks. Nineteen were excluded from the study because of protocol violation. The HAMD score was significantly lower over time with SJW. Depression scores improved significantly in the SJW group compared with the placebo group (23).

◆ In a double-blind study using SJW extract to treat acute severe depression, 251 adults were randomly assigned to 900 mg SJW (SJW extract labeled as WS 5570) or 300 mg SJW three times/day or paroxetine daily for 6 weeks. In this study, after 42 days of supplementation, the WS 5570 was as effective as the prescribed medication in reducing depression score (HAMD), and the supplement was associated with fewer adverse events (24).

◆ In a double-blind, parallel-design, multicenter study in Germany, 324 subjects were randomly assigned to receive 500 mg hypericum extract ZE 117 or 150 mg imipramine (antidepressant drug) for 6 weeks. Main outcome measures included HAMD, Clinical Global Impression-Severity scale (CGI-S), and patient's global impression scale. Both groups improved on the main outcome measures, with no significant differences between groups. However, the mean score on the anxiety-somatization subscale of the HAMD reported a significant improvement with SJW compared with imipramine. Tolerability was also significantly better with SJW. The authors concluded that SJW is therapeutically equivalent to imipramine in treating mild to moderate depression, but SJW seems to be better tolerated (25).

◆ In a double-blind, placebo-controlled multicenter trial in Germany, 263 individuals with moderate depression were randomly assigned to receive 1,050 mg SJW extract (divided into three doses/day), 100 mg imipramine (in three doses/day), or a placebo daily for 8 weeks. SJW was significantly more effective in reducing HAMD scores than the placebo, and as effective as imipramine. No differences between SJW and imipramine were found for Hamilton Rating Scale for Anxiety (HAMA) scores, Clinical Global Impression scales, or the Zung self-rating depression scale. Quality of life was more improved with both active treatments compared with the placebo. The rates of adverse events were similar between SJW and the placebo, which were less than that of the imipramine group (26).

◆ In a double-blind, parallel-design study, 240 subjects were randomly assigned to receive 500 mg SJW extract (Hypericum ZE 117) or 40 mg of the serotonin reuptake inhibitor fluoxetine (Prozac) for 6 weeks. Both groups had reductions in mean HAMD scores, with no significant differences between the treatments. However, SJW use was associated with a significantly superior score on the mean Clinical Global Impression Severity scale. Incidence of adverse events was significantly less with SJW (8%) compared with fluoxetine (23%) (27).

◆ In a double-blind, parallel, placebo-controlled study, 147 outpatients with clinically diagnosed mild or moderate depression were randomly assigned to receive one of three treatments: (*a*) a placebo, (*b*) 300 mg standardized SJW extract (5% hyperforin), or (*c*) 300 mg extract (0.5% hyperforin) for 42 days. Depressive symptoms were assessed using the HAMD on days 0, 7, 14, 28, and 42. Depression was also rated by the investigators at the beginning and end of the study using the Clinical Global Impression scale. In the group taking extract containing 5% hyperforin, depressive symptoms improved significantly (according to HAMD scores) compared with the placebo, whereas the clinical impact of 0.5% hyperforin extract did not differ from the placebo. The authors concluded that the therapeutic effect of SJW depends on its hyperforin content (28).

◆ In a double-blind, comparative study, 165 subjects with mild to moderate depression were randomly assigned to receive 900 mg standardized SJW or 75 mg tricyclic amitriptyline (antidepressant) for 6 weeks. There were no significant differences between groups on the HAMD response rate, although there was a tendency for a better response in the amitriptyline group. Decreases in the total HAMD and

Montgomery-Asberg scores showed a significant advantage for amitriptyline, but only at week 6. Fewer adverse events occurred with subjects using SJW (37% of subjects) compared with amitriptyline (64%), specifically in relation to anticholinergic and central nervous system side effects (dry mouth, drowsiness, dizziness). Other reported side effects included headache, constipation, and nausea/vomiting (29).

St John's Wort and Major Depression

◆ In a double-blind, placebo-controlled, multicenter study in the United States, 200 patients with major depression were randomly assigned to receive either SJW extract (900 mg/day for 4 weeks, increased to 1,200 mg/day in the absence of response), or a placebo for 8 weeks. All subjects completed a 1-week, single-blind, run-in of placebo use prior to treatment. The main outcome measure was rate of change on HAMD and secondary measures included the Beck Depression Inventory, (HAMA), the Global Assessment of Function scale, and the Clinical Global Impression-Severity and Improvement scales. There were no significant differences in any of the assessment scales. The proportion of subjects responding was not different between groups. The number reaching remission of illness was significantly higher with SJW (14.3%) than the placebo (4.9%) group, although overall numbers were considered low. Treatment was well-tolerated, with the exception of significantly greater occurrence of headache with SJW compared with the placebo. The authors concluded that SJW was not effective for major depression in this study (30).

◆ In a double-blind, comparative, multicenter study, 209 patients (ages 18 to 70 years) with clinically diagnosed severe depression were randomly assigned to receive 1,800 mg standardized SJW extract divided into three doses or 150 mg imipramine (antidepressant)/day for 6 weeks. Response was defined as a reduction of at least 50% of the HAMD score. Both treatments were effective, as measured by a reduction in the scale, but not statistically equivalent within an a priori–defined 25% interval of deviation (imipramine was more effective). Both treatments were statistically equivalent, as measured by global assessment of efficacy by the investigators and patients. The percentage of adverse effects (ie, dry mouth, gastric symptoms, sedation, sweating, constipation) was statistically significantly greater in imipramine-treated subjects (41% of subjects) than in SJW-treated subjects (23%). The authors acknowledged the need for more studies in this population but suggested that SJW may be an alternative to synthetic tricyclic antidepressant imipramine in the majority of severe forms of depression (31).

◆ Results from a study of the efficacy of SJW for major depressive disorder, which was funded by the National Center for Complementary and Alternative Medicine at NIH in 1998, were published in the *Journal of the American Medical Association* by the Hypericum Depression Trial Study Group in 2002 (32). A total of 340 adult outpatients with major depression were randomly assigned in a 1:1:1 ratio to SJW (dosages ranging from 900 to 1500 mg/day), placebo, or sertaline (dosages ranging from 50 to 100 mg/day) for a period of 8 weeks. Subjects responding to treatment at 8 weeks remained on study treatment for an additional 18 weeks. Efficacy of study treatments was assessed using the HAMD. Response to treatment did not differ across treatment groups or as compared with baseline in any group.

References

1. Nathan PJ. *Hypericum perforatum* (St John's Wort): a non-selective reuptake inhibitor? A review of the recent advances in its pharmacology. *J Psychopharmacol.* 2001;15:47–54.
2. Blumenthal M, ed. *The Complete German Commission E Monographs Therapeutic Guide to Herbal Medicines.* Austin, Tex: American Botanical Council; 1998.
3. De Smet PA, Nolen WA. St John's wort as an antidepressant. *BMJ.* 1996;313:241–242.
4. Knuppel L, Linde K. Adverse effects of St. John's wort: a systematic review. *J Clin Psychiatry.* 2004;65:1470–1479.
5. Kobak KA, Taylor L, Futterer R, et al. St John's wort in generalized anxiety disorder: three more case reports. *J Clin Psychopharmacol.* 2003;23:531–532.
6. Obach RS. Inhibition of human cytochrome P450 enzymes by constituents of St John's wort, an herbal preparation used in the treatment of depression. *J Pharmacol Exp Ther.* 2000;294:88–95.
7. Muller RS, Breitkreutz J, Groning R. Interactions between aqueous *Hypericum perforatum* extracts and drugs: in vitro studies. *Phytother Res.* 2004;18:1019–1023.
8. Mills, E, Montori VM, Wu P, et al. Interaction of St. John's wort with conventional drugs: systematic review of clinical trials. *BMJ.* 2004;329:27–30.
9. Mannel M. Drug interactions with St John's wort: mechanisms and clinical implications. *Drug Saf.* 2004;27:773–797.
10. Karliova M, Treichel U, Malago M, et al. Interaction of Hypericum perforatum (St. John's wort) with cyclosporin A metabolism in a patient after liver transplantation. *J Hepatol.* 2000;33:853–855.
11. Mai I, Kruger H, Budde K, et al. Hazardous pharmacokinetic interaction of Saint John's wort (Hypericum perforatum) with the immunosuppressant cyclosporin. *Int J Clin Pharamcol Ther.* 2000;38:500–502.
12. Barone GW, Gurley BJ, Ketel BL, et al. Drug interaction between St. John's wort and cyclosporine. *Ann Pharmacother.* 2000;34:1014–1016.
13. Breidenbach T, Kliem V, Burg M, et al. Profound drop of cyclosporin A whole blood trough levels caused by St. John's wort (*Hypericum perforatum*). *Transplantation.* 2000;27:2229–2230.
14. Ruschitzkaa F, Meier PJ, Turina M, et al. Acute heart transplant rejection due to Saint John's wort. *Lancet.* 2000;355:1912.
15. Johne A, Brockmoller J, Bauer S, et al. Pharmacokinetic interaction of digoxin with an herbal extract from St John's wort (Hypericum perforatum). *Clin Pharmacol Ther.* 1999;66:338–345.
16. Piscitelli SC, Burstein AH, Chaitt D, et al. Indinavir concentrations and St John's wort. *Lancet.* 2000;355:547–548.

17. Pfrunder A, Schiesser M, Gerber S, et al. Interaction of St. John's wort with low-dose oral contraceptive therapy: a randomized controlled study. *Br J Clin Pharmacol.* 2003:26:683–690.

18. Gordon JB. SSRIs and St. John's wort: possible toxicity? *Am Fam Physician.* 1998;57: 950,953.

19. Gurley BJ, Gardner SF, Hubbard MA, et al. Clinical assessment of effects of botanical supplementation on cytochrome P450 phenotypes in the elderly: St. John's wort, garlic oil, Panax ginseng and Ginkgo biloba. *Drugs Aging.* 2005;22:525–539.

20. Staffeldt B, Kerb R, Brockmoller J, et al. Pharmacokinetics of hypericin and pseudo-hypericin after oral intake of the *Hypericum perforatum* extract LI 160 in healthy volunteers. *J Geriatr Psychiatry Neurol.* 1994;7(Suppl 1):S47-S53.

21. Linde K, Berner M, Egger M, et al. St. John's Wort for depression: meta-analysis of randomised controlled trials. *Br J Psychiatry.* 2005;186:99–107.

22. Werneke U, Horn O, Taylor DM. How effective is St. John's wort? The evidence revisited. *J Clin Psychiatry.* 2004;65:611–617.

23. Uebelhack R, Gruenwald J, Graubaum HJ, et al. Efficacy and tolerability of Hypericum extract STW 3-VI in patients with moderate depression: a double-blind, randomized, placebo-controlled clinical trial. *Adv Ther.* 2004;21:265–275.

24. Szegedi A, Kohnen R, Dienel A, et al. Acute treatment of moderate to severe depression with hypericum extract WS 5570 (St. John's wort); randomised controlled double blind non-inferiority trial versus paroxetine [errata in *BMJ.* 2005;330:759. Dosage error in text.]. *BMJ.* 2005;330:503. Epub 2005 Feb.

25. Woelk H. Comparison of St. John's wort and imipramine for treating depression: randomized controlled trial. *BMJ.* 2000;321:536–539.

26. Philipp M, Kohnen R, Hiller KO. Hypericum extract versus imipramine or placebo in patients with moderate depression: randomized multicenter study of treatment for eight weeks. *BMJ.* 2000;319:1534–1538.

27. Schrader E. Equivalence of St John's wort extract (Ze 117) and fluoxetine: a randomized, controlled study in mild-moderate depression. *Int Clin Psychopharmacol.* 2000;15:61–68.

28. Laakmann G, Schule C, Baghai T, et al. St. John's wort in mild to moderate depression: the relevance of hyperforin for the clinical efficacy. *Pharmacopsychiatry.* 1998;31 (Suppl 1):54–59.

29. Wheatley D. LI 160, an extract of St. John's wort, versus amitriptyline in mildly to moderately depressed outpatients—a controlled 6 week clinical trial. *Pharmacopsychiatry.* 1997;30(Suppl 2):77–80.

30. Shelton RC, Keller MB, Gelenberg A, et al. Effectiveness of St John's wort in major depression: a randomized controlled trial. *JAMA.* 2001;285:1978–1986.

31. Vorbach EU, Arnoldt KH, Hubner WD. Efficacy and tolerability of St. John's wort extract LI 160 versus imipramine in patients with severe depressive episodes according to ICD-10. *Pharmacopsychiatry.* 1997;30(Suppl 2):81–85.

32. Hypericum Depression Trial Study Group. Effect of *Hypericum perforatum* (St John's Wort) in major depressive disorder: a randomized controlled trial. *JAMA.* 2002;287: 1807–1814.

Saw Palmetto *(Serenoa repens)*

Native to the southern regions of North America, the berries of the saw palmetto plant were once used to treat conditions such as cystitis and bronchitis. Possible active constituents in saw palmetto include free fatty acids, sitosterols, flavonoids, and polysaccharides. The liposterolic (fatty acids and sterols) extract of saw palmetto has been investigated for its potential role in treating benign prostatic hyperplasia (BPH). Increasing amounts of research provide support that the mechanism of action of saw palmetto may be related to the inhibition of 5a-reductase, which limits the conversion of testosterone to dihydrotestosterone (DHT) (1–4), and it seems to do this without altering PSA levels (5). Because DHT is associated with hyperplasia, it has been implicated in the pathogenesis of BPH. Studies have also shown that saw palmetto inhibits the binding of DHT to androgen receptors in prostate cell lines, and that it may exert antioxidant and anti-inflammatory effects (6–8).

Media and Marketing Claims	Efficacy
Improves symptoms of enlarged prostate	↔
Prevents prostate cancer	NR
Prevents male-pattern baldness/hair loss	NR

Safety

- In the research cited, 320-mg daily doses of saw palmetto extracts were well tolerated for studies lasting as long as 12 months. However, there are no controlled studies testing the safety of long-term supplementation.

- According to the German Commission E monograph on saw palmetto, in rare cases this herb may be associated with gastrointestinal discomfort. The monograph also notes that consultation with a physician at regular intervals is recommended during use of this herb (9).

- Patients scheduled for surgery should discontinue use of saw palmetto at least 2 weeks before surgery due to the herb's anticoagulant effects.

Drug/Supplement Interactions

- Saw palmetto may interfere with blood clotting and increase bleeding time in patients taking anticoagulant medications.

- Theoretically, saw palmetto may interfere with hormone and contraceptive drug therapies.

Key Points

- ◆ Evidence from clinical trials is limited because of the short duration of studies as well as variability in study design, formulations, and reports of outcomes. The available research suggests that saw palmetto may improve urologic symptoms and urine flow measures. However, not all studies have shown benefits. More research using standardized supplements is needed to determine long-term efficacy.

- ◆ There is currently no evidence that saw palmetto prevents prostate cancer in human trials. Preliminary cell culture research suggests that saw palmetto may inhibit cancer growth in prostate cancer cell lines.

- ◆ Currently, there is no research testing the effectiveness of saw palmetto on male-pattern baldness.

Food Sources

None

Dosage Information/Bioavailability

Saw palmetto is available in capsules, tablets, or tinctures from the liposterolic portion of the berry in hexane or ethanol extract. Manufacturers suggest taking 160 to 320 mg of the extract daily (equivalent to 2 to 4 mL of tincture or 3 to 4 g of dried berries). Some products are standardized to contain 85% to 95% fatty acids. Most studies used the liposterolic extract of *Serenoa repens* available in Europe and the United States. In a study comparing 14 brands of *S. repens,* extracts showed wide variability in fatty acid content; high fatty acid content has been associated with reduced clinical efficacy (10). Similar findings were reported by Feifer et al, who identified select saw palmetto products that had no active ingredient (11).

Relevant Research

Saw Palmetto and Benign Prostatic Hyperplasia (BPH)

- ◆ A meta-analysis was conducted of 13 studies: 7 randomized, placebo-controlled trials, four studies that were randomized and included saw palmetto vs one of four known prescription medications, and two large open-label studies. The authors concluded that BPH symptoms—including peak urinary flow rate (reported in 10 of 13 studies) and night-time urinary frequency (all 13 studies), comparing baseline frequency to frequency at the end of treatment—decreased significantly with saw palmetto use (12). However, comparison across studies is difficult because no symptom score was consistently applied across all studies and the study designs were somewhat heterogeneous.

- ◆ A 1-year, single-blind, randomized, parallel intervention trial in which 64 men with prostatitis were randomly assigned to receive 325 mg saw palmetto or 5 mg finasteride daily showed that saw palmetto supplementation was ineffective in treating prostatitis, based on scores on the NIH Chronic Prostatitis Symptom Index taken at baseline, 3, 6 and 12 months. Finasteride was effective in reducing related symptoms with the exception of NIH-Chronic Prostatitis Symptom Index scores for urination (13).

♦ Similarly, negative results for saw palmetto were found in a trial recently reported by Willetts et al, who treated 100 men who had been previously diagnosed with prostatitis with saw palmetto (320 mg/day) or placebo in a randomized, double-blind study that lasted 12 weeks. There was a small improvement in symptoms, but the change did not reach significance nor was it different across treatment groups (14). The duration of intervention may have been too short, but otherwise this is among the better-designed trials testing efficacy of saw palmetto for BPH.

♦ Permixon, a medication developed from lipidosterolic extract of *S. repens*, was used to treat prostatitis among 150 men for 2 years (15). In this study, the International Prostate Symptom Score, Sexual Function Score, quality of life and urination were each assessed at 6, 12, 18, and 24 months. Significant improvements were reported for all measured outcomes. However, this study lacked placebo control and was unblinded, limiting interpretation, especially considering the subjectivity of the outcomes measured.

♦ In a double-blind, placebo-controlled US study, 44 men with symptomatic BPH, ages 45 to 80 years, were randomly assigned to receive saw palmetto herbal blend (318 mg saw palmetto lipoidal extract, 240 mg nettle root extract, 480 mg pumpkin seed extract, 99 mg lemon bioflavonoid extract, and 570 IU vitamin A) or a placebo daily for 6 months. Endpoints included routine clinical measurements (symptom score, uroflowmetry, and postvoid residual urine volumes), blood analyses (prostate-specific antigen [PSA], sex hormones, and multiphasic analysis), prostate volumetrics by magnetic resonance imaging, and prostate biopsy. Both groups experienced clinical improvements, with a slight nonsignificant advantage for the saw palmetto blend group. There were no changes in PSA or prostate volume in either group. A significant decrease in the percentage prostate epithelium (from 17.8% at baseline to 10.7% at study's end) occurred after saw palmetto–blend treatment. Histological studies also indicated a significant increase in percentage of atrophic glands (from 25.2% to 40.9%) with saw palmetto. No adverse effects were noted (16).

Saw Palmetto and Prostate Cancer

♦ Cell culture research using three different prostate cancer cell lines exposed to saw palmetto extract showed an inhibition of cellular growth of 20% to 25%, as well as reduced Cyclo-oxygenase-2 (COX-2) expression, indicating reduced inflammatory response, an effect that should be protective against cancer formation (17).

References

1. Niederprum HJ, Schweikert HU, Zanker KS. Testosterone 5a-reductase inhibition by free fatty acids from Sabal serrulata fruits. *Phytomedicine.* 1994;1:127–133.
2. Di Silverio F, Monti S, Sciarra A, et al. Effects of long-term treatment with *Serenoa repens* (Permixon) on the concentrations and regional distribution of androgens and epidermal growth factor in benign prostatic hyperplasia. *Prostate.* 1998;37:77–83.

3. Gerber GS. Saw palmetto for the treatment of men with lower urinary tract symptoms. *J Urol.* 2000;163:1408–1412.

4. Marks LS, Hess DL, Dorey FJ, et al. Tissue effects of saw palmetto and finasteride: use of biopsy cores for in situ quantifications of prostatic androgens. *Urology.* 2001;57: 999–1005.

5. Habib FK, Ross M, Ho CK, et al. Serenoa repens (Permixon) inhibits the 5a-reductase activity of human prostate cancer cell lines without interfering with PSA expression. *Int J Cancer.* 2005;114:190–194.

6. Plosker GL, Brogden RN. *Serenoa repens* (Permixon). A review of its pharmacology and therapeutic efficacy in benign prostatic hyperplasia. *Drugs Aging.* 1996;9:379–395.

7. Ravenna L, Di Silverio F, Russo MA, et al. Effects of the lipidosterolic extract of *Serenoa repens* (Permixon) on human prostatic cell lines. *Prostate.* 1996;29:219–230.

8. Schulz V, Hansel R, Tyler VE. *Rational Phytotherapy: A Physician's Guide to Herbal Medicine.* 3rd ed. Berlin, Germany: Springler-Verlag; 1998.

9. Blumenthal M, ed. *The Complete German Commission E Monographs Therapeutic Guide to Herbal Medicines.* Austin, Tex: American Botanical Council; 1998.

10. Habib FK, Wylie MG. Not all brands are created equal: a comparison of selected components of different brands of *Serenoa reopens* extract. *Prostate Cancer Prostatic Dis.* 2004;7:195–200.

11. Feifer AH, Fleshner NE, Klotz L. Analytical accuracy and reliability of commonly used nutritional supplements in prostate disease. *J Urol.* 2002;168:150–154.

12. Boyle P, Robertson C, Lowe F, et al. Meta-analysis of clinical trials of Permixon in the treatment of symptomatic benign prostatic hyperplasia. *Urology.* 2000;55:533–539.

13. Kaplan SA, Volpe MA, Te AE. A prospective, 1-year trial using saw palmetto versus finasteride in the treatment of category III prostatitis/chronic pelvic pain syndrome. *J Urol.* 2004;171:284–288.

14. Willetts KE, Clements MS, Champion S, et al. *Serenoa repens* extract for benign prostatic hyperplasia: a randomized controlled trial. *BJU Int.* 2003;92:267–270.

15. Pytel YA, Vinarov A, Lopatkin N, et al. Long-term clinical and biologic effects of the lipidosterolic extract of Serenoa repens in patients with symptomatic benign prostatic hyperplasia. *Adv Ther.* 2002;19:297–306.

16. Marks LS, Partin AW, Epstein JI, et al. Effects of saw palmetto herbal blend in men with symptomatic benign prostatic hyperplasia. *J Urol.* 2000;163:1451–1456.

17. Goldmann WH, Sharma AL, Currier SJ, et al. Saw palmetto berry extract inhibits cell growth and Cox-2 expression in prostatic cancer cells. *Cell Biol Int.* 2001;25:1117–1124.

Selenium

Selenium, an essential trace mineral, was first recognized as important to human nutrition in the 1970s. As part of a number of selenoproteins in the body, selenium forms the active site of the potent antioxidant enzyme glutathione peroxidase. Functioning synergistically with vitamin E, selenium protects against cellular damage from oxygen radicals. Selenium also plays a role in the function of the thyroid and male reproductive system. Several organic and inorganic forms exist in nature: selenomethionine (predominant form in food); selenocysteine; selenate, selenite, and methylselenocysteine. Low selenium intakes caused by selenium-deficient soil or long-term total parenteral nutrition with inadequate selenium have been associated with Keshan disease (cardiomyopathy), aspermatogenesis, cataracts, and growth retardation. Although the functions and requirements of selenium are not fully understood, recent research has focused on the potential role of selenium in cancer and cardiovascular disease prevention (1).

Media and Marketing Claims	Efficacy
Protects against cancer (only in selenium-deficient adults)*	↑?
Reduces risk of cardiovascular disease	↔
Enhances immune function	↑?
Improves athletic performance	NR
Reduces symptoms of rheumatoid arthritis	NR
Reduces symptoms of asthma	NR

New research has reported an increase in the rate of cancer in subjects with elevated plasma selenium levels.

Safety

- The Tolerable Upper Intake Level (UL) for most adults is 400 µg/day (2).

- Limited evidence suggests that selenium supplementation (200 µg selenium yeast) in individuals with normal (or elevated) plasma selenium values may increase cancer risk. Until more is known, evaluation of selenium status should be completed before supplementing with more than the RDA (55 µg the RDA for most adults, excluding pregnant and lactating women).

- A review of the toxicity of selenomethionine has been published (3).

- In a dose-toxicity study conducted in 24 men receiving either 1,600 (n = 8) or 3,200 µg (n = 16) selenium/day for 12 months, no clear selenium-related toxicity was found at either dose. More subjects taking 3,200 µg reported symptoms associated with toxicity; however, their plasma levels did not indicate elevated selenium exposure (4).

- Toxicity has been documented at doses more than the UL. Selenium toxicity is manifested by alopecia, mild nerve damage, white blotchy spots on nails, and immunosuppression.

Drug/Supplement Interactions

- One report suggests that selenium may help prevent cytotoxicity from the chemotherapeutic drug cisplatin, but another report suggests the opposite, that selenium may enhance cytotoxicity of this drug.

- Selenium may reduce efficacy of statin medications (HMG-CoA-reductase inhibitors).

Key Points

- Selenium is an essential trace mineral important in human health. Individuals should be encouraged to consume a balanced diet including foods rich in selenium (red meat [including organ meat], seafood, whole grains). If dietary selenium is not adequate, a multivitamin/mineral supplying no more than the adult RDA (55 μg) is suggested.

- Epidemiological research and evidence from a large multicenter trial suggest that selenium supplements may reduce cancer risk. Additional controlled clinical trials are needed to confirm the results of this study. The largest prospective, randomized, placebo-controlled clinical trial to assess the role of selenium in primary cancer prevention (SELECT; n ≥ 32,000 men) is currently underway to test the hypothesis that selenium supplementation will significantly reduce the incidence of prostate cancer (5). It is important to note that one study showed an increased risk of cancer in subjects with elevated plasma selenium who took selenium supplements (200 μg). Clearly, more research is needed to determine the safety of supplementing with selenium. In light of this finding, it may be advisable to test plasma selenium levels before using supplements.

- Results from epidemiological studies conflict regarding the relationship between selenium status and heart disease. Controlled clinical trials are required to determine the potential efficacy of selenium in preventing heart disease.

- Increasing amounts of evidence suggest that selenium supplementation may improve health outcomes in immunosuppressed individuals. More studies are needed to determine the specific patient populations, dosage, and duration of selenium supplementation needed to achieve the optimal clinical benefit in immunocompromised individuals.

- In the few studies reported, selenium did not enhance exercise performance. One study assessing the role of selenium and exercise-induced oxidative stress in humans suggests that a combined antioxidant supplement containing selenium has no significant effect on oxidative stress associated with exercise.

- There is limited evidence that selenium supplementation may protect against rheumatoid arthritis.

- One well-designed study has investigated the role of selenium in asthma; however, the evidence for evaluating efficacy in clinical practice is insufficient.

- Much of the evidence regarding selenium and health is observational and is based on the correlation of plasma selenium levels, not supplements, to a particular disease or condition in humans (6). This includes studies associating low selenium intake with recurrent pregnancy miscarriage (7), cardiomyopathy associated with selenium deficiency induced by the ketogenic diet (8), cystic fibrosis (9), and gestational hyperglycemia (10). More research specifically testing the efficacy and safety of selenium supplements is needed.

Food Sources

Because of the differences in the selenium content of soil, the selenium content of plant foods vary substantially. Meats, seafood, and whole-grains are good sources of selenium. Brazil nuts are also a significant source. Several supplementation trials have used selenelized yeast. The typical US diet supplies an average of 70 to 100 μg selenium per day (1).

Food	Selenium, μg/Serving
Tuna, canned in water (3 oz)	56
Beef, lean ground (4 oz)	18
Sunflower seeds, with hulls (1 cup)	22
Chicken breast, skinless (½)	24
Egg (1)	16
Bread, whole-wheat (1 slice)	9.5
Wheat germ, toasted (2 Tbsp)	9.2
Cheese, cheddar (1½ oz)	6.0
Cocoa powder (1 Tbsp)	0.8

Source: Data are from reference 11.

Dosage Information/Bioavailability

Selenium is sold as inorganic sodium selenite or organic selenomethionine in tablets and capsules in doses ranging from 25 to 200 μg. High-selenium yeast (organic) is also available in capsules. Selenium is sold in individual supplements or as part of antioxidant formulas that also include vitamins E and C, and beta carotene. The RDA for selenium is 55 μg/day for men and for women who are neither pregnant or lactating (2). Most ingested selenium is almost completely absorbed. Excretion is the primary homeostatic mechanism for selenium (1). Data from cohort studies of selenium and cancer risk suggest that there may be substantial variability in selenium bioavailability between males and females when comparing dietary reported intake to levels of selenium measured in toenail samples (4).

Dietary measurement of selenium is generally thought to be unreliable because of variance in levels in food related to selenium levels in soil.

Relevant Research

Selenium and Cancer

♦ Many publications connecting selenium with cancer outcomes have been published as a result of the Nutritional Prevention of Cancer Trial conducted in the 1980s and early 1990s. In this double-blind, placebo-controlled, multicenter trial, 1,312 subjects (ages 18 to 80 years) diagnosed with basal/squamous cell carcinomas of the skin were randomly assigned to receive selenium-enriched yeast (200 µg/day) or a low-selenium yeast placebo. Subjects were recruited from 1983 to 1990 and followed up through 1993. Regular dermatologic exams and plasma selenium concentrations were recorded. Selenium did not affect the primary endpoint: incidence of recurrent skin carcinomas. However, selenium supplementation was correlated with significant reductions in secondary endpoints: mortality from all cancers combined (29 deaths in the selenium group vs 57 deaths in placebo group), incidence of all cancers combined (77 in the selenium group vs 119 in the placebo group), and incidence of lung cancer, colorectal cancer, and prostate cancers, specifically. The blinded phase of the trial was stopped early because of the apparent reductions in mortality and cancer incidence with selenium treatment. The authors concluded: "These effects of selenium require confirmation in an independent trial of appropriate design before new public health recommendations can be made" (12). The follow-up analysis published in 2002, for which all cases were included that had occurred at the time of unblinding, showed that selenium supplementation reduced overall mortality (Hazards Ratio [HR] = 0.75; 95% CI = 0.58–0.97) and prostate cancer incidence (HR = 0.48; 95% CI = 0.28–0.80), but in this analysis previous associations with lung and colorectal cancer were not seen (13). Of importance, subjects with low baseline plasma selenium levels had reduced cancer incidence over time with supplementation, whereas those within the highest tertile of plasma selenium at baseline had an increased risk for cancer with selenium supplementation. This suggests that supplementation should be considered only among those with low plasma levels.

♦ A separate analysis of the data set using all cases of nonmelanoma skin cancers at the time of unblinding supported earlier findings that suggested that supplementation with 200 µg selenium per day was associated with protection from basal cell cancers, but also with increased risk for squamous cell skin cancer and total nonmelanoma skin cancer (14).

♦ Several trials are underway to follow up findings from the previous study. These trials will attempt to assess the effects of 200 µg selenium per day on the prevention and treatment of prostate cancer (15). Among these trials is the large NCI SELECT study testing the efficacy of selenium, selenium plus vitamin E, or placebo in reducing prostate cancer risk (16).

♦ A study of the relationship between serum selenium levels and non-Hodgkin's lymphoma assessed baseline selenium levels in 100 individuals treated from 1986 to 1999. In this study, higher serum selenium levels were associated with higher chemotherapeutic dosing (tolerance) as well as initial response and long-term remission and, finally, overall survival (HR = 0.76; 95% CI = 0.60–0.95) for every 0.2 mmol/L increase in selenium levels. The authors suggest: "serum selenium concentration at presentation is a prognostic factor, predicting positively for dose delivery, treatment response and long-term survival in aggressive non-Hodgkin's lymphoma" (17). What is unclear is whether serum selenium levels are specific prognostic indicators for non-Hodgkin's lymphoma or if, instead, it reflects a generally improved nutritional and medical status, making response to treatment more plausible as well as increasing tolerance to larger chemotherapy doses.

♦ In a double-blind, placebo-controlled study, 33 subjects with head and neck cancer were randomly assigned to receive 200 µg/day of sodium selenite on the first day of treatment (ie, surgery, radiation, or both) for 8 weeks. Immune functions were monitored. Selenium therapy resulted in significantly enhanced cell-mediated immune response as measured by the patient's lymphocyte response to stimulation with mitogen, to generate cytotoxic lymphocytes, and to destroy tumor cells. In contrast, immune responsiveness decreased in the placebo group. Additionally, patients in the study had significantly lower plasma selenium levels than did healthy individuals (18).

♦ In a randomized controlled trial (Linxian study), 29,584 Chinese adults (age 40 to 69 years) were randomly assigned to receive one of four dietary supplements for 5 years, providing dosages ranging from one to two times the US RDA: (*a*) beta carotene, vitamin E, and selenium; (*b*) riboflavin and niacin; (*c*) vitamin C and molybdenum; or (*d*) retinol and zinc. Mortality and cancer incidence were assessed from March 1986 to May 1991. A total of 2,127 deaths occurred during the trial period (32% of all deaths were attributed to esophageal or stomach cancer). There was a significantly lower total mortality (relative risk = 0.91) in subjects in the beta carotene, vitamin E, and selenium supplement group. The reduction was mainly due to lower cancer rates, with the reduced risk emerging 1 to 2 years after the start of supplementation. No significant effects on mortality rates were apparent with the other three treatments. However, the study design does not permit the attribution of cancer reduction to selenium alone (19).

Selenium and Cardiovascular Disease

♦ A study of the association between C-reactive protein (CRP) levels (a prognostic indicator in cardiovascular disease) and plasma selenium conducted in 14,519 US adults showed that CRP levels were significantly inversely associated with plasma selenium levels (20), suggesting that selenium reduces the level of inflammation. Whether this has relevance to cardiovascular events has not been demonstrated.

♦ A randomized, placebo-controlled supplemental selenium study was conducted in New Zealanders (n = 189) who had suboptimal selenium status and found that 200 µg/day for 20 weeks vs placebo was associated with a significant increase in selenium levels as compared to plasma selenium levels at baseline. Supplementation with selenium did not modulate plasma homocysteine levels, a biomarker of cardiovascular disease risk (21). The article does not clearly describe whether the study was blinded.

♦ In a nested, case-control study, prospective plasma levels of selenium were measured in subjects in the Physicians' Health Study. Within the study, 251 subjects who had myocardial infarctions (MIs) were matched to 251 healthy control subjects to explore whether plasma selenium predicted the risk of MI. There were no significant differences between groups for mean plasma selenium levels or in cardiovascular events when comparing highest with lowest quintiles of plasma levels after adjusting for other cardiovascular risk factors. According to the authors: "these data provide no evidence for an association between increased plasma selenium and reduced risk of MI at the current levels of selenium intake within the United States" (22).

♦ In a prospective cohort study, 3,387 Danish men (age 53 to 74 years) without cardiovascular disease were followed up for 3 years. Subjects completed questionnaires, underwent clinical exams, and had blood samples drawn. Three years later, data were collected on the number of ischemic heart disease (IHD) events. Men with serum selenium levels in the lowest tertile had a 70% increased risk of IHD as compared with those in the highest tertile. (23).

♦ In a cross-sectional study of 1,132 eastern Finnish men (mean age 54 years), serum selenium concentrations had a strong significant inverse relationship with platelet aggregation and a weak positive relationship with plasma HDL cholesterol levels, suggesting that selenium may be associated with reduced platelet aggregation and increased HDL levels important to maintaining cardiovascular health. Furthermore, men with ischemic electrocardiogram findings during exercise had lower mean selenium levels than men with normal electrocardiograms (24).

♦ A review article summarizing possible mechanisms whereby selenium may protect against heart disease suggested that selenium is associated with reduction of LDL oxidation, modulation of prostaglandin synthesis and platelet aggregation, and protection against toxic heavy metals. However, the author noted: "The therapeutic benefit of selenium administration in the prevention and treatment of cardiovascular diseases still remains insufficiently documented" (25).

Selenium and Immunity

♦ In a pilot study, selenium supplentation (200 mg/day) was given to 17 immunosuppressed individuals with asthma and 17 patients with low plasma selenium levels on corticosteroid therapy. After 96 weeks (and at several intermediate timepoints) of selenium supplementation, subjects showed significant improvements in several immune parameters, including both cellular and humoral immunity (26).

♦ In a randomized, double-blind, placebo-controlled trial of 186 individuals with HIV, 200 µg selenium supplementation per day for 2 years was associated with a significant reduction in the number of hospitalizations as compared with placebo (27). However, it seems this was a secondary analysis conducted retrospectively after the study; prospective studies in this population are needed. Selenium deficiency also has been reported in individuals with HIV. A review article noted that selenium deficiency is a significant predictor of HIV-related mortality independent of CD4 count and antiretroviral treatment (28).

♦ In a prospective, observational study of 134 surgical and medical intensive care unit (ICU) patients, researchers assessed plasma selenium concentrations and presence or absence of systemic inflammatory response syndrome (SIRS), sepsis, or direct ischemia-reperfusion during their ICU stay. Patients with SIRS had lower mean plasma selenium concentrations than those without SIRS. Mean plasma selenium was also less in all patients with severe sepsis and septic shock, and in patients with ischemia-reperfusion from aortic cross-clamping. The frequency of ventilator-associated pneumonia, organ system failure, and mortality was three-fold greater in patients with low plasma selenium concentrations at time of admission (≤ 0.70 μmol/L) than for the other patients. The authors concluded that the decrease in plasma selenium concentrations reached deficiency status and may be associated with the increase in morbidity and mortality of these patients (29).

♦ In a review of research on the efficacy of selenium supplementation in reducing the acute inflammatory response associated with burn and trauma, the authors concluded that, "selenium supplementation seems to improve the outcome of patients with systemic inflammatory response syndrome" (30). This review included a description of four supplementation trials using variable doses of selenium, all of which suggested reduced infection and/or mortality rates with selenium supplementation; however, more prospective intervention trials are warranted.

Selenium and Exercise

♦ In a double-blind, placebo-controlled study, 24 healthy, untrained, male subjects were given 180 μg selenium (selenomethionine) or a placebo during a 10-week endurance training program (three times a week). A maximum endurance treadmill test was completed before and after the training. Maximal oxygen uptake and plasma and erythrocyte glutathione peroxidase activity were measured before and after the test. Training significantly increased plasma glutathione peroxidase activity and aerobic power and capacity. Selenium supplementation caused a significant increase in the basal plasma glutathione level but had no effect on physical performance parameters (31).

♦ Selenium- and/or vitamin E–deficient rats were found to have oxidative free radical generation in lung tissue as measured by electron spin resonance spectra. The oxidative generation increased when rats were subjected to exhaustive exercise. Selenium-and/or vitamin E–supplemented rats did not experience free radical generation during exercise. The authors suggested that these supplements may offer protection against exercise-induced oxidative stress (32).

Selenium and Rheumatoid Arthritis

♦ In Belgium, a multicenter study used a randomized, placebo-controlled design to test the hypothesis that regular selenium supplementation would reduce symptoms of arthritis in a sample population of 50 adults. Subjects were randomly assigned to 200 μg selenized yeast or placebo daily for 3 months. Subjective measures of symptoms, including the visual analogue scale and self-reported frequency and number of swollen joints, improved significantly over time for both the selenium and placebo groups (33). The improvement was thought to be a placebo effect associated with the increased attention provided to subjects who participated in this clinical trial. Limitations of the study include the lack of reporting of baseline selenium status of the participants and the multiple comparisons, which made may have resulted in the significant findings by chance alone.

Selenium and Asthma

♦ A Cochrane Database Review of selenium supplementation for asthma indicates that only one study met inclusion criteria as being randomized and blinded. In the study, 24 individuals with asthma were randomized to daily selenium supplementation in addition to asthma medication or asthma medication plus placebo in a 1:1 ratio. Patients taking selenium reported more subjective improvements in clinical status than those taking the placebo, a difference that was statistically significant. However, no objective clinical parameters, such as lung function, were assessed (34). More research with larger population samples and more objective indicators of response is needed.

References

1. Burk RF, Levander OA. Selenium. In: Shils ME, Olson JA, Shike M, et al, eds. *Modern Nutrition in Health and Disease.* 9th ed. Baltimore, Md: Williams & Wilkins; 1999: 265–276.
2. Institute of Medicine. *Dietary Reference Intakes: Vitamin C, Vitamin E, Selenium, and Carotenoids.* Washington, DC: National Academy Press; 2000.
3. Schrauzer GN. The nutritional significance, metabolism and toxicology of selenomethionine. *Adv Food Nutr Res.* 2003;47:73–112.
4. Reid ME, Stratton MS, Lillico AJ, et al. A report of high-dose selenium supplementation: response and toxicities. *J Trace Elem Med Biol.* 2004;18:69–74.
5. Klein EA, Thompson IM, Lippman SM, et al. SELECT: the Selenium and Vitamin E Cancer Prevention Trial: rationale and design. *Prostate Cancer Prostatic Dis.* 2000;3: 145–151.
6. Wei WQ, Abnet CC, Qiao YL, et al. Prospective study of serum selenium concentrations and esophageal and gastric cardia cancer, heart disease, stroke, and total death. *Am J Clin Nutr.* 2004;79:80–85.
7. Kumar KS, Kumar A, Prakash S, et al. Role of red cell selenium in recurrent pregnancy loss. *J Obstet Gynaecol.* 2002;22:181–183.
8. Bergqvist AG, Chee CM, Lutchka L, et al. Selenium deficiency associated with cardiomyopathy: a complication of the ketogenic diet. *Epilepsia.* 2003;44:618–620.
9. Michalke B. Selenium speciation in human serum of cystic fibrosis patients compared to serum from healthy persons. *J Chromatogr A.* 2004;1058:203–208.
10. Bo S, Lezo A, Menato G, et al. Gestational hyperglycemia, zinc, selenium, and antioxidant vitamins. *Nutrition.* 2005;21:186–191.
11. US Department of Agriculture. Agricultural Research Service. Nutrient Data Laboratory. Available at: http://www.ars.usda.gov/main/site_main.htm?modecode=12354500. Accessed October 31, 2005.
12. Clark LC, Combs GF, Turnbull BW, et al. Effects of selenium supplementation for cancer prevention in patients with carcinoma of the skin. A randomized controlled trial. Nutritional Prevention of Cancer Study Group. *JAMA.* 1996;276:1957–1963.
13. Duffield-Lillico AJ, Reid ME, Turnbull BW, et al. Baseline characteristics and the effect of selenium supplementation on cancer incidence in a randomized clinical trial: a sum-

mary report of the Nutritional Prevention of Cancer Trial. *Cancer Epidemiol Biomarkers Prev.* 2002;11:630–639.

14. Duffield-Lillico AJ, Slate EH, Reid ME, et al; Nutritional Prevention of Cancer Study Group. Selenium supplementation and secondary prevention of nonmelanoma skin cancer in a randomized trial. *J Natl Cancer Inst.* 2003;95:1477–1481.

15. Clark LC, Marshall JR. Randomized, controlled chemoprevention trials in populations at very high risk for prostate cancer: elevated prostate-specific antigen and high-grade prostatic intraepithelial neoplasia. *Urology.* 2001;57(4 Suppl 1):185–187.

16. Lippman SM, Goodman PJ, Klein EA, et al. Designing the Selenium and Vitamin E Cancer Prevention Trial (SELECT). *J Natl Cancer Inst.* 2005;97:94–102.

17. Last KW, Cornelius V, Delves T, et al. Presentation serum selenium predicts for overall survival, dose delivery, and first treatment response in aggressive non-Hodgkin's lymphoma. *J Clin Oncol.* 2003;21:2335–2341.

18. Kiremidjian-Schumacher L, Roy M, Glickman R, et al. Selenium and immunocompetence in patients with head and neck cancer. *Biol Trace Elem Res.* 2000;73:97–111.

19. Blot WJ, Li JY, Taylor PR, et al. Nutrition intervention trials in Linxian, China: supplementation with specific vitamin/mineral combinations, cancer incidence, and disease-specific mortality in the general population. *J Natl Cancer Inst.* 1993;85:1483–1492.

20. Ford ES, Liu S, Mannino DM, et al. C-reactive protein concentration and concentrations of blood vitamins, carotenoids, and selenium among United States adults. *Eur J Clin Nutr.* 2003;57:1157–1163.

21. Venn BJ, Grant AM, Thomson CD, et al. Selenium supplements do not increase plasma total homocysteine concentrations in men and women. *J Nutr.* 2003;133:418–420.

22. Salvini S, Hennekens CH, Morris JS, et al. Plasma levels of the antioxidant selenium and risk of myocardial infarction among U.S. physicians. *Am J Cardiol.* 1995;76:1218–1221.

23. Suadicani P, Hein HO, Gyntelberg F. Serum selenium concentration and risk of ischemic heart disease in a prospective cohort study of 3000 males. *Atherosclerosis.* 1992;96:33–42.

24. Salonen JT, Salonen R, Seppanen K, et al. Relationship of serum selenium and antioxidants to plasma lipoproteins, platelet aggregability and prevalent ischemic heart disease in Eastern Finnish men. *Atherosclerosis.* 1988;70:155–160.

25. Neve J. Selenium as a risk factor for cardiovascular diseases. *J Cardiovasc Risk.* 1996;3:42–47.

26. Gazdik F, Horvathova M, Gazdikova K, et al. The influence of selenium supplementation on the immunity of corticoid-dependent asthmatics. *Bratisl Lek Listy.* 2002;103:17–21.

27. Burbano X, Miquez-Burbano MJ, McCollister K, et al. Impact of a selenium chemoprevention clinical trial on hospital admissions of HIV-infected participants. *HIV Clin Trials.* 2002;3:483–491.

28. Baum MK, Shor-Posner G. Micronutrient status in relationship to mortality in HIV-1 disease. *Nutr Rev.* 1998;56:S135-S139.

29. Forceville X, Vitoux D, Gauzit R, et al. Selenium, systemic immune response syndrome, sepsis, and outcome in critically ill patients. *Crit Care Med.* 1998;26:1536–1544.

30. Gartner R, Albrich W, Angstwurm MW. The effect of a selenium supplementation on the outcome of patients with severe systematic inflammation, burn and trauma. *Biofactors.* 2001;14:199–204.

31. Tessier F, Margaritis I, Richard MJ, et al. Selenium and training effects on the glutathione system and aerobic performance. *Med Sci Sports Exerc.* 1995;27:390–396.

32. Reddy KV, Kumar TC, Prasad M, et al. Pulmonary lipid peroxidation and antioxidant defenses during exhaustive physical exercise: the role of vitamin E and selenium. *Nutrition.* 1998;14:448–451.

33. Peretz A, Siderova V, Neve J. Selenium supplementation in rheumatoid arthritis investigated in a double blind, placebo-controlled trial. *Scand J Rheumatol.* 2001;30:208–212.

34. Allam MF, Lucane RA. Selenium supplementation for asthma. *Cochrane Database Syst Rev.* 2004;(2):CD003538.

Senna

Senna is a shrub native to China, India, and Pakistan. It has been used medicinally since the ninth century. The functional parts of the plant are the leaves, pods, and fruit (1). Traditionally, senna was used to "cleanse" the body of impurities. Today, it is marketed and used as a treatment for constipation. Senna is also available as SennaKot, an over-the-counter medication for the treatment of constipation.

Media and Marketing Claims	Efficacy
Relieves constipation	NR

Safety

- Senna has been shown to be safe when taken for short periods of time (up to several days). As with many laxative supplements, dependence can develop with prolonged use. Therefore, senna should only be used intermittently when needed (1).

- Mild side effects have been reported, including cramping, diarrhea, and discoloration of the urine (1).

- Senna should not be taken for more than 10 consecutive days. Prolonged use can lead to chronic diarrhea, weight loss, electrolyte imbalance, hypokalemia, changes in heart rhythm, and clubbing of the fingers and toes (2).

- A case of hepatic toxicity was reported for a 28 year old woman who was drinking senna tea. A rechallenge with senna suggested that the liver enzymes rose within 7 days and that the toxicity appeared to be related to slow metabolism of the active metabolites due to the patient's p450 genetic variant (3).

Drug/Supplement Interactions

♦ Senna should not be taken with other stimulant laxatives or diuretics because of the increased risk of hypokalemia.

♦ High doses of senna may increase the risk of adverse side effects from digoxin.

♦ Based on the case report described under Safety, there may be concern that senna taken concurrently with medications that are metabolized using cytochrome p450 enzymes may reduce the drugs' efficacy.

Key Points

♦ Senna is marketed as an effective treatment for constipation; however, a recent review of the safety and efficacy of traditional medical therapies for chronic constipation revealed a lack of quality data supporting the use of senna for chronic constipation (4).

Food Sources

None

Dosage Information/Bioavailability

Senna is most commonly taken as a liquid or tea. Capsules, powder, tablets, and softgels containing between 15 and 30 g of sennoside B are also available. Taken as a tea, 1 to 2 g dried senna is steeped in 1 cup of warm water for 10 minutes. Manufacturers generally recommend consuming tea in the morning and at bedtime, although a single daily dose may be adequate to reduce constipation in some individuals (2). It is possible to become dependent on senna in that the laxative effects will reduce the body's own ability to produce regular bowel movements; therefore, it should not be consumed for more than 10 consecutive days.

Relevant Research

Senna and Constipation

♦ A systematic review of the role of herbal therapies for the treatment of constipation that included three separate studies with senna plus a bulking agent vs lactulose suggested that there is insufficient and conflicting evidence for senna as an effective laxative agent. Although none of the reviewed studies included senna as a single agent to treat constipation, there were several studies that compared the efficacy of senna combined with a bulking agent to other treatments such as lactulose or sodium picosulphate. Generally, senna-containing supplements resulted in a slight increase in the number of bowel movements produced on a weekly basis as compared with lactulose, but senna also was more frequently associated with loose stools (4). The studies reviewed included small numbers of patients (30 to 77 patients) and were frequently unblinded (4).

♦ In a prospective case-control study to investigate the safety of anthranoid laxatives, 202 individuals with colorectal carcinoma, 114 with adenomatous polyps, and 238 without colorectal neoplasms were interviewed on the day of colonoscopy. Specific information gathered included use of laxative and other anthranoids. Anthranoid use was not significantly associated with risk for or protection from the development of colorectal neoplasms (5).

♦ In a randomized, open, parallel-group study to compare senna with lactulose in the treatment of constipation in individuals with terminal cancer being treated with opiods, 91 subjects (mean age 67.8 years) received either senna (n = 43) or lactulose (n = 48) for 27 days. Dosing started at 12 mg for senna and 10 g or 15 mL for lactulose and was increased every 3 days (by providing an additional daily dose of the same amount), depending on the patient's clinical response. The maximum dosage was set at 48 mg for senna and 40 g for lactulose. Subjects were evaluated for laxative effects after 7 days of treatment and for an additional 20 days to determine mean morphine dose that resulted in a need for constipation treatment. Outcome measurement included the number of 72-hour defecation-free episodes, days with defecation, general health, and cost. Among the 75 patients that completed the trial, there was no difference in response between senna and lactulose in terms of number of days with defecation or defecation-free 72-hour intervals. No comparison between baseline bowel frequency and end study bowel frequency was assessed. Treatment with senna was much less expensive than lactulose (6). Adverse events, including diarrhea, vomiting and abdominal cramping, were reported in 6 patients on senna and 3 on lactulose.

References

1. Covington TR, et al. *Handbook of Nonprescription Drugs*. 11th ed. Washington, DC: American Pharmaceutical Association; 1996.
2. Senna drug information. Available at: http://www.drugs.com. Accessed May 31, 2005.
3. Seybold U, Landauer N, Hillebrand S, et al. Senna-induced hepatitis in a poor metabolizer. *Ann Intern Med*. 2004;141:650–651.
4. Ramkumar D, Rao SS. Efficacy and safety of traditional medical therapies for chronic constipation: systematic review. *Am J Gastroenterol*. 2005;100:936–971.
5. Nusko G, Schneider B, Schneider I, et al. Anthranoid laxative use is not a risk factor for colorectal neoplasia: results of a prospective case control study. *Gut*. 2000;46:651–655.
6. Agra, Y, Sacristan A, Gonzalez M, et al. Efficacy of senna versus lactulose in terminal cancer patients treated with opioids. *J Pain Symptom Manage*. 1998;15:1–7.

Shark Cartilage

Shark cartilage is thought to contain a substance that may inhibit angiogenesis (the formation of new blood vessels typically seen in malignant tumors). Because the shark skeleton is made up of cartilage (a nonvascularized tissue) and sharks rarely develop neoplasms, consumption of shark cartilage supplements has been marketed as a way to slow tumor growth. Although the active component(s) have not been fully elucidated, a potent angiogenesis inhibitor composed of two single peptides from blue shark cartilage has been isolated. One inhibitor, SCF2, seems to be a heat-stable proteoglycan that contains keratan sulfate units and peptides. A few compounds from shark cartilage, including AE-941, have been developed for pharmacokinetic testing (1). AE-941, for which orphan drug status has been awarded, is also currently being tested for efficacy in lung cancer (2) and renal cell cancer (3). Findings from preliminary in vitro studies (4–6) as well as a popular consumer book, *Sharks Don't Get Cancer,* have helped fuel the popular belief that shark cartilage could cure cancer in humans.

Note: Shark cartilage is also a source of chondroitin sulfate. (*See* Chondroitin Sulfate.)

Media and Marketing Claims	Efficacy
Cures cancer	NR
Stops cancer spread (prevents tumor from developing a blood supply—ie, angiogenesis)	NR
Prevents blood clotting	NR
Treats psoriasis	NR

Safety

- There is speculation that dietary supplements that contain shark cartilage may have contributed to the development of hypercalcemia in cancer patients (7).
- Safety has been demonstrated with daily use for as long as 40 months for the shark cartilage-derived compound Neovastat (AE-941; Dupont, US patent no. 5618925) in a study of renal cancer patients who took 240 mL daily (3).

Drug/Supplement Interactions

No reported adverse interactions

Key Points

- There is currently no evidence from controlled trials that shark cartilage cures cancer in animals or humans. Although the media have reported on a few human trials in cancer patients outside the United States (4), these studies have not been published in peer-reviewed journals; thus, their validity is difficult to assess.
- In vitro and animal studies suggest that shark cartilage decreases tumor vascularization (5,6). One of the first controlled human studies that suggested that shark cartilage

inhibits angiogenesis was conducted in healthy men with experimentally induced wounds. An open clinical trial of cancer patients did not show any benefit with supplementation, although controlled trials are needed to substantiate these results.

♦ Studies for the use of shark cartilage to treat blood clots have not been conducted in humans, and data on shark cartilage treatment for psoriasis are limited. Efficacy cannot be determined until more research is completed.

♦ Current studies in cancer primarily use the experimental drug AE-941 (Neovastat, Les Laboratories-Quebec, Canada) (8), a product derived from shark cartilage that is not available for public use.

Food Sources

None

Dosage Information/Bioavailability

♦ Shark cartilage is sold in capsule, tablet, and powder forms. Manufacturers suggest taking doses ranging from 5-mg to 20-g doses three to four times per day. Manufacturers suggest mixing the powder with water and taking it orally or as an enema. Some of the potentially bioactive components of shark cartilage (AE-941) are being investigated in Phase I/II trials. These trials have advanced our understanding of bioavailability, but the intestinal absorption of crude shark cartilage extract needs to be studied.

Relevant Research

Shark Cartilage and Angiogenesis/Cancer

♦ A phase II, open-label, open-ended, non-randomized trial of the shark cartilage-derived drug Neovastat was conducted at a doses of either 60 mL/day or 240 mL/day in 144 patients with solid tumors that were previously unresponsive to standard cancer therapy. No untreated group was included for comparison. Subjects received the experimental drug until death, intolerance, or withdrawal from the study. Patients took the supplement orally in a divided dose, twice daily until an endpoint was reached. Survival analysis showed a dose-response effect in the 22 subjects with refractory renal cell cancer with less liver metastasis in the high-dose group as compared with the low-dose group, but also greater frequency of bone metastasis in the high-dose vs the low-dose group. Overall survival time was significantly longer in subjects receiving 240 mL/day (16.3 months) vs those receiving 60 mL/day (7.1 months). Taste alterations were reported in 13.6% of subjects, 1 in the 60 mL/d dose group and 2 in the 240 mL/d dose group, otherwise tolerance was good (8). Further studies are warranted for renal cell cancer and other cancers with poor survival rates.

♦ In a prospective, randomized, double-blind, placebo-controlled study, 29 healthy male subjects were randomly assigned to one of three intervention groups for 23 days: (*a*) 7 mL liquid shark cartilage extract; (*b*) 21 mL liquid shark cartilage extract;

or (*c*) placebo. On day 12, a polyvinyl alcohol sponge threaded in a perforated silicone tubing was inserted subcutaneously in the arm; this was removed on day 23. Researchers indirectly measured angiogenesis by assessing of endothelial cell density with factor VIII immunostaining on histological sections of the implant. Mean endothelial cell density was significantly lower in groups that had received either dose of shark cartilage extract. There were no differences among groups in side-effects, blood chemistry, urine analysis, or bleeding times. The authors concluded: "These results demonstrate that the liquid cartilage extract contains an antiangiogenic component bioavailable in humans by oral administration. This is the first report of an inhibition of wound angiogenesis in healthy men" (9).

- In an open clinical trial, 60 subjects with advanced previously treated cancers (several sites) were given 1 g shark cartilage/kg/day divided into three doses for 12 weeks. Extent of disease, quality of life, and hematologic, biochemical, and selected immune function were evaluated at baseline, and after 6 and 12 weeks. Twenty-three patients did not complete the study. No complete or partial positive responses were noted. Twenty percent of the 50 assessable patients (or 16.7% of the 60 intent-to-treat patients) had stable disease for 12 weeks or more. The authors concluded: "Under the specific conditions of this study, shark cartilage as a single agent was inactive in patients with advanced-stage cancer and had no salutary effect on quality of life" (10). However, stable disease might be considered as "activity" by some clinicians and researchers.

- In a randomized, placebo-controlled, double-blind trial of Benefin (LaneLabs, Allendale, NJ), 88 individuals diagnosed with advanced breast or colorectal cancer (43 assigned to supplement and 45 on placebo) were recruited to evaluate the efficacy of shark cartilage on overall survival (11). In this study, subjects received 24 g of supplement initially followed by escalation of dose to a maximum of 96 g/day. Dropout rates were high, with 27% of subjects on Benefin and 39% of subjects on placebo discontinuing within 1 week, and only 10% remaining on supplement or placebo at 6 months. No significant survival benefit was shown, with approximately 45% of subjects alive at 6 months, regardless of treatment group assignment.

Shark Cartilage and Blood Clotting

- There have been no human studies to determine whether shark cartilage reduces blood clot formation or increases clotting time.

- Direct activity of shark cartilage extract against fibrinogen and fibrin clotting capacity has been demonstrated in vitro and suggests a role of shark cartilage extract in vascular disorders (12). Endothelial cell-specific apoptosis has also been demonstrated with AE-941. This research initially has focused on cancer therapeutics, but it may lead to additional clinical research using this compound for vascular disease (13).

Shark Cartilage and Psoriasis

- In the only trial published to date regarding the therapeutic potential of shark cartilage extract for psoriasis, 49 individuals with psoriasis were randomly assigned to AE-941 at a dosage of 30, 60, 120, or 240 mL/day for 12 weeks in a randomized, open-label, dose-comparison trial (14). Thirty-three (67.3%) of patients completed the 12-week trial. Treatment efficacy with AE-941 was demonstrated, with 12.2% of patients showing a 30% reduction in Psoriasis Area and Severity Index scores and 30.6% showing a 20% improvement. No dose response was seen. The 30 mL/day dose was ineffective. Adverse effects were generally limited to gastrointestinal complaints in this Phase I/II trial.

References

1. FDA grants orphan-drug status to AEterna's Neovastat for kidney cancer. *Expert Rev Anticancer Ther.* 2002;2:618.
2. Dredge K. AE 941(AEterna). *Curr Opin Investig Drugs.* 2004;5:668–677.
3. Bukowski RM. AE-941, a multifunctional antiangiogenic compound: trials in renal cell carcinoma. *Expert Opin Investig Drugs.* 2003;12:1403–1411.
4. Hunt TJ, Connelly JF. Shark cartilage for cancer treatment. *Am J Health Syst Pharm.* 1995;52:1756,1760.
5. Sheu JR, Fu CC, Tsai ML, et al. Effect of U-995, a potent shark cartilage-derived angiogenesis inhibitor, on anti-angiogenesis and anti-tumor activities. *Anticancer Res.* 1998;18:4435–4441.
6. Liang JH, Wong KP. The characterization of angiogenesis inhibitor from shark cartilage. *Adv Exp Med Biol.* 2000;476:209–223.
7. Lagman R, Walsh D. Dangerous nutrition? Calcium, vitamin D, and shark cartilage nutritional supplements and cancer-related hypercalcemia. *Support Care Cancer.* 2003;11:232–235.
8. Batist G, Patenaude F, Champagne P, et al. Neovastat (AE-941) in refractory renal cell carcinoma patients: report of a phase II trial with two dose levels. *Ann Oncol.* 2002;13; 1259–1263.
9. Berbari P, Thibodeau A, Germain L, et al. Antiangiogenic effects of the oral administration of liquid cartilage extract in humans. *J Surg Res.* 1999;87:108–113.
10. Miller DR, Anderson GT, Stark JJ, et al. Phase I/II trial of the safety and efficacy of shark cartilage in the treatment of advanced cancer. *J Clin Oncol.* 1998;16:3649–3655.
11. Loprinzi CL, Levitt R, Barton DL, et al. Evaluation of shark cartilage in patients with advanced cancer A north central cancer treatment group trial. *Cancer.* 2005;104: 176–182.
12. Ratel D, Glazier G, Provencal M, et al. Direct-acting fibrinolytic enzymes in shark cartilage extract: potential therapeutic role in vascular disorders. *Thromb Res.* 2005;115: 143–152.
13. Boivin D, Gendron S, Beaulieu E, et al. The antiangiogenic agent Neovastat (AE-941) induces endothelial cell apoptosis. *Mol Cancer Ther.* 2002;1:795–802.
14. Sauder DN, Dekoven J, Champagne P, et al. Neovastat (AE-941), an inhibitor of angiogenesis: randomized phase I/II clinical trial results in patients with plaque psoriasis. *J Am Acad Dermatol.* 2002;47:535–541.

Silymarin. *See* Milk Thistle *(Silybum marianum).*

Sodium Bicarbonate

Sodium bicarbonate (baking soda) is an alkaline salt that buffers metabolic acids in the body. Because exhaustion during high-intensity exercise has been attributed to lactic acidosis and an increase in hydrogen ions (H^+), bicarbonate supplementation has been proposed to enhance the buffering capacity of the blood. Metabolic demands of high-intensity activity are met mainly by the anaerobic breakdown of glucose, resulting in the production of metabolic acids (lactic acid), which decrease the pH of exercising muscle. Bicarbonate may reduce the acidity of muscle cells by drawing out H^+ and lactic acid. Theoretically, increasing the body's buffering capacity may delay the onset of fatigue and improve exercise performance (1).

Media and Marketing Claims	Efficacy
Enhances power and strength (for anaerobic exercise) and reduces fatigue in trained athletes	↑?

Safety

◆ Ingestion of sodium bicarbonate is contraindicated for individuals with dietary sodium restriction. A typical dose (15 to 22 g) contains 4 to 6 g sodium.

◆ Doses of 300 mg/kg body weight have not been associated with any reported serious adverse effects.

◆ Some subjects report gastrointestinal distress, including diarrhea, cramps, and bloating after ingestion of sodium bicarbonate. This is attributed to the sodium load, which pulls additional fluid into the intestine to create an isotonic solution. Drinking sufficient water may alleviate these side effects (1).

Drug/Supplement Interactions

No reported adverse interactions

Key Points

◆ Laboratory studies of high-intensity exercise show that sodium bicarbonate (300 mg/kg/day) may exert an ergogenic effect under conditions of anaerobic exercise lasting from 1 to 7 minutes. Evidence is also supportive in terms of prolonged intermittent exercise (cycling). However, not all studies support this, and the available studies are relatively small in terms of the numbers of subjects enrolled.

◆ Sodium bicarbonate supplementation is not recommended for recreational athletes because of possible gastrointestinal side effects and because the potential benefits are limited to near-maximal exercise lasting 1 to 7 minutes.

Food Sources

Sodium bicarbonate is household baking soda.

Dosage Information/Bioavailability

Sodium bicarbonate is sold in capsules, usually combined with other alkaline salts (sodium phosphate and sodium citrate). Most manufacturers recommend taking 15 to 22 g sodium bicarbonate with water 1 to 2 hours before exercise.

Relevant Research

Sodium Bicarbonate and Exercise Performance

♦ In a meta-analysis, 29 randomized, placebo-controlled, double-blind trials (total n = 285 subjects) of bicarbonate supplementation during anaerobic exercise (sprints on a cycle or row ergometer, or track run) were analyzed. Studies provided bicarbonate in dosages ranging from 100 to 400 mg sodium bicarbonate/kg body weight (approximately 7 to 28 g for a 70-kg person) via capsules, solution, or intravenous injection. Endpoints included time to exhaustion, changes in power, and/or total work accomplished over a given period of time. Sixteen of the trials showed no effect with treatment compared with 19 studies that reported benefits. Sodium bicarbonate ingestion resulted in a more alkaline blood pH, with the dose only moderately related to the increase in pH and bicarbonate. Overall, there was a positive effect on performance with bicarbonate (weighted mean effect size = 0.44), indicating that the mean performance of the bicarbonate trials was 0.44 standard deviations better than the placebo trial. However, the range of effect was large. The authors attributed this to differences in dosages, intensity and duration of exercise, and conditions of ingestion. Studies involving performance trials with a large anaerobic segment, large doses of bicarbonate, or repetitive work bouts showed the most powerful ergogenic effect (2).

♦ A review article concluded that bicarbonate-loading (300 mg/kg) delays fatigue during exhaustive exercise lasting 1 to 7 minutes, but studies using other exercise protocols and lower dosages have not consistently improved performance (1).

♦ In a study assessing the role of sodium bicarbonate supplementation on VO_2 capacity, 10 active subjects performed 6-minute cycling bouts on two separate days at 25 watts more than their ventilatory threshold (3), one day with sodium bicarbonate supplementation and the other without. Pre-exercise sodium bicarbonate was associated with an increase in blood pH. It also was associated with slowed release of oxygen to the working muscle, which led to reduced muscle fatigue during the slow component of exercise.

♦ A study of the effect of sodium bicarbonate on prolonged intermittent cycling exercise was conducted in eight healthy male athletes. Subjects were randomly assigned to take either sodium chloride (0.045 g/kg^{-1}) or sodium bicarbonate (0.3 g/kg^{-1}) one hour prior to the intermittent cycling exercise. Subjects were blinded to the intervention, but investigators were not. The intermittent exercise included 10 3-minute blocks that included 90 seconds of cycling at 40% VO_{2max}, 60 seconds at 60% VO_{2max}, and 14 seconds at maximal sprint followed by 16 seconds of active rest. Results showed that sodium bicarbonate supplementation increased pH resulting in alkalosis that was maintained throughout the exercise bout; similar effects on pH were not shown in the group taking sodium chloride. Oxygen consumption and heart rate were comparable across groups throughout the study. Sodium bicarbonate supplementation prior to exercise was also associated with improved sprint performance in that the subjects taking sodium bicarbonate were able to maintain the same level of performance throughout the exercise period, a pattern of performance not sustained in the sodium chloride group (4).

◆ In a placebo-controlled study in professional cyclists to assess the role of pre-activity sodium bicarbonate intake on exercise performance, seven subjects consumed sodium bicarbonate at a dose of 0.3 g/kg^{-1} or placebo and then 1 hour later completed two 6-minute bouts of high intensity activity (90% VO_{2max}) interspersed with 8 minutes of active recovery. Slow component VO_2 was the primary outcome. Because the slow component of VO_2 (defined as the difference between end-exercise VO_2 and the VO_2 at the end of the third minute) was not significantly different between sodium bicarbonate and placebo treatments, the authors concluded that sodium bicarbonate did not significantly improve performance (5).

◆ In a double-blind, randomized trial, seven endurance-trained males ingested 0.3 g/kg^{-1} body mass sodium bicarbonate or calcium carbonate (control) divided into four equal doses and consumed 120, 110, 100 and 90 minutes before exercise (6). Both fine-needle muscle sampling and plasma samples were collected before and throughout the study. Subjects completed a standardized ergometer bout, which included a 5 minute warm-up, then a 30-minute exercise at 80% VO_{2max}, followed by a 30-minute linear mode where subjects were asked to complete as much work as possible. Supplementation with sodium bicarbonate was not associated with improved endurance exercise performance: the time and average power output were similar between the two groups. Oxygen consumption, heart rate, perceived exertion were also not significantly different between groups. The treatment with sodium bicarbonate was associated with a small degree of muscular alkalosis, but no significant difference in muscle lactate formation or muscle glycogen formation. Previously, it was thought that sodium bicarbonate might cause increased muscle glycogenolysis and glycolysis, leading to reduced performance. This did not occur in this study, but no benefit was demonstrated either.

References

1. Linderman JK, Gosselink KL. The effects of sodium bicarbonate ingestion on exercise performance. *Sports Med.* 1994;18:75–80.
2. Matson LG, Tran ZV. Effects of sodium bicarbonate ingestion on anaerobic performance: a meta-analytic review. *Int J Sport Nutr.* 1993;3:2–28.
3. Kolkhorst FW, Rezende RS, Levy SS, et al. Effects of sodium bicarbonate on VO_2 kinetics during heavy exercise. *Med Sci Sports Exerc.* 2004;36:1895–1899.

4. Price M, Moss P, Rance S. Effects of sodium bicarbonate ingestion on prolonged inter-
    mittent exercise. *Med Sci Sports Exerc.* 2003;35:1303–1308.
5. Santalla A, Perez M, Montilla M, et al. Sodium bicarbonate ingestion does not alter the
    slow component of oxygen uptake kinetics in professional cyclists. *J Sports Sci.* 2003;21:
    39–47.
6. Stephens TJ, McKenna MJ, Canny BJ, et al. Effect of sodium bicarbonate on muscle
    metabolism during intense endurance cycling. *Med Sci Sports Exerc.* 2002;34:614–621.

Soy Protein and Isoflavones

Soy protein and isoflavones (a type of flavonoid found primarily in soy products) are
found naturally in food and packaged in supplements. They are being investigated primarily for their potential to treat symptoms of menopause and to prevent heart disease,
cancer, and osteoporosis; recent research has also focused on their role in improved renal
health in individuals with diabetes. Isoflavones are naturally occurring weak estrogens
(also called "phytoestrogens") that may exert both estrogenic and antiestrogenic properties. Genistein, daidzein, and glycetein are the principle isoflavones in the soybean (1).

In 1999, the FDA approved a soy protein health claim for use on food packaging. The
claim states that "Diets low in saturated fat and cholesterol that include 25 grams of soy
protein a day may reduce the risk of heart disease. One serving of [name of food] provides
[number of] grams of soy protein" (2). For a soy food to bear the health claim, one serving
must contain at least 6.25 g soy protein; the food must also be low in fat, saturated fat, and
cholesterol, and it must have a low sodium value (specific values vary depending on the
type of food). The basis of this health claim was derived from a meta-analysis conducted
in 1995 by Anderson et al, which established that 25 g soy protein per day could reduce
cholesterol in individuals with hypercholesterolemia (3).

In 2006 the American Heart Association (AHA) published a scientific advisory for
health care professionals regarding soy protein and isoflavones and cardiovascular disease
(4). The review of the literature conducted included 22 trials and estimated mean reductions in LDL cholesterol to be 3% when mean daily intake of soy protein is 50 g. Data for
soy isoflavone effects showed no clinical efficacy. Thus, the AHA suggests that soy should
not be considered as an effective supplement for prevention of heart disease, but rather soy
foods should be considered as cardioprotective because they are low in fat and saturated
fat and high in fiber and minerals.

Media and Marketing Claims	Efficacy
Reduces cholesterol levels in individuals with hypercholesterolemia	↑?
Reduces risk of cancer	↔
Reduces menopausal symptoms	↔
Reduces risk of osteoporosis	↔
Improves kidney function in people with both diabetes and renal impairment	NR

Safety

♦ Women with breast cancer should avoid using soy protein and concentrated isoflavone supplements. There is some concern that soy protein and isoflavones, which possess weak estrogenic activity, may stimulate cancer proliferation in women with breast cancer (5,6). Genistein stimulated tumor growth in ovariectomized mice with experimentally induced breast cancer (7).

♦ There is some concern that soy protein or isoflavone supplements may adversely affect thyroid hormone levels (8,9), especially in individuals without adequate iodine intake. A review of 14 studies (thyroid function was not main outcome) found that in people with normal thyroid function, soy intake had no adverse effects on thyroid levels(10). However, soy supplements may interfere with the absorption of synthetic thyroid medication. Also, in people who have compromised thyroid function or inadequate iodine status, soy supplements could induce hypothyroidism (10).

♦ Long-term use (up to 5 years) of 150 mg soy isoflavone supplements daily in post-menopausal women has been associated with endothelial hyperplasia (11).

Drug/Supplement Interactions

♦ Soy supplements may reduce the absorption of thyroid medications (levothyroxine) when taken concurrently.

♦ Theoretically, the potential estrogenic properties of soy could interfere with estrogen replacement therapy. There is concern that soy may have antagonist effects on tamoxifen binding to estrogen receptors, which could lead to reduced drug efficacy.

Key Points

♦ There is evidence that soy protein may reduce cholesterol levels in individuals with hypercholesterolemia, but not in individuals with normal cholesterol levels. Whether these effects are specifically related to isoflavones or other compounds in soy protein (eg, saponins, phytic acid) or an interaction between soy protein and isoflavones needs further study. Therefore, at present, soy foods are preferable to concentrated supplements of isolated genistein, daidzein, or soy protein.

♦ The potential relationship between soy protein and specific isoflavones in human cancer is inconclusive. In vitro and animal studies are promising; however, studies specifically testing soy protein supplements or genistein in cancer prevention studies or cancer treatment in humans are lacking. The notion that age at administration may be a critical factor in how soy protein or isoflavones affect cancer is intriguing and requires further study. Currently, several trials are underway testing the effects of soy on the development of breast and prostate cancer. There are also a few studies underway to assess the relationship between soy and other cancers such as bladder and endometrial cancers.

♦ A recent meta-analysis of 13 parallel-design trials examining hot flashes and soy in 1,746 women found that initial hot flash frequency explained approximately 46% of the treatment effect (12). Hot flash frequency decreased approximately 5% (more than the placebo/control effects) for each additional hot flash per day in women whose initial hot flash frequency was 5 or more. This is less than hormone replacement therapy (HRT), but for women with contraindications to HRT, soy isoflavones may provide some relief, particularly for women who experience several hot flashes per day. Doses required for efficacy are relatively high.

◆ Increasing amounts of research suggest that soy protein–containing isoflavones increase bone mineral density and may attenuate losses in postmenopausal women. Earlier studies using the synthetic isoflavone ipriflavone found a reduction in bone loss in postmenopausal women. However, a large-scale, well-controlled trial of ipriflavone supplements reported no benefit in women with osteoporosis and was associated with significant decreases in lymphocyte concentrations.

◆ General findings from a published review of soy and bone mineral density suggest that soy isoflavones are more effective in preventing bone loss in younger women than in postmenopausal women, and that the amount needed to attenuate bone loss is approximately 80 mg/day (13).

◆ Women with estrogen receptor positive (ER+) breast cancer are advised to not increase their soy intake because there is some evidence that genistein may stimulate breast cancer growth; women with ER+ tumors who take tamoxifen are advised to avoid soy (14). Isoflavone supplements are not recommended for women with breast cancer (15).

◆ Preliminary evidence suggest plant proteins may improve renal function in people with diabetes. However, the effect of soy supplementation on renal function has not been adequately studied in this patient population.

◆ Although people in certain cultures have been consuming soy foods for centuries, the efficacy and safety of concentrated sources of isolated isoflavones in pill form is not known. As with other phytochemicals, the composition of isoflavones in plants with other nutrients and numerous other phytochemicals occur in certain proportions. Until the research is clear, soy products such as miso, soy milk and soy-based beverages, tofu, and whole soybeans will continue to be the preferred source of soy protein, isoflavones, and other potentially bioactive compounds in soy.

Food Sources

Food	Soy Protein, g	Genistein, mg	Daidzein, mg
Soy protein isolates (isolated soy protein—92% protein)	23 per oz	51 per ½ cup	19 per ½ cup
Soy flour (½ cup)	22	94	56
Natto (fermented soybeans) (½ cup)	15	32	23
Tofu (4 oz)	17	19	9
Tempeh (½ cup)	16	32	23

Food	Soy Protein, g	Genistein, mg	Daidzein, mg
Soy protein, dry textured (½ cup) (70% protein)	11	72	43
Soybeans (½ cup)	11	6	20
Soy milk (1 cup)	7	6	4
Soy nuts, roasted (2 Tbsp)	5	26	16

Source: Data are from references 16 and 17.

Most soy products (soybean, tofu, soy milk, tempeh, soy flour) contain isoflavones. Soy foods processed by techniques that use excessive water, alcohol, or organic washings may have lower levels of isoflavones. For example, textured soy protein or soy protein concentrates made by aqueous alcohol extraction are very low in isoflavones because the isoflavones are soluble in alcohol and are thus removed during processing. However, some manufacturers add isoflavones after processing. The isoflavone content of some soy products may be diluted by added ingredients (eg, water in soy milk). Soy oil and soy sauce contain no appreciable soy protein or isoflavones (18).

In general, a 7- to 10-g serving of soy protein supplies 30 to 50 mg isoflavones (1 to 2 mg genistein per 1 g soy protein). Three servings of soy foods (eg, 2 cups soy milk plus 4 oz tofu) provide approximately 20 to 30 g soy protein.

In the United States, daily soy consumption is typically less than 1 g soy protein and 0.1 to 3.0 mg isoflavones (17). In contrast, daily soy intake in Japan and China is estimated to be between 30 and 50 mg isoflavones (12,19), 5 to 10 g soy protein (19,20), and 50 to 80 g soy foods/day (19,20).

Dosage Information/Bioavailability

Soy protein powders provide 1 to 10 mg isoflavones in 1.0 to 3.5 g of soy protein. A typical serving of a commercial soy protein supplement provides approximately 20 to 25 g protein. Soy isoflavones are available in tablets, capsules, powders, drinks, and bars. Genistein supplements provide 30 to 55 mg genistein. Mixed isoflavonoid supplements typically provide 25 to 100 mg total isoflavones. The bioavailability of isoflavones varies from 13% to 35%, depending on gut microflora (21). Ingestion of 60 g soy protein resulted in increased plasma concentrations of genistein (plasma peak after 6 to 8 hours) and daidzein (plasma peak after 1.5 hours) (22). In a study describing the pharmacokinetics of single isoflavone doses of 1, 2, 4, 8, and 16 mg/kg body weight, half-lives of free genistein and diadzein were 3.2 and 4.2 hours, respectively, and tolerance was good (23).

Relevant Research

Soy Protein/Isoflavones and Lipid Levels and Cardiovascular Disease

- The American Heart Association Nutrition Committee published a Science Advisory for Professionals regarding soy protein, isoflavones and cardiovascular health in 2006. This advisory suggests that review of well-designed studies does not support the use of soy isoflavones for cardiovascular disease risk reduction and that soy protein is estimated to be associated with only a 3% reduction in LDL cholesterol at intakes, on average, of 50 g/day (4).

◆ A prospective epidemiological study (EPIC) assessed the relationship between dietary phytoestrogen intake and cardiovascular disease (CVD) in 16,165 women from the general population living in European countries (some with and some without cardiovascular disease) ages 49 to 70 years. Five hundred nineteen subjects experienced a cardiovascular event during the 5.2-year study period. The results indicate that the Cox Hazards Ratio for having a cardiovascular event was not significantly associated with isoflavone or lignan intake (24).

◆ A meta-analysis of 38 controlled clinical trials (total n = 730 subjects) evaluated the effects of soy protein consumption on serum lipid levels in humans. Twenty studies used isolated soy protein, 15 used textured soy protein, and three used a combination of the two. There was a significant association between soy protein intake (mean intake = 47 g/day) and improved serum lipids. Thirty-four of 38 trials reported decreases in serum cholesterol. Overall, daily soy protein consumption was associated with a 9.3% decrease in total cholesterol, 12.9% decrease in LDL cholesterol, and 10.5% decrease in serum triglycerides. There was a nonsignificant increase in HDL cholesterol (3).

◆ A study compared the lipid-reduction effects of daily milk protein (42 g/day) vs soy protein (42 g/day) in 94 postmenopausal women with baseline elevated serum cholesterol levels. Subjects taking the soy supplement included one group that received soy protein with isoflavone supplementation (80 mg aglycone) and a second group that received soy protein with only trace amounts of isoflavones. Subjects took the randomly assigned supplement daily for a period of 12 weeks. Over time, lipid levels decreased more in the group receiving soy with isoflavones than in the group taking soy protein without isoflavones; however, neither change was significantly different than the change for the milk protein group. This unexpected reduction in serum LDL and total cholesterol in all three groups suggests that a change in body weight may have contributed to the reduction in cholesterol independent of soy protein or isoflavone effects. However, weight remained stable in all three groups. This study was unblinded and not placebo-controlled (25).

◆ A double-blind, placebo-controlled study was conducted in 36 postmenopausal women with moderately elevated serum cholesterol levels who were randomly assigned to receive either a phytoestrogen supplement (150 mg) or placebo daily for 8 weeks. An additional follow-up assessment of triglycerides and total cholesterol was conducted at 6 months (26). Phytoestrogen supplementation had no significant effect on lipids at any time point of measurement. This study suggests that the specific phytoestrogens found in soy foods do not play a role in lipid modulation, but other soy constituents are responsible for this biological effect. It is important to note, however, that supplementation of 150 mg/day is much less than the recommended 25 g/day for reducing lipid levels. In addition, the supplement used was reportedly a phytoestrogen supplement, and thus soy protein allocation could have been substantially less.

- In a double-blind, parallel-design trial, 156 men and women with hypercholes-terolemia who had been given instruction in a National Cholesterol Education Program (NCEP) Step I diet were randomly assigned for 9 weeks to one of five diets: 25 g isolated soy protein per day with 3, 27, 37, or 62 mg isoflavones, or 25 g casein (for isoflavone-free comparison). Compared with casein, soy protein with 62 mg of isoflavones significantly reduced total and LDL cholesterol levels by 4% and 6%, respectively. Soy protein with 37 mg isoflavones reduced total and LDL cholesterol by 8%. There was a dose-response effect of increasing amounts of isoflavones on total and LDL cholesterol levels. Triglycerides and HDL cholesterol were not affected. Soy protein with 3 mg isoflavones had no significant effect on lipid levels (28).

- In a double-blind, placebo-controlled trial, 156 subjects with hypercholesterolemia on an NCEP Step I cholesterol-reducing diet were randomly assigned to consume one of five beverages for 9 weeks: (*a*) 25 g soy protein containing 62 mg isoflavones, (*b*) 25 g soy protein containing 37 mg isoflavones, (*c*) 25 g soy protein containing 27 mg isoflavones, (*d*) 25 g soy protein containing 3 mg isoflavones, or (*e*) a placebo beverage with 25 g casein and 0 mg isoflavones. Prior to randomization to treatment, subjects completed a 4-week run-in using the NCEP Step I Diet. In subjects with a baseline LDL more than 160 mg/dL, LDL cholesterol was significantly reduced by 10% in those sub-jects ingesting the 62-mg isoflavone dosage and by 10% in subjects ingesting the 37-mg isoflavone dosage compared with the placebo, but not with lower dosages of isoflavone. In subjects with baseline LDL between 140 and 160 mg/dL, there was no significant effect on cholesterol associated with any soy protein beverage (28).

- In a randomized, blinded controlled trial among hyperlipidemic postmenopausal women, 40 women were randomly assigned to either 90 mg isoflavones per day or placebo for 6 weeks (29). Vascular function was tested using flow-mediated vasodila-tion and response to nitroglycerin (endothelial-independent). Although lipid levels were not modulated by isoflavone supplementation, nitroglycerine responsiveness was greater in the isoflavone-supplemented group. Flow-mediated vasodilation was also not affected by supplementation. The inconsistent results suggest that select compo-nents in soy foods may have different mechanisms of action. If research is not appro-priately designed to "match" soy constituents with appropriate outcome measures that are mechanistic-specific, it is unlikely that any such studies will show efficacy.

- In a double-blind, placebo-controlled trial, 213 healthy (normotensive, normolipi-demic) men and women (ages 50 to 75 years) were randomly assigned to receive either soy protein isolate (40 g soy protein, 118 mg isoflavones) or placebo (casein) daily for 3 months. One-hundred seventy-nine subjects completed the study. Dietary compliance was measured by urinary phytoestrogen levels. Blood pressure, lipids, hormone profiles, vascular function, and endothelial function were assessed. Soy was associated with a significant reduction in mean blood pressure (–4.2 mm Hg) com-pared with placebo. Soy also resulted in significant reductions in LDL:HDL ratios and triglycerides (TG), but resulted in an increase in lipoprotein a (Lp[a]). Both groups experienced improved total, LDL, and HDL cholesterol with no significant differences between groups. There were no significant changes in any hormone level (follicle-stimulating hormone [FSH], luteinizing hormone [LH], testosterone) in male or female subjects with either soy supplementation or placebo. Arterial function also did not differ between groups, as both groups improved. Peripheral vascular resistance significantly improved with soy, whereas flow-mediated vasodilation (measure of endothelial function) actually decreased in men consuming soy compared with men consuming the placebo. The authors noted that soy supplementation had both beneficial (improved blood pressure, cholesterol ratios, TG, peripheral vascular resistance) and negative cardiovascular effects (increase in Lp(a) and decrease in endothelial function in men) (30).

♦ In a double-blind, placebo-controlled trial, 104 postmenopausal women were randomly assigned to receive 60 g isolated soy protein or a placebo (caseinate) daily for 12 weeks. Seventy-seven subjects (44 were dyslipidemic) completed the trial. Both the soy and placebo groups experienced significant reductions in total and LDL cholesterol, but only those consuming soy had a significant reductions in apolipoprotein B and LDL:HDL ratios. Lp(a) plasma levels were not significantly changed by either treatment. The authors concluded that isolated soy protein is slightly better than caseinate in favorably modifying the lipoprotein metabolism of postmenopausal women, and this effect is greatest in those with hypercholesterolemia (31).

♦ In a randomized, placebo-controlled, double-blind study was conducted in 202 postmenopausal women ranging in age from 60 to 75 years. Subjects were overweight (mean BMIs of 25.9 and 26.4 in the placebo and soy groups, respectively) and inactive. At the time of enrollment, approximately 20% of subjects were on lipid-lowering medications, but mean serum cholesterol levels were elevated (236.2 mg/dL and 240.2 mg/dL in the placebo and soy groups, respectively) at baseline. Most subjects were nonsmokers. During the trial, subjects consumed either a 99-mg isoflavone supplement or placebo daily for 12 months. The soy intervention resulted in a significant increase in systolic blood pressure, a change that was significantly greater than the small increase in the placebo group. Changes in endothelial function did not differ significantly between the placebo and soy supplementation groups (32).

♦ Two review articles discussed potential mechanisms by which soy protein and/or isoflavones may reduce risk of heart disease. Animal and in vitro studies have demonstrated that soy may (*a*) increase bile acid excretion, (*b*) promote estrogenic activity, (*c*) improve vascular reactivity, and/or (*d*) inhibit LDL cholesterol oxidation and exhibit antioxidant activity. Alternatively, soy protein may displace foods high in saturated fat and cholesterol and thus have an indirect effect on reducing blood cholesterol levels (33,34).

Soy Protein/Isoflavones and Cancer

♦ Several epidemiological studies in China and Japan have found that consumption of soy foods is associated with lower risk of breast, colon, and prostate cancers. Consumption of nonfermented soy products (soy milk and tofu) tended to be either protective or not associated with cancer risk, whereas no consistent pattern was apparent with fermented soy foods (miso). In the studies that demonstrated a protective effect, a single serving of soy (4 oz tofu or 1 cup soy milk) daily throughout the lifespan was associated with reduced cancer risk (35).

♦ A mixed-ethnicity case-control study of 500 women with endometrial cancer and 470 age-matched control subjects living in the San Francisco, California, area showed the odds ratio of developing endometrial cancer was significantly less in women in the highest quintile of phytoestrogen intake as compared with the lowest quintile (OR = 0.59; 95% CI = 0.37–0.93), particularly in women with normal BMIs, whereas obese, postmenopausal women with low phytoestrogen intake had an approximately seven-fold increased risk for endometrical cancer (36). The findings from case-control studies, however, have not always held up when prospective intervention trials have been conducted in follow-up, probably because these studies rely on retrospective recall of diet and other lifestyle data.

♦ In two small studies assessing the effect of soy supplementation on PSA levels, no significant effects were identified. The first was a substudy of the Soy Isoflavone Prevention Trial, which was a randomized, controlled, double-blind dietary intervention trial to evaluate the effects of soy on colorectal cancer risk and colonic epithelial cells. This study enrolled 81 males who were randomly assigned to 12 months of supplementation with either isoflavone-rich or -deplete soy protein drinks containing 83 mg isoflavones per day or less than 5 mg per day. In this study, the association between PSA and soy was assessed as a secondary hypothesis (37). Subjects were men between the ages of 57 and 72.5 years, predominantly well-educated whites, with mean baseline PSA levels of 1.7 ng/mL. Regardless of beverage consumed, PSA levels increased by approximately 16% during the 12-month time frame and change in PSA correlated significantly with serum genistein concentrations (marker of soy exposure).

♦ The second study, an unblinded pilot study where no control group was included, recruited 41 men with increasing PSA levels in "watchful-waiting" status (ie, their PSA levels were elevated, indicating a new prostate cancer diagnosis, but not high enough to consider surgical or other medical interventions to treat) or men who had rising PSA levels after previous treatment for prostate cancer, including local or hormone therapy (38). Thirty nine patients completed the intervention, which consisted of 100 mg soy isoflavone twice daily for 3 to 6 months (median of 5.5 months). Soy supplementation did not result in a sustained reduction in PSA levels, but PSA levels did stabilize in 83% of subjects who had previously received androgen-ablation therapy. Additional randomized, blinded, placebo-controlled studies are needed with particular attention not only to PSA but also tissue-specific changes that may support a chemopreventive role of soy.

♦ In the European Prospective Investigation of Cancer (EPIC), a large epidemiological study, 280 cases of breast cancer were diagnosed in a cohort of 15,555 women during a 4-year time frame (39). The Hazard Ratio (HR) for developing breast cancer when comparing high consumers of isoflavones with low consumers of isoflavones was 1.0, indicating no protective effect. Major limitations of this study include the lack of wide variability in isoflavone intake as well as low median intake (0.4 mg/day).

◆ The timing of soy consumption may help reduce breast cancer risk. Exposure during prepubescent and pubescent years may be of particular biological importance because that is when mammary gland differentiation takes place. In an epidemiological study conducted in Chinese women, 1,459 women with breast cancer and 1,556 control women provided dietary data based on recall of intake between the ages of 13 and 15 years (40). The data support that exposure to soy foods during adolescence was protective against the development of breast cancer later in life and a dose-response was demonstrated. Self-reported data about dietary intake were also verified by comparing each mother's report of her child's pattern of soyfood intake during adolescence and subsequent breast cancer risk as well. This study provides an interesting hypothesis upon which intervention trials should be developed to test prospectively the relationship between early soy food exposure and breast cancer risk later in life.

◆ Research is not conclusive, but most clinicians do not recommend soy to treat postmenopausal symptoms in women with a history of breast cancer because there is concern that soy may increase estradiol levels and/or interfere with the clinical efficacy of select estrogen receptor modulators or aromatase inhibitors. A review of the topic that was published in 2001 presents issues to consider (41).

◆ An unblinded pilot study that included no control group assigned 16 postmenopausal women to receive 20 g soy protein and 20 g isoflavones as genistein daily for 24 weeks. Women ranged in age from 51 to 61 years and demonstrated baseline follicular stimulating hormone levels greater than 40 mIU/mL. Results showed no increase in estradiol or gonadotropin levels with supplementation (42). However, given the small sample size and weak study design, these results need to be interpreted cautiously.

Soy Protein/Isoflavones and Menopause

◆ Numerous small studies assessing the effects of soy supplementation on menopausal symptoms have yielded variable findings. In a randomized, double-blind, placebo-controlled study of the role of soy in modulating cognitive decline associated with menopause (SOPHIA study), 56 postmenopausal women received 110 mg soy isoflavones or placebo daily for 6 months. Soy supplementation was associated with a significant improvement above baseline in cognitive function (as measured by Trails A and B, category fluency testing, and logical memory and recall) and also with significantly higher scores than were shown in the placebo group (43). Another randomized, double-blinded, placebo-controlled study was conducted among 26 postmenopausal women drinking an isoflavone-enriched beverage containing 134.4 mg total isoflavones or a placebo beverage daily for 12 weeks. At the end of study, there were no significant differences between groups for Greene Menopause Symptom Scores, vaginal maturation, hot flashes, or follical stimulating hormone or sex hormone binding globulin levels (44). Women in the soy-supplemented group reported more adverse events and more frequently reported "bad taste," which suggests that blinding may have been compromised.

◆ A randomized, double-blind, placebo-controlled study of 80 postmenopausal women, randomly assigned 40 to receive placebo and 40 to receive isoflavones (100 mg/day). The study reported that isoflavone supplementation for 4 months was associated with significant improvements in perimenopausal symptom scores (Kupperman Index) from baseline and between groups at the end of intervention (45).

◆ In the randomized, double-blind, placebo-controlled Soy Estrogen Alternative Study, vasomotor symptoms (hot flashes and night sweats recorded in a symptom diary) decreased in the 241 peri- and postmenopausal women receiving 25 g of soy protein daily for 2 years, regardless of isoflavone levels in the supplement (0, 42, or 58 mg/day). These results suggest that either a significant placebo effect exists or that some compound other than isoflavones found in soy protein supplements and placebo may improve vasomotor symptoms associated with menopause (46).

◆ A randomized, double-blind, multicenter study evaluated the effects of isoflavones and melatonin on menopausal symptoms in 232 women. The Greene Climacteric Scale was used to quantify symptoms at baseline and 3 months in a 2 × 2 factorial design. Symptoms decreased 39% from baseline with 80 mg isoflavones plus 3 mg melatonin, 38% with isoflavones alone, 26% with melatonin, and 38% with placebo. The author stated that "placebo effect was much higher than planned, making it meaningless to perform any statistical test" (47).

◆ In a randomized, double-blind, placebo-controlled study, 90 healthy post-menopausal women received either estrogen/progesterone replacement therapy, genistein (54 mg/day), or placebo for 1 year (48). There was a consistent reduction in daily hot flashes at 3, 6, and 12 months in both the group receiving genistein and the HRT group as compared with those receiving placebo. HRT was more significantly more effective than genistein in reducing hot flashes, but genistein was not associated with detrimental effects on endometrial tissue thickness, a common clinical sequelae associated with HRT use.

◆ In a prospective cohort study of 1,106 Japanese women (ages 41 to 60 years), soy food intake was measured by a food-frequency questionnaire. Compared with the lowest tertile of intake, the highest tertile for the study population had a significantly lower report rate of hot flashes, as measured using the Kupperman test of menopausal distress (HR = 0.47; 95% CI = 0.28–0.79) (19).

◆ In a double-blind, placebo-controlled study, 69 menopausal women were randomly assigned to one of three groups for 24 weeks: (*a*) isolated soy protein with 80.4 mg isoflavones per day; (*b*) isolated soy protein with 4.4 mg of isoflavones/day; or (*c*) whey protein control. A menopausal index assessed changes in hot flashes and night sweats and other symptoms at baseline, week 12, and week 24. There were no differences between groups in hot flash or night sweat frequency. However, there was a significant decrease in hot flash and night sweat frequency with time in all treatment groups. The authors concluded that this indicated a placebo effect or simply an improvement in symptoms during the course of the trial (49).

◆ In a double-blind, placebo-controlled, multicenter study, 177 postmenopausal women (mean age 55 years) who were experiencing five or more hot flashes per day were randomly assigned to receive either soy isoflavone extract (total of 50 mg genistin and daidzin per day) or a placebo daily for 12 weeks. Both groups experienced relief of vasomotor symptoms; however, in the soy group hot flashes decreased significantly during the first 2 weeks whereas hot flashes did not decrease in the placebo group until week 4. Throughout 12 weeks, the frequency and severity of hot flashes decreased more in the soy group, but this difference was not significant. Endometrial thickness (measured by ultrasound), lipoproteins, bone markers, sex hormone-binding globulin and follicle-stimulating hormone, and vaginal cytology did not change in either group (50).

♦ In a double-blind, placebo-controlled, crossover study, 177 women with a history of breast cancer and substantial hot flashes received, in random order, soy tablets (150 mg soy isoflavones—similar to amount in three glasses of soy milk) or a placebo each day for 4 weeks, after a 1-week baseline period with no treatment, but no washout. Patients completed a daily questionnaire documenting hot flash frequency and intensity and perceived side effects. At the end of the study, use of soy tablets demonstrated no effect on the frequency of hot flashes (51).

♦ In a double-blind, placebo-controlled study, 104 postmenopausal women were randomly assigned to receive 60 g soy protein isolate containing 40 g protein and 76 mg isoflavones daily or a placebo (60 g casein, no isoflavones) for 12 weeks. Twenty-five patients dropped out of the study (11 in the soy group, 14 in the placebo group) because of gastrointestinal side effects such as constipation and bloating. Changes from baseline in self-reported mean number of moderate to severe hot flashes and night sweats were measured during treatment. Compared with subjects in the placebo group, subjects consuming soy protein reported significantly fewer mean number of hot flashes per 24 hours after 4, 8, and 12 weeks. Specifically, in the soy group, the mean number of hot flashes decreased 26% by week 3, 33% by week 4, and 45% by week 12 compared with 30% reduction in the placebo group by week 12. The overall rates of adverse effects were similar for soy and casein (placebo) (52).

Soy Protein/Isoflavones/Ipriflavone and Osteoporosis

♦ Numerous studies have assessed the relationship between soy intake and bone health, yielding mixed results.

♦ In an randomized, double-blind, placebo-controlled study of 202 postmenopausal women, 87 received placebo and 88 received 25.6 g soy protein containing 99 mg isoflavones daily for the entire 12 month intervention period. DXA scans of the hip and lumbar spine showed that 12 months of supplementation with soy did not significantly change bone mineral density (BMD) compared with placebo (53).

♦ A prospective cohort study comparing the effects of dietary soy exposure on BMD in premenopausal (n = 293) and postmenopausal (n = 357) Chinese women showed that soy intake at the highest tertile as compared with the lowest favorably modulated lumbar and Ward's triangle BMD in post menopausal (54). No association between dietary soy phytoestrogen intake and BMD was seen in premenopausal women. In this population of Chinese women, soy phytoestrogens are commonly consumed throughout the lifespan, but the positive effects on BMD are only shown here in postmenopausal women.

◆ In a double-blind, randomized, controlled pilot study of 65 postmenopausal women, subjects were randomly assigned to (*a*) soy protein with 96 mg isoflavones, (*b*) soy protein with 52 mg isoflavones, or (*c*) soy without isoflavones for 9 months, with a final assessment 6 months posttreatment (55). Trochanter BMD improved only in the group taking soy protein without isoflavones. Soy supplementation was not associated with improved spinal or femoral neck BMD in any of the groups.

◆ In a randomized, double-blind, placebo-controlled study conducted in 64 men (ages 42 to 77 years) with no known history of osteoporosis and who were between the ages of 42 and 77 years, 40 g intake of soy protein (88 mg total isoflavones) or milk-based protein (placebo) daily for 3 months did not significantly modulate bone growth and/or turnover (56).

◆ In a crossover design, double-blind study, 19 women were randomly assigned to first receive 110 mg/day of soy isoflavones or placebo for 6 months to determine the effect on BMD. Type I collagen alpha 1-chain helical peptide (a biomarker of bone resorption) was significantly increased with soy isoflavone therapy as compared with baseline or placebo (57). Spinal BMD at lumbar 2 and lumbar 3 was also significantly increased, but total spinal BMD showed an only borderline significant improvement ($P \leq .05$).

◆ In a double-blind, placebo-controlled study, 69 perimenopausal subjects were randomly assigned to one of three groups for 24 weeks: (*a*) soy protein isolate with isoflavones (80.4 mg/day); (*b*) soy protein isolate with poor isoflavone content; or (*c*) control (whey protein). Treatment was given in the form of a muffin and protein powder to be mixed into a drink. Subjects were told to stop taking any of their own supplements and were provided with a vitamin and mineral supplement containing 160 mg calcium (all treatments provided 650 mg calcium daily). Lumbar spine BMD and bone mineral content (BMC) were assessed at baseline and at the end of the trial. BMD did not change in either soy group, but significant BMD losses occurred in the control group. When various factors were controlled for (such as body composition, alcohol intake, smoking history, and hormone levels), the soy protein with isoflavones had a significant positive effect on the percentage of change (loss) in both BMD and BMC (58).

◆ In a double-blind, placebo-controlled study, 66 free-living, hypercholesterolemic, postmenopausal women were randomly assigned to one of three groups for 6 months (*a*) NCEP Step I diet with 40 g protein/day from casein and nonfat dry milk, (*b*) NCEP Step I diet with 40 g protein from isolated soy protein containing 1.39 mg isoflavones per gram of protein, or (*c*) NCEP Step I diet with 40 g isolated soy protein containing 2.2 mg isoflavones per gram of protein. Prior to randomization, all subjects followed a 14-day run-in period on the NCEP Step I diet. Total and regional bone mineral content and density of the lumbar spine, proximal femur, and total body were assessed by dual-energy x-ray absorptiometry at baseline and after 6 months. Blood lipids were also analyzed at the baseline and every 2 weeks during the study. Of the skeletal sites tested, lumbar-spine BMC and BMD increased significantly after 6 months of treatment with soy protein containing 2.2 mg isoflavones per gram of protein compared with the control group. The lower dose (1.39 mg isoflavones/g protein) was not associated with any significant changes in bone density. Compared with the control group, both soy protein treatments were associated with a significant increase in HDL cholesterol and improvement in the ratio of total to HDL cholesterol (59).

◆ Several studies conducted in Europe and Asia found ipriflavone (600 mg), a synthetic isoflavone derivative available as a dietary supplement, reduced bone loss in animal models of experimental osteoporosis and in postmenopausal women (60–62).

◆ In a double-blind, placebo-controlled, multicenter study in Europe, 475 post-menopausal women with osteoporosis of the lumbar spine were randomly assigned to receive 600 mg ipriflavone or a placebo daily for 3 years. Both groups also received 500 mg calcium/day. Spine, hip, and forearm BMD were assessed by dual-energy radiograph absorptiometry, and biomarkers of bone resorption were measured every 6 months. The number of new vertebral fractures was assessed each year. There were no differences in the yearly percentage of change in BMD at any site compared with baseline between groups. There were also no differences in biochemical markers and vertebral fractures. Subjects receiving ipriflavone had a significant reduction in lymphocyte concentrations that began 6 months after treatment. Lymphocytopenia developed in 31 subjects; this resolved in 81% of the subjects after 2 years (63).

◆ In a double-blind, placebo-controlled, multicenter study in Italy, 198 post-menopausal women (age 50 to 65 years) with vertebral bone density less than the mean value for normal were randomly assigned to receive 600 mg ipriflavone or a placebo for 2 years. All subjects also received a daily 1-g calcium supplement as calcium carbonate. One hundred thirty-four subjects completed the trial. Bone density and markers of bone turnover were measured at baseline and every 6 months. Analysis of liver and kidney function and routine hematological blood tests were measured before and at the end of treatment. Vertebral bone density increased significantly in the group taking ipriflavone (mean increase of 1.4% after 1 year, and 1% after 2 years). The difference in bone density between the placebo and ipriflavone groups was significant. Urinary hydroxyproline decreased significantly in ipriflavone-treated subjects, suggestive of a reduction in bone turnover rate. Patient compliance assessed by residual tablet count revealed a compliance of more than 80% of study pills after 2 years in 92% of all subjects (62).

Soy and Renal Function in Individuals with Diabetes

◆ In a randomized, crossover design dietary trial conducted among 14 patients (10 men, 4 women) with renal disease associated with a diagnosis of diabetes, patients ate a low-protein diet (0.8 g/kg/day, 70% animal protein/30% plant protein) for 7 weeks, followed by usual diet for 4 weeks (washout period), and then switched to a diet with 30% energy as soy protein and 30% as other plant protein for an additional 7 weeks (64). Urinary nitrogen and protein excretion was significantly reduced in subjects consuming the soy plus other plant protein diet as compared with the 70% animal and 30% plant protein diet. Renal function was also improved, but the change was not significant.

♦ In a randomized, placebo-controlled, crossover design study, 32 postmenopausal women with type 2 diabetes, mean BMI of 32, and mild elevated creatinine levels were randomly assigned and completed the study, taking 30 g soy protein with 132 mg isoflavones or placebo for 12 weeks, after which they completed a 2-week washout and then switched to the alternate supplementation plan (65). As compared with placebo, soy supplementation was associated with significant improvements in glycemic control and in blood lipid levels, but not with improvements in renal function. However, serum creatinine was the only marker of renal function measured. Given the favorable effects on glucose control, indirect effects related to improved renal function could be expected and warrant further study.

References

1. Anderson RL, Wolf WJ. Compositional changes in trypsin inhibitors, phytic acid, saponins, and isoflavones related to soybean processing. *J Nutr.* 1995;125(3 Suppl):S581-S588.
2. Food and Drug Administration Proposed Rule. Food labeling: health claims; soy protein and coronary heart disease. *Fed Regist.* November 10, 1998;63:62977–63015.
3. Anderson JW, Johnstone BM, Cook-Newell ME. Meta-analysis of the effects of soy protein intake on serum lipids. *N Engl J Med.* 1995;333:276–282.
4. Sacks FM, Lichtenstein A, Van Horn L, et al. Soy protein, isoflavones and cardiovascular health. An American Heart Association Science Advisory for professionals from the Nutrition Committee. *Circulation.* 2006;113;1034–1044.
5. McMichael-Phillips DF, Harding C, Morton M, et al. Effects of soy-protein supplementation on epithelial proliferation in the histologically normal human breast. *Am J Clin Nutr.* 1998;68(6 Suppl):S1431-S1435.
6. Petrakis NL, Barnes S, King EB, et al. Stimulatory influence of soy protein isolate on breast secretion in pre- and postmenopausal women. *Cancer Epidemiol Biomarkers Prev.* 1996;5:785–794.
7. Hsieh CY, Santell RC, Haslam SZ, et al. Estrogenic effects of genistein on the growth of estrogen-receptor-positive human breast cancer (MCF-7) cells in vitro and in vivo. *Cancer Res.* 1998;58:3833–3838.
8. Persky VW, Turyk ME, Wang L, et al. Effect of soy protein on endogenous hormones in postmenopausal women. *Am J Clin Nutr.* 2002;75:145–153.
9. Divi RL, Chang HC, Doerge DR. Anti-thyroid isoflavones from soybeans: isolation, characterization, and mechanism of action. *Biochem Pharmacol.* 1997;54:1087–1096.
10. Messina M, Redmond G. Effects of soy protein and soybean isoflavones on thyroid function in healthy adults and hypothyroid patients: a review of the relevant literature. *Thyroid.* 2006;16:249–258.
11. Unfer V, Casinin ML, Costabile L, et al. Endometrial effects of long-term treatment with phytoestrogens: a randomized, double-blind, placebo-controlled study. *Fertil Steril.* 2004;82:145–148.
12. Messina M, Hughes C. Efficacy of soyfoods and soybean isoflavone supplements for alleviating menopausal symptoms is positively related to initial hot flush frequency. *J Medical Foods.* 2003;6:1–11.

13. Messina M, Ho S, Alekel DL. Skeletal benefits of soy isoflavones: a review of the clinical trial and epidemiologic data. *Curr Opin Clin Nutr Metab Care.* 2004;7:649–658.

14. Messina MJ, Loprinzi CL. Soy for breast cancer survivors: a critical review of the literature. *J Nutr.* 2001;131(11 Suppl):S3095–S3108.

15. Block KI, Constantinou A, Hilakivi-Clarke L, et al. Point-counterpoint: soy intake for breast cancer patients. *Integr Cancer Ther.* 2002;1:90–100.

16. US Department of Agriculture, Agricultural Research Service. USDA Nutrient Data Laboratory. Available at: http://www.nal.usda.gov/fnic/cgi-bin/nut_search.pl. Accessed August 23, 1999.

17. US Soyfoods Directory. Soyfood descriptions. Available at: http://www.soyfoods.com/soyfoodsdescriptions/texturedsoyprotein.html. Accessed August 23, 1999.

18. Lusas EW, Riaz MN. Soy protein products: processing and use. *J Nutr.* 1995;125 (3 Suppl):S573–S580S.

19. Nagata C, Takatsuka N, Kawakami N, et al. Soy product intake and hot flashes in Japanese women: results from a community-based prospective study. *Am J Epidemiol.* 2001;153:790–793.

20. Chen YM, Ho SC, Lam SS, et al. Beneficial effects of soy isoflavones on bone mineral content was modified by years since menopause, body weight, and calcium intake: a double-blind, randomized, controlled trial. *Menopause.* 2004;11:246–254.

21. Xu X, Harris KS, Wang HJ, et al. Bioavailability of soybean isoflavones depends upon gut microflora in women. *J Nutr.* 1995;125:2307–2315.

22. Watanabe S, Yamaguchi M, Sobue T, et al. Pharmacokinetics of soybean isoflavones in plasma, urine, and feces of men after ingestion of 60 g baked soybean powder (Kinako). *J Nutr.* 1998;128:1710–1715.

23. Busby MG, Jeffcoat AR, Bloedon LT, et al. Clinical characteristics and pharmacokinetics of purified soy isoflavones: single-dose administration to healthy men. *Am J Clin Nutr.* 2002;75:126–136.

24. van der Schouw YT, Kreijkamp-Kaspers S, Peeters PH, et al. Prospective study on usual dietary phytoestrogen intake and cardiovascular disease risk in Western women. *Circulation.* 2005;111:465–471.

25. Gardner CD, Newell KA, Cherin R, et al. The effect of soy protein with or without isoflavones relative to milk protein on plasma lipids in hypercholesterolemic postmenopausal women. *Am J Clin Nutr.* 2001;73:728–735.

26. Dewell A, Hollenbeck CB, Bruce B. The effects of soy-derived phytoestrogens on serum lipids and lipoproteins in moderately hypercholesterolemic postmenopausal women. *J Clin Endocr Metab.* 2002;87:118–121.

27. Crouse JR, Morgan T, Terry JG, et al. A randomized trial comparing the effect of casein with that of soy protein containing varying amounts of isoflavones on plasma concentrations of lipids and lipoproteins. *Arch Intern Med.* 1999;159:2070–2076.

28. Crouse JR III, Morgan T, Terry JG, et al. A randomized trial comparing the effect of casein with that of soy protein containing varying amounts of isoflavones on plasma concentrations of lipids and lipoproteins. *Arch Intern Med.* 1999;159:2070–2076.

29. Lissin LW, Oka R, Lakshmi S, et al. Isoflavones improve vascular reactivity in postmenopausal women with hypercholesterolemia. *Vasc Med.* 2004;9:26–30.

30. Teeded HJ, Dalais FS, Kosopoulos D, et al. Dietary soy has both beneficial and potentially adverse cardiovascular effects: a placebo-controlled study in men and postmenopausal women. *J Clin Endocrinol Metab.* 2001;86:3053–3060.
31. Vigna GB, Pansini F, Bonaccorsi G, et al. Plasma lipoproteins in soy-treated postmenopausal women: a double-blind, placebo-controlled trial. *Nutr Metab Cardiovasc Dis.* 2000;10:315–322.
32. Kreijkamp-Kaspers S, Kok L, Bots ML, et al. Randomized controlled trial of the effects of soy protein containing isoflavones on vascular function in postmenopausal women. *Am J Clin Nutr.* 2005;81:189–195.
33. Lichtenstein AH. Soy protein, isoflavones, and cardiovascular disease risk. *J Nutr.* 1998;128:1589–1592.
34. Potter SM. Soy protein and cardiovascular disease: the impact of bioactive components in soy. *Nutr Rev.* 1998;56:231–235.
35. Messina MJ, Persky V, Setchell KD, et al. Soy intake and cancer risk: a review of the in vitro and in vivo data. *Nutr Cancer.* 1994;21:113–131.
36. Horn-Ross PL, John EM, Canchola AJ, et al. Phytoestrogen intake and endometrial cancer risk. *J Natl Cancer Inst.* 2003;95:1158–1164.
37. Adams KF, Chen C, Newton KM, et al. Soy isoflavones do not modulate prostate-specific antigen concentrations in older men in a randomized controlled trial. *Cancer Epidemiol Biomarkers Prev.* 2004;13:644–648.
38. Hussain M, Banerjee M, Sarkar FH, et al. Soy isoflavones in the treatment of prostate cancer. *Nutr Cancer.* 2003;47:111–117.
39. Keinan-Boker L, van Der Schouw YT, Grobbee DE, et al. Dietary phytoestrogens and breast cancer risk. *Am J Clin Nutr.* 2004;79:282–288.
40. Shu XO, Jin F, Dai Q, et al. Soyfood intake during adolescence and subsequent risk of breast cancer among Chinese women. *Cancer Epidemiol Biomarkers Prev.* 2001;10:483–488.
41. This P, De La Rochefordiere A, Clough K, et al. Phytoestrogens after breast cancer. *Endocr Relat Cancer.* 2001;8:129–134.
42. Foth D, Nawroth F. Effect of soy supplementation on endogenous hormones in postmenopausal women. *Gynecol Obstet Invest.* 2003;55:135–138.
43. Kritz-Silverstein D, Von Muhlen D, Barrett-Connor E, et al. Isoflavones and cognitive function in older women: the SOy and Postmenopausal Health in Aging (SOPHIA) study. *Menopause.* 2003;10:196–202.
44. Knight DC, Howes JB, Eden JA, et al. Effects on menopausal symptoms and acceptability of isoflavone-containing soy powder dietary supplementation. *Climacteric.* 2001;4:13–18.
45. Han KK, Soares JM Jr, Haidar MA, et al. Benefits of soy isoflavone therapeutic regimen on menopausal symptoms. *Obstet Gynecol.* 2002;99:389–394.
46. Burke GL, Legault C, Anthony M, et al. Soy protein and isoflavone effects on vasomotor symptoms in peri- and postmenopausal women: the Soy Estrogen Alternative Study. *Menopause.* 2003;10:147–153.
47. Secreto G, Chiechi LM, Amadori A, et al. Soy isoflavones and melatonin for the relief of climacteric symptoms: a multicenter, double-blind, randomized study. *Maturitas.* 2004;47:11–20.

48. Crisafulli A, Marini H, Bitto A, et al. Effects of genistein on hot flushes in early post-menopausal women: a randomized, double-blind EPT- and placebo-controlled study. *Menopause.* 2004;11:400–404.

49. St Germain A, Peterson CT, Robinson JG, et al. Isoflavone-rich or isoflavone-poor soy protein does not reduce menopausal symptoms during 24 weeks of treatment. *Menopause.* 2001;8:17–26.

50. Upmalis DH, Lobo R, Bradley L, et al. Vasomotor symptom relief by soy isoflavone extract tablets in postmenopausal women: a multicenter, double-blind, randomized, placebo-controlled study. *Menopause.* 2000;7:236–242.

51. Quella SK, Loprinzi CL, Barton DL, et al. Evaluation of soy phytoestrogens for the treatment of hot flashes in breast cancer survivors: a North Central Cancer Treatment Group Trial. *J Clin Oncol.* 2000;18:1068–1074.

52. Albertazzi P, Pansini F, Bonaccorsi G, et al. The effect of dietary soy supplementation on hot flushes. *Obstet Gynecol.* 1998;91:6–11.

53. Kreijkamp-Kaspers S, Kok L, Grobbee DE, et al. Effect of soy protein containing isoflavones on cognitive function, bone mineral density, and plasma lipids in post-menopausal women: a randomized controlled trial. *JAMA.* 2004;292:65–74.

54. Mei J, Yeung SS, Kung AW. High dietary phytoestrogen intake is associated with higher bone mineral density in postmenopausal but not premenopausal women. *J Clin Endocrinol Metab.* 2001;86:5217–5221.

55. Gallagher JC, Satpathy R, Rafferty K, et al. The effect of soy protein isolate on bone metabolism. *Menopause.* 2004;11:290–298.

56. Khalil DA, Lucas EA, Juma S, et al. Soy protein supplementation increases serum insulin-like growth factor-I in young and old men but does not affect markers of bone metabolism. *J Nutr.* 2002;132:2605–2608.

57. Harkness LS, Fiedler K, Sehgal AR, et al. Decreased bone resorption with soy isoflavone supplementation in postmenopausal women. *J Womens Health (Larchmt).* 2004;13:1000–1007.

58. Alekel DL, St Germain A, Peterson CT, et al. Isoflavone-rich soy protein attenuates bone loss in the lumbar spine of perimenopausal women. *Am J Clin Nutr.* 2000;72:844–852.

59. Potter SM, Baum JA, Teng H, et al. Soy protein and isoflavones: their effects on blood lipids and bone density in postmenopausal women. *Am J Clin Nutr.* 1998;68(6 Suppl):S1375–S1379.

60. Brandi ML. Natural and synthetic isoflavones in the prevention and treatment of chronic diseases. *Calcif Tissue Int.* 1997;61:5–8.

61. Agnusdei D, Crepaldi G, Isaia G, et al. A double-blind, placebo-controlled trial of ipri-flavone for prevention of postmenopausal spinal bone loss. *Calcif Tissue Int.* 1997;61:142–147.

62. Agnusdei D, Bufalino L. Efficacy of ipriflavone in established osteoporosis and long-term safety. *Calcif Tissue Int.* 1997;61(Suppl 1):S23-S27.

63. Alexandersen P, Toussaint A, Christiansen C, et al. Ipriflavone in the treatment of postmenopausal osteoporosis. *JAMA.* 2001;285:1482–1488.

64. Azadbakht L, Shakerhosseini R, Atabak S, et al. Beneficiary effect of dietary soy protein on lowering plasma levels of lipid and improving kidney function in type II diabetes with nephropathy. *Eur J Clin Nutr.* 2003;57:1292–1294.
65. Jayagopal V, Albertazzi P, Kilpatrick ES, et al. Beneficial effects of soy phytoestrogen intake in postmenopausal women with type 2 diabetes. *Diabetes Care.* 2002;25:1709–1714.

Spirulina/Blue-Green Algae

One of many forms of blue-green algae, spirulina (*Spirulina platensis* or *Spirulina maxima*) is a multicellular organism classified as a group of cyanobacteria. Spirulina grows wild in highly alkaline lakes. Other forms of algae used in supplements include *Aphanizomenon flos aquae* (blue-green algae) and *Chlorella pyrenoidosa* (green algae). The characteristic blue-green color in spirulina is due to the chlorophyll and phycocyanin content. These pigments and other compounds (glycolipids and sulfolipids) have been studied for their potential anti-inflammatory, antioxidant, and antiviral properties. *Spirulina platensis* has a history of use in an African village in Chad where dried cakes of spirulina (called *dihe*) are harvested from Lake Chad and are eaten with meals and in sauces. *Spirulina maxima* is also found abundantly in Lake Texcoco near Mexico City. It is thought that spirulina was harvested, dried, and sold for human consumption by the Aztecs during the time of Spanish conquest (1–4).

Dried spirulina contains 60% to 70% protein, 10% to 20% carbohydrate, 9% to 14% lipids (including gamma-linolenic acid and some cholesterol), 4% nucleic acids, and 4% to 6% ash (minerals). In general, microalga are viewed as having a protein quality value greater than other vegetable sources, but poorer than animal sources because alga are somewhat low in methionine, cysteine, and lysine (2). Spirulina is also a source of beta carotene and iron. It was originally thought to be a source of vitamin B-12, but the B-12 analogues present in algae are not considered biologically active (5). Spirulina has been used commercially in feed for animals, as a coloring agent in Japanese foods, and in dietary supplements (1–3,6,7). Three polysaccharides with immunostimulatory effects have been isolated from *Spirulina platensis* (8,9).

Media and Marketing Claims	Efficacy
Improves immunity	NR
Reduces cholesterol	NR
Reduces cancer risk	NR
Improves intestinal health	NR
Aids weight loss	NR

Safety

- Although no long-term studies have evaluated the safety of spirulina, this algae along with others has been ingested in different areas of the world as a food for hundreds of years with few reports of adverse effects (1,2).

- Serious adverse effects have not been reported.

- Mice fed spirulina at high levels (10%, 20%, and 30% of diet) for 13 weeks experienced no adverse affects on behavior, food and water intake, growth or survival, blood chemistries, and gross or microscopic findings from postmortem examinations. The algae levels tested were higher than any anticipated human consumption (10). In addition, reproductive toxicity and mutagenicity tests in rodents reported no toxic effects with spirulina (11,12).

- There is concern that some spirulina products may be contaminated with microbes or heavy metals. Also, some blue-green algae (such as *Aphanizomenon flos aquae*, but not *Spirulina platensis, maxima,* or *fusiformis*) contain toxins that could pose a danger if they are inadvertently included in supplements. Ingestion could cause allergic reactions, mild liver enzyme elevation, and gastroenteritis in humans (13). Manufacturers have drafted voluntary guidelines to detect and control exposure to cyanotoxins in supplements (2).

- Individuals following vegan and macrobiotic diets should not rely on spirulina as their sole source of vitamin B-12 because vitamin B-12 found in algae may not have adequate biological activity. In one study, vitamin B-12–deficient vegetarian children did not respond to therapy with spirulina (5).

- Patients with phenylketonuria should be avoid consuming spirulina due to potential phenylalanine content.

Drug/Supplement Interactions

No reported adverse interactions

Key Points

- Like other microbial cells, spirulina is a source of protein and some vitamins and minerals. These nutrients are found in concentrated amounts, which is why companies promote spirulina as a "superfood." As a protein source, however, spirulina is considerably more expensive than an equivalent amount of protein from eggs, dairy, meat, or soy products. Although rich in certain nutrients, spirulina supplements are not a substitute for the fiber and variety of nutrients and phytochemicals in fruits and vegetables. Consumers must decide whether the cost differential is worth supplementing with spirulina.

- Preliminary evidence from in vitro and animal studies suggests that isolated sulfolipids and sulfated polysaccharides in spirulina provide immune-enhancing and antiviral activity. Controlled clinical trials are needed to determine whether spirulina enhances immune function and resistance to infection in humans.

- Preliminary studies in rodents have reported a lipid-lowering effect with high doses of spirulina. Controlled clinical trials are needed to determine whether this effect is apparent in humans.

- Preliminary evidence from one human study in India and from animal studies suggests that spirulina inhibits oral cancers. Additional controlled clinical trials are needed.

- Research on spirulina's effect on digestion and elimination is lacking. However, some strains of spirulina promote the growth of lactic acid bacteria in vitro, which may have a positive effect on the gastrointestinal tract. (For effects on intestinal health, *see* Acidophilus/Lactobacillus Acidophilus [LA].)

- Some have suggested that spirulina may play a role in weight control, but no studies have been published to date.

Food Sources

Spirulina (in the form of dried cakes) harvested from Lake Chad is consumed in Africa.

Dosage Information/Bioavailability

Spirulina is available in tablets, capsules, powders, and in processed foods such as snack bars providing approximately 500 mg/dose. Product labels recommend consuming 3 to 10 g of the algae per day. Spirulina, along with other microalgae, are cultivated both in human-made environments (photostats) and in natural environments (2). Ten grams of dried spirulina contains 29 kcal, 0.7 g fat, 5.7 g protein, 2.4 g carbohydrate, 5.7 RE (57 IU) vitamin A, 0.24 mg thiamin, 0.38 mg riboflavin, 1.3 mg niacin, 0.4 mg vitamin B-6, 0 mg vitamin B-12, 9.4 µg folate, 1 mg vitamin C, 0.5 mg vitamin E, 104 mg sodium, 136 mg potassium, 12 mg calcium, 20 mg magnesium, 2.8 mg iron, and 0.2 mg zinc (14). Manufacturers' analyses report variable levels of these nutrients, and some report significantly higher levels of vitamin A, iron, and calcium for the same quantity of spirulina. *Note:* Spirulina is not a reliable source of vitamin B-12.

The bioavailability of carotenes from spirulina is comparable with other food sources such as carrots (15). In East Indian children with vitamin A deficiency, spirulina (2 g/day) increased serum retinol levels significantly (15). Studies in rats suggest that beta carotene from spirulina is absorbed and thus can be a source of vitamin A (16). In addition, the absorption of iron from spirulina was less than that of ferrous sulfate from whole egg, but more than that from whole-wheat (17).

Initial analysis of the vitamin B-12 content of spirulina using bioassay methods presented values that were not accurate. More sensitive measures (radioassays and newer microbiological methods) have produced data indicating that much of the vitamin B-12 amounts previously reported were actually B-12 analogues (2). Vitamin B-12 analogues are thought to possess minimal biological activity in humans (18).

Relevant Research

Spirulina and Immunity

- In a non-randomized, uncontrolled pilot study conducted among 12 healthy male volunteers given hot water extract of spirulina (50 mL taken orally daily for 8 weeks), supplementation was associated with increased natural killer cell activity in more than 50% of subjects. In a subset of four subjects, supplementation was also associated with improved in vitro interferon gamma production (19). Although this study provides preliminary evidence of immune-modulating effects of spirulina, the limitations in study design and sample size make interpretation difficult. Further blinded, placebo-controlled trials are needed.

- In one animal study, spirulina enhanced humoral and cell-mediated immune functions in chickens (20). In another study, spirulina stimulated macrophage function, phagocytosis, and interleukin-1 in mice (21).

- A sulfated polysaccharide (calcium spirulan) isolated from spirulina inhibited herpes simplex virus type 1, human cytomegalovirus, measles virus, mumps virus, influenza A virus, and HIV in vitro (22,23).

- Sulfolipids isolated from blue-green algae (type not specified) demonstrated antiviral activity against the AIDS virus in vitro (24).

Spirulina and Cholesterol

- Animal studies conducted by one research group found a hypocholesterolemic effect of *Spirulina platensis* (25,26). In one study, spirulina prevented the fructose-induced increase in liver triglyceride levels in rats fed a 60% fructose diet (27).

Spirulina and Cancer

- In a placebo-controlled, single-blind (details of blinding of subjects not sufficiently described) study, 87 subjects with oral leukoplakia and a history of tobacco-chewing from a fishing village in India were randomly assigned to receive 1 g *Spirulina fusiformis* (containing 2 mg beta carotene, 4 mg total carotenes, 1 µg vitamin B-12, 1 mg iron, 0.35 mg zinc, and 0.06 mg vitamin B-complex) or a placebo daily for 1 year. Subjects were advised to stop using tobacco and alcohol. Subjects had normal plasma concentrations of vitamin A at baseline and did not have vitamin A deficiency. Biopsies from lesions were taken at baseline and at the end of the study. Subjects were assessed every 2 months by a dentist and physician who were blinded to treatment groups. Complete response was defined as total disappearance of the lesions. The complete response rates of homogenous lesions were 11% with the placebo and 57% with spirulina; the difference was statistically significant. None of the nodular and ulcerated leukoplakias (n = 4) responded to treatment. There was no difference between groups in plasma retinol, beta carotene, or alpha tocopherol. The authors summarized: "More human trials with hard endpoints in different settings and different populations are required to further establish the effectiveness of spirulina algae before any conclusions can be made" (28).

♦ Spirulina extracts have been shown to inhibit chemically induced buccal cancers in animal studies by one group of investigators (29–31).

Spirulina and Intestinal Health

♦ An in vitro study reported that spirulina (platensis) promoted the growth of lactic acid bacteria *(Lactobacillus bulgaricus, L. casei, L. acidophilus, L. lactis, Streptococcus thermophilus)* in media with pH adjusted to 5.3, 6.3, and 7.0. The authors concluded that further experiments in animals and humans are needed to determine whether spirulina may be used as a type of prebiotic to improve lactic acid bacteria colonization and human health (32).

References

1. Ciferri O. Spirulina, the edible microorganism. *Microbiol Rev.* 1983;47:551–578.
2. Kay RA. Microalgae as food and supplement. *Crit Rev Food Sci Nutr.* 1991;30:555–573.
3. Maranesi M, Barzanti V, Carenini G, et al. Nutritional studies on *Spirulina maxima. Acta Vitaminol Enzymol.* 1984;6:295–304.
4. Romay C, Armesto J, Remirez D, et al. Antioxidant and anti-inflammatory properties of C-phycocyanin from blue-green algae. *Inflamm Res.* 1998;47:36–41.
5. Dagnelie PC, van Staveren WA, van den Berg H. Vitamin B12 from algae appears not to be bioavailable [erratum in *Am J Clin Nutr.* 1991;53:988]. *Am J Clin Nutr.* 1991;53:695–697.
6. Ciferri O, Tiboni O. The biochemistry and industrial potential of spirulina. *Annu Rev Microbiol.* 1985;39:503–526.
7. Clement G, Giddey C, Menzi R. Amino acid composition and nutritive value of the alga spirulina maxima. *J Sci Food Agric.* 1967;18:497–501.
8. Pugh N, Ross SA, ElSohly MA, et al. Isolation of three high molecular weight polysaccharide preparations with potent immunostimulatory activity from Spirulina platensis, aphanizomenon flos-aquae and Chlorella pyrenoidosa. *Planta Med.* 2001;67:737–742.
9. Ozdemir G, Karabay NU, Dalay MC, et al. Antibacterial activity of volatile component and various extracts of Spirulina platensis. *Phtother Res.* 2004;18:754–757.
10. Salazar M, Martinez E, Madrigal E, et al. Subchronic toxicity study in mice fed *Spirulina maxima. J Ethnopharmacol.* 1998;62:235–241.
11. Chamorro G, Salazar M. Dominant lethal study of *Spirulina maxima* in male and female rats after short-term feeding. *Phytother Res.* 1996;10:28–32.
12. Chamorro G, Salazar S, Favila-Castillo L, et al. Reproductive and peri- and postnatal evaluation of *Spirulina maxima* in mice. *J Appl Phycol.* 1997;9:107–112.
13. Spoerke DG, Rumack BH. Blue-green algae poisoning. *J Emerg Med.* 1985;2:353–355.
14. Pennington JA. *Bowes and Church's Food Values of Portions Commonly Used.* 17th ed. Philadelphia, Pa: Lippincott-Raven Publishers; 1998.
15. Annapurna V, Shah N, Bhaskaram P, et al. Bioavailability of Spirulina carotenes in pre-school children. *J Clin Biochem Nutr.* 1991;10:145–151.

16. Annapurna VV, Deosthale YG, Bamji MS. Spirulina as a source of vitamin A. *Plant Foods Hum Nutr.* 1991;41:125–134.
17. Kapoor R, Mehta U. Iron bioavailability from *Spirulina platensis,* whole egg, and whole wheat. *Indian J Exp Biol.* 1992;30:904–907.
18. Herbert V, Drivas G. Spirulina and vitamin B12. *JAMA.* 1982;248:3096–3097.
19. Hirahashi T, Matsumoto M, Hazeki K, et al. Activation of the human innate immune system by Spirulina: augmentation of interferon production and NK cytotoxicity by oral administration of hot water extract of *Spirulina platensis. Int Immunopharmacol.* 2002;2:423–434.
20. Qureshi MA, Garlich JD, Kidd MT. Dietary *Spirulina platensis* enhances humoral and cell-mediated immune functions in chickens. *Immunopharmacol Immunotoxicol.* 1996;18: 465–476.
21. Hayashi O, Katoh T, Okuwaki Y. Enhancement of antibody production in mice by dietary *Spirulina platensis. J Nutr Sci Vitaminol (Tokyo).* 1994;40:431–441.
22. Hayashi K, Hayashi T, Kojima I. A natural sulfated polysaccharide, calcium spirulan, isolated from *Spirulina platensis:* in vitro and ex vivo evaluation of anti-herpes simplex virus and anti-human immunodeficiency virus activities. *AIDS Res Hum Retroviruses.* 1996;12:1463–1471.
23. Hayashi T, Hayashi K, Maeda M, et al. Calcium spirulan, an inhibitor of enveloped virus replication, from blue-green alga *Spirulina platensis. J Nat Prod.* 1996;59:83–87.
24. Gustafson KR, Cardellina JH, Fuller RW, et al. AIDS-Antiviral sulfolipids from cyanobacteria (blue-green algae). *J Natl Cancer Inst.* 1989;81:1254–1258.
25. Devi MA, Venkataraman LV. Hypocholesterolemic effect of blue green algae *Spirulina platensis* in albino rats. *Nutr Rep Int.* 1983;28:519–530.
26. Devi MA, Venkataraman LV, Rajasekaran T. Hypocholesterolemic effect of diets containing algae on albino rats. *Nutr Rep Int.* 1979;20:83–90.
27. Gonzalez de Rivera C, Miranda-Zamora R, Diaz-Zagoya JC, et al. Preventive effect of *Spirulina maxima* on the fatty liver induced by a fructose-rich diet in the rat, a preliminary report. *Life Sci.* 1993;53:57–61.
28. Mathew B, Sankaranarayanan R, Nair PP, et al. Evaluation of chemoprevention of oral cancer with *Spirulina fusiformis. Nutr Cancer.* 1995;24:197–202.
29. Schwartz J, Shklar G. Regression of experimental hamster cancer by beta-carotene and algae extracts. *J Oral Maxillofac Surg.* 1987;45:510–515.
30. Schwartz J, Shklar G, Reid S, et al. Prevention of experimental oral cancer by extracts of Spirulina-Dunaliella algae. *Nutr Cancer.* 1988;11:127–134.
31. Shklar G, Schwartz J. Tumor necrosis factor in experimental cancer regression with alpha-tocopherol, beta-carotene, canthaxanthin and algae extract. *Eur J Cancer Clin Oncol.* 1988;24: 839–850.
32. Parada JL, Zulpa de Caire G, Zaccaro de Mule MC, et al. Lactic acid bacteria growth promoters from *Spirulina platensis. Int J Food Microbiol.* 1998;45:225–228.

Thiamin. *See* Vitamin B-1 (Thiamin).

Turmeric (*Curcuma longa*)

Turmeric, a close relative of ginger, has been used in India for centuries as a spice and medicine. It is most commonly known as the spice that gives flavor and color to curry. Turmeric is derived from the *Curcuma longa* plant. The rhizome is boiled, dried, and pounded into a fine powder. Its active constituents are curcuminoids, which include curcumin. Curcumin has antioxidant properties that may be as strong as vitamins C and E. Both turmeric and curcumin have been shown to have anti-inflammatory, anti-angiogenic and even wound healing effects (1).

Media and Marketing Claims	Efficacy
Treats dyspepsia	NR
Treats anterior uveitis (inflammation of the eye)	NR
Protects against cancer	NR

Safety

Turmeric has Generally Recognized as Safe (GRAS) status in the United States (2).

Drug/Supplement Interactions

Use of turmeric with anticoagulant or antiplatelet medications could theoretically increase the risk of bleeding due to increased platelet aggregation.

Key Points

- ◆ Most research studies of turmeric have used the major biologically active constituent, curcumin, and have been completed using cell lines and animal models; it is unclear how these results will translate to humans.

- ◆ In a few small and poorly designed clinical trials, curcumin was found to be effective in treating dyspepsia (3,4).

- ◆ A small preliminary study on the role of curcumin in the treatment of chronic anterior uveitis indicated that curcumin is effective in improving vision (5).

- ◆ Cell line studies (6–8) indicate that turmeric extract (curcumin) has several antitumor effects. More study is needed to determine curcumin's chemoprotective effects, particularly in humans.

Food Sources

The only natural food source of turmeric is the spice itself, which can be added to a variety of foods. When used as to flavor food, turmeric provides less curcumin than the dose in supplements; however, the smaller amounts in food preparations may still be of biological importance. Research is needed to determine whether this is true.

Dosage Information/Bioavailability

Turmeric is available as a tincture, tablet, powder, ointment, lotion, liquid, tea, cream, or capsule. To be most effective, a supplement should contain at least 95% curcumin. For dyspepsia, 500 mg four times per day was the dose used in one study (4); for anterior uveitis, 375 mg capsules were taken 3 times daily (5). One study in patients with advanced colorectal cancer suggests that systemic bioavailability of curcumin is limited: supplementation resulted in a measurable presence of curcumin metabolites in feces only, not in blood or urine (7).

Relevant Research

Turmeric and Dyspepsia

- In a small phase II clinical trial investigating the efficacy of turmeric in the treatment of peptic ulcer, 45 subjects (24 men and 21 women) with peptic ulcers between 0.5 and 1.5 cm in diameter were given 300 mg of turmeric in capsule form five times daily (1,500 mg total) for 12 weeks. More than half of the subjects improved substantially, with no ulcer seen on follow-up endoscope. All subjects reported satisfactory reduction in abdominal pain and discomfort after 2 weeks of treatment (3). Larger studies should be conducted to confirm these results.

- In a multicenter, randomized, placebo-controlled, double-blind study conducted in Thailand, 116 adults with dyspepsia were randomized to receive curcumin *(Curcuma domestica Val)* (n = 39), flatulence (n = 36), or placebo (n = 41) four times daily for 7 days. At the end of 7 days, 9.5% of patients did not return for follow up evaluation. Subjects were asked to self-report improvements in symptoms. Significant improvements in clinical symptoms were reported by 87%, 83%, and 53% of patients in the curcumin, flatulence, and placebo groups, respectively, as compared with baseline. The difference in efficacy between curcumin and placebo was also significant (4).

Turmeric and Anterior Uveitis

- In a small nonrandomized, unblinded clinical trial of the efficacy of curcumin for the management of anterior uveitis (a condition characterized by inflammation of the eye and more specifically the anterior area where the macula is located), 32 subjects were divided into two groups. The first group (n = 18) received only curcumin supplements at a dose of 375 mg 3 times daily, and the second group with more severe disease by clinical examination (n = 14) received the same dosage of curcumin plus antitubercular treatments. Improvements in visual response were first detected within 2 weeks of starting treatment and this improvement was sustained throughout the 12 weeks of supplementation. All subjects in the first group improved, whereas 86% of patients who also received antitubercular treatment showed a clinical response. Three-year follow-up showed a recurrence rate of 55% and 36% in groups 1 and 2 respectively. Because this study was not blinded, the results should be viewed with caution (5).

Turmeric and Cancer

◆ In an investigation into the antitumor effects of curcumin, mouse melanoma cells (B16) were used for in vitro and in vivo experiments. The B16 cells were selected for doxorubicin resistance prior to study. The effects of curcumin on these cells was investigated using a cell survival assay with a curcumin-supplemented (ranging from 1–100 μM) medium and analysis for apoptosis. B16-R cells (those resistant to doxorubicin) were subcutaneously injected into the flanks of mice, which were then treated with 25 mg/kg curcumin injections daily. In parallel experiments, mice were injected with tumor cell lysates to stimulate an immune response against the B16-R cells. Tumor growth was assessed weekly. Survival was estimated in mice who received either curcumin alone or in those that had been immune stimulated with tumor cell lysates. In these experiments, curcumin was cytotoxic to the melanoma cells and induced the typical DNA fragmentation associated with apoptosis and TUNEL-positive assays in a time- and dose-dependent manner. In vivo studies found that the combination of curcumin and immune stimulation inhibited tumor growth and increased survival, but neither treatment alone was effective (6).

◆ To investigate pharmacological aspects of curcumin in terms of safety and efficacy and excretion in humans with colorectal cancer, 15 subjects with advanced disease that was not responsive to previous treatment were given daily P54FP capsules containing 20 mg curcuminoids at one of five dose levels: 2, 4, 6, 8, or 10 capsules daily (36, 72, 108, 144, or 180 mg curcumin) until disease progression occurred or patients withdrew. Tumor progression was evaluated with tumor markers CEA and CA19.9 and by radiologic imaging throughout the 29 days of treatment. Curcumin and its metabolites were analyzed from blood, urine, and feces by high performance liquid chromatography (HPLC) and showed that curcumin was not measurable in the plasma or urine, regardless of dose, but it was present in feces at escalating doses based on amount consumed. The P54FP extracts were well tolerated at all doses. Five subjects exhibited stable disease (based on CT scan) at 3 months while taking 36, 72, and 144 mg curcumin daily. Two others, taking 72 and 108 mg/day, exhibited stable disease on CT scan for 4 months (7). Other patients experienced some evidence of disease progression (increased CEA or CA19.9, or exhibited on CT scan).

◆ Cyclooxygenase-2 (COX-2) is an enzyme that is known to cause an inflammatory response within the body. Reducing or blocking the activity of this enzyme might also reduce the risk of chronic illnesses characterized by inflammation, such as cancer. To investigate whether curcumin could inhibit the activity of COX-2–associated inflammation induced by chenodeoxycholate (CD) or phorbol 12-myristate 13-acetate (PMA) in gastrointestinal cell lines, several in vitro experiments were conducted in which cultured cells were treated with various levels of curcumin. SK-GT-4, SCC450, IEC-18, and HCA-7 cell lines were exposed to CD or PMA and cytotoxicity was eval-

uated using lactate dehydrogenase release, trypan blue exclusion, and dimethylthia-
zole (MTT) analysis. COX-2 expression was determined by Western and Northern
blot analysis. COX-2 activity was evaluated by analysis of PGE_2 production. In these
experiments, curcumin inhibited COX-2 expression and activity in a dose-dependent
manner at 1, 5, 10 and 20 micromolar concentration in all gastrointestinal cell lines
tested (8). This suggests that curcumin may provide anti-inflammatory effects
against cancer.

References

1. Maheshwari RK, Singh AK, Gaddipati J, et al. Multiple biological activities of curcumin: a short review. *Life Sci.* 2006;78:2081–2087.
2. FDA. Center for Food Safety and Applied Nutrition, Office of Premarket Approval,
   EAFUS: a food additive database. Available at: vm.cfsan.fda.gov/~dms/eafus.html.
   Accessed August 13, 2005.
3. Prucksunand C, Indrasukhsri B, Leethochawalit M, et al. Phase II clinical trial on
   effect of the long turmeric (Curcuma longa Linn) on healing of peptic ulcer. *Southeast
   Asian J Trop Med Public Health.* 2001;32:208–215.
4. Thamlikitkul V, Bunyapraphatsara N, Dechatiwongse T, et al. Randomized double-
   blind study of Curcuma domestica Val. for dyspepsia. *J Med Assoc Thai.* 1989;72:
   613–620.
5. Lal B, Kapoor AK, Asthana OP, et al. Efficacy of curcumin in the management of
   chronic anterior uveitis. *Phytother Res.* 1999;13:318–322.
6. Odot J, Albert P, Carlier A, et al. In vitro and in vivo anti-tumoral effect of curcumin
   against melanoma cells. *Int J Cancer.* 2004;111:381–387.
7. Sharma RA, McLelland HR, Hill KA, et al. Pharmacodynamic and pharmacokinetic
   study of oral *Curcuma* extract in patients with colorectal cancer. *Clin Cancer Res.*
   2001;7:1894–1900.
8. Zhang F, Altorki NK, Mestre JR, et al. Curcumin inhibits cyclooxygenase-2 transcrip-
   tion in bile acid- and phorbol ester-treated human gastrointestinal epithelial cells.
   Carcinogenesis. 1999;20:445–451.

Ubiquinone. *See* Coenzyme Q_{10}.

Valerian *(Valeriana officinalis)*

Valerian, the common name for plants belonging to the genus *Valeriana,* has been used for
centuries as a sleep aid. *Valeriana officinalis* is the species most often used for traditional
medicinal purposes. Originally carried on the US National Formulary, valerian was omit-
ted in the 1950s as use of barbiturates increased. In Europe, it is widely prescribed for its

mild sedative effects. Valerian is thought to act by depressing the central nervous system and promoting muscle relaxation. Although the active components have not been identified, researchers have suggested that the valepotriates, volatile oils (valerenic acid), or a combination of these may be responsible for the sedative properties. The valepotriate and volatile oil levels have been found to vary considerably in the native plant and different types of preparations (1,2).

Media and Marketing Claims	Efficacy
Enhances sleep	↔
Reduces stress and anxiety	NR

Safety

+ Valerian has a Generally Recognized As Safe (GRAS) rating from the FDA.

+ There are no long-term trials testing the safety of valerian in humans. Data from short-term studies suggest that valerian preparations are well-tolerated (2).

+ Individuals may experience serious withdrawal symptoms if valerian is abruptly discontinued; doses should be tapered slowly. In a case study, a man with a history of coronary artery disease, hypertension, and congestive heart failure experienced cardiac complications and delirium after abruptly stopping valerian. He had been self-medicating with valerian (530 to 2,000 mg/dose) five times daily for several years to aid sleep (3).

+ Some individuals have reported feeling drowsy the morning following ingestion of higher doses of valerian (900 mg). However, a randomized, controlled, double-blind trial of 102 subjects reported that a single or repeated evening administration of 600 mg valerian extract had no relevant negative impact on reaction time, alertness, or concentration the morning after intake (4). Similarly, a study conducted among 10 young healthy males administered escalating doses of valerian ranging from 600 to 1,800 mg showed no reduction in psychomotor skills whereas diazepam did (5).

+ Because of the possible risk of drowsiness, users should avoid driving or operating heavy machinery while taking valerian.

+ The herb has been linked to a few cases of liver damage, which has been attributed to contamination (6). Valerian preparations should be avoided by individuals with liver disease (2).

Drug/Supplement Interactions

+ A multi-night time dose study of valerian where 12 healthy volunteers took 1,000 mg valerian (11 mg valerinic acid) for 14 days showed no significant reduction in

CYP3A4 or CYP2D6 activity in healthy volunteers, suggesting it will not interfere with drug efficacy for common medications metabolized via this pathway (7).

♦ Valerian should not be used concomitantly with barbiturates, benzodiazepine, or other sedatives because excessive sedative effects may occur (8).

♦ Valerian potentially may increase sedative effect of anesthetics. One review suggested that valerian be tapered several weeks before surgery due to the potential excessive sedation when combined with anesthetics. Additionally, long-term use of valerian could increase anesthesia requirements (9). More research is needed.

♦ Valerian should not be used in combination with St John's wort, kava, L-tryptophan, or alcohol due to additive sedative effects.

Key Points

♦ Preliminary research conflicts about whether valerian improves sleep quality. However, one reviewer cautioned: "It is difficult to adequately quantify the sleep promoting effects of valerian based on these trials because the study designs, subject characteristics, dosage, and content of the various preparations differed" (2).

♦ Studies comparing the effects of valerian with sleep-promoting drugs (benzodiazepines, barbiturates) suggest prescribed medications are more effective, but these studies are limited in number and sample size. There is currently no evidence that valerian is habit-forming, as is the case for some sedative medications.

♦ The sedative effects of valerian were too mild to be picked up by electroencephalogram (EEG) studies.

♦ More clinical trials are needed to evaluate the potential role of valerian in reducing everyday tension and anxiety.

♦ Overall, much more controlled research is needed to examine the efficacy, long-term safety, and potential active components of valerian.

Food Sources

None

Dosage Information/Bioavailability

Valerian is sold as capsules, tablets, teas, and tinctures. Many products are standardized to different levels of valerenic acid. Some labels recommend taking 200 to 1,500 mg 1 hour before bedtime or during "stressful" days. It is often combined with other herbs such as skullcap, passion flower, chamomile, and hops. It should not be combined with kava kava due to additive effects. The unpleasant smell associated with aqueous valerian results from enzyme hydrolysis of some of the plant components (2).

Relevant Research

Valerian and Sleep

- ♦ Researchers conducted a systematic review of clinical trials of valerian extract with subjects experiencing insomnia. Nine randomized, placebo-controlled, double-blind studies using single preparations of valerian were examined for methodological quality. The authors reported that the study findings were contradictory and had many inconsistencies in terms of subjects, experimental design and procedures, and methodological quality. They concluded that evidence for valerian as a treatment for insomnia is inconclusive and more rigorous trials are needed (10).

- ♦ In a study conducted in five children with sleep difficulties, children were randomly assigned to valerian or placebo in a double-blind, placebo-controlled study lasting 8 weeks (11). Over time and as compared with placebo, valerian was effective in reducing time to sleep and nighttime awakening as well as reported sleep quality. Further research in this population should be considered because the results of this study are extremely preliminary given that only five children were enrolled.

- ♦ In a double-blind, placebo-controlled study conducted using sleep EEG and psychometric tests as outcome markers, 16 subjects with sleep disturbances were randomly assigned to 300 mg or 600 mg valerian, or placebo (single dose). Subjects who took valerian showed no clinically significant improvement in sleep parameters with treatment (12). The investigators suggested that valerian may not be effective for acute sleep problems. However, this does not preclude its potential efficacy with more chronic sleep problems, for which supplementation would be used for a longer duration. It should be noted that subjects were admitted to a sleep laboratory for this study, which may have altered their ability to sleep.

- ♦ In a randomized, double-blind, comparative, multicenter study (n = 202 adults with insomnia) that was among the first to compare valerian to oxazepam therapy for insomnia, valerian (LI 156, Sedonium) administered at a dosage of 600 mg/day for 6 weeks resulted in a significant improvement in several measures of sleep quality and quantity and it was as effective as oxazepam (13).

- ♦ In a double-blind, placebo-controlled, randomized, crossover study, 16 subjects with previously established psychophysiological insomnia (ages 22 to 55 years) had their sleep assessed after a single dose and a multiple dose of valerian (14 days). Subjects received 600 mg valerian extract doses 1 hour before bedtime. Eight polysomnographic recordings were done during the study. The main outcome was effect on sleep efficiency ([total sleep time/time in bed] × 100). Sleep time, sleep onset latency, slow-wave sleep, REM sleep, as well as subjective parameters of sleep quality were assessed. A single dose of valerian had no effect on polysomnography readings or subjective sleep parameters. After the multiple-dose treatment, sleep efficiency increased significantly for both the placebo and valerian treatments compared with baseline polysomnography, indicating a placebo effect. However, slow-wave sleep latency decreased significantly with valerian, shifting it to the beginning of the sleep period. The authors suggested that this result may indicate a reconstruction of slow-wave sleep back to its proper physiological time. Overall, however, the authors concluded that in comparison with the immediate effects of other sleep-inducing substances such as benzodiazepines, the influence of valerian on sleep is slight and delayed. (14).

♦ In a double-blind, placebo-controlled trial, 14 elderly poor sleepers were randomly assigned to receive 1,215 mg valerian extract (divided into three doses) or a placebo for 7 days. Sleep polysomnography was conducted on 3 nights, at 1-week intervals (before, during, and after treatment) in a sleep laboratory. In valerian-treated subjects, slow-wave sleep increased and stage 1 sleep decreased compared with the placebo. There was no effect on REM sleep, sleep onset time, or time awake after sleep onset. There was also no effect on self-rated sleep quality (15).

♦ In a double-blind, placebo-controlled study, 128 subjects were given valerian extract (400 mg) prepared in the laboratory, a commercial valerian product (400 mg valerian plus hop flower extract), or a placebo in random order before bedtime during 9 nonconsecutive nights at home. Subjects completed postsleep questionnaires each morning. Valerian extract significantly decreased subjective sleep latency scores and improved sleep quality. When subjects were divided into self-reported "poor" vs "good" sleepers, valerian extract significantly improved sleep quality in poor sleepers compared with the placebo, but not for good sleepers. There was no change in night awakenings, hangover effect, or dream recall (16).

♦ In a placebo-controlled, double-blind, crossover study, 27 patients with self-reported sleep difficulties were given 400 mg of a commercial standardized valerian extract or a placebo for 1 night each, with no washout period. Subjects were randomly assigned with regard to which treatment was taken first. The morning after taking the second treatment (valerian or placebo), subjects rated their sleep after each preparation. The difference between ratings of the two preparations was statistically significant: 21 of 27 subjects rated valerian as better than the control. No adverse effects were reported (17).

Valerian and Anxiety

♦ In a double-blind, 2 × 2 factorial design study, 50 healthy subjects were randomly assigned to receive 100 mg valerian extract, 20 mg propranolol (beta-blocker), valerian plus propranolol, or a placebo. Ninety minutes after administration, subjects were asked to stand up and complete as many arithmetic calculations as possible in front of a group. Changes in physiological activation (pulse frequency), in performance, and in mood variables were assessed before and after the test. As expected, both propranolol treatments prevented the normal increase in pulse induced by the social stress situation. Valerian had no effect on pulse frequency, but did lead to less intensive subjective feelings of somatic arousal compared with the placebo. The authors concluded that valerian influences feelings of somatic arousal despite high physiological activation during an induced stress situation (18).

References

1. Wagner J, Wagner ML, Hening WA. Beyond benzodiazepines: alternative pharmacologic agents for the treatment of insomnia. *Ann Pharmacother.* 1998;32:680–691.
2. Houghton PJ. The biological activity of valerian and related plants. *J Ethnopharmacol.* 1988;22:121–142.
3. Garges HP, Varia I, Doraiswamy PM. Cardiac complications and delirium associated with valerian root withdrawal. *JAMA.* 1998;280:1566–1567.
4. Kuhlmann J, Berger W, Podzuweit H, et al. The influence of valerian treatment on "reaction time, alertness and concentration in volunteers." *Pharmacopsychiatry.* 1999;32:235–241.
5. Gutierrez S, Ang-Lee MK, Walker DJ, et al. Assessing subjective and psychomotor effects of the herbal medication valerian in healthy volunteers. *Pharmacol Biochem Behav.* 2004;78:57–64.
6. Shepherd C. Sleep disorders. Liver damage warning with insomnia remedy. *BMJ.* 1993;306:1477.
7. Donovan JL, DeVane CL, Chavin KD, et al. Multiple night-time doses of valerian (Valeriana officinalis) had minimal effects on CYP3A4 activity and no effect on CYP2D6 activity in healthy volunteers. *Drug Metab Dispos.* 2004;32:1333–1336.
8. Miller LG. Herbal medicinals: selected clinical considerations focusing on known or potential drug-herb interactions. *Arch Intern Med.* 1998;158:2200–2211.
9. 5. Ang-Lee, MK, Moss J, Yuan CS. Herbal medicines and perioperative care. *JAMA.* 2001;286:208–216.
10. Stevinson C, Ernst E. Valerian for insomnia: a systematic review of randomized clinical trials. *Sleep Med.* 2000;1:91–99.
11. Francis AJ, Dempster RJ. Effect of valerian, Valeriana edulis, on sleep difficulties in children with intellectual deficits: randomised trial. *Phytomedicine.* 2002;9:273–279.
12. Diaper A, Hindmarch I. A double-blind, placebo-controlled investigation of the effects of two doses of a valerian preparation on the sleep, cognitive and psychomotor function of sleep-disturbed older adults. *Phytother Res.* 2004;18:831–836.
13. Ziegler G, Ploch M, Miettinen-Baumann A, Collet W. Efficacy and tolerability of valerian extract LI 156 compound with oxazepam in the treatment of non-organic insomnia—a randomized, double-blind, comparative clinical study. *Eur J Med Res.* 2002;7: 480–486.
14. Donath F, Quispe S, Diefenbach K, et al. Critical evaluation of the effect of valerian extract on sleep structure and sleep quality. *Pharmacopsychiatry.* 2000;33:47–53.
15. Schulz H, Stolz C, Muller J. The effect of valerian extract on sleep polygraphy in poor sleepers: a pilot study. *Pharmacopsychiatry.* 1994;27:147–151.
16. Leathwood PD, Chauffard F, Heck E, et al. Aqueous extract of valerian root (*Valeriana officinalis L*) improves sleep quality in man. *Pharmacol Biochem Behav.* 1982;17: 65–71.
17. Lindahl O, Lindwall L. Double blind study of a valerian preparation. *Pharmacol Biochem Behav.* 1989;32:1065–1066.

18. Kohnen R, Oswald WD. The effects of valerian, propranolol, and their combination on activation, performance, and mood of healthy volunteers under social stress conditions. *Pharmacopsychiatry.* 1988;21:447–448.

Valine. *See* Branched-Chain Amino Acids (BCAA).

Vanadium

Vanadium (vanadyl sulfate, or VS) is a trace mineral present in nature and mammalian cells. Because its physiological role is not clearly defined, vanadium is presently not deemed essential in human nutrition. Vanadium deficiency has not been identified in humans, but it has been reported in goats and rats. Research in the last 30 years has found that vanadium exists in several forms, each with varying actions. Because animal studies have shown vanadium helps facilitate glucose uptake into muscle and converts glucose into fat, researchers are investigating the potential role of vanadium supplements in the management of diabetes (1–3).

Media and Marketing Claims	Efficacy
Reduces insulin requirements in diabetes	NR
Increases muscle mass	NR
Improves muscular strength	NR

Safety

- The Tolerable Upper Intake Level (UL) from foods and supplements is 1.8 mg elemental vanadium per day (3).

- Prolonged use at high doses may cause renal dysfunction; renal function should be monitored if vanadium is taken long-term (more than 6 months).

- Vanadium can be a relatively toxic element. The high amounts of vanadium used in the human studies discussed here were pharmacological doses that have been associated with toxicity in animals. These doses far exceed amounts available from the diet.

- Toxicity studies in animals have shown that inorganic vanadium can induce hematological and biochemical changes; reproductive and developmental toxicity; excess vanadium retention in bone, kidney, and liver; and prooxidative effects on glutathione, ascorbic acid, lipids, and NADPH (4). More recent data have shown that organic vanadium compounds are much safer than inorganic vanadium salts and do not cause gastrointestinal discomfort or liver or kidney toxicity (5).

- Side effects associated with VS therapy in the studies discussed here included cramping, diarrhea, and abdominal pain (6).

- Excess vanadium consumption (4 to 18 mg for 6 to 10 weeks) may cause green discoloration of the tongue (6).

- The safety of 0.5 mg/kg/day in 31 weight-training athletes was assessed throughout 12 weeks. VS had no effect on hematological indexes, blood viscosity, or biochemistry (7).

Drug/Supplement Interactions

- VS may have blood-thinning effects, and thus may heighten the anti-clotting effects of anticoagulant drugs.

- There is a potential additive effect on reducing blood glucose levels if VS is combined with diabetes medications.

Key Points

- According to preliminary findings in very small numbers of patients, VS seems to improve insulin sensitivity. However, according to one review article: "It is still too early to conclude whether vanadium salts will be used therapeutically in the future care of diabetes. It is more likely that vanadium research will assist in a better understanding of the backup systems involved, and eventually lead to the development of more potent and less toxic vanadium substitutes" (1).

- Preliminary research shows VS has little or no effect on strength training and body composition. Much more research is needed to evaluate the impact of VS supplementation in athletes.

- At this time, routine supplementation of vanadium is not supported by scientific evidence. Supplements containing more than 1.8 mg/day (the UL) of vanadium should be avoided because of potential toxicity.

Food Sources

The average American diet provides 15 to 30 µg vanadium per day. Rich sources of vanadium are shellfish, parsley, mushrooms, and dill seed (4). Vanadium is also present in wine (7 to 90 µg/L) (8).

Dosage Information/Bioavailability

Vanadium is sold in the form of VS or vanadate providing 7 to 15 mg/capsule ($\approx$ 1 to 5 mg elemental vanadium). Some manufacturers suggest taking very high doses of vanadium (15 to 60 mg VS [$\approx$ 5 to 20 mg elemental vanadium] per day). Although the metabolism of vanadium is not well understood, it is estimated that 5% to 30% is absorbed from the intestine and then binds to iron-containing proteins in the blood (6).

A biological role of vanadium has not been identified. Therefore, the National Academy of Sciences has not set an RDA or AI (3).

Relevant Research

VS and Diabetes

♦ Compounds of the element vanadium seem to exert antidiabetic insulin-like activity in both animal and human subjects with both type 1 and type 2 diabetes. A review of these insulin-modulating effects of vanadium has recently been published. It suggests that as early as 1899 oral vanadium was used to reduce glucose levels in the urine of patients with diabetes. Further, vanadium has been shown to reduce fasting insulin levels in patients with type 2 diabetes, increase glucose transport into muscle cells, and potentially reduce appetite by modulating neuropeptide Y levels (9).

♦ In a single-blind, placebo-controlled (not randomized) study, eight patients with type 2 diabetes received 100 mg VS daily for 4 weeks. Six patients continued the study and received a placebo for an additional 4 weeks. Daily glucose tests were self-recorded and four euglycemic-hyperinsulinemic clamps were administered before, during, and after the study. VS was associated with a significant 20% decrease in fasting glucose compared with no effect during the placebo phase. VS also caused a decrease in hepatic glucose output during hyperinsulinemia that was sustained through the placebo phase. There was no effect on peripheral (muscle) insulin resistance, glycogen synthesis, glycolysis, or lipolysis. The authors concluded: "VS resulted in modest reductions of fasting plasma glucose and hepatic insulin resistance" (10).

♦ Five subjects with type 2 diabetes and five with type 1 diabetes were given 125 mg sodium metavanadate/day for weeks 2 and 3 of a 4-week study. During week 1 and week 4 of the study, subjects received no treatment. Subjects recorded blood glucose four times daily, as well as insulin doses and diet throughout the study. Glucose metabolism measured by a 2-step euglycemic-hyperinsulinemic clamp was not significantly increased by vanadate in subjects with type 1 diabetes. However, in subjects with type 2 diabetes, glucose metabolism improved by 29% during low-dose insulin infusion, and 39% in high-dose insulin infusion. Basal hepatic glucose production and suppression of hepatic glucose production were unaffected by vanadate; however, insulin requirements decreased in subjects with type 1 diabetes. Cholesterol levels decreased significantly in all subjects. The authors concluded: "Vanadate or related agents may have a potential role as adjunctive therapy in patients with diabetes mellitus" (11).

♦ In a single-blind, placebo-controlled study, 7 obese subjects with type 2 diabetes and six nondiabetic obese subjects underwent euglycemic-hyperinsulinemic clamps after 2 weeks of placebo and after 3 weeks of 100 mg VS per day. All subjects were instructed to keep diet and exercise constant, but this was not monitored. Glucose turnover, glycolysis, glycogen synthesis, and carbohydrate and lipid oxidation were measured. Fasting plasma glucose and A1C decreased significantly in subjects with type 2 diabetes using VS, but not in nondiabetic control subjects. However, A1C has a turnover rate of 60 to 90 days, and the duration of VS supplementation was only 21 days; thus, changes in A1C would not reflect an effect of VS. During VS supplementation, the glucose infusion rate required to maintain euglycemia significantly increased in subjects with type 2 diabetes but not in control subjects. This improvement in insulin sensitivity was attributed to a significant increase of glucose disposal and enhanced suppression of hepatic glucose output in these subjects. VS also was associated with a significant suppression of plasma free fatty acids and lipid oxidation during clamps. All subjects experienced transient gastrointestinal symptoms (nausea, mild diarrhea, cramps) during VS supplementation. The authors concluded: "VS does not alter insulin sensitivity in nondiabetic subjects, but it does improve both hepatic and skeletal muscle insulin sensitivity in NIDDM [type 2] subjects in part by enhancing insulin's inhibitory effect on lipolysis. These data suggest that VS may improve a defect in insulin signaling specific to NIDMM" (12).

VS and Muscle Mass/Muscle Strength

♦ In a double-blind, placebo-controlled trial, 40 trained subjects were randomly assigned to receive 0.5 mg vanadyl sulfate/kg/day or a placebo for 12 weeks. Subjects were pair-matched based on sex, age, weight, height, and training program. Measurements included body weight, skinfold thickness, body circumference, and 1- and 10-repetition maximum tests for the bench press and leg extension at weeks 0, 4, 8, and 12. Blood tests and a subjective questionnaire were also given. Thirty-one subjects completed the trial (two subjects in the VS group withdrew as a result excessive tiredness and mood changes). Anthropometric measures and body composition did not differ between the groups. Both groups improved in performance, but the only significant effect of treatment was a treatment × time interaction in the leg extension, which the authors attributed to the vanadyl subjects having a lower performance at the baseline. The authors concluded: "Vanadyl sulfate was ineffective in changing body composition in weight training athletes, and any modest performance-enhancing effect requires further investigation" (13).

References

1. Shechter Y, Li J, Meyerovitch J, et al. Insulin-like actions of vanadate are mediated in an insulin-receptor-independent manner via non-receptor protein tyrosine kinases and protein phosphotyrosine phosphates. *Mol Cell Biochem*. 1995;153:39–49.
2. Moore RJ, Friedl KE. Physiology of nutritional supplements: chromium picolinate and vanadyl sulfate. *Natl Strength Cond Assoc J*. 1992;14:47–51.
3. Institute of Medicine. *Dietary Reference Intakes for Vitamin A, Vitamin K, Chromium, Copper, Iodine, Iron, Manganese, Molybedenum, Nickel, Silicon, Vanadium, and Zinc.* Washington, DC: National Academy Press; 2001.
4. Domingo JL, Gomez M, Sanchez DJ, et al. Toxicology of vanadium compounds in diabetic rats: the action of chelating agents on vanadium accumulation. *Mol Cell Biochem*. 1995;153:233–240.

5. Srivastava AK. Anti-diabetic and toxic effects of vanadium compounds. *Mol Cell Biochem.* 2000;206:177–182.

6. Nielsen FH. Ultratrace Minerals. In: Shils ME, Olson JA, Shike M, Ross AC, eds. *Modern Nutrition in Health and Disease.* 9th ed. Baltimore, Md: Williams & Wilkins; 1999:286–288.

7. Fawcett JP, Farquhar SJ, Thou T, et al. Oral vanadyl sulphate does not affect blood cells, viscosity, or biochemistry in humans. *Pharmacol Toxicol.* 1997;80:202–206.

8. Teissedre PL, Krosniak M, Portet K, et al. Vanadium levels in French and Californian wines: influence on vanadium dietary intake. *Food Addit Contam.* 1998;15:585–591.

9. Srivastava AK, Mehdi MZ. Insulino-mimetic and anti-diabetic effects of vanadium compounds. *Diabet Med.* 2005;22:2–13.

10. Boden G, Chen X, Ruiz J, et al. Effects of vanadyl sulfate on carbohydrate and lipid metabolism in patients with non-insulin-dependent diabetes mellitus. *Metabolism.* 1996;45:1130–1135.

11. Goldfine AB, Simonson DC, Folli F, et al. Metabolic effects of sodium metavanadate in humans with insulin-dependent and non-insulin-dependent diabetes mellitus in vivo and in vitro studies. *J Clin Endocrinol Metab.* 1995;80:3311–3320.

12. Halberstam M, Cohen N, Shlimovich P, et al. Oral vanadyl sulfate improves insulin sensitivity in NIDDM but not in obese nondiabetic subjects. *Diabetes.* 1996;45:659–666.

13. Fawcett JP, Farquhar SJ, Walker RJ, et al. The effect of oral vanadyl sulfate on body composition and performance in weight-training athletes. *Int J Sport Nutr.* 1996;6: 382–390.

Vitamin A/Beta Carotene

Vitamin A is the general term used to describe retinoids that have the biologic activity of retinol. This fat-soluble, essential vitamin exists in three oxidative states: retinol (alcohol), retinal (aldehyde), and retinoic acid. Vitamin A plays a role in cell differentiation and morphogenesis, thus affecting growth, reproduction, bone development, skin, and immunity. As part of rhodopsin, the retinal form of vitamin A has a major function in vision (1).

Beta carotene, a precursor to vitamin A, is the most abundant provitamin-A carotenoid found in fruits and vegetables. Carotenoids act as electron-transport agents during photosynthesis and also protect plants from oxygen radicals. Of the approximately 600 carotenoids that have been identified, only 50 show provitamin A activity (1). Approximately six of the many carotenoids in nature are found in significant amounts in human plasma (1). Other provitamin A carotenoids that have been studied in depth include alpha carotene and beta cryptoxanthin. Lutein and lycopene are carotenoids that are not converted into vitamin A (2).

Beta carotene and other carotenoids are being investigated for their possible antioxidant activity in cancer, cardiovascular diseases, and other conditions of oxidative stress (3). The National Academy of Sciences Food and Nutrition Board panel on Antioxidants and Related Compounds reviewed data to determine whether DRIs could be set for beta carotene and other carotenoids. In 2000, when evidence was reviewed, the panel concluded that values could not presently be determined to set required levels of intake. However, the panel did support recommendations to increase intake of carotenoid-rich fruits and vegetables (4).

Media and Marketing Claims	Efficacy
Beta carotene	
Reduces risk of cancer	Supplement ↓
	Dietary ↑
Prevents cardiovascular disease	↓
Enhances immunity in poorly nourished subjects	↑?
Improves eye health and reduces risk for cataracts	↓?
Vitamin A	
Enhances immunity in poorly nourished subjects	↑?
Improves vision (if vitamin A–deficient)	↑
Treats skin disorders (OTC supplements)	NR
Treats acne (prescription form)	↑
Reverses signs of aging in skin	NR

Safety

Vitamin A

- Vitamin A, but not beta carotene, is toxic in doses at 10 times the RDA (900 µg/day for men; 700 µg/day for nonpregnant, nonlactating women).

- The Tolerable Upper Intake Level (UL) for men and women is 3,000 µg/day (10,000 IU) preformed vitamin A. There is no established UL for carotenoids.

- The UL is 3,000 µg preformed vitamin A per day for pregnant women, and 2,000 µg/day for pregnant teenagers. Excessive amounts of vitamin A and other retinoids have been found to be teratogenic in experimental animals and in women. Ingestion of 20,000 IU (6,000 µg) during early pregnancy can cause spontaneous abortion and birth defects. Healthy pregnant women eating well-balanced diets containing fruits and vegetables do not need supplemental vitamin A. However, if a supplement is required it should not exceed 10,000 IU (3,000 µg) during pregnancy (1).

- Hypervitaminosis A has been associated with increased risk for bone fracture in rats (5). The researcher states, "our results suggest that long-term ingestion of modest excesses of vitamin A may contribute to fracture risk." An epidemiological study assessing the relationship between serum retinol levels and bone fracture supports the animal model findings (6). In the sample population of 2,322 males, 266 fractures were adjudicated during a 30-year follow-up period. The hazard ratio for any fracture was 1.64 (95% CI = 1.12–2.41) and increased to 2.47 (95% CI = 1.15–5.28) for hip fracture. Thus, study subjects with a mean serum retinol level more than 75.62 µg/dL had a 64% increased risk of fracture as compared with those with mean serum levels ranging between 62.16 and 67.60 µg/dL. A third report assessing fracture risk and vitamin A intake from food and supplements among postmenopausal women also supports a contraindication for long-term supplementation with vitamin A (7). In this study, 603 hip fractures were diagnosed in a cohort of more than 72,000 women participating in the Nurses' Health Study between 1980 and 1998. The relative risk for hip fracture was 1.48 (95% CI = 1.05–2.07) for women consuming more than 3,000 µg retinol equivalents (RE) per day as compared with those consuming less than 1,250 µg RE per day.

- Acute, high doses of vitamin A (> 200,000 µg RE in adults) are associated with nausea, vomiting, increased cerebrospinal fluid pressure, vertigo, blurred vision, and loss of muscular coordination. The median lethal dose (LD_{50}) of vitamin A extrapolated from studies in monkeys is 500 mg (500,000 µg RE) for a 70-kg adult (1).

- Chronic toxicity can result from ingested doses of vitamin A at 10 times the RDA. Adverse effects include alopecia, ataxia, bone and muscle pain, cheilitis, conjunctivitis, headache, hepatotoxicity, hyperlipemia, membrane dryness, pruritis, skin disorders, and visual impairment (1).

Beta Carotene

- There are no known acute negative effects with high doses of food sources of beta carotene. High doses of either food or supplemental sources of beta carotene may cause hypercarotenemia, resulting in an orange-yellow tint of the skin, especially on palms, soles of feet, and cheeks, where local fat deposits exist (1).

- Long-term ingestion of high dose beta carotene supplements has been associated with increased lung cancer risk in men who smoke and asbestos workers, increased mortality in male smokers with heart disease, and increased risk of intracerebral hemorrhage in smokers without a history of stroke (8–12). In more recent analyses, supplemental beta carotene has been associated with an increase in coronary event risk in male smokers and in increase in gastrointestinal cancer (13,14).

Drug/Supplement Interactions

- HMG-CoA reductase inhibitors used to reduce cholesterol (eg, atorvastatin, lovastatin, fluvastatin) and oral contraceptives are associated with increased blood levels of vitamin A.

- Other medications, including bile acid sequestrants such as cholestyramine and colestipol, as well as mineral oil, orlistat, and neomycin may reduce vitamin A absorption. Patients taking these medications should be advised to take a multivitamin supplement that contains vitamin A.

- Isotretinoin (Accutane) is similar in structure to vitamin A. Using vitamin A supplements with this drug may result in toxicity.

- Antacids (eg, lansoprazole, omeprazole) may interfere with vitamin A and beta carotene absorption.

Key Points

+ Beta carotene supplements have not been associated with reduced risk of most types of cancer, and there is evidence of an increase in risk for lung cancer among smokers and asbestos workers taking beta carotene supplements. Many researchers agree that nutrients in food work synergistically and that the cancer-protective effects of diets rich in carotenoid-containing fruits and vegetables are not due to any one carotenoid.

+ Similarly, beta carotene supplements have not demonstrated any benefit in preventing or treating cardiovascular disease and in fact may increase risk of death from myocardial infarction in male smokers with a history of heart disease and also the risk of intracerebral hemorrhage in male smokers without a history of stroke. The American Heart Association statement concurs that antioxidant supplementation does not prevent cardiovascular disease (15).

+ Vitamin A deficiency has a negative effect on immune status. Supplementation will improve immune status in people with deficiencies, especially children. However, most studies evaluating the effects of beta carotene supplements on immune function showed no benefit. Although individuals with AIDS tend to have reduced plasma carotenoid levels, more research is needed to determine whether beta carotene supplements improve overall health and survival in these individuals.

+ The role of vitamin A in vision is well-known. An overt deficiency of vitamin A can result in permanent or night blindness. Pilot data also suggest vitamin A supplementation may improve clinical response to photorefractory keratectomy (PK) surgery. Preliminary evidence is not suggestive of a benefit of beta carotene supplementation in reducing incidence of cataracts and age-related maculopathy. Other carotenoids (lutein, zeaxanthin) are being investigated for their potential protective effect on degenerative vision disorders.

+ High doses of synthetic vitamin A are currently used in prescription medications to treat acne (isotretinoin) and other skin disorders. While using these medications, patients are closely monitored for adverse affects by their physician. Self-dosing with equivalent amounts of over-the-counter vitamin A is not recommended because of the severe side effects associated with pharmacological doses. Although topical vitamin A analogues (tretinoin [Retin A]) are used in the treatment of acne, blemishes, and wrinkles, there is no evidence that oral vitamin A or beta carotene supplements reverse the signs of aging.

+ Long-term moderately elevated intakes of vitamin A in women have been preliminarily associated with increased risk of hip fracture and osteoporosis. Beta carotene supplementation, however, did not seem to contribute to fracture risk (7).

+ At this time, there is much controversy surrounding the benefits and possible adverse effects of supplementing with beta carotene and/or other carotenoids. The Institute of Medicine report on carotenoids concluded that beta carotene supplements are not advisable, other than as a provitamin A source and to control vitamin A deficiency in at-risk populations (4). Until further evidence is gathered, individuals should be encouraged to consume a variety of fruits and vegetables rich in carotenoids (*see* Food Sources section).

Food Sources

Good sources of preformed vitamin A include liver, eggs, and fortified milk. Rich sources of beta carotene include bright orange and yellow fruits and vegetables. Data for the specific carotenoid contents of foods are limited because calculation methods are fairly new (16,17). Mild heat treatment, mixing foods in a blender, and dietary fat enhance carotenoid absorption, whereas soluble fiber interferes with carotenoid uptake (18).

Food	Beta carotene, mg/3.5 oz	Alpha carotene, mg/3.5 oz	Beta cryptoxanthin, mg/3.5 oz	Lutein and Zeaxanthin, mg/3.5 oz	Lycopene, mg/3.5 oz
Apricot	176	—	—	—	8.64
Carrot	98.0	37.0	—	—	—
Collard greens	54.0	—	—	—	—
Spinach, raw	41.0	—	—	102.0	—
Beet greens	25.6	0.03	—	—	—
Broccoli	13.0	—	—	18.0	—
Mango	13.0	0.01	0.54	—	—
Tomato juice, canned	9.0	—	—	—	8.58
Corn	0.51	0.50	—	7.8	—

Source: Data are from reference 17.

Food	Vitamin A, Retinol Equivalents (RE)	Vitamin A, IU
Liver, beef (3.5 oz)	10,602	37,679
Potato, sweet (1)	2,487	24,877
Carrot (1)	2,025	20,253
Spinach (½ cup)	737	7,371
Mango (1)	805	8,061
Milk, nonfat (1 cup)	149	500
Papaya (1)	85	863
Egg (1)	84	280

Source: Data are from reference 19.

Dosage Information/Bioavailability

The current RDA for vitamin A is 900 µg (3,000 IU) for men and 700 µg (2,333 IU) for women (4). This differs from the previous 1989 RDA for vitamin A of 1,000 RE (5,000 IU) for men and 800 RE (4,000 IU) for women (20). The Institute of Medicine has not set a DRI for beta carotene or other carotenoids (4). The new DRI report did note that the

National Cancer Institute's recommendations for five fruits and vegetables daily would provide approximately 5 to 6 mg provitamin A carotenoids per day, and that this amount from foods is similar to the quantity needed to maintain plasma beta carotene levels in the range associated with a lower risk of various chronic diseases (4).

Beta carotene is sold individually or with other carotenoids or with vitamin C or E in doses ranging from 15,000 IU to 50,000 IU (≈ 90 to 300 mg beta carotene). Beta carotene is bottled in either the synthetic form (all-*trans*-beta carotene) or the natural form (all-*trans*-beta carotene and 9-*cis*-beta carotene) derived from *Dunaliella* alga. Most studies have used the synthetic form of beta carotene. Beta carotene from supplements has a much higher bioavailability than from foods. For instance, 30 mg of supplemental all-*trans*-beta carotene per day increased plasma beta carotene levels five times more than beta carotene from carrots (4). Although the synthetic all-*trans*-beta carotene may be more efficiently absorbed, the tendency of the synthetic form to alter normal serum *trans/cis* ratios in favor of the *trans* isomer may not be a beneficial effect (21).

Vitamin A is available in single preparations or multivitamin/mineral supplements typically providing 5,000 to 10,000 IU (≈ 1,500 to 3,000 µg vitamin A) as retinol or retinyl palmitate. Many supplements contain both retinyl palmitate and beta carotene, which are represented on the label as "total vitamin A activity." Although most supplement labels list vitamin A and beta carotene in international units (IU), the preferred unit of measure is micrograms or retinol activity equivalents (RAE), where 1 RAE = 1 µg retinol = 12 µg of all-*trans*-beta carotene = 24 µg all other provitamin A carotenoids.

RAE is the new interconversion unit used in place of RE, which was used in the 1989 RDA values: 1 IU vitamin A activity = 0.3 µg of all-*trans*-retinol = 3.6 µg all-*trans*-beta carotene = 7.2 µg other provitamin A carotenoids.

Relevant Research

Beta Carotene's Effect on Plasma Carotenoids

- In a 4-year, placebo-controlled study of 108 subjects, supplementation with 25 mg beta carotene resulted in a 151% increase in serum beta carotene but did not significantly change serum retinol, alpha tocopherol, or other serum carotenoids (lycopene, lutein, or alpha carotene) (22).

- In a 5-year study with 259 subjects taking 50 mg supplemental beta carotene daily, beta and alpha carotene plasma concentrations increased by 9- to 10-fold and 2-fold, respectively. Supplementation had no effect on plasma lycopene, lutein/zeaxanthin, retinol, or alpha tocopherol levels (23). After taking a single beta carotene supplement of 12 to 30 mg, plasma levels increased more than after consuming a similar amount of beta carotene from carrots (24,25).

Beta Carotene/Vitamin A and Cancer

- Understanding that beta carotene is a precursor for vitamin A, particularly among those with vitamin A–deficient diets, several observational and intervention studies have examined the effects of dietary beta carotene and beta carotene supplements (and other micronutrients) in cancer prevention. These studies were developed because of the known biological properties of beta carotene and because of substantial epidemiological evidence suggesting that high intakes of fruits and vegetables are associated with reduced risk of several types of cancer. Both epidemiological and intervention trials are described here.

Beta Carotene/Vitamin A and Breast Cancer

♦ In a prospective cohort study in the Netherlands, 65,573 women were followed up for 4.3 years for incidence of breast cancer. After adjusting for risk factors, breast cancer risk was not influenced by the intake of beta carotene, vitamin E, fiber, vitamin C supplements, vegetables, or potatoes. For dietary retinol, a weak positive association with breast cancer was observed (26).

♦ In a population-based, case-control study, 3,543 subjects with breast cancer and 9,406 control subjects were evaluated for food and supplement use. Eating carrots or spinach more than twice per week compared with not eating any carrots or spinach was associated with a 44% reduced risk of breast cancer. However, there was no association between estimated preformed vitamin A intake from foods and supplements and risk of breast cancer across all categories of intake (27).

♦ In a retrospective cohort study, 273 women with breast cancer and 371 matched control subjects were interviewed about their diet at different ages throughout their life. Women were at lower risk of developing breast cancer with increasing levels of reported dietary intake of beta carotene. There was also no association for supplemental beta carotene or vitamin A and breast cancer risk (28).

Beta Carotene and Other Cancers in Women

♦ In the double-blind, placebo-controlled, Women's Health Study, 29,876 women (age > 45 years) were randomly assigned to receive beta carotene (50 mg on alternate days), vitamin E, aspirin, or a placebo. The beta carotene arm was terminated early after a median treatment duration of 2.1 years plus 2 years follow-up. Beta carotene had no effect on cancer incidence, nor did it have any significant effects for any site-specific cancer. Additionally, beta carotene had no effect on all-cause mortality or cardiovascular disease incidence (29). No data on supplemental sources of these nutrients were provided.

Beta Carotene/Vitamin A and Lung Cancer

♦ In the Alpha Tocopherol Beta Carotene (ATBC) Cancer Prevention Study, 29,133 male cigarette smokers, ages 50 to 69, years were randomly assigned to receive 20 mg beta carotene, 50 mg alpha tocopherol, both vitamins, or a placebo daily for 5 to 8 years. Beta carotene did not cause a decrease in cancer at any site and was associated with a significant 18% increased risk in lung cancer. However, lower lung cancer rates were observed in men in the placebo group who had higher amounts of both serum and dietary beta carotene and vitamin E at the baseline (8).

♦ In a follow-up analysis, results from the ATBC Cancer Prevention Study were examined to determine whether the pattern of intervention effects across subgroups would provide further interpretation of the main ATBC study results. The beta carotene effect seemed stronger in subjects who smoked 20 or more cigarettes per day than in those who smoked 5 to 19 cigarettes daily and in those with higher alcohol intake (> 11 g ethanol per day). The authors concluded: "Beta carotene at pharmacologic levels may modestly increase lung cancer incidence in cigarette smokers, and this effect may be associated with heavier smoking and higher alcohol intake" (9).

◆ In the prospective, double-blind, placebo-controlled Beta-Carotene and Retinol Efficacy Trial (CARET), 18,314 men and women at risk of developing lung cancer (asbestos workers and smokers) were randomly assigned to receive 30 mg beta carotene plus 25,000 IU vitamin A (retinyl palmitate) or a placebo. The study was stopped 21 months early because of "clear evidence of no benefit and substantial evidence of possible harm." An analysis of subgroups revealed a greater risk of lung cancer in subjects in the highest quartile of alcohol intake. The authors noted that the excess lung cancer incidence and mortality with beta carotene and vitamin A were highly consistent with the results found in the ATBC study (10).

Beta Carotene/Vitamin A and Gastrointestinal Cancers

◆ A Cochrane Database Systemic Review of 14 trials (total n = 170,525 study participants), of which nine included beta carotene analysis and four included vitamin A analysis, showed a general pattern of increased risk for gastrointestinal cancers with supplementation. Use of beta carotene and vitamin A resulted in a combined study relative risk (RR) of 1.29 (95% CI = 1.01–1.20), suggesting an almost 30% increase in risk with supplementation (30). A separate meta-analysis conducted by the same group (14) also suggested a statistically significant increase in overall mortality associated with supplementation with beta carotene and vitamin A (RR = 1.29; CI = 1.14–1.45).

◆ In the ATBC study (see earlier paragraph for details), beta carotene supplements (50 mg/day for 5 to 8 years) had no effect on colorectal cancer incidence (9).

Beta Carotene/Vitamin A and Oral Cancer

◆ In a trial of 214 subjects diagnosed with early-stage squamous cell cancer of the head and neck, subjects were randomly assigned to no supplementation or 75 mg beta carotene per day for 3 months, 1 month off, repeat cycles for 3 years total duration (31). After a median 59 months of treatment, with a dropout rate of 31%, the disease-free survival times were essentially equal across groups, and 10-year survival also did not differ significantly.

◆ In a prospective cohort study (ATBC Cancer Prevention Study), 409 men who smoked were randomly assigned to receive 20 mg beta carotene, 50 mg vitamin E, a mixture of both, or a placebo daily for 5 to 7 years. There was no significant difference between groups in the prevalence of oral mucosal lesions or in the cells of unkeratinized epithelium of the tongue (32).

◆ In a double-blind, placebo-controlled study, 264 subjects who had been curatively treated for a recent early-stage squamous cell carcinoma of the oral cavity, pharynx, or larynx were randomly assigned to receive 50 mg beta carotene or a placebo daily for up to 90 months. After a median follow-up of 51 months, there were no differences between groups in the development of a second primary tumor plus local recurrence. When analyzed by specific site of cancer, beta carotene had no effect on second occurrence of head and neck cancer or lung cancer. The vitamin also had no effect on total mortality (33).

Beta Carotene and Skin Cancer

♦ In a double-blind study based on mechanistic research suggesting that UV light–induced oxidative damage is the primary pathway to skin cancer formation, researchers provided 16 subjects with vitamin E (400 IU) or beta carotene (15 mg) daily for 8 weeks in an unblinded design. Skin biopsies from ultraviolet light exposed and unexposed skin were taken before and after supplementation. Assessment of plasma beta carotene levels indicated good compliance with supplementation over time with a 2.25-fold increase in levels. Neither supplement was effective in reducing oxidative stress (34).

♦ In a randomized intervention trial, 1,621 adults residing in Australia (where skin cancer rates are among the highest in the world) took supplemental beta carotene (30 mg/day) or placebo for 2 years. Beta carotene efficacy was also compared with daily sunscreen use. Sunscreen was associated with a 24% reduction in solar keratoses, a precursor lesion for skin cancer, whereas beta carotene showed no efficacy (35).

♦ In a parallel-design placebo-controlled study to evaluate the protective effects of beta carotene and mixed carotenoids against UV-associated erythema, 36 subjects were randomly assigned to placebo, beta carotene (24 mg/day), or mixed carotenoids (24 mg/day) for 12 weeks. Participants were subjected to irradiation with a solar light simulator at baseline, and at 6 and 12 weeks. Subjects' carotenoid levels and skin erythema values were taken before and 24 hours after irradiation. At week 12, skin carotenoid values had increased significantly and both beta carotene and mixed carotenoids were associated with reduced skin erythema (36). It is not known whether this association translates to reduced risk of skin cancer.

♦ In a double-blind, placebo-controlled Physician's Health Study, 22,071 healthy male physicians (ages 40 to 82 years) were randomly assigned to receive 50 mg beta carotene or placebo every other day for 12 years. After adjusting for age and aspirin assignment, beta carotene supplements had no significant effect on incidence of nonmelanoma skin cancer (basal cell carcinoma and squamous cell carcinoma). There was also no evidence of a harmful or beneficial effect of beta carotene on skin cancer incidence when subjects were separated by smoking status (current, past, or never) (37).

Beta Carotene and Cardiovascular Disease

♦ The American Heart Association Science Advisory published in 2004 provides a detailed review of evidence regarding the use of antioxidants, including beta carotene, in reducing cardiovascular risk and adverse clinical outcomes (15). This summary provides no evidence that beta carotene supplementation reduces cardiovascular events. In fact, the ATBC suggests slight increases in ischemic heart disease, hemorrhagic stroke, and ischemic stroke mortality in those receiving beta carotene supplementation. The position states, "at this time, the scientific data do not justify the use of antioxidant vitamin supplements for CVD risk reduction."

◆ The Heart Protection Study (HPS), a multicenter randomized, double-blind, placebo-controlled clinical trial, was initiated among 20,536 adults (ages 40 to 80 years), with a minimum total cholesterol of 3.5 mmol/L, to determine the efficacy of statins, with or without antioxidants, or placebo in modulating cardiovascular morbidity and mortality (38). Whereas statins were highly effective in reducing total mortality (–12%), and coronary heart disease events (–24%), there was no significant benefit associated with daily "antioxidant cocktail" supplementation that provided 250 mg vitamin C, 650 mg vitamin E, and 20 mg beta carotene.

◆ The US Preventive Task Force paper on antioxidant supplementation to prevent cardiovascular disease suggests that while some epidemiological evidence suggests a protective effect, insufficient randomized prospective controlled trials are available to support generalized recommendations for antioxidant supplementation for the prevention of cardiovascular disease (39).

◆ Although beta carotene supplementation trials have not been supportive, epidemiological data assessing *dietary* beta carotene in reducing coronary artery disease (CAD) have shown a protective effect. A study of 998 CAD cases prospectively identified in a cohort of 73,286 female nurses showed the relative risk for CAD was 26% less for women at the highest quintile of beta carotene intake as compared with the lowest quintile of beta-carotene intake (40).

◆ In a prospective, double-blind, placebo-controlled study, 27,271 male smokers from the ATBC Cancer Prevention Study with no history of myocardial infarction were randomly assigned to receive 20 mg beta carotene, 50 mg alpha tocopherol, a mixture of both, or a placebo daily for 5 to 8 years. The endpoint was the first nonfatal or fatal major coronary event. Beta carotene supplementation had no significant effect on the incidence of nonfatal or fatal coronary events or incidence of myocardial infarction (MI) compared with other groups. The authors concluded: "Supplementation with beta carotene has no primary preventive effect on major coronary events" (41).

◆ A follow-up analysis conducted at the end of 2002 among ATBC study participants (n = 25,563) showed that for the 7,261 men who died between May 1, 1993, and April 30, 2001, mortality was significantly greater for those assigned to the beta carotene group (hazards ratio = 1.07; 95% CI = 1.02–1.12), primarily associated with cancer during the first 4 years, but then shifted to cardiovascular events (42). A second follow-up focused on major coronary events among at-risk men (previous MI patients) showed that those receiving beta carotene during the ATBC study were at a 14% increased risk for a major coronary event (43) and risk for nonfatal MI also increased 16% among those with no previous MI. Again, this population included men who smoked, and the interaction between smoking and supplementation is thought to have significant effects on oxidative status. Follow-up data related to stroke risk did not support an increased risk associated with beta carotene supplementation (RR = 0.97; 95% CI = 0.86–1.09) (13).

♦ In a double-blind placebo-controlled study, a subgroup of 1,862 male smokers with previous myocardial infarction from the ATBC Cancer Prevention Study were randomly assigned to receive 20 mg beta carotene, 50 mg alpha tocopherol, both, or a placebo daily for a mean of 5 years. There were no significant differences in the number of major coronary events between any supplementation group and the placebo group. There was a significant increase in deaths from coronary heart disease in the beta carotene and the combined alpha tocopherol and beta carotene groups than the placebo group. The authors concluded that alpha tocopherol or beta carotene supplements are not recommended in male smokers with heart disease (11).

♦ In a prospective, double-blind, placebo-controlled study, 1,759 male smokers with angina pectoris from the ATBC Cancer Prevention Study were randomly assigned to receive 20 mg beta carotene, 50 mg vitamin E, mixture of both, or a placebo daily for 5 to 7 years. Recurrence of angina pectoris at annual follow-up visits, progression from mild to severe angina, and incidence of major coronary events were measured. There were no significant differences between groups. The authors concluded: "There was no evidence of beneficial effects for alpha tocopherol or beta carotene supplements in male smokers with angina pectoris, indicating no basis for therapeutic or preventive use of these agents in such patients" (44).

Beta Carotene or Vitamin A and Immunity

♦ Male smokers hospitalized with pneumonia were included in a subgroup analysis conducted within the ATBC trial. In this double-blind, randomized, placebo-controlled study, subjects were randomly assigned to daily antioxidant supplementation with 50 mg vitamin E, 20 mg beta carotene, a combination of both, or placebo for a median follow-up of 6.1 years. Overall, beta carotene was not associated with risk for pneumonia. In fact, it was associated with increased risk for pneumonia among those who reported starting smoking at a later age (older than 21 years) (45). However, vitamin E supplementation was associated with a significant decrease risk for pneumonia in this subgroup of later-onset smokers (RR = 0.65; 95% CI = 0.49–0.86). This study did not provide objective data on related illnesses or immune status biomarkers that would support a direct role for these antioxidants in modulating the immunity of this study population.

♦ In a double-blind placebo-controlled study, 58 healthy subjects with adequate nutritional status and who were older than 65 years of age were randomly assigned to receive 8.2 mg beta carotene, 13.3 mg lycopene, or a placebo daily for 12 weeks. Markers of immune function (total lymphocytes, T-cell subsets including CD4 and CD8 and the expression of functionally associated cell surface molecules using lectin-stimulated lymphocyte proliferation) were measured at baseline and at 12 weeks. No significant differences were seen in any of the immunity parameters measured in any group (46).

◆ In a double-blind, placebo-controlled study, 54 healthy, elderly men randomly selected from the Physician's Health Study were randomly assigned to receive 50 mg beta carotene every other day for 10 to 12 years. In a second study, 25 elderly women were given 90 mg beta carotene per day for 3 weeks. In both studies, subjects taking supplements had greater plasma beta carotene levels than placebo subjects after supplementation. Delayed hypersensitivity skin test responses given before and after the intervention did not differ between beta carotene and placebo groups in either the short-term or long-term study. Short-term or long-term beta carotene had no effect on T cell–mediated immune responses as measured by lymphocyte proliferation, interleukin-2 and prostaglandin E_2 production, and composition of lymphocyte subsets (47).

◆ In a double-blind, placebo-controlled, crossover study, 25 healthy male nonsmokers were randomly assigned to receive 15 mg beta carotene daily or a placebo for 26 days each. After beta carotene supplementation, there were significant increases in plasma beta carotene levels. There was a significant association between beta carotene supplementation and elevated expression of peripheral blood monocyte surface molecules (involved in initiating immune responses) and with an increase in the secretion of TNF-alpha (plays a role in host resistance to infection) by blood monocytes. The authors concluded: "Moderate increases in the dietary intake of beta-carotene can enhance cell-mediated immune responses within a relatively short period of time, providing a potential mechanism for the anticarcinogenic properties attributed to beta-carotene" (48).

◆ In a controlled depletion-repletion study, nine healthy women lived in a metabolic unit for 100 days and consumed a basal diet supplemented with 1.5 mg beta carotene for 4 days (baseline), followed by the basal diet without supplements for 68 days (depletion), followed by 15 mg beta carotene/day for the last 28 days (repletion). Neither beta carotene depletion nor repletion significantly affected proliferation of peripheral blood mononuclear cells cultured with phytohemagglutinin or concanavalin A, in vitro production of interleukin 2 receptor, or the concentration of circulating lymphocytes and their subsets. The authors concluded that in healthy adults consuming adequate vitamin A, beta carotene depletion had no apparent adverse effects and that modest beta carotene supplementation had no beneficial effects (49).

◆ In a double-blind, placebo-controlled study, 17 subjects with HIV were randomly assigned to receive 180 mg beta carotene or a placebo for 4 weeks. Supplementation statistically significantly increased total white blood cells and percentage of CD4 lymphocytes (50).

◆ Vitamin A supplementation historically has been shown to enhance immunity through increased antibody formation in children living in developing countries who are provided immunizations. However, in a prospective, randomized, placebo-controlled study conducted among approximately 400 children in India, vitamin A supplementation was not associated with increased antibody levels or sustained levels of antibodies at 6 months (78% with high titer of measles at 6 months in vitamin

A group, 85% in placebo group, but it was not statistically significant) (51). Subjects were excluded if they had clinical signs of vitamin A deficiency. In most studies showing a therapeutic benefit of vitamin A in immunization response, children were vitamin A–deficient at the time of supplementation. Another difference is that this study provided a single dose of 100,000 IU vitamin A, whereas other studies have provided higher doses once or twice per day for 1 to 7 days.

Beta Carotene/Vitamin A and Eye Health

♦ Photorefractory keratectomy (PK) is becoming a common eye surgery to correct vision. In a pilot study, investigators randomly assigned two groups of 20 people each who were scheduled for PK to either retinol (25,000 IU) plus 230 mg alpha tocopherol (Group 1) or placebo (Group 2) from surgical day 1 through 1-year follow-up. Re-epithelialization of eye tissue occurred significantly sooner in the vitamin-supplemented group than in the placebo group ($P = .035$). The vitamin-supplemented group also showed significantly greater correction of myopathy as compared with the placebo group ($P = .043$), a clinical response that was sustained in terms of the reduced need for vision at 1 year as compared with the placebo group. Given the pilot nature of this study and small sample size, follow-up studies are needed (52).

♦ A prospective, randomized, controlled blinded study of the efficacy of a mixed antioxidant supplement (400 IU vitamin E, 15 mg beta carotene, and 500 mg vitamin C daily) for age-related cataract and vision loss was conducted for 11 years among 4,757 adults ages 55 to 80 years (53). Among the 4,629 participants who had intact lenses at study onset and were followed up for 6.3 years, there was no significant effect of supplementation on visual acuity loss or age-related lens opacities as measured by nuclear, cortical, or posterior subscapsular opacity grades.

♦ A secondary analysis completed using data from the Nurses' Health Study, including 129 subjects with a cataract diagnosis, indicated that beta carotene supplementation for a mean of 2.1 years at a dosage of 50 mg every other day was not associated with cataract prevention or risk (54).

♦ In a double-blind, placebo-controlled study, a random sample of 1,828 male smokers from the ATBC Cancer Prevention Study were randomly assigned to receive 20 mg beta carotene, 50 mg alpha tocopherol, a mixture of both, or a placebo daily for 5 to 8 years. Supplementation did not affect the end-of-trial prevalence of nuclear, cortical, or posterior subscapsular cataract or affect the median lens opacity meter value (measure of cataract severity) (55). It should be noted that subjects were smokers and the trial was not prospectively designed to test hypotheses relating antioxidant supplementation to eye health.

♦ In a double-blind, placebo-controlled study, a subgroup of 941 male smokers from the ATBC Cancer Prevention Study were randomly assigned to receive 20 mg beta carotene, 50 mg alpha tocopherol, a mixture of both, or a placebo daily for 5 to 8 years. Subjects had an ophthalmologic exam at the end of the trial. There were 269 cases of age-related maculopathy, and no benefit was associated beta carotene or vitamin E supplements (56).

Vitamin A and Skin Health

♦ Natural and synthetic analogues of vitamin A (isotretinoin, etretinate, acitretin) have been used successfully in the treatment of skin disorders, including acne vulgaris and psoriasis (57). Individuals undergoing retinoid therapy are monitored for adverse effects typical of hypervitaminosis A, including liver toxicity, abnormal lipid profiles, teratogenic effects, and mucocutaneous side effects (58).

References

1. Shils ME, Olson JA, Shike M, Ross AC, eds. *Modern Nutrition in Health and Disease.* 9th ed. Baltimore, Md: Williams & Wilkins; 1999.
2. Vainio H, Rautalahti M. An international evaluation of the cancer preventive potential of carotenoids. *Cancer Epidemiol Biomarkers Prev.* 1998;7:725–728.
3. Mayne ST. Beta-carotene, carotenoids, and disease prevention in humans. *FASEB J.* 1996;10:690–701.
4. Institute of Medicine. *Dietary Reference Intakes: Vitamin C, Vitamin E, Selenium, and Carotenoids.* Washington, DC: National Academy Press; 2000.
5. Johansson S, Lind PM, Hakansson H, et al. Subclinical hypervitaminosis A causes fragile bones in rats. *Bone.* 2002;31:685–689.
6. Michaelsson K, Lithell H, Vessby B, et al. Serum retinol levels and the risk of fracture. *N Engl J Med.* 2003;348:287–294.
7. Feskanich D, Singh V, Willett WC, et al. Vitamin A intake and hip fractures among postmenopausal women. *JAMA.* 2002;287:47–54
8. Albanes D, Heinonen OP, Huttunen JK, et al. Effects of alpha-tocopherol and beta-carotene supplements on cancer incidence in the Alpha Tocopherol Beta-Carotene Cancer Prevention Study. *Am J Clin Nutr.* 1995;62(6 Suppl):S1427-S1430.
9. Albanes D, Heinonen OP, Taylor PR, et al. Alpha-tocopherol and beta-carotene supplements and lung cancer incidence in the Alpha-Tocopherol, Beta-Carotene cancer prevention study: effects of base-line characteristics and study compliance. *J Natl Cancer Inst.* 1996;88:1560–1570.
10. Omenn GS, Goodman GE, Thornquist MD, et al. Risk factors for lung cancer and for intervention effects in CARET, the Beta-Carotene and Retinol Efficacy Trial. *J Natl Cancer Inst.* 1996;88:1550–1559.
11. Rapola JM, Virtamo J, Ripatti S, et al. Randomized trial of alpha-tocopherol and beta-carotene supplements on incidence of major coronary events in men with previous myocardial infarction. *Lancet.* 1997;349:1715–1720.
12. Leppala JM, Virtamo J, Fogelholm R, et al. Controlled trial of alpha-tocopherol and beta-carotene supplements on stroke incidence and mortality in male smokers. *Arterioscler Thromb Vasc Biol.* 2000;20:230–235.
13. Tornwall ME, Virtamo J, Korhonen PA, et al. Effect of alpha-tocopherol and beta-carotene supplementation on coronary heart disease during the 6-year post-trial follow up in the ATBC study. *Eur Heart J.* 2004;25:1171–1178.

14. Bjelakovic G, Nikolava D, Simonetti RG, et al. Antioxidant supplements for prevention of gastrointestinal cancers: a systematic review and meta-analysis. *Lancet.* 2004;364:1219–1228.

15. Kris-Etherton PM, Lichtenstein AH, Howard BV, et al. Antioxidant vitamin supplements and cardiovascular disease. *Circulation.* 2004;110:637–641.

16. Chug-Ahuja, Holden JM, Beecher GR, et al. The development and application of a carotenoid database for fruits, vegetables, and selected multicomponent foods. *J Am Diet Assoc.* 1993;93:318–323.

17. Mangels AR, Holden JM, Beecher JR, et al. Carotenoid content of fruits and vegetables: an evaluation of analytic data [erratum in *J Am Diet Assoc.* 1993;93:527]. *J Am Diet Assoc.* 1993;93:284–296.

18. Rock CL. Carotenoids: biology and treatment. *Pharmacol Ther.* 1997;75:185–197.

19. Pennington JA. *Bowes and Church's Food Values of Portions Commonly Used.* 17th ed. Philadelphia, Pa: Lippincott-Raven Publishers; 1998.

20. Food and Nutrition Board. *Recommended Dietary Allowances.* 10th ed. Washington, DC: National Academy Press; 1989.

21. Patrick L. Beta-carotene: the controversy continues. *Altern Med Rev.* 2000;5:530–545.

22. Nierenberg DW, Dain BJ, Mott LA, et al. Effects of 4 y of oral supplementation with beta-carotene on serum concentrations of retinol, tocopherol, and five carotenoids. *Am J Clin Nutr.* 1997;66:315–319.

23. Mayne ST, Cartmel B, Silva F, et al. Effect of supplemental beta-carotene on plasma concentrations of carotenoids, retinol, and alpha-tocopherol in humans. *Am J Clin Nutr.* 1998;68:642–647.

24. Brown ED, Micozzi MS, Craft NE, et al. Plasma carotenoids in normal men after a single ingestion of vegetables or purified beta-carotene. *Am J Clin Nutr.* 1989;49:1258–1265.

25. Micozzi MS, Brown ED, Edwards BK, et al. Plasma carotenoid response to chronic intake of selected foods and beta-carotene supplements in men. *Am J Clin Nutr.* 1992;55:1120–1125.

26. Verhoeven DT, Assen N, Goldbohm RA, et al. Vitamin C and E, retinol, beta-carotene, and dietary fibre in relation to breast cancer risk: a prospective cohort study. *Br J Cancer.* 1997;75:149–155.

27. Longnecker MP, Newcomb PA, Mittendorf R, et al. Intake of carrots, spinach, and supplements containing vitamin A in relation to risk of breast cancer. *Cancer Epidemiol Biomarkers Prev.* 1997;6:887–892.

28. Jumaan AO, Holmberg L, Zack M, et al. Beta-carotene intake and risk of postmenopausal breast cancer. *Epidemiology.* 1999;10:49–53.

29. Lee IM, Cook NR, Manson JE, et al. Beta-carotene supplementation and incidence of cancer and cardiovascular disease: the Women's Health Study. *J Natl Cancer Inst.* 1999;91:2102–2106.

30. Bjelakovic G, Nikolova D, Simonetti RG, et al. Antioxidant supplements for preventing gastrointestinal cancers. *Cochrane Database Syst Rev.* 2004;18(4):CD004183.

31. Toma S, Bonelli L, Sartoris A, et al. Beta-carotene supplementation in patients radically treated for stage I-II head and neck cancer: results of a randomized trial. *Oncol Rep.* 2003;10:1895–1901.

32. Liede K, Hietanen J, Saxen L, et al. Long-term supplementation with alpha-tocopherol and beta-carotene and prevalence of oral mucosal lesions in smokers. *Oral Dis.* 1998;4:78–83.

33. Mayne ST, Cartmel B, Baum M, et al. Randomized trial of supplemental beta-carotene to prevent second head and neck cancer. *Cancer Res.* 2001;61:1457–1463.

34. McArdle F, Rhodes LE, Parslew RA, et al. Effects of oral vitamin E and beta-carotene supplementation on ultraviolet radiation-induced oxidative stress in human skin. *Am J Clin Nutr.* 2004;80:1270–1275.

35. Darlington S, Williams G, Neale R, et al. A randomized controlled trial to assess sunscreen application and beta carotene supplementation in the prevention of solar keratoses. *Arch Dermatol.* 2003;139:451–455.

36. Heinrich U, Gartner C, Wiebusch M, et al. Supplementation with beta-carotene or a similar amount of mixed carotenoids protect human from UV-induced erythema. *J Nutr.* 2003;133:98–101.

37. Frieling UM, Schaumberg DA, Kupper TS, et al. A randomized, 12-year primary-prevention trial of beta carotene supplementation for nonmelanoma skin cancer in the physician's health study. *Arch Dermatol.* 2000;136:179–184.

38. Collins R, Peto R, Armitage J. The MRC/BHF Heart Protection Study: preliminary results. *Int J Clin Pract.* 2002;56:53–56.

39. Morris CD, Carson S. Routine vitamin supplementation to prevent cardiovascular disease: a summary of the evidence for the U.S. Preventive Services Task Force. *Ann Intern Med.* 2003;139:56–70.

40. Osganian SK, Stampfer MJ, Rimm E, et al. Dietary carotenoids and risk of coronary artery disease in women. *Am J Clin Nutr.* 2003;77:1390–1399.

41. Virtamo J, Rapola JM, Ripatti S, et al. Effect of vitamin E and beta-carotene on the incidence of primary nonfatal myocardial infarction and fatal coronary heart disease. *Arch Intern Med.* 1998;158:668–675.

42. Virtamo J, Pietinen P, Huttunen JK, et al. Incidence of cancer and mortality following alpha-tocopherol and beta-carotene supplementation: a postintervention follow-up. *JAMA.* 2003;290:476–485.

43. Tornwall ME, Virtamo J, Korhonen PA, et al. Postintervention effect of alpha tocopherol and beta carotene on different strokes: a 6 year follow up of the Alpha Tocopherol, Beta Carotene Cancer Prevention Study. *Stroke.* 2004;35:1908–1913.

44. Rapola JM, Virtamo J, Ripatti S, et al. Effects of alpha tocopherol and beta carotene supplements on symptoms, progression, and prognosis of angina pectoris. *Heart.* 1998;79:454–458.

45. Hemila H, Virtamo J, Albanes D, et al. Vitamin E and beta-carotene supplementation and hospital-treated pneumonia incidence in male smokers. *Chest.* 2004;125:557–565.

46. Corridan BM, O'Donoghue M, Hughes DA, et al. Low-dose supplementation with lycopene or beta carotene does not enhance cell-mediated immunity in healthy free-living elderly humans. *Eur J Clin Nutr.* 2001;55:627–635.

47. Santos MS, Leka LS, Ribaya-Mercado JD, et al. Short- and long-term beta-carotene supplementation do not influence T cell-mediated immunity in healthy elderly persons. *Am J Clin Nutr.* 1997;66:917–924.

48. Hughes DA, Wright AJ, Finglas PM, et al. The effect of beta-carotene supplementation on the immune function of blood monocytes from healthy male nonsmokers. *J Lab Clin Med.* 1997;129:309–317.

49. Daudu PA, Kelley DS, Taylor PC, et al. Effect of a low-beta-carotene diet on the immune functions of adult women. *Am J Clin Nutr.* 1994;60:969–972.

50. Coodley GO, Nelson HD, Loveless MO, et al. Beta-carotene in HIV infection. *J Acquir Immune Defic Syndr.* 1993;6:272–276.

51. Cherian T, Varkki S, Raghupathy P, et al. Effect of vitamin A supplementation on the immune response to measles vaccination. *Vaccine.* 2003;21:2418–2420.

52. Vertrugno M, Maino A, Cardia G, et al. A randomised, double masked, clinical trial of high dose vitamin A and vitamin E supplementation after photorefractive keratectomy. *Br J Opthamol.* 2001;85:537–539.

53. Age-Related Eye Disease Study Research Group. A randomized, placebo-controlled, clinical trial of high-dose supplementation with vitamins C and E and beta carotene for age-related cataract and vision loss: AREDS report no. 9. *Arch Opthalmol.* 2001;119:1439–1452.

54. Christen W, Glynn R, Sperduto R, et al. Age-related cataract in a randomized trial of beta-carotene in women. *Opthamol Epidemiol.* 2004;11:401–412.

55. Teikari JM, Virtamo J, Rautalahti M, et al. Long-term supplementation with alpha-tocopherol and beta-carotene and age-related cataract. *Acta Ophthalmol Scand.* 1997;75:634–640.

56. Teikari JM, Laatikainen L, Virtamo J, et al. Six-year supplementation with alpha-tocopherol and beta-carotene and age-related maculopathy. *Acta Ophthalmol Scand.* 1998;76:224–229.

57. Hartmann D, Bollag W. Historical aspects of the oral use of retinoids in acne. *J Dermatol.* 1993;20:674–678.

58. David M, Hodak E, Lowe NJ. Adverse effects of retinoids. *Med Toxicol Adverse Drug Exp.* 1988;3:273–288.

Vitamin B-1 (Thiamin)

The water-soluble vitamin thiamin, as part of thiamin pyrophosphate (TPP) and thiamin triphosphate (TTP), acts as a coenzyme in the metabolism of carbohydrates and branched-chain amino acids. Thiamin works synergistically with lipoic acid, niacin (NAD+), and pantothenic acid in energy production. The body contains a total of 30 mg of thiamin (80% as TPP) with higher concentrations found in muscles including the heart, and in the liver, kidneys, and brain. Because thiamin is not stored in large amounts in any tissue, a regular dietary supply is needed to prevent deficiency. Beriberi, the clinical deficiency of thiamin, is characterized by peripheral neuropathy, muscle atrophy, and/or cardiovascular problems (edema, cardiomegaly, congestive heart failure). Although an overt deficiency is rare, aging, alcoholism, dialysis, and hypermetabolism increase the risk for thiamin deficiency (1).

Media and Marketing Claims	Efficacy
Increases energy, prevents fatigue, enhances exercise performance	NR
Reduces dementia, improves mental status in individuals with Alzheimer's disease or alcoholism, or those on renal dialysis	↔
Reduces stress	NR
Prevents mouth ulcers, canker sores	NR
Reduces risk for cataracts	NR

Safety

- No serious adverse effects have been reported. Thiamin is an FDA-approved prescription product and is available at lower dosage levels in over-the-counter products.
- Thiamin in excessive doses is rapidly cleared by the kidneys and has no apparent toxic effects (1). A Tolerable Upper Intake Level (UL) has not been set because data for quantitative risk assessment is lacking.
- The lethal dose (LD_{50}) in mice and dogs is 125 mg to 350 mg/kg body weight.

Drug/Supplement Interactions

- Loop diuretics (eg, furosemide) increase urinary thiamin losses and may result in thiamin deficiency.
- Thiamin deficiency has been documented in patients on phenytoin; multivitamin or B-complex vitamin supplementation is advised.

Key Points

- There is little evidence suggesting that thiamin supplements improve exercise performance or reduce fatigue and increase the perception of "energy" in healthy individuals without thiamin deficiency. Well-controlled trials are needed to assess these claims.
- The elderly may be at risk for several nutrient deficiencies, including thiamin deficiency. Preliminary research in individuals with Alzheimer's disease on high-dose thiamin therapy is equivocal. One small study showed reduced plasma thiamin levels in individuals with Alzheimer's disease, but thiamin in cerebral spinal fluid was not decreased as compared with control subjects (2). Elderly patients may need to modify their diets to ensure adequate consumption of thiamin (and other B vitamins). If intake is low, a multivitamin/mineral supplement providing 100% of the RDA could be helpful.
- Patients with a history of alcohol abuse at risk for Wernicke-Korsakoff syndrome show improved mental function and awareness from thiamin supplementation, but

specifics regarding the optimal dose, duration, and administration routes have not been formulated (3). However, treatment of this clinical condition requires a medical diagnosis and is thus under the practice of medicine. Other health care professionals should be aware that those who abuse alcohol could be at risk of thiamin deficiency.

♦ Thiamin supplementation may be advisable in individuals receiving chronic peritoneal dialysis to prevent encephalopathy.

♦ Although thiamin and other B-vitamin requirements increase with intense physical exertion or physical trauma, there is currently no controlled research indicating that thiamin supplements improve the body's ability to cope with daily emotional stress or anxiety.

♦ Preliminary evidence suggests that a subclinical thiamin deficiency is associated with recurrent mouth ulcers. Research is needed to determine the possible role of thiamin supplements in ameliorating this condition.

♦ Diets sufficient in thiamin may protect against the development of cataracts, but additional research is needed, including randomized controlled trials in at-risk subjects using supplemental thiamin.

Food Sources

Meat, legumes, whole grains (germ), and seeds are good sources of thiamin. Thiamin is easily oxidized by heat (cooking, baking, pasteurization, spray-drying milk), sulfites (in dried fruit), irradiation, refining whole-wheat, and sodium bicarbonate (added to canned legumes) (1). In addition, the presence of thiaminases in raw fish (sushi) and rice bran or thiamin antagonists in tea, coffee, and rice bran interfere with thiamin absorption (1).

Food	Thiamin, mg/serving
Pork loin (3.5 oz)	0.92
Peas, green (½ cup)	0.23
Rice, brown (1 cup)	0.19
Beans, pinto (½ cup)	0.16
Potato, baked	0.16
Peanuts (1 oz)	0.12
Chicken breast (3.5 oz)	0.07
Beef, ground, lean (3.5 oz)	0.05
Broccoli (½ cup)	0.04

Source: Data are from reference 4.

Dosage Information/Bioavailability

The RDA is 1.1 mg for women and 1.2 mg for men (5). Thiamin is available in multivitamin/mineral supplements, B-complex supplements, and single preparations in the form of thiamin hydrochloride in doses ranging from 1 to 500 mg. Some studies have used a fat-soluble thiamin derivative (thiamin tetrahydrofurfuryl disulfide) that is absorbed more efficiently than the water-soluble form and is readily converted into thiamin (6). Ingested thiamin is fairly well absorbed and is converted to phosphorylated forms (TPP and TTP) (1). Thiamin status depends on its bioavailability from foods, alcohol consumption, presence of antithiamin factors, and folate and protein status (1).

Relevant Research

Thiamin and Exercise

- In a short-term, double-blind, placebo-controlled crossover study, 14 subjects were randomly assigned to receive 1,000 mg of a thiamin derivative (thiamin tetrahydrofurfuryl disulfide) or a placebo for 4 days each. There was a 10-day washout between trials. On day 3, subjects completed a progressive exercise test to exhaustion on a cycle ergometer to determine $VO_{2submax}$, VO_{2peak}, lactate concentration, lactate threshold, and heart rate. On day 4, subjects performed a maximal timed trial on the cycle. There were no significant differences between trials on any of the parameters measured, indicating that supplementation did not prevent fatigue or enhance exercise performance (6).

Thiamin for the Elderly and for Dementia or Encephalopathy

- There have been several reports of low plasma and brain thiamin levels in individuals with Alzheimer's disease and frontal lobe degeneration of the non-Alzheimer's type (5–7); however, not all show decreased thiamin levels in cerebrospinal fluid (2).

- A 2001 Cochrane Database Review addressing the association between thiamin and Alzheimer's disease concluded that the number of studies was insufficient and the design of studies poor, making it difficult and inappropriate at this time to draw conclusions regarding the role of thiamin status or thiamin supplementation in preventing or improving symptoms of Alzheimer's disease (7).

- In a double-blind, placebo-controlled study, 76 elderly subjects (35 subjects with low erythrocyte concentrations of TPP on two measurements [3 months apart] and 41 subjects with one low TPP level) were randomly assigned to 10 mg thiamin or a placebo daily for 3 months. Blood pressure, hand-grip strength, height, and weight, were measured and BMI calculated before and after the study. Cognition, functional ability, and general health were assessed by the Mini-Mental State Examination (MMSE), the 45-point Frenchay Activities Index, and the Nottingham Health Profile, respectively. Daily alcohol and food intake was assessed as part of a dietary survey with a validated food frequency questionnaire. Thiamin supplementation was associated with a significant increase in erythrocyte TPP concentrations compared with the placebo. Mean daily alcohol intake was significantly higher in subjects with persistently low TPP levels than in those with only one low TPP level. Only thiamin-treated subjects with persistently low TPP levels (n = 18) showed subjective benefits, with significant improvements in quality of life, and significant decreases in systolic blood pressure and weight compared with placebo subjects with persistently low TPP (n = 17). Thiamin supplementation had no effect on grip strength, functional ability, cognition, or general health (8).

♦ In a double-blind, placebo-controlled, crossover trial, 18 subject with Alzheimer's type dementia were randomly assigned to receive 3,000 mg thiamin or a placebo daily for 1 month each with no washout period. A second, single-blind experiment used 4,000 to 8,000 mg thiamin per day for 5 to 13 months in 17 patients (6 from the first trial). Doses were increased monthly throughout this second trial. Neuropsychological tests (Alzheimer's Disease Assessment Scale [ADAS]; MMSE), electrocardiogram, complete blood count, and liver function tests were done at the baseline and at the end of each treatment phase in the first trial and every 4 weeks in the second trial. A physician assessment (Clinical Global Impression of Change [CGIC]) was included only in the second experiment. In the first experiment, ADAS scores improved significantly in the thiamin group compared with the placebo group after 1 month. Placebo scores, but not thiamin treatment scores, on ADAS and MMSE were significantly worse after 1 month compared with the baseline. In the second trial, high-dose thiamin significantly improved ADAS scores compared with the baseline at months 1, 6, and 7. MMSE scores did not differ. CGIC scores tended to improve with thiamin but did not reach significance. The authors concluded: "In our opinion, high-dose thiamin offers only a mildly beneficial symptomatic therapy" (9).

♦ In a double-blind, placebo-controlled crossover study, 11 individuals with moderate cognitive impairment and "probable Alzheimer's disease" were given 3,000 mg thiamin or a placebo (niacinamide) daily for 3 months each. Subjects were well-nourished with no evidence of thiamin deficiency. Global cognitive scores on the MMSE improved significantly with thiamin therapy compared with the niacinamide placebo. There was no effect on behavioral ratings or the subjective judgment of clinical state between therapies (10).

♦ A pilot study investigating the etiology of peritoneal dialysis–associated encephalopathy was conducted among 30 subjects. Seven of 10 subjects with unknown etiology for their altered mental status were highly responsive to administration of thiamin, with a significant improvement in clinical status. Three subjects died, which the author suggested was related to a delay in thiamin supplementation or more severe disease. Pretreatment thiamin levels were not available for all 10 subjects. Among those with measured thiamin levels (n = 7), deficiencies were shown, and the remaining three patients showed significant clinical response to thiamin therapy, suggesting a deficiency was present prior to supplementation (11). Further research in this potentially vulnerable group is needed.

Thiamin and Mouth Ulcers

♦ Low erythrocyte thiamin levels have been associated with recurrent aphthous stomatitis (mouth ulcers), independent of age, sex, or underlying disease causing the stomatitis (12).

◆ A study of 60 individuals with recurrent mouth ulcers found that 28.2% were deficient in at least one of the following: thiamin, riboflavin, and pyridoxine. Replacement therapy of these vitamins was given to a group of deficient and nondeficient subjects for 1 month. At the end of the study and 3 months after, subjects with a deficiency had a significant sustained clinical improvement. However, it is not possible to attribute the benefits to thiamin supplements alone (13).

Thiamin and Cataracts

In the Blue Mountains Eye Study of Australia, which included 2,900 adults ranging in age from 49 to 97 years, increased dietary intake of thiamin was associated with a significant 40% reduction in risk for cataract development (14). Lens photographs were used to verify events. This is the first study to identify an association between thiamin and cataracts, and the association was made for dietary thiamin, not thiamin supplementation. In addition, thiamin intake may be a surrogate marker of an overall healthful diet. Further research is needed.

References

1. Tanphaichitr V. Thiamin. In: Shils ME, Olson JA, Shike M, et al, eds. *Modern Nutrition in Health and Disease.* 9th ed. Baltimore, Md: Williams & Wilkins; 1999:381–389.
2. Molina JA, Jimenez-Jimenez FJ, Hernanz A, et al. Cerebrospinal fluid levels of thiamine in patients with Alzheimer's disease. *J Neural Transm.* 2002;109:1035–1044.
3. Day E, Bentham P, Callaghan R, et al. Thiamine for Wernicke-Korsakoff Syndrome in people at risk from alcohol abuse. *Cochrane Database Syst Rev.* 2004;(1):CD004033.
4. Pennington JA. *Bowes & Church's Food Values of Portions Commonly Used.* 17th ed. Philadelphia, Pa: Lippincott; 1998.
5. Institute of Medicine. *Dietary Reference Intakes for Thiamin, Riboflavin, Niacin, Vitamin B-6, Folate, Vitamin B-12, Pantothenic Acid, Biotin, and Choline.* Washington, DC: National Academy Press; 1998.
6. Webster MJ, Scheett TP, Doyle MR, et al. The effect of a thiamin derivative on exercise performance. *Eur J Appl Physiol.* 1997;75:520–524.
7. Rodriquez-Martin JL, Qizilbash N, et al. Thiamine for Alzheimer's disease. *Cochrane Database Syst Rev.* 2001;(2):CD001498.
8. Wilkinson TJ, Hanger HC, Elmslie J, et al. The response to treatment of subclinical thiamine deficiency in the elderly. *Am J Clin Nutr.* 1997;66:925–928.
9. Meador K, Loring D, Nichols M, et al. Preliminary findings of high-dose thiamine in dementia of Alzheimer's type. *J Geriatr Psychiatry Neurol.* 1993;6:222–229.
10. Blass JP, Gleason P, Brush D, et al. Thiamine and Alzheimer's disease. A pilot study. *Arch Neurol.* 1988;45:833–835.
11. Hung SC, Hung SH, Tarng DC, et al. Thiamine deficiency and unexplained encephalopathy in hemodialysis and peritoneal dialysis patients. *Am J Kidney Dis.* 2001;38:941–947.

12. Haisraeli-Shalish M, Livneh A, Katz J, et al. Recurrent aphthous stomatitis and thiamine deficiency. *Oral Surg Oral Med Oral Pathol Oral Radiol Endod.* 1996;82:634–636.
13. Nolan A, McIntosh WB, Allam BF, et al. Recurrent aphthous ulceration: vitamin B-1, B-2 and B-6 status and response to replacement therapy. *J Oral Pathol Med.* 1991;20: 389–391.
14. Cumming RG, Mitchell P, Smith W. Diet and cataract: The Blue Mountains Eye Study. *Ophthalmology.* 2000;107:450–456.

Vitamin B-2 (Riboflavin)

As part of the coenzymes FAD (flavin adenine dinucleotide) and FMN (flavin adenine mononucleotide), riboflavin is involved in numerous oxidation/reduction reactions. Riboflavin, along with other water-soluble B vitamins, is used in the oxidation of glucose and fatty acids to produce ATP. FAD and FMN also act together to convert vitamin B-6 to its functional coenzyme, which then converts tryptophan into niacin. The thyroid gland is responsible for regulating an enzyme that phosphorylates riboflavin to its active form. Although rare in Western cultures, riboflavin deficiency is characterized by photophobia, vascularization of the cornea, magenta tongue, cheilitis, and seborrheic dermatitis of the nose and scrotum. Elderly individuals and people with alcoholism are at increased risk for subclinical riboflavin deficiency (1,2). Less than 5% of individuals in all genders and life stage groups have intakes less than the Estimated Average Requirement for riboflavin (3).

Media and Marketing Claims	Efficacy
Prevents migraine headaches	NR
Reduces risk for cataracts	NR

Safety

- No reported serious adverse effects.
- Because excess riboflavin is excreted by the kidneys, toxicity is rare (1,3).
- Due to lack of data, a Tolerable Upper Intake Level (UL) has not been determined for riboflavin (4).

Drug/Supplement Interactions

Chlorpromazine, doxorubicin, and possibly oral contraceptive medications reduce the conversion of riboflavin to its active form.

Key Points

- A preliminary controlled study in 55 subjects suggested that high-dose riboflavin reduces the frequency, incidence, and duration of migraine headaches in the short-term. Additional studies are needed to examine the potential beneficial role of riboflavin in migraine headaches.

- Riboflavin is necessary for energy production; however, there is no evidence that healthy individuals have increased "energy" or less fatigue from supplements.

- Diets sufficient in riboflavin may protect against the development of cataracts, but additional research is needed, including randomized controlled trials of supplemental riboflavin use in at-risk subjects.

Food Sources

Good sources of riboflavin include dairy products, meats, eggs, and green leafy vegetables. Although riboflavin is heat stable, it is easily destroyed by light and alkali (baking soda). Sixty percent of the vitamin is lost during milling of flour. However, breads and cereals are enriched to replace losses (1,2).

Food	Riboflavin, mg/serving
Milk, nonfat (1 cup)	0.34
Egg (1)	0.26
Spinach (½ cup)	0.21
Spaghetti (1 cup)	0.14
Salmon (3.5 oz)	0.11
Chicken (½ breast)	0.11
Broccoli (½ cup)	0.09

Source: Data are from reference 5.

Dosage Information/Bioavailability

The RDA for riboflavin is 1.3 mg/day for men and 1.1 mg/day for women (4). Riboflavin is available in multivitamin/mineral supplements, B-complex supplements, and individual preparations as pure riboflavin in doses ranging from 1.1 to 100 mg. One study reported that the maximal amount of riboflavin absorbed from a single dose (40 to 60 mg) in eight healthy subjects was 27 mg (6). However, even though intestinal absorption of riboflavin is a saturable process, there is evidence that prolonged retention of the vitamin in the small intestine can increase the total amount absorbed (7).

Relevant Research

Riboflavin and Migraine

♦ An open-label, nonrandomized, noncontrolled study using 400 mg riboflavin daily in 23 subjects with chronic migraines with or without aura (according to the International Headache Society criteria) suggested that riboflavin treatment was associated with a significant reduction in headache frequency (8). Subjects were recruited from a single clinic and had reported a history of two to eight migraines during the previous 6 months. The study was initiated with a 1-month baseline period followed by 3 months of treatment and an additional 3 months of treatment for "responders." Headaches were evaluated using a patient diary of number and duration of headaches, quality and pain distribution, related symptoms such as nausea/vomiting or photophobia, as well as a headache intensity scale (0, indicating no pain, to 5, unbearable pain). Patients also recorded the use of other medications to treat the migraines. Mean migraine attack frequency was reduced by 50% (from four to two attacks/month) during supplementation and remained 50% lower at 6 months. Secondary outcome measures of migraine burden, including duration or intensity, were not significantly changed with riboflavin supplementation. Use of medications to treat symptoms was significantly reduced with riboflavin supplementation, likely because the number of days with migraines was reduced. Although this study is limited by its nonrandomized, unblinded design, it provides preliminary evidence for further research to assess the role of riboflavin in migraine treatment.

♦ In a randomized, double-blind, placebo-controlled Kaiser Permanente study, 52 individuals with a history of migraine were randomly assigned to a supplement containing a combination of riboflavin (440 mg), magnesium (300 mg), and feverfew (100 mg standardized to 0.7% parthenolide) or placebo (25 mg riboflavin to match color changes in urine associated with riboflavin supplementation). Forty-nine subjects completed a 1-month run-in followed by a 3-month intervention (9). Compared with baseline, 42% of subjects in the supplement group and 44% of patients in the placebo group had a 50% reduction in number of migraines at 3 months. The difference between the two groups was not significant. Also compared with baseline, both groups reported fewer migraines, shorter duration, and lower migraine intensity. The author noted that "the placebo response exceeds that reported for any other placebo in trials of migraine prophylaxis and suggest riboflavin 25 mg may be an active comparator." Further research is needed using a true placebo as well as variable dosing of riboflavin and more objective measures of migraine activity.

♦ In a double-blind, placebo-controlled trial, 55 subjects with migraine were randomly assigned to receive 400 mg riboflavin or a placebo for 3 months. All participants received a placebo for 1 month prior to the study. Migraine attack frequency, number of headache days, and duration of migraines decreased significantly with riboflavin treatment compared with the placebo. In a comparison of the proportion of subjects with favorable responses, the riboflavin group (59% improved) had a statistically greater improvement compared with placebo (15% improved) (7).

Riboflavin and Cataracts

♦ The Blue Mountains Eye Study of Australia, a population-based cross-sectional study, which included 2,900 adults ranging in age from 49 to 97 years, showed that subjects in the highest quintile of dietary riboflavin intake (median 2.6 mg/day, as measured by a food-frequency questionnaire) were 50% less likely to develop cataracts than individuals in the lowest quintile of riboflavin intake (median 1.2 mg/day) (10). Lens photographs were used to verify events. This is the first study to identify an association between riboflavin and cataracts, and the association is for diet not supplementation. In addition, riboflavin intake may be a surrogate marker of overall improved diet. Further research is needed.

References

1. McCormick DB. Riboflavin. In: Shils ME, Olson JA, Shike M, et al, eds. *Modern Nutrition in Health and Disease.* 9th ed. Baltimore, Md: Williams & Wilkins; 1999:391–399.
2. Madigan SM, Tracey F, McNulty H, et al. Riboflavin and vitamin B-6 intakes and status and biochemical response to riboflavin supplementation in free-living elderly people. *Am J Clin Nutr.* 1998;68:389–395.
3. Bates CJ. Bioavailability of riboflavin. *Eur J Clin Nutr.* 1997;51(Suppl 1):S38–S42.
4. Institute of Medicine. *Dietary Reference Intakes for Thiamin, Riboflavin, Niacin, Vitamin B-6, Folate, Vitamin B-12, Pantothenic Acid, Biotin, and Choline.* Washington, DC: National Academy Press; 1999.
5. Pennington JA. *Bowes and Church's Food Values of Portions Commonly Used.* 17th ed. Philadelphia, Pa: Lippincott; 1998.
6. Zempleni J, Galloway JR, McCormick DB. Pharmacokinetics of orally and intravenously administered riboflavin in healthy humans. *Am J Clin Nutr.* 1996;63:54–66.
7. Schoenen J, Jacquy J, Lenaerts M. Effectiveness of high-dose riboflavin in migraine prophylaxis. A randomized controlled trial. *Neurology.* 1998;50:466–470.
8. Boehnke C, Reuter U, Flach U, et al. High-dose riboflavin treatment is efficacious in migraine prophylaxis: an open study in a tertiary care centre. *Eur J Neurol.* 2004;11:475–477.
9. Maizels M, Blumenfeld A, Burchette R. A combination of riboflavin, magnesium, and feverfew for migraine prophylaxis: a randomized trial. *Headache.* 2004;44:885–890.
10. Cumming RG, Mitchell P, Smith W. Diet and cataract: the Blue Mountain Eye Study. *Ophthalmology.* 2000;107:450–456.

Vitamin B-3 (Niacin)

Niacin is the collective term used to describe nicotinic acid and nicotinamide (or nicotinate and niacinamide, respectively). The metabolically active forms of niacin are the coenzymes nicotinamide adenine dinucleotide (NAD) and NAD phosphate (NADP). Hundreds of enzymes are dependent on NAD and NADP in the synthesis and/or degradation of carbohydrates, fatty acids, and amino acids. The classic deficiency of niacin is pellagra, characterized by dermatitis, diarrhea, and dementia, commonly referred to as the three Ds. Pharmacologic doses of nicotinic acid has been used as an effective therapy for reducing blood lipids since 1955 (1). Mechanisms of action in modulating blood lipids include inhibition of diacylglycerol acyltransferase 2, and inhibition of HDL apo AI catabolism (2).

Media and Marketing Claims	Efficacy
Reduces risk for heart disease by reducing cholesterol and other lipid levels (prescription nicotinic acid form)	↑
Reduces lipid levels in individuals with diabetes	↔
Reduces glucose levels in individuals with diabetes	↓
Reduces symptoms associated with arthritis	NR

Safety

- The Tolerable Upper Intake Level (UL) for adults is 35 mg niacin equivalents per day (3).

- Due to potential serious adverse effects, pharmacologic doses of niacin should only be used while under the care of a physician.

- High doses of nicotinic acid can cause skin flushing and pruritis, gastrointestinal discomfort, and abnormal liver function tests. Taking regular niacin with meals in divided doses or with aspirin may reduce flushing (4). Individuals taking high-dose nicotinic acid should be monitored by their physician because of these serious adverse effects (5). In contrast, nicotinamide has not been associated with vasodilative effects.

- Previously, sustained- or time-released niacin (nicotinic acid) supplements that reduced skin flushing were associated with liver toxicity (6). However, newer prescription time-released niacin preparations approved by the FDA for treating lipid disorders are reported to be safe and well-tolerated (7,8).

- High doses of nicotinamide have also inconsistently been associated with minor insulin resistance (9). An acute oral dose of nicotinamide (2 g) was associated with an increase in insulin resistance in patients at risk for developing type 1 diabetes (10). Nicotinic acid was associated with diminished glycemic control in individuals with type 2 diabetes (11).

- Niacin therapy should not be used by individuals with active peptic ulcers or gastroesophageal reflux, liver disease, or alcohol abuse (5).

- The oral median lethal dose (LD_{50}) for rats is 4.5 to 5.2 g/kg for nicotinic acid and 3.5 g/kg for nicotinamide (1).

Drug/Supplement Interactions

- Niacin may potentially contribute to hyperglycemic events in diabetes.

- Niacin may increase risk of myopathy if combined with lovastatin (HMG-CoA reductase inhibitor for hypercholesterolemia).
- Niacin may increase levels of carbamazepine (antiseizure drug).
- Bile acid sequestrants or isoniazid may reduce niacin levels.

Key Points

- Self-administration of nicotinic acid is not recommended. For most individuals, a balanced diet in accordance with the 2005 Dietary Guidelines should provide sufficient niacin to meet daily recommendations. Because of the side effects and risk of hepatoxicity, individuals should be under medical supervision while they are taking gram quantities of niacin.
- High-dose niacin (nicotinic acid) is an accepted medical therapy for treating hyperlipidemia. Nicotinic acid therapy has been found to significantly reduce the risk of cardiovascular disease endpoints and all-cause mortality. Niaspan is the medication used in several newer studies. This formulation has both immediate- and extended-release properties.
- Nicotinamide does not produce lipid-lowering effects.
- More research is needed to clarify possible benefits, dosage, and safety of using nicotinamide in the possible prevention of type 1 diabetes for individuals at risk. According to animal studies, nicotinamide has a protective effect on beta cells in the pancreas. Although a meta-analysis of 16 clinical trials also reported a protective effect on beta cells with nicotinamide, there was no improvement in glycemic control in subjects with diagnosed type 1 diabetes. Trials are investigating the effects of nicotinamide therapy in individuals at risk for developing type 1 diabetes. Of the completed clinical studies, one reported no benefit in preventing or delaying diabetes onset.
- The efficacy of nicotinic acid in people with established diabetes is unclear. Although nicotinic acid can be effective in treating dyslipidemia, it may also worsen glycemic control.
- One preliminary research study suggests a possible benefit of nicotinamide therapy for osteoarthritis. Large, controlled clinical trials are needed to verify these results.

Food Sources

Meats, fish, legumes, some cereals, and products containing enriched flours (breads, cereals, pastas) are good sources of niacin (1 to 40 mg/100 g). Coffee beans also have a high niacin content (40 mg/100 g). Niacin is unique in that the essential amino acid tryptophan, a niacin precursor, can contribute significantly to meeting dietary niacin requirements. Therefore, a diet containing 100 g protein (approximately 1% tryptophan) and no preformed niacin could meet the RDA (1,12).

Food	Niacin, mg/serving
Chicken breast (½)	11.8
Tuna, canned (3 oz)	11.3
Beef, ground, lean (3.5 oz)	4.3
Peanuts, roasted (1 oz)	3.8
Avocado (1 medium)	3.3
Bagel (3½ inch)	3.2
Potato, baked, no skin (medium)	2.2
Beans, navy (1 cup)	1.3
Mango (1)	1.2
Milk, nonfat (1 cup)	0.2

Source: Data are from reference 13.

Dosage Information/Bioavailability

The RDA for niacin is represented as milligrams of niacin equivalents (NE) because tryptophan can contribute to total niacin intake. The revised RDA is 16 mg NE for adult men and 14 mg NE for adult women, with the UL set at 35 mg NE for adults older than 18 years (3). Niacin is available in single preparation supplements or in multivitamin/mineral or B-complex supplements as nicotinic acid (nicotinate) or nicotinamide (niacinamide) supplements in doses ranging from 14 to 1,000 mg.

In many foods, niacin has low bioavailability because it is bound to macromolecules of carbohydrate or protein. Food processing or mild alkaline treatment during cooking releases much of the bound niacin (1,3).

Relevant Research

Niacin (Nicotinic Acid/Nicotinate) and Cardiovascular Disease

- Nicotinic acid at pharmacologic dosages (1 to 3 g/day divided into three or four doses) is well known as a drug used to decrease levels of triglycerides, decrease total and LDL cholesterol, and increase HDL cholesterol levels. Because these large dosages have been associated with flushing of the skin (vasodilation), hyperuricemia, abnormal liver function, and hyperglycemia, pharmacologic niacin should be administered under the supervision of a physician. New formulations have allowed for more effective dosing with reduced side effects. Nicotinamide does not affect blood lipids or cause these side effects (1).

- A position paper from the European Consensus Panel on HDL-C suggests that "nicotinic acid is not only the most potent agent for raising HDL-C but is also effective in reducing key atherogenic lipid components including triglyceride-rich lipoproteins, LDL-C and lipoprotein (a)" (14).

- A review of clinical trials that were published in MEDLINE between 1996 and 2004 using extended-release nicotinic acid (Niaspan) showed that in the four randomized, placebo-controlled studies (522 subjects total), LDL cholesterol decreased by a mean of 13%, triglycerides by 26%, and lipoprotein(a) by 17%, whereas HDL cholesterol increased by 18% (15). Controlled clinical trials that combined nicotinic acid and statin therapy showed an even greater lipid-reduction response, with LDL cholesterol decreasing by 36%, triglycerides by 34%, and lipoprotein(a) by 23%. Flushing was reported in 69% of patients despite the extended-release formulation.

◆ In a pilot study, low-dose niacin (50 mg twice daily) combined with statin therapy was shown to be effective in increasing HDL cholesterol (16). In this study, 50 patients were initially recruited after 3 months of statin therapy; 39 completed the trial. HDL cholesterol levels increased significantly after 3 months of therapy with 50 mg niacin twice per day as compared with placebo. The low retention rate, which was associated with changes in statin medications, incomplete follow-up data, and/or noncompliance with medication, is of concern in interpretation of these results.

◆ A review article summarized six major randomized, placebo-controlled trials of niacin with cardiovascular endpoints. The Coronary Drug Project (n = 8,341 men) reported significant decreases in recurrent myocardial infarction and cerebrovascular events with niacin monotherapy (3 g/day). The other five trials used varying combinations of niacin with other pharmacologic agents. These trials reported significant reductions in coronary and total mortality, coronary events, and angiographic progression of atherosclerosis in all trials except for one in patients with normal blood cholesterol levels at entry (17).

Niacin and Diabetes

◆ In a retrospective review of medical records of 32 patients with type 2 diabetes who had been prescribed variable dosages of Niaspan (1,000, 1,500, or 2000 mg/day) to treat hyperlipidemia over the previous 6 months indicated that A1C, an indicator of glucose control, was significantly reduced by a mean of 0.5 mg/dL (a magnitude that may be limited in clinical relevance) during 6 months of Niaspan therapy. However, one patient reported an increase in blood glucose levels with therapy, causing him to discontinue the study. Niaspan use was also associated with a significant increase (34%) in HDL cholesterol concurrent with a significant reduction in serum triglycerides (36%) (18). However, LDL and total cholesterol were not significantly modulated by treatment at any dose. This study is limited by the small sample size, retrospective design, and lack of a placebo control group. In addition, of the 32 patients, only 22 were included in the final analysis because 10 had incomplete laboratory data and another 3 did not complete 6 months of Niaspan therapy due to side effects.

◆ In a 16-week, randomized, double-blind, placebo-controlled study of 148 subjects with type 2 diabetes and hyperlipidemia, extended-release niacin at a dosage of 1,000 or 1,500 mg/day was associated with a significant increase in HDL cholesterol, with HDL levels increasing by an average of 19% in those assigned to 1,000 mg/day and by 24% in subjects assigned to 1,500 mg/day (19). As hypothesized by the investigators, serum triglycerides decreased with niacin supplementation by a mean of 13%

for the group taking 1,000 mg/day and 28% for the group taking 1,500 mg/day. The 1,500-mg dose, but not the 1,000-mg dose, resulted in a significant increase in A1C levels at the 16-week measurement, but not at the earlier 4-, 8-, and 12-week measurements. The increase in A1C above baseline, from 7.2% to 7.5%, is likely not of clinical relevance in terms of glucose control.

♦ In a placebo-controlled trial (Deutsche Nicotinamide Intervention Study), 55 children (ages 3 to 12 years) at risk of developing type 1 diabetes were randomly assigned to receive 1.2 g/m^2 body surface area sustained-release nicotinamide or a placebo for a maximum of 3.8 years. Subjects at risk for developing diabetes were identified by screening siblings (ages 3 to 12 years) of patients with type 1 diabetes for the presence of high titer islet cell antibodies. Rates of diabetes onset were similar in both groups. The trial was terminated after 3 years after the eleventh case of diabetes showed that no reduction of the cumulative diabetes incidence was detectable. The authors concluded: "In this subgroup of diabetes-prone individuals at very high risk and with an assumed rapid disease progression, nicotinamide treatment did not cause a major decrease or delay of diabetes development" (20).

♦ A 1996 meta-analysis of 16 trials (10 randomized, 5 of which were placebo-controlled) testing nicotinamide treatment in patients with recent-onset type 1 diabetes reported no differences in the insulin dose required or glycated hemoglobin values between subjects taking nicotinamide and control subjects (21).

♦ In a controlled crossover trial, 13 individuals with type 2 diabetes and dyslipidemia were assigned in random order to receive nicotinic acid (1.5 g three times/day) or no therapy for 8 weeks each. Compared with no therapy, nicotinic acid supplements significantly reduced blood lipids (total cholesterol, triglycerides, VLDL cholesterol, LDL cholesterol) and increased HDL cholesterol; however, therapy resulted in a deterioration of glycemic control (16% increase in mean plasma glucose, 21% increase in A1C levels, and glycosuria in some patients). The authors concluded: "Despite improvement in lipid and lipoprotein concentrations, because of worsening hyperglycemia and the development of hyperuricemia, nicotinic acid must be used with caution in patients with non-insulin-dependent diabetes. We suggest that the drug not be used as a first-line hypolipidemic drug in patients with non-insulin-dependent diabetes mellitus" (11).

Niacin and Arthritis

♦ In double-blind, placebo-controlled trial, 72 patients with osteoarthritis were randomly assigned to receive 3 mg nicotinamide (divided into six doses) or a placebo daily for 12 weeks. Global arthritis impact and pain, joint range of motion and flexibility, erythrocyte sedimentation rate, complete blood count, liver function tests, cholesterol, uric acid, and fasting blood sugar were measured. There was a significant 29% improvement in global arthritis impact with nicotinamide compared with a 10% reduction with the placebo. Pain levels did not differ between groups. There was a significant 13% reduction of anti-inflammatory medication use, reduced erythrocyte sedimentation, and increased joint mobility associated with nicotinamide treatment. Nicotinamide had no effect on fasting blood glucose, uric acid, cholesterol, or hematologic values. The authors concluded that nicotinamide may play a role in the treatment of osteoarthritis and that more extensive evaluation is warranted (22).

References

1. Cervantes-Laurean D, McElvaney NG, Moss J. Niacin. In: Shils ME, Olson JA, Shike M, eds. *Modern Nutrition in Health and Disease.* 9th ed. Baltimore, Md: Williams & Wilkins; 1999:401–411.
2. Malik S, Kashyap ML. Niacin, lipids, and heart disease. *Curr Cardiol Rep.* 2003;5: 470–476.
3. Institute of Medicine. *Dietary Reference Intakes for Thiamin, Riboflavin, Niacin, Vitamin B-6, Folate, Vitamin B-12, Pantothenic Acid, Biotin, and Choline.* Washington, DC: National Academy Press; 1998.
4. Jungnickel PW, Maloley PA, Vander Tuin EL, et al. Effect of two aspirin pretreatment regimens on niacin-induced cutaneous reactions. *J Gen Intern Med.* 1997;12:591–596.
5. Schuna AA. Safe use of niacin. *Am J Health Syst Pharm.* 1997;54:2803.
6. Henkin Y, Oberman A, Hurst DC, et al. Niacin revisited: clinical observations on an important but underutilized drug. *Am J Med.* 1991;91:239–246.
7. Capuzzi DM, Guyton JR, Morgan JM, et al. Efficacy and safety of an extended-release niacin (Niaspan): a long-term study. *Am J Cardiol.* 1998;82(12A):74U-81U.
8. McKenney J. New perspectives on the use of niacin in the treatment of lipid disorders. *Arch Intern Med.* 2004;164:697–705.
9. Knip M, Douek IF, Moore WP, et al. Safety of high-dose nicotinamide: a review. *Diabetologia.* 2000;43:1337–1345.
10. Greenbaum CJ, Kahn SE, Palmer JP. Nicotinamide's effect on glucose metabolism in subjects at risk for IDDM. *Diabetes.* 1996;45:1631–1634.
11. Garg A, Grundy SM. Nicotinic acid as therapy for dyslipidemia in non-insulin-dependent diabetes mellitus. *JAMA.* 1990;264:723–726.
12. van den Berg H. Bioavailability of niacin. *Eur J Clin Nutr.* 1997;51(Suppl 1):S64-S65.
13. Pennington JA. *Bowes and Church's Food Values of Portions Commonly Used.* 17th ed. Philadelphia, Pa: Lippincott-Raven Publishers; 1998.
14. Chapman MJ, Assmann G, Fruchart JC, et al. Raising high density lipoprotein cholesterol with reduction of cardiovascular risk: the role of nicotinic acid—a position paper developed by the European Consensus Panel on HDL-C. *Curr Med Res Opin.* 2004;20:1253–1268.
15. Birjmohun RS, Hutten BA, Kastelein JJ, et al. Increasing HDL cholesterol with extended-release nicotinic acid: from promise to practice. *Neth J Med.* 2004;62: 229–234.
16. Wink J, Giacoppe G, King J. Effect of very-low-dose niacin on high-density lipoprotein in patients undergoing long-term statin therapy. *Am Heart J.* 2002;143:514–518.
17. Guyton JR. Effect of niacin on atherosclerotic cardiovascular disease. *Am J Cardiol.* 1998;82(12A):18U–23U.
18. Kane MP, Hamilton RA, Addesse E, et al. Cholesterol and glycemic effects of Niaspan in patients with type 2 diabetes. *Pharmacotherapy.* 2001;21:1473–1478.

19. Grundy SM, Vega GL, McGovern ME, et al. Efficacy, safety, and tolerability of once-daily niacin for the treatment of dyslipidemia associated with type 2 diabetes: results of the assessment of diabetes control and evaluation of the efficacy of Niaspan trial. *Arch Intern Med.* 2002;162:1568–1576.

20. Lampeter EF, Klinghammer A, Scherbaum WA, et al. The Deutsche Nicotinamide Intervention Study: an attempt to prevent type 1 diabetes. DENIS Group. *Diabetes.* 1998;47:980–984.

21. Pozzilli P, Browne PD, Kolb H. Meta-analysis of nicotinamide treatment in patients with recent-onset IDDM. The Nicotinamide Trialists. *Diabetes Care.* 1996;19:1357–1363.

22. Jonas WB, Rapoza CP, Blair WF. The effect of niacinamide on osteoarthritis: a pilot study. *Inflamm Res.* 1996;45:330–334.

Vitamin B-6 (Pyridoxine)

Vitamin B-6 is the collective term used to describe pyridoxine (found in plant foods), and the phosphorylated forms pyridoxal and pyridoxamine (found in animal foods). The coenzyme forms of vitamin B-6 are pyridoxal 5'phosphate (PLP) and pyridoxamine 5'phosphate (PMP). PLP, the active form, is involved in more than 100 enzymatic reactions. After absorption, the liver releases vitamin B-6 as pyridoxal into the blood plasma with the majority bound to hemoglobin in red blood cells. The other major pool of vitamin B-6 is found in the muscle, where PLP is bound to glycogen phosphorylase. Vitamin B-6 plays a role in the synthesis, catabolism, and transport of amino acids; gluconeogenesis; niacin formation; neurotransmitter synthesis; erythrocyte metabolism; hormone modulation; and lipid metabolism (1,2).

Media and Marketing Claims	Efficacy
Relieves pain of carpal tunnel syndrome	↓?
Relieves symptoms of PMS	↔
Reduces risk for heart disease related to C-reactive protein and homocysteine levels	↑?
Improves asthma symptoms	↓?
Treats autism	NR
Improves cognition among the elderly	↓

Safety

♦ Long-term use of very high dosages (500 to 5,000 mg/day) is associated with neuropathy that is reversible with discontinuation.

♦ The Tolerable Upper Intake Level (UL) for vitamin B-6 is 100 mg/day for adults. For children the UL is 80 mg/day for ages 14 to 18 years, 60 mg/day for ages 9 to 13 years, and 40 mg/day for ages4 to 8 years (3).

♦ In 5- to 10-year studies, large populations of subjects with carpal tunnel syndrome using 100 to 150 mg vitamin B-6 per day have reported little or no toxicity. However, neurological symptoms (numbness, tingling, bone pain, muscle weakness) were reported in 103 of 172 (60%) of women who took a mean daily dosage of 117 mg vitamin B-6 for 3 years. After 6 months' cessation, symptoms resolved and serum vitamin B-6 levels returned to normal (4).

Drug/Supplement Interactions

♦ Combining vitamin B-6 with amiodarone may increase risk for photosensitivity.

♦ Pyridoxine increases levodopa clearance, which reduces the drug's efficacy in Parkinson's disease treatment.

♦ Pyridoxine may also increase clearance of phenobarbital and phenytoin.

♦ The following drugs interfere with vitamin B-6 status: isoniazid (antibiotic); hydralazine (for hypertension); phenelzine, cycloserine (antibiotic); penicillamine (for Wilson's disease); conjugated estrogens (oral contraceptives); theophylline (bronchodilator); corticosteroids (anti-inflammatory); erythromycin (antibiotic); gentamicin, neomycin, sulfonamides (antibiotics); alcohol; and caffeine. Alternatively, high-dose vitamin B-6 supplements (500 to 1,000 mg/day) could potentially interfere with these drugs (1). Consult with a physician regarding these drug-nutrient interactions.

Key Points

♦ Vitamin B-6 supplementation for carpal tunnel syndrome (CTS) remains controversial, but research generally does not support its use. Most of the studies to date have been small, uncontrolled, and lacking in randomization and double-blind design. Large, well-controlled studies are required before supplement use can be recommended. Some researchers suggest using vitamin B-6 simply because of the low toxicity when taken at doses less than the UL and the potential for an individual response.

♦ Evidence from studies using high-dose supplements of vitamin B-6 in subjects with PMS is equivocal. Although there is evidence of some beneficial effects, most positive trials have been criticized for poor quality.

♦ Epidemiological data suggest that low serum levels of vitamin B-6 are associated with increased CVD risk. Vitamin B-6 supplementation has been shown to reduce homocysteine levels, and patients with elevated C-reactive protein levels (a risk factor for CVD) are more likely to demonstrate lower serum levels of vitamin B-6. However, controlled clinical trials are required to fully evaluate the effect of vitamin B-6 supplements on CVD morbidity and mortality.

- Individuals with asthma who take theophylline, a vitamin B-6 antagonist, may have reduced vitamin B-6 status. High-dose supplementation does not seem to improve asthmatic symptoms.

- Studies suggesting the efficacy of vitamin B-6 for autistic disorders have been criticized for serious methodological flaws. A well-controlled, small study did not support the use of vitamin B-6 in treating autism. Larger, controlled trials are needed to substantiate this finding.

- One review assessed the relationship between vitamin B-6 supplementation and improved cognition and found that there were not enough well-designed studies with large enough sample sizes to test this hypothesis at this time.

- Individuals who may be at risk for low vitamin B-6 status (*see* Safety) should be encouraged to consume whole grains, legumes, and nuts rich in vitamin B-6 as part of a varied, healthful eating plan. Vitamin supplements may be used if needs are not met through diet, but care must be taken not to exceed the UL.

Food Sources

Good food sources of vitamin B-6 are whole grains, legumes, nuts, meat, and poultry. Most of the vitamin is removed from the grain during milling and processing.

Food	Vitamin B-6, mg/serving
Potato with skin, baked	0.540
Garbanzo beans (½ cup)	0.535
Turkey, roasted (3 oz)	0.480
Seeds, sunflower (⅓ cup)	0.459
Banana (1 medium)	0.369
Avocado (½ cup)	0.332
Soybeans (½ cup)	0.295
Rice, brown (½ cup)	0.231
Beef, ground (3 oz)	0.224
Carrots, raw, chopped (½ cup)	0.109
Peas, frozen (½ cup)	0.088
Milk, nonfat (8 oz)	0.012
Peaches, canned (½ cup)	0.011

Source: Data are from reference 5.

Dosage Information/Bioavailability

The RDA for adults is 1.3 mg for men and women ages 19 to 50 years, 1.5 mg for women older than 50 years, and 1.7 mg for men older than 50 years (3). The typical daily intake of vitamin B-6 is approximately 2 mg for men and 1.5 mg for women (3). The average bioavailability of vitamin B-6 is 75% from most foods (1). Vitamin B-6 is sold in capsules or tablets in the form of pyridoxine hydrochloride or PLP. Supplements range in doses from 10 to 500 mg per pill.

Relevant Research

Vitamin B-6 and Carpal Tunnel Syndrome

+ Two review papers have suggested that the evidence for recommending vitamin B-6 supplementation to reduce pain associated with carpal tunnel syndrome is insufficient and generally does not support a therapeutic role for B-6 supplements (6,7). Another reports suggest that risk is low, and thus vitamin B-6 supplementation (200 mg/day) should be used on a trial basis to reduce pain with CTS (8). It should be noted the UL for vitamin B-6 is 100 mg/day.

+ In a cross-sectional study, 125 randomly selected active workers underwent electro-diagnostic testing for CTS and were assessed for vitamin B-6 status. Vitamin B-6 status (red blood cell and plasma levels) was unrelated to self-reported symptoms of CTS, electrophysiologically determined nerve function, and CTS (defined by self-report and electrophysiological results). The authors concluded: "Empiric prescription of vitamin B-6 to patients with CTS is unwarranted and potentially hazardous" (9).

+ In a cross-sectional study, 441 self-selected subjects from six industries and a university setting participated in study comparing plasma vitamin B-6 concentrations with the prevalence and severity of nerve slowing, self-reported hand/wrist symptoms, and the prevalence of CTS. Dietary vitamin B-6 intake was not assessed. There were no significant differences in plasma PLP concentrations between subjects with no CTS symptoms (control subjects) and subjects with nerve slowing, CTS symptoms, or both. However, in men who do not use vitamin supplements, higher PLP levels were associated with reduced prevalence and frequency of CTS symptoms (10). The data analyses, and discussion of results in this study have been criticized for poor design by other researchers (11). However, the study is included here because it is cited to support marketing claims.

+ There has been considerable debate regarding the efficacy of vitamin B-6 for CTS (11,12). A review article (13) concluded that research has not provided convincing evidence for the use of vitamin B-6 as the sole treatment for patients with CTS. However, the authors noted that vitamin B-6 may be of value as adjunct therapy because of its potential benefit on pain perception and increasing pain threshold.

Vitamin B-6 and Premenstrual Syndrome (PMS)

+ A meta-analysis of 10 randomized, placebo-controlled, double-blinded studies that examined supplemental vitamin B-6 (50 mg to 600 mg/day) for PMS reported a relief in overall PMS and depressive PMS symptoms. However, of the 10 studies, only one was scored by the authors as high-quality, and this trial reported no effect of B-6 on PMS. The remaining nine studies were considered to be poor quality (14).

◆ A review article summarized 12 controlled trials on supplemental vitamin B-6 (ranging from 50 to 500 mg/day) in the treatment of PMS. The authors noted that the major drawbacks of the trials were the limited number of subjects and varying dosages. They concluded that the existing evidence of positive effects of vitamin B-6 is weak and that well-designed trials are needed (15).

◆ In a double-blind, placebo-controlled, crossover study, 63 women (age 18 to 49 years) were randomly assigned to receive 50 mg pyridoxine or a placebo for 3 months each (no washout period). Subjects kept a daily menstrual diary grading the severity of nine symptoms 1 month prior to baseline, followed by 6 months treatment. Only 32 subjects completed the entire study. Of these women, a significant benefit of pyridoxine was observed on emotional symptoms (depression, irritability, tiredness), but not on any other PMS symptoms measured (16).

◆ In a double-blind, placebo-controlled study, 55 women with self-reported moderate to severe PMS were randomly assigned to receive 150 mg pyridoxine or a placebo for 2 months. Subjects kept daily logs 1 month prior to the baseline, followed by 2 months of treatment. Vitamin B-6 improved autonomic symptoms (dizziness, vomiting) and behavioral symptoms; however, it did not improve symptoms of depression and anxiety during the premenstrual phase. The authors concluded: "Because depression and anxiety are more likely than other premenstrual symptoms, such as water retention, to interfere with daily activities, we conclude that B-6 is not the treatment of choice for the symptoms most women present" (17).

◆ In a retrospective study, the effect of pyridoxine was assessed by the response to treatment (defined as none, partial, or good) in 630 women attending a PMS clinic during the period of 1976 to 1983. The daily doses of pyridoxine varied from 40 to 100 mg during the early years to 120 to 200 mg in the later years examined. The response to treatment was "good" (no significant residual complaints) in 40% of patients treated with 100 to 150 mg vitamin B-6, and 60% in patients treated with 160 to 200 mg. No symptoms of peripheral neuropathy were noted (18).

◆ In a double-blind, placebo-controlled, crossover study, 44 women (mean age 32 years) were given, in random order, one of four treatments for one menstrual cycle: (*a*) 200 mg magnesium (oxide); (*b*) 50 mg vitamin B-6; (*c*) magnesium with B-6; or (*d*) a placebo. During the study, each subject recorded daily symptoms on a 5-point scale in a menstrual diary of 30 symptoms that were grouped into categories (anxiety, craving, depression, hydration, other). Urinary magnesium output was not affected by treatment, suggesting poor absorption of the magnesium. There were no overall differences in symptoms among the treatments; however, a modest significant reduction in premenstrual anxiety-related symptoms was associated with the magnesium plus vitamin B-6 combination (19).

Vitamin B-6 and Cardiovascular Disease

◆ In a randomized, double-blind, placebo-controlled study, investigators randomly assigned overweight but otherwise healthy subjects (ages 63 to 80 years) with 1.6 mg vitamin B-6 supplementation (n = 11) or placebo (n = 11) for 12 weeks (20). All subjects had previously demonstrated favorable decreases in homocysteine (tHcy) levels in response to 6 weeks of folic acid supplementation and 18 weeks of riboflavin supplementation. After supplementation, subjects demonstrated a significant increase in vitamin B-6 status as assessed by plasma pyridoxal-*P* and a concomitant significant reduction in homocysteine as compared with baseline and with the placebo group. These data suggest that vitamin B-6 should be considered in conjunction with other B vitamin supplementation for reduction in tHcy levels.

♦ Data from the Framingham Heart Study indicate that among 891 participants for which plasma B-6 levels were assessed in association with C-reactive protein (CRP), vitamin B-6 levels were significantly lower in those subjects demonstrating an elevated CRP (21). CRP is an established risk factor for cardiovascular disease. The researchers suggest that inflammatory processes indicative of elevated CRP may result in increased vitamin B-6 utilization and possibly an increased requirement.

♦ A meta-analysis of 12 randomized trials of the effect of vitamin supplements on homocysteine levels reported that folic acid and vitamin B-12 reduced homocysteine levels, but vitamin B-6 did not have any significant effect (22).

Vitamin B-6 and Asthma

♦ In a case-control study, 22 patients with asthma and vitamin B-6 deficiency using theophylline (vitamin B-6 antagonist) and 24 matched control subjects with normal vitamin B-6 status were given oral methionine load tests. Methionine loading resulted in significantly higher homocysteine and cystathionine concentrations in vitamin B-6–deficient patients than in control subjects. All subjects were then supplemented with 20 mg vitamin B-6 per day for 6 weeks. Supplementation significantly reduced homocysteine levels in deficient subjects but did not affect levels in control subjects. The authors concluded: "A vitamin B-6 deficiency may contribute to impaired transulfuration and an abnormal methionine load test, which is associated with premature vascular disease" (23).

♦ It has been suggested that vitamin B-6 corrects an abnormality in tryptophan metabolism occurring in people with steroid-dependent bronchial asthma (24).

♦ In a double-blind, placebo-controlled study, 31 subjects taking steroid medication for asthma were randomly assigned to receive 300 mg pyridoxine or a placebo daily for 9 weeks. There was no difference between groups on pulmonary function tests, asthma symptom scores, 24-hour urinary 5-hydroxy-indole acetic acid (serotonin metabolite), skin test reactivity, and blood serotonin levels. Patients treated with the bronchodilator theophylline had lower plasma pyridoxine levels at the baseline than did nonmedicated subjects. The authors concluded; "Prescription or usage of oral pyridoxine for the treatment of asthma cannot be justified in such patients" (24).

♦ In a double-blind, placebo-controlled, crossover study, 20 healthy subjects were put on theophylline and received in random order 15 mg pyridoxine hydrochloride or a placebo for 7 weeks each, with a 6-week washout period. Evaluation of central nervous system (CNS) stimulation and side effects were recorded at the baseline, after a 2-week run-in period, after a series of tests (hand steadiness, electrophysiological tests, the Sternberg Test of information processing), after the administration of a single 7-mg/kg dose of rapid-release theophylline, and after 4 weeks of 8 mg/kg of slow-release theophylline. Five subjects did not complete the study because of theophylline-associated headaches. During vitamin B-6 supplementation, subjects had significantly reduced theophylline-related hand tremors after a single dose of theophylline and a similar but insignificant trend was observed with repeated doses when compared with the placebo. Compared with the placebo, vitamin B-6 supplementation had no significant effect on CNS symptoms, electroencephalography, the Sternberg Test of information processing, or questionnaires of sleep quality and daytime sleepiness (25).

Vitamin B-6 and Autism

◆ In a double-blind, placebo-controlled, crossover study, 10 children with autism were randomly assigned to receive pyridoxine (30 mg/kg) and magnesium (10 mg/kg) supplements or a placebo for 4 weeks each. The mean dose ingested was 638.9 mg of pyridoxine and 216 mg magnesium oxide. Prior to the study, subjects took a 2-week supply of a placebo and baseline parameters were measured. Teachers, parents, and clinicians evaluated autistic behavior with the Children's Psychiatric Rating Scale (CPRS), the Clinical Global Impression Scale, and the NIMH Global Obsessive Compulsive Scale. Pyridoxine and magnesium supplements had no effect on autistic behavior compared with the placebo. During the placebo run-in phase of the study, 5 of 10 subjects had a 30% greater reduction in CPRS scores. The authors concluded that their study "raises the issue of whether a 'placebo' or 'study' effect may be present in patients with autism disorder" (26).

◆ A critical analysis of 12 studies using vitamin B-6 and magnesium combinations for individuals with autism was reported. Although most of the research reported favorable responses to vitamin treatment, the authors noted that these findings need to be interpreted with caution because of methodological shortcomings in many of the studies. Specific problems included imprecise outcome measures, small sample sizes, repeat use of the same subjects in more than one study, lack of adjustment for regression effects in measuring improvement, and failure to collect long-term follow-up data (27).

Vitamin B-6 and Cognition in the Elderly

◆ A review assessing the relationship between vitamin B-6 supplementation and cognition found that evidence was lacking in this area, with no studies conducted among people with cognitive impairment. Only two trials have been done in healthy elderly subjects: one in men and one in women, with neither study showing a significant effect over placebo (28).

◆ A cross-sectional analysis of vitamin B-6 status conducted among 499 functional community-based elderly showed that among those with the lowest plasma levels of vitamin B-6 there was a significant reduction in cognitive function (29). Studies using supplementation with vitamin B-6 should be developed in follow-up to this finding before recommendations can be made for use of B-6 in enhancing cognitive function in the elderly.

References

1. Leklem JE. Vitamin B-6. In: Shils ME, Olson JA, Shike M, et al, eds. *Modern Nutrition in Health and Disease.* 9th ed. Baltimore, Md: Williams & Wilkins; 1999;413–421.
2. Linder MC, ed. *Nutritional Biochemistry and Metabolism.* 2nd ed. New York, NY: Elsevier; 1991.
3. Institute of Medicine. *Dietary Reference Intakes for Thiamin, Riboflavin, Niacin, Vitamin B-6, Folate, Vitamin B-12, Pantothenic Acid, Biotin, and Choline.* Washington, DC: National Academy Press; 1998.
4. Dalton K, Dalton MJ. Characteristics of pyridoxine overdose neuropathy syndrome. *Acta Neurol Scand.* 1987;76:8–11.
5. USDA National Nutrient Database for Standard Reference. Available at: http://www.nal.usda.gov/fnic/foodcomp/search. Accessed March 29, 2006.
6. Gerritsen AA, de Krom MC, Struijs MA, et al. Conservative treatment options for carpal tunnel syndrome: a systematic review of randomised controlled trials. *J Neurol.* 2002;249:272–280.
7. Goodyear-Smith F, Arroll B. What can family physicians offer patients with carpal tunnel syndrome other than surgery? A systematic review of nonsurgical management. *Ann Fam Med.* 2004;2:267–273.
8. Aufiero E, Stitik TP, Foye PM, et al. Pyridoxine hydrochloride treatment of carpal tunnel syndrome: a review. *Nutr Rev.* 2004;62:96–104.
9. Franzblau A, Rock CL, Werner RA, et al. The relationship of vitamin B-6 status to median nerve function and carpal tunnel syndrome among active industrial workers. *J Occup Environ Med.* 1996;38:485–491.
10. Keniston RC, Nathan PA, Leklem JE, et al. Vitamin B-6, vitamin C, and carpal tunnel syndrome. A cross-sectional study of 441 adults. *J Occup Environ Med.* 1997;39:949–959.
11. Franzblau A, Rock CL, Werner RA, et al. Vitamin B-6, vitamin C, and carpal tunnel syndrome [letter]. *J Occup Environ Med.* 1998;40:305–309.
12. Keniston RC, Leklem JE, Nathan PA. Vitamin B-6 in carpal tunnel syndrome [letter]. *J Occup Environ Med.* 1996;38:959–960.
13. Jacobson MD, Plancher KD, Kleinman WB. Vitamin B-6 (pyridoxine) therapy for carpal tunnel syndrome. *Hand Clin.* 1996;12:253–257.
14. Wyatt KM, Dimmock PW, Jones PW. Poor-quality studies suggest that vitamin B-6 use is beneficial in premenstrual syndrome. *BMJ.* 1999;318:1375–1381.
15. Kleijnen J, Ter Riet G, Knipschild P. Vitamin B-6 in the treatment of the premenstrual syndrome—a review. *Br J Obstet Gynaecol.* 1990;97:847–852.
16. Doll H, Brown S, Thurston A, et al. Pyridoxine (vitamin B-6) and the premenstrual syndrome: a randomized crossover trial. *J R Coll Gen Pract.* 1989;39:364–368.

17. Kendall KE, Schnurr PP. The effects of vitamin B-6 supplementation on premenstrual symptoms. *Obstet Gynecol.* 1987;70:145–149.

18. Brush MG, Bennett T, Hansen K. Pyridoxine in the treatment of premenstrual syndrome: a retrospective survey in 630 patients. *Br J Clin Pract.* 1988;42:448–452.

19. De Souza MC, Walker AF, Robinson PA, et al. A synergistic effect of a daily supplement for one month of 200 mg magnesium plus 50 mg vitamin B-6 for the relief of anxiety-related premenstrual symptoms: a randomized, double-blind, crossover study. *J Womens Health Gend Based Med.* 2000;9:131–139.

20. McKinley MC, McNulty H, McPartlin J, et al. Low-dose vitamin B-6 effectively lowers fasting plasma homocysteine in healthy elderly persons who are folate and riboflavin replete. *Am J Clin Nutr.* 2001;73:759–764.

21. Friso S, Jacques PF, Wilson PW, et al. Low circulating vitamin B(6) is associated with elevation of the inflammation marker C-reactive protein independently of plasma homocysteine levels. *Circulation.* 2001;103:2788–2791.

22. Clarke R, Armitage J. Vitamin supplements and cardiovascular risk: review of the randomized trials of homocysteine-lowering vitamin supplements. *Semin Thromb Hemost.* 2000;26:341–348.

23. Ubbink JB, van der Merwe A, Delport R, et al. The effect of subnormal vitamin B-6 status on homocysteine metabolism. *J Clin Invest.* 1996;98:177–184.

24. Sur S, Camara M, Buchmeier A, et al. Double-blind trial of pyridoxine (vitamin B6) in the treatment of steroid-dependent asthma. *Ann Allergy.* 1993;70:147–152.

25. Bartel PR, Ubbink JB, Delport R, et al. Vitamin B-6 supplementation and theophylline-related effects in humans. *Am J Clin Nutr.* 1994;60:93–99.

26. Findling RL, Maxwell K, Scotese-Wojtila L, et al. High-dose pyridoxine and magnesium administration in children with autistic disorder: an absence of salutary effects in a double-blind, placebo-controlled study. *J Autism Dev Disord.* 1997;27:467–479.

27. Pfeiffer SI, Norton J, Nelson L, et al. Efficacy of vitamin B-6 and magnesium in the treatment of autism: a methodology review and summary of outcomes. *J Autism Dev Disord.* 1995;25:481–493.

28. Malouf R, Grimley Evans J. The effect of vitamin B6 on cognition. *Cochrane Database Syst Rev.* 2003;(4):CD004393.

29. Kado DM, Karlamangla AS, Huang MH, et al. Homocysteine versus the vitamins folate, B6, and B12 as predictors of cognitive function and decline in older high-functioning adults: MacArthur Studies of Successful Aging. *Am J Med.* 2005;118:161–167.

Vitamin B-12 (Cobalamin)

Vitamin B-12 is a water-soluble vitamin containing cobalt. The active forms of vitamin B-12, methylcobalamin and adenosylcobalamin, function as part of the enzymes methionine synthase and methylmalonyl-CoA mutase, respectively. As part of methionine synthase, methylcobalamin is used to regenerate the folate cofactor back to tetrahydrofolate, allowing folate to biosynthesize purines and pyrimidines necessary for DNA formation. Additionally, methylcobalamin recycles homocysteine to methionine, providing methyl groups necessary for the biosynthesis of many structures including myelin. The mutase allows catabolism of fatty acids with odd chain lengths and some amino acids (1,2).

A deficiency of vitamin B-12 impairs these enzymatic reactions. Pernicious anemia, characterized by neurological damage and megaloblastic anemia, is the classic vitamin B-12 deficiency that occurs when there is a lack of intrinsic factor secretion (IF). However, a more prevalent cause of mild deficiency is because of food-bound cobalamin malabsorption. This malabsorption, the inability to absorb food-bound but not free (supplemental) cobalamin, occurs in 10% to 30% of people older than age 50 years because of achlorhydria (3). Therefore, neuropsychiatric symptoms may be present without overt macrocytic anemia or reduced serum cobalamin levels diagnosed by elevated methylmalonic acid with or without elevated total homocysteine concentrations in combination with low or low-normal serum vitamin B-12. Those at risk for B-12 deficiency include the elderly; those with chronic alcoholism; patients on long-term therapy with gastric acid inhibitors; vegans; patients with partial gastrectomy, atrophic gastritis, autoimmune disorders (type 1 diabetes, AIDS/HIV, and thyroid disorders), or dementia; and patients undergoing nitrous oxide anesthesia (1,2,4).

Media and Marketing Claims	Efficacy
Corrects B-12 deficiency in the elderly	↑
Reduces symptoms of dementia unrelated to B-12 deficiency	↓
Improves sleep quality	NR
Helps treat AIDS-related dementia	NR
Improves immunity in HIV patients	NR
Reduces risk for heart disease	NR
Improves overall health of people with diabetes	NR
Reduces fatigue	NR

Safety

◆ No adverse effects have been associated with excess vitamin B-12 intake from food or supplements in healthy people (3).

◆ Due to the low toxicity of vitamin B-12, a Tolerable Upper Intake Level (UL) has not been determined.

◆ Individuals with vitamin B-12 deficiency and who are at risk for Leber's optic atrophy (genetic disorder caused by chronic cyanide intoxication) should not be treated with the cyanocobalamin form of vitamin B-12 because it can increase the risk of neurologic damage. Hydroxocobalamin is a cyanide antagonist and, thus, is not associated with adverse effects in this population (3).

Drug/Supplement Interactions

♦ Several drugs may interfere with vitamin B-12 absorption and reduce blood levels: zidovudine (Retrovir, AZT) (HIV therapy); antacids (only food-bound B-12, not supplemental); clofibrate (for hypercholesterolemia), colchicines (for gout); cycloserine, erythromycin (antibiotic); isoniazid (antibiotic for tuberculosis); metformin (for diabetes); aldomet (antihypertensive); neomycin (antibiotic prior to surgery); nitrous oxide (anesthetic gas); oral contraceptives; sulfanamides (antibiotic); tetracycline (antibiotic).

♦ Folic acid supplementation may mask vitamin B-12 deficiency.

♦ Supplemental vitamin C or iron may interfere with the bioavailability of vitamin B-12.

Key Points

♦ Individuals older than 50 years are at increased risk for preclinical vitamin B-12 deficiency because of possible malabsorption of food-bound cobalamin. Classic deficiency symptoms such as pernicious anemia are not usually present in this population. The DRI for vitamin B-12, released in 1998, advises that individuals older than 50 years old meet the RDA mainly by consuming foods fortified with vitamin B-12 or a B-12–containing supplement (3). One review article noted that for those with a documented deficiency, large amounts of oral vitamin B-12 (100 to 1,000 µg/day) are effective; thus, the quantity usually found in multivitamin supplements (< 6 µg) is not adequate. There is currently some controversy regarding the most effective method of screening for deficiency and the minimum effective dose of oral vitamin B-12 needed to correct deficiency in elderly subjects.

♦ Vitamin B-12 deficiency can progress to produce signs of dementia. Controlled studies verifying clinical improvement in dementia from vitamin B-12 supplementation are limited and have not demonstrated a benefit. The role of supplements in treating Alzheimer's-type dementia or neurological disturbances unrelated to deficiency has not been adequately tested in controlled trials. However, the Institute of Medicine recommends that adults older than 50 years consume the RDA for vitamin B-12 from fortified foods or vitamin supplements. Because individuals with Alzheimer's disease and dementia are typically elderly, they are included in this recommendation.

♦ The first randomized, placebo-controlled study of vitamin B-12 in subjects with delayed sleep phase syndrome reported no benefit. This conflicts with previous open trials and case studies of vitamin B-12 (not described here). Additional controlled research is needed to determine what role, if any, vitamin B-12 plays in sleep disorders.

♦ Controlled trials evaluating the effect of B-12 supplements on AIDS-related dementia have not been conducted. However, because decreased blood cobalamin levels occur in 20% of patients with AIDS and drugs used to treat the infection may reduce B-12 levels, this population should be evaluated for vitamin B-12 deficiency and treated if needed.

♦ Because vitamin B-12 reduces serum levels of homocysteine (a possible risk factor for cardiovascular disease), the vitamin may be indirectly involved in cardiovascular health. Longer term controlled trials are needed to determine whether vitamin B-12 supplements reduce cardiovascular risk and mortality, particularly in individuals with hyperhomocysteinemia.

♦ Increased homocysteine levels have been associated in some studies with diabetic complications in individuals with type 2 diabetes. Long-term, controlled trials of vitamin B-12 are needed to determine whether, in fact, reducing homocysteine concentrations reduces the risk or treats neuropathy, nephropathy, and other chronic conditions related to diabetes.

♦ Vitamin B-12 injections are sometimes given to patients complaining of fatigue. Controlled trials have not been conducted to evaluate the efficacy of this treatment in subjects with normal cobalamin status.

♦ In general, healthy individuals aged younger than 50 years who eat a diet including animal products or an adequate amount of foods fortified with vitamin B-12 do not require B-12 supplements. However, vegans and healthy people older than 50 years may need to take a vitamin B-12 supplement, especially if they do not consume enough B-12–fortified foods to meet the RDA.

Food Sources

Vitamin B-12 is present in significant quantities in animal foods only. Fermented soybeans and legumes contain an insignificant amount of vitamin B-12. Seaweed contains a form of vitamin B-12 that is not thought to be bioavailable. The function and effects of cobalamin analogues present in foods are not known.

Food	Vitamin B-12, µg/serving
Oysters (6)	14.34
Crab, Alaskan (3 oz)	9.78
Beef, ground (3.5 oz)	2.90
Salmon, Atlantic (3 oz)	2.38
Egg (1)	0.56
Chicken (½ breast)	0.29
Milk, nonfat (1 cup)	0.10

Source: Data are from reference 5.

Dosage Information/Bioavailability

The RDA for vitamin B-12 for men and women is 2.4 µg/day (3). The mean daily intake is estimated to be 5.0 µg in the United States (1). Vitamin B-12 is available as cyanocobalamin (not active) and methylcobalamin (active form) in tablets and capsules in doses ranging from 2 to 1,000 µg. It is included in multivitamin/mineral and B-complex formulations.

The absorption of vitamin B-12 is dependent on intestinal intrinsic factor. In healthy subjects, a maximal amount of 1.5 to 2.0 µg of dietary and supplemental vitamin B-12 is absorbed per meal with the intrinsic factor system. Approximately 1% of high doses of supplemental vitamin B-12 can be absorbed by passive diffusion, which does not require intrinsic factor (2). The methylcobalamin form is thought to be more efficiently absorbed and used than the cyanocobalamin form (6). In one study, vitamin B-12 was destroyed and therefore was not bioavailable if coingested with supplemental vitamin C or iron (7).

Documented vitamin B-12 deficiency due to lack of intrinsic factor is routinely treated with vitamin B-12 injections. In one study of individuals with vitamin B-12 deficiency, however, daily oral administration of 2 mg of cyanocobalamin was as effective as 1 mg administered intramuscularly on a monthly basis (8). One reviewer considered the route of oral, high-dose vitamin B-12 supplements for deficiency states "an underused alternative to parenteral treatment" (9).

Relevant Research

Vitamin B-12 Deficiency in the Elderly

- Approximately 10% to 30% of the population older than 50 years have vitamin B-12 deficiency (3), diagnosed by elevated methylmalonic acid with or without elevated total homocysteine concentrations in combination with low or low-normal serum vitamin B-12 levels. Deficiency is most often due to malabsorption of dietary cobalamin caused by atrophic gastritis (most often due to *Helicobacter pylori*) and hypochlorhydria. Clinical signs and symptoms of deficiency in elderly patients can be masked by the presence of other conditions, making diagnosis and responses to therapy difficult to evaluate. Some experts expressed concern that the federally mandated food folate-fortification program could present a problem in the elderly because folate reduces hyperhomocysteinemia (a diagnostic marker of vitamin B-12 deficiency) and thus could mask macrocytic anemia (10,11).

Vitamin B-12 and Dementia in the Elderly

- In some reports, low serum cobalamin levels have been associated with Alzheimer's disease and dementia, but the data are not consistent (12–14). However, normal serum cobalamin concentrations do not rule out the possibility of deficiency (1,15).

- A Cochrane Database System Review that was focused on the role of vitamin B-12 in reducing loss of cognitive function associated with aging included only two studies of adequate scientific rigor. The systematic review concluded that, "there was no statistically significant evidence of treatment effect, vitamin B-12 supplementation compared with placebo, on cognitive function" (16).

- In an open, prospective study, serum vitamin B-12 levels were measured in 181 patients (mean age 77.5 years) with diagnosed dementia. The frequency of vitamin

B-12 deficiency (defined as < 200 pg/mL) was 25% (46 of 181; 36 subjects without anemia or macrocytosis). Treatment outcome of vitamin B-12 injections (1 mg repeated five times at 5-day intervals and a maintenance dose of 1 mg every 3 months) was obtained in 19 of 46 patients throughout 3 to 24 months. Sixteen of these 19 patients had persistent declines in mental functioning at follow-up visits despite cobalamin injections. Of the three patients who showed some improvement, all had mild dementia for less than 2 years. The authors concluded that true vitamin B-12 dementia is rare, but that screening for low serum vitamin B-12 levels should be considered in patients with recent onset of mild mental status changes (17).

Vitamin B-12 and Sleep Disorders

♦ In a double-blind, placebo-controlled study, 50 patients (ages 13 to 55 years) with delayed sleep phase syndrome were randomly assigned to receive 3,000 μg methylcobalamin or a placebo divided into three oral doses daily for 4 weeks. There were no significant differences between groups over time in subjective evaluations of mood or drowsiness during the daytime or night sleep by sleep-log evaluation (18).

Vitamin B-12 and HIV/AIDS

♦ Several studies have reported the presence of vitamin B-12 malabsorption and deficiency in individuals with HIV (19,20). Low serum cobalamin levels were associated with faster progression of HIV type 1 disease during a 9-year period as determined by CD4 cell count (21,22).

♦ In an in vitro study, methylcobalamin inhibited HIV-1 infection of healthy human blood monocytes and lymphocytes (23).

♦ Controlled trials evaluating the effect of B-12 supplements on AIDS-related dementia have not been conducted.

Vitamin B-12 and Cardiovascular Disease

♦ Several studies have reported that the B vitamins, particularly supplemental vitamin B-12 (≈ 0.5 mg/day) and folic acid (0.5 to 5 mg/day), are associated with reductions in homocysteine levels (a risk factor for heart disease) by up to 30% (24).

♦ In a double-blind study of 50 subjects with known coronary artery occlusion, patients were randomly assigned to receive either placebo, variable doses of vitamin B-6, or 5 mg folic acid combined with 0.25 mg vitamin B-12 for 12 weeks (25). No group received only vitamin B-12. Homocysteine levels decreased significantly in the group receiving folic acid plus vitamin B-12, but not in the groups taking vitamin B-6 or placebo. The modulating effect of folic acid alone could likely have accounted for the reduction of tHcy. In addition, the per group sample sizes were extremely small and thus limit any interpretation of the findings.

♦ In a double-blind, placebo-controlled trial, 89 men with coronary heart disease were randomly assigned to receive 5 mg folic acid plus 1 mg vitamin B-12 or a placebo daily for 8 weeks. Brachial artery flow-mediated dilatation (endothelium dependent) and nitroglycerin-induced dilatation (endothelium independent) were measured before and after treatment. After treatment, flow-mediated dilatation improved significantly with vitamin supplementation, but not with the placebo. The vitamins had no effect on nitroglycerin-induced dilatation. Additionally, the B vitamins were significantly associated with reductions in plasma total homocysteine, protein-bound homocysteine, and free homocysteine, and elevations in serum folate and vitamin B-12. In regression analysis, the improved flow-mediated dilatation was significantly correlated with reduction in free plasma homocysteine. From this, the authors concluded that folic acid and vitamin B-12 supplementation seems to improve vascular endothelial function, and this effect is likely mediated through reduced homocysteine levels (26).

Vitamin B-12 and Diabetes

- Increased homocysteine levels have been associated in some studies with complications such as neuropathy and nephropathy in individuals with type 2 diabetes (27–29). Because vitamin B-12 seems to reduce homocysteine levels, some propose that supplemental vitamin B-12 may reduce the risk among patients with diabetes of developing these conditions.

- In a double-blind, placebo-controlled Saudi Arabian study, 50 subjects with diabetic neuropathy (11 subjects with type 1 diabetes and 39 subjects with type 2 diabetes) were randomly assigned to receive 1,500 mg methylcobalamin divided into three doses or a placebo daily for 4 months. The researchers did not evaluate vitamin B-12 status. Clinical and neurophysiologic (nerve conduction studies) were completed before and at the end of the study. There was a significant improvement in the somatic and autonomic symptoms, with regression of signs of neuropathy after vitamin B-12 treatment. However, motor and sensory nerve conduction studies showed no improvement (30).

References

1. Weir DG, Scott JM. Vitamin B-12 Cobalamin. In: Shils ME, Olson JA, Shike M, Ross AC, eds. *Modern Nutrition in Health and Disease.* 9th ed. Baltimore, Md: Williams & Wilkins; 1999:447–459.
2. Scott JM. Bioavailability of vitamin B-12. *Eur J Clin Nutr.* 1997;51(Suppl 1):S49–S53.
3. Institute of Medicine. *Dietary Reference Intakes for Thiamin, Riboflavin, Niacin, Vitamin B-6, Folate, Vitamin B-12, Pantothenic Acid, Biotin, and Choline.* Washington, DC: National Academy Press; 1998.
4. Nilsson-Ehle H. Age-related changes in cobalamin (vitamin B-12) handling. Implications for therapy. *Drugs Aging.* 1998;12:277–292.
5. Pennington JA. *Bowes and Church's Food Values of Portions Commonly Used.* 17th ed. Philadelphia, Pa: Lippincott-Raven Publishers; 1998.
6. Methylcobalamin. *Altern Med Rev* [erratum in *Altern Med Rev.* 1999;4:9]. 1998;3: 461–463.

7. Herbert V. The elderly need oral vitamin B-12. *Am J Clin Nutr.* 1998;67:739–752.
8. Kuzminski AM, Del Giacco EJ, Allen RH, et al. Effective treatment of cobalamin deficiency with oral cobalamin. *Blood.* 1998;92:1191–1198.
9. Delva MD. Vitamin B-12 replacement. To B-12 or not to B-12. *Can Fam Physician.* 1997;43:917–922.
10. Stabler SP, Lindenbaum J, Allen RH. Vitamin B-12 deficiency in the elderly: current dilemmas. *Am J Clin Nutr.* 1997;66:741–749.
11. Carmel R. Cobalamin, the stomach, and aging. *Am J Clin Nutr.* 1997;66:750–759.
12. Cole MG, Prchal JF. Low serum vitamin B-12 in Alzheimer-type dementia. *Age Ageing.* 1984;13:101–105.
13. Basun H, Fratiglioni L, Winblad B. Cobalamin levels are not reduced in Alzheimer's disease: results from a population based study. *J Am Geriatr Soc.* 1994;42:132–136.
14. Bell IR, Edman JS, Marby DW, et al. Vitamin B-12 and folate status in acute geropsychiatric inpatients: affective and cognitive characteristics of a vitamin nondeficient population. *Biol Psychiatry.* 1990;27:125–137.
15. Hutto BR. Folate and cobalamin in psychiatric illness. *Compr Psychiatry.* 1997;38:305–314.
16. Malouf R, Areosa Sastre A. Vitamin B12 for cognition. *Cochrane Database Syst Rev.* 2002;(3):CD004326.
17. Cunha UG, Rocha FL, Peixoto JM, et al. Vitamin B-12 deficiency and dementia. *Int Psychogeriatr.* 1995;7:85–88.
18. Okawa M, Takahashi K, Egashira K, et al. Vitamin B-12 treatment for delayed sleep phase syndrome: a multi-center double-blind study. *Psychiatry Clin Neurosci.* 1997;51:275–279.
19. Paltiel O, Falutz J, Veilleux M, et al. Clinical correlates of subnormal vitamin B-12 levels in patients infected with the human immunodeficiency virus. *Am J Hematol.* 1995;49:318–322.
20. Herzlich BC, Schiano TD, Moussa Z, et al. Decreased intrinsic factor secretion in AIDS: relation to parietal cell acid secretory capacity and vitamin B-12 malabsorption. *Am J Gastroenterol.* 1992;87:1781–1788.
21. Tang AM, Graham NM, Chandra RK, et al. Low serum vitamin B-12 concentrations are associated with faster human immunodeficiency virus type 1 (HIV-1) disease progression. *J Nutr.* 1997;127:345–351.
22. Baum MK, Shor-Posner G, Lu Y, et al. Micronutrients and HIV-1 disease progression. *AIDS.* 1995;9:1051–1056.
23. Weinberg JB, Sauls DL, Misukonis MA, et al. Inhibition of productive human immunodeficiency virus-1 infection by cobalamins. *Blood.* 1995;86:1281–1287.
24. Clarke R, Armitage J. Vitamin supplements and cardiovascular risk: review of the randomized trials of homocysteine-lowering vitamin supplements. *Semin Thromb Hemost.* 2000;26:341–348.
25. Lee BJ, Huang MC, Chung LJ, et al. Folic acid and vitamin B12 are more effective then vitamin B6 in lowering fasting plasma homocysteine concentration in patients with coronary artery disease. *Eur J Clin Nutr.* 2004;58:481–487.

26. Chambers JC, Ueland PM, Obeid OA, et al. Improved vascular endothelial function after oral B vitamins: an effect mediated through reduced concentrations of free plasma homocysteine. *Circulation.* 2000;102:2479–2483.
27. Ambrosch A, Dierkes J, Lobmann R, et al. Relation between homocysteinaemia and diabetic neuropathy in patients with type 2 diabetes mellitus. *Diabet Med.* 2001;18: 185–192.
28. Buysschaert M, Dramais AS, Wallemacq PE, et al. Hyperhomocyteinemia in type 2 diabetes: relationship to macroangiopathy, nephropathy, and insulin resistance. *Diabetes Care.* 2000;23:1816–1822.
29. Stabler SP, Estacio R, Jeffers BW, et al. Total homocysteine is associated with nephropathy in non-insulin-dependent diabetes mellitus. *Metabolism.* 1999;48:1096–1101.
30. Yaqub BA, Siddique A, Sulimani R. Effects of methylcobalamin on diabetic neuropathy. *Clin Neurol Neurosurg.* 1992;94:105–111.

Vitamin C

Vitamin C is the term used to describe two biologically active forms of the nutrient: ascorbic acid (reduced form) and dehydroascorbic acid (oxidized form). Vitamin C acts as an electron donor for eight enzymes. Specifically, vitamin C is involved in reactions needed to synthesize collagen, neurotransmitters (dopamine, tyramine), carnitine, tyrosine, and catecholamines. Vitamin C's electron-donating function also makes it an effective antioxidant. The vitamin scavenges reactive oxygen species, singlet oxygen, hypochlorite, and hydroxyl, peroxyl, superoxide, peroxynitrite, nitroxide radicals. High tissue levels of ascorbate provide significant antioxidant protection in the eye, neutrophils, semen, and lipoproteins. The vitamin may also provide indirect antioxidant protection by regenerating other antioxidants, including glutathione and vitamin E. Of particular interest is how supplemental doses of vitamin C may play a beneficial role in conditions and diseases resulting from oxidative damage (1,2).

Media and Marketing Claims	Efficacy
Treats the common cold	↔
Reduces symptoms of asthma	↔
Enhances immunity	↑?
Enhances exercise performance by reducing oxidative stress	↓
Reduces risk of heart disease	↔
Reduces blood pressure in people with hypertension	↑?
Protects against cancer	↔
Reduces risk of cataracts	↑?

Safety

- The Tolerable Upper Intake Level (UL) for adults is 2,000 mg/day from food and supplements (2).
- According to a review of clinical studies of the safety of vitamin C supplementation, high levels of intake from supplements was not associated with adverse responses except for occasional gastrointestinal upset or mild diarrhea (3).
- In the same review (3), the authors also state that high-level vitamin C supplementation does not seem to lead to iron toxicity in humans. However, because vitamin C facilitates nonheme iron absorption, large supplemental doses of vitamin C should be avoided by individuals with hemachromatosis, while iron supplementation should be avoided all together (1,2).
- Vitamin C is generally considered safe even in large doses because the kidneys efficiently excrete any excess. Several double-blind, controlled trials supplementing up to 10 g vitamin C daily for more than 1 year or up to 5 g/day for more than 3 years reported no serious adverse effects (4).
- Diarrhea and nausea can occur with very large doses (3–10 g/day) because of the osmotic effects of the unabsorbed vitamin. These side effects may be minimized by a gradual increase in vitamin C dose over time (1,2).
- Excess amounts of vitamin C in urine and feces from supplementation can interfere with certain diagnostic tests by causing glycosuria and fecal occult blood. Additionally, excess vitamin C can interfere with blood tests based on redox chemistry, including cholesterol and glucose (1).
- It is generally accepted that high vitamin C intakes do not cause kidney stone formation. In the Health Professional's Follow-Up Study, a cohort of 45,251 men age 40 to 75 years with no history of kidney stones, no association was found between high daily intake of vitamin C (> 1,500 mg) and the risk of stone formation (5). However, individuals with recurrent kidney stones or renal disease are advised not to supplement with dosages exceeding 100 mg/day (6).
- There has been concern about the possible prooxidant effects of high doses of vitamin C. In a placebo-controlled study, 500 mg vitamin C supplementation increased 8-oxoadenine (marker of DNA damage) and decreased 8-oxoguanine levels in DNA isolated from lymphocytes. The authors concluded: "Our discovery of an increase in a potentially mutagenic lesion, 8-oxo-adenine, following a typical vitamin C supplementation should therefore be of some concern although at doses of < 500 mg/day the antioxidant effect may predominate" (7). The results and conclusions drawn from this study are controversial because a reduction in 8-oxoguanine levels has been associated with lower mutation rates (8).

Drug/Supplement Interactions

- Vitamin C increases iron absorption (ferric acid).
- Vitamin C may prolong clearance time for acetaminophen.

- ◆ Vitamin C may increase activity of anticoagulants.

- ◆ Vitamin C may interfere with activity of vitamin B-12, although doses up to 4 g of vitamin C per day do not induce B-12 deficiency.

- ◆ Excessive vitamin C intake may interfere with copper and chromium absorption and metabolism.

- ◆ When taken with aluminum-containing antacids, vitamin C may increase aluminum absorption.

- ◆ Aspirin, corticosteroids, and indomethacin (NSAID) increase urinary vitamin C losses.

- ◆ High doses of vitamin C may reduce efficacy of select chemotherapeutic medications, including cyclophospahmide, chlorambucil, busulfan and doxorubicin. Supplementation above the DRI (or > 70 to 90 mg/day) is not recommended.

- ◆ Vitamin C may increase plasma estrogen levels in individuals taking exogenous hormones or oral contraceptives.

- ◆ Large doses of vitamin C may interfere with anticoagulant medications (1). However, in healthy males, 2,000 mg vitamin C had no effect on hemostatic parameters (5).

Key Points

- ◆ According to research to date, certain subpopulations tend to have low plasma vitamin C levels, particularly men, elderly, smokers, individuals with diabetes, and oral contraceptive users. These individuals should be encouraged to increase their consumption of vitamin C–rich foods and beverages. For those who do not consume adequate vitamin C through the diet, a vitamin C supplement (up to 250 mg/day) may be appropriate to increase plasma levels (9).

- ◆ After 30 years of research on vitamin C as a rhinovirus treatment, results are equivocal. However, it is possible that some further protection may be offered by supplements to individuals with low plasma vitamin C stores or in subjects undergoing oxidative stress from physical exercise (ultramarathon runners). In addition, efficacy may be influenced by dose, duration, and timing of supplementation as well as specific outcome measured (frequency of colds, length, severity, etc).

- ◆ Similarly, the results from clinical studies of the effects of vitamin C on asthma are equivocal. Additional research is needed in this area. Individuals with asthma should be encouraged to increase dietary sources of vitamin C.

- ◆ There is evidence that vitamin C has a positive effect on some markers of immune function.

- ◆ There is no evidence that people undergoing physical or mental stress have increased vitamin C needs. With regard to reducing exercise-induced oxidative damage, more research is needed to determine whether single preparations of vitamin C supplements affect markers of oxidative status and whether this improves performance and long-term health in athletes. Limited evidence suggests a potential role for vitamin C supplementation in reducing upper respiratory tract infections in ultraendurance athletes.

♦ Epidemiological data are conflicting regarding the relationship between vitamin C intake or supplementation and cardiovascular disease. Sufficient data from controlled clinical trials are lacking; thus, more research is needed in this area.

♦ Studies generally support vitamin C supplements and diets high in vtamin C to help control blood pressure.

♦ Epidemiological evidence linking fruit and vegetable intake to lower rates of cancer suggests that vitamin C may have a possible protective effect against certain cancer, but other studies have found no effect. Well-controlled clinical research is needed to further examine the potential role of vitamin C supplementation in cancer prevention.

♦ Epidemiological data suggest that vitamin C may reduce cataract risk. Most of this data assessed dietary, not supplemental, intake. A few trials using supplemental vitamin C also suggest a benefit; however, additional well-designed studies are needed.

Food Sources

The mean daily dietary vitamin C intake in the United States is 90 mg/day for women and 105 mg/day for men (2). Eating at least five servings of fruits and vegetables per day may provide more than 200 mg vitamin C (1). Vitamin C content is reduced by cooking, exposing foods to air and light, and prolonging storage and transport of fresh fruits and vegetables.

Food	Vitamin C, mg/serving
Papaya (1 medium)	188
Strawberries (1 cup)	84
Orange, navel (1)	75
Broccoli (½ cup)	58
Mango (1)	57
Brussels sprouts (½ cup)	48
Sweet pepper, raw (½ cup)	45
Grapefruit (½ medium)	42
Raspberries (1 cup)	31
Pineapple (1 cup)	24
Tomato (1 medium)	23
Russet potato (medium), baked, with skin	22

Source: Data are from reference 10.

Dosage Information/Bioavailability

Vitamin C is available in tablets, capsules, chewable tablets, and powders ranging from 60 to 1,000 mg/serving. Vitamin C is sold in a variety of forms, including pure ascorbic acid, vitamin C from rose hips, chelated to sodium or other minerals, or bound to bioflavonoids. One study found that vitamin C in supplements from pure ascorbic acid was more bioavailable than other, more expensive commercial vitamin C preparations (8). Bioavailability of vitamin C from foods and from supplements is not significantly different (2). Plasma vitamin C concentrations in people who regularly consume vitamin C supplements are approximately 60% to 70% higher than in those who do not take supplements (6). An excellent review was done by Carr and Frei (9).

The Institute of Medicine released DRIs for vitamin C in the year 2000. The new adult RDA for vitamin C is 75 mg/day for women and 90 mg/day for men (2). The report also stated that smokers require an additional 35 mg/day to obtain a steady-state ascorbate body pool similar to nonsmokers. These values were based on the amount of vitamin C intake needed to maintain near-maximal neutrophil concentrations with minimal urinary excretion of ascorbate.

The effectiveness of mega-dosing on tissue saturation has been the subject of debate (11,12). Some researchers report that tissue and plasma saturation levels of vitamin C are reached with an approximate intake of 200 to 300 mg/day (9,13,14). However, it has also been suggested that a daily intake near 1,000 mg is necessary to maintain plasma vitamin C levels at high concentrations (75 to 80 µmol) (6). Maximal absorption is achieved by ingesting several spaced doses of less than 1,000 mg, rather than one large dose (1).

Relevant Research

Vitamin C and the Common Cold

- Many review articles and meta-analyses have been written since Linus Pauling first published his research in the 1970s suggesting that 1,000 mg vitamin C reduced rhinovirus symptoms in school children in a skiing camp in the Swiss Alps (15).

- A Cochrane Database Systematic Review (16) conducted in 2004 suggests that response to vitamin C therapy depends on several factors. Findings from meta-analyses are summarized in the following table:

No. of Trials	No. of Subjects	Descriptors	RR (95% CI) or *t* test
29	11,077	Developing a cold while on prophylaxis	0.96 (0.92–1.00) (4% reduced risk)
6	642 athletes	Developing a cold while on prophylaxis	0.50 (0.38–0.66) (50% reduced risk)
30	9,676	Cold duration while on prophylaxis vitamin C (study A)	Adults: 0.92 (0.67–0.87) (8% reduced risk) Children: 0.86 (0.79–0.95) (14% reduced risk)

No. of Trials	No. of Subjects	Descriptors	RR (95% CI) or *t* test
7	3,294	Cold duration while on prophylaxis vitamin C (study B)	No difference between vitamin C and placebo
15	7,045	Severity while on prophylaxis	Days off-work for illness vs at-work (healthy); significant protection ($P = .02$)

- In a prospective study, 400 adults were instructed to initiate supplementation with placebo or variable amounts of vitamin C after 4 hours of the onset of cold symptoms, the 149 subjects who returned records reported on 184 cold events. No significant difference in duration or severity of cold was seen with 1,000, 2,000, or 3,000 mg vitamin C supplementation or as compared with placebo (17).

- In a double-blind, placebo-controlled study, 92 ultramarathon runners and 92 control subjects (nonrunners) took either 600 mg supplemental vitamin C or a placebo for 21 days before an ultramarathon race. (Control subjects did not run the race.) Symptoms of upper respiratory tract (URT) infection were monitored for 14 days after the race. Sixty-eight percent of the runners in the placebo group reported development of symptoms of URT infection, which was significantly more than vitamin C–supplemented runners. The duration and severity of URT symptoms reported in control subjects taking vitamin C supplements was significantly less than control subjects taking placebos (18).

Vitamin C for Asthma and Pulmonary Function

- A study of 2,526 adults randomly selected from the first National Health and Nutrition Examination Survey (NHANES I) between 1971 and 1974 found that dietary vitamin C was positively and significantly associated with forced expiratory volume in 1 second (FEV_1) of the lung. The authors hypothesized that vitamin C intake may have a protective effect on pulmonary function (19).

- In a review of 21 studies on the role of vitamin C on asthma and allergy, evidence was conflicting. The authors noted that the majority of studies were short-term and only assessed immediate effects of vitamin C supplementation. They concluded that long-term supplementation with vitamin C and delayed effects both need to be studied (20).

Vitamin C and Immune Function

- In a double-blind, placebo-controlled trial, 57 elderly patients admitted to the hospital with acute respiratory infections (bronchitis and bronchopneumonia) were randomly assigned to receive 200 mg vitamin C/day or a placebo. Patients were assessed biochemically on admission and at weeks 2 and 4 in the study. Severity of illness was scored on a scale of 1 to 10 on three main diagnostic features of respiratory infections: cough; breathlessness; and radiological evidence of chest infection. Supplementation led to a significant increase in plasma and white blood cell vitamin C concentrations. When evaluated using a clinical scoring system based on major symptoms, vitamin C–supplemented subjects fared significantly better than did the placebo group, with a pronounced effect seen in the most serious cases (21).

Vitamin C and Exercise-Induced Oxidative Stress

- In a double-blind, placebo-controlled study, 12 experienced marathon runners were randomly assigned to receive 1,000 mg vitamin C/day or a placebo for 8 days. Blood samples were taken before and 6 hours after subjects completed a 2.5-hour treadmill run at 75% to 80% VO_{2max}. Vitamin C had no effect on hormonal (cortisol, catecholamines) or immune measures (leukocyte subsets, interleukin-6, natural killer cell activity, lymphocyte proliferation, granulocyte phagocytosis, and activated oxidative burst) during recovery (22).

- In a double-blind, placebo-controlled study, 16 ultramarathon athletes were randomly assigned to receive vitamin C (500 mg twice daily) or a placebo for 7 days prior to a 90-km run, as well as on race day and 2 days after the run. Blood was drawn 16 hours before the race and at 30 minutes, 24 hours, and 48 hours after finishing. Prerace vitamin C levels in the supplemented group were unchanged after the race, whereas levels increased in the placebo group immediately postrace, and then returned to baseline after 24 hours. Immediately after the run, both groups experienced elevations in circulating neutrophils, monocytes and platelets, interleukin-6, cortisol, C-reactive protein (CRP), and creatine kinase. However, in the vitamin C-supplemented group, CRP levels were significantly higher at each time point and cortisol levels were significantly lower only 30 minutes postrace. The authors concluded that these observations suggest that vitamin C may blunt the adaptive mobilization of the vitamin from adrenals during exercise-induced oxidative stress and may be associated with an enhancement of the acute phase protein response and attenuation of the exercise-induced increase in cortisol (23).

- In a double-blind, placebo-controlled trial of 184 healthy subjects, vitamin C (500 mg/day) had no significant effect or interaction effect on oxidative DNA damage as measured by urinary 8-hydroxy-2'deoxyguanosine. However, fruit and vegetable intake (at least three servings daily) was associated with lower oxidative damage (24).

Vitamin C and Cardiovascular Disease

- The US Preventive Task Force paper on antioxidant supplementation to prevent cardiovascular disease suggests that although some epidemiological evidence suggests a protective effect, the evidence from randomized, prospective, controlled trials is insufficient to support generalized recommendations for antioxidant supplementation for the prevention of CVD (25).

- The Nurses' Health Study cohort provides evidence suggesting that vitamin C supplementation, but not dietary vitamin C, is associated with a 28% reduction in relative risk for coronary heart disease (26). This epidemiological study included analysis of diet and supplement data from 85,118 nurses for 16 years of follow-up, including 1,356 incident cases of coronary heart disease.

- A study among postmenopausal women with diabetes participating in the Iowa Women's Health Study (n = 1,923) evaluated vitamin C intake from diet and supplements in relation to CVD (27). After 15 years of follow-up, 513 subjects experienced CVD, coronary artery disease, or stroke. Relative risk for CVD increased with increasing vitamin C "exposure," a result that was significantly associated only with supplemental vitamin C "exposure" when diet and supplement intake were analyzed separately. This is one of the first studies to demonstrate an increased risk for CVD with vitamin C supplementation. One explanation may be that ascorbic acid enhances iron absorption and the excess iron could act as a pro-oxidant. Mean supplementation in the highest quintile was more than 300 mg vs 0 mg in the lowest quintile.

- The Antioxidant Supplementation in Atherosclerosis Prevention (ASAP) Trial was initiated in the late 1990s to test the hypothesis that daily supplementation with vitamin E (136 IU) and 500 mg vitamin C would significantly reduce atherosclerosis in men and postmenopausal women, including both smokers and nonsmokers (n = 520) (28). All had elevated serum total cholesterol levels on enrollment. At the 3-year time point, men showed a beneficial effect in terms of carotid atherosclerosis but women did not. The 6-year evaluation using carotid artery intima-media thickness as measured by ultrasound showed supplementation reduced progression of disease in all subjects by a mean of 26%, with mean change in slope among men measured at a 33% reduction (as compared with placebo) and mean change in slope among women at a 14% reduction; the change in women was assessed to be statistically nonsignificant. Efficacy tended to be higher in those with lower baseline ascorbic acid levels and less initial plaque build-up.

- In a study designed to test the use of vitamins C and E in improving endothelial function in children with hyperlipidemia, a randomized, placebo-controlled design was used. Fifteen children with familial disease were recruited and randomly assigned to either 500 mg vitamin C plus 400 IU vitamin E or placebo for 6 weeks concurrent with the NCEP Step II diet, which was initiated 4.5 months before supplementation started and continued during supplementation. This study suggested a significant difference in flow-mediated dilation of the brachial artery with antioxidant use as compared with placebo, despite no significant improvements in inflammatory or oxidative stress biomarkers (29). Although this was a pilot study, these findings support conducting further research about the application of antioxidant supplementation in children with high-risk disease.

- The Heart Protection Study (HPS) was initiated among 20,500 at-risk adults to determine the efficacy of statin drugs with or without antioxidants or placebo in modulating cardiovascular morbidity and mortality (30). Although statins were proven to be highly effective in reducing total mortality (–12%), and coronary heart disease events (–24%), there was no significant benefit associated with daily supplementation with a single supplement containing 250 mg vitamin C, 650 mg vitamin E, and 20 mg beta carotene.

◆ A systematic review assessed all ecological, case-control, and prospective studies from 1980 to 1996 examining vitamin C intake or status with cardiovascular disease. For coronary heart disease four of seven ecological, one of four case-control, and three of 12 cohort studies found a significant protective effect. For total circulatory disease, two of three cohort studies reported a significant protective correlation with vitamin C intake. For strokes, two of two epidemiological studies, zero of one case-control study, and two of seven cohort studies found a significant protective effect (31).

◆ In an epidemiological study of 1,605 randomly selected Finnish men age 42, 48, 54, or 60 years without cardiovascular disease, a higher incidence of myocardial infarction correlated with low plasma vitamin C levels (32). Another study of a randomly selected cohort of 730 elderly people revealed that subjects with the lowest vitamin C status had a higher mortality rate from stroke, but not mortality from coronary heart disease (33).

◆ Animal and human studies have investigated the role of vitamin C in cholesterol metabolism, in the maintenance of vascular integrity, in the synthesis of prostacyclin (vasodilator and antiplatelet agent), and its antioxidant role in lipid oxidation (via reductive regeneration of vitamin E). A comprehensive review article noted that although there seems to be a possible protective association between vitamin C and CVD, conclusive evidence is lacking. The authors note that human data have been inconsistent, but "taken together indicate that for individuals with high cholesterol concentrations (> 200 mg/dL) and less than full tissue saturation [of vitamin C], increasing the concentration of vitamin C may have a salutary effect on total cholesterol" (34).

Vitamin C and Hypertension

◆ In a systematic review of cross-sectional and prospective studies from 1980 to 1996 on vitamin C and blood pressure, 10 of 14 cross-sectional studies reported an inverse association between plasma vitamin C and blood pressure. Three of four reported an inverse relationship with dietary vitamin C intake. The authors noted that none of the cross-sectional studies adequately controlled for potential confounding dietary factors. Of four randomized, controlled trials, only one reported a significant decrease in blood pressure with vitamin C supplementation (250 to 1,000 mg), whereas two studies were considered "uninterpretable" (35).

◆ In a double-blind, placebo-controlled, crossover study, 40 men and women (ages 60 to 80 years) were given, in random order, 500 mg vitamin C and a placebo for 3 months each, with a 1-week washout period. Blood pressure and blood lipid levels were measured at baseline and at the end of each phase. Blood pressure measured at the clinic did not differ between groups. However, daytime ambulatory blood pressure showed a small but significant reduction in systolic, but not diastolic, blood pressure with vitamin C supplementation. Regression analysis revealed that the higher the baseline daytime pressure, the greater the decrease in blood pressure observed with vitamin C. There were no differences between groups in cholesterol levels. However, when women were analyzed alone, there was a significant increase in HDL cholesterol with vitamin C supplementation (36).

♦ In a randomized, controlled, blinded study of vitamin C and blood pressure, 439 Japanese adults consumed either 50 or 500 mg supplemental vitamin C for 5 years (37). Dropout rates were more than 30%, limiting interpretation of the data. At baseline there was no association between serum vitamin C levels and systolic or diastolic blood pressure. This lack of association was also shown at the end of 5 years when change in blood pressure over time was compared across treatment groups. In fact, blood pressure increased over time, which is thought to be associated mainly with aging. This report suggests that low or high levels of vitamin C supplementation, even over 5 years, are ineffective in reducing blood pressure.

♦ In a controlled feeding study conducted among 68 men with hypertension, subjects participated in a 1-month vitamin C depletion phase followed by a 1-month vitamin C supplement phase (117 mg/day), a second vitamin C depletion phase, and a second supplementation phase. Dietary vitamin C intake was controlled throughout the study. Plasma ascorbic acid levels were significantly inversely related to diastolic blood pressure and to a lesser extent with systolic blood pressure (38). This study is strengthened by the tight control on vitamin C exposure throughout.

♦ In a small, randomized, double-blind, placebo-controlled study, 30 patients (ages 45 to 70 years) with type 2 diabetes and systolic blood pressure greater than 95 mm Hg were randomly assigned to oral administration of 500 mg supplemental vitamin C daily (n= 15) or placebo (n = 15). After 1 month, arterial blood pressure was less and arterial stiffness was significantly reduced with supplementation (39). Additional larger studies seem warranted.

Vitamin C and Cancer

♦ Cancer mortality was investigated in the 25-year Seven Countries Study. Vitamin C intake was inversely correlated with stomach cancer mortality, even after correcting for smoking and sodium and nitrate intake (40). Review articles have also summarized evidence that suggests lower risk of esophagus, oral cavity, and pharynx cancers with vitamin C intake (approximately 70 to 100 mg/day) (8). However, in the Linxian Nutrition Intervention Trial, daily supplementation of 120 mg vitamin C and 30 μg molybdenum for 5 years did not reduce mortality from stomach cancer in 29,584 Chinese subjects (41).

♦ A review article specifically addressing supplement use and epidemiological research on cancer risk reported an inverse relationship between bladder cancer and vitamin C supplements in case-control studies (42).

♦ The US Cancer Prevention Study II cohort of more than 990,000 adults, of whom 1,289 cases of bladder cancer were diagnosed in a 16-year period, showed no significant association between self-reported vitamin C supplementation and bladder cancer risk (RR = 0.91; 95% CI = 0.68–1.20) (43).

Vitamin C and Cataracts

♦ In the Nurses' Health Study, 50,828 women age 45 to 67 years were evaluated for incidence of cataract extraction during an 8-year prospective study. Those who reported using vitamin C supplements for 10 or more years had a significant 45% reduction in cataract risk (RR = 0.55; 95% CI = 0.32–0.96). In those not using supplements, dietary vitamin C intake had no correlation with risk (44).

♦ In a cross-sectional study, a subset of 240 women with very high or very low vitamin C intakes were selected from the Nurses' Health Study cohort (no history of diabetes or diagnosed cataract). All subjects received a detailed eye exam. Women who took vitamin C supplements for 10 or more years (n = 26) had a significant 77% lower incidence of early age-related lens opacities and a significant 83% lower incidence of moderate lens opacities at any lens compared with women not taking vitamin C (n = 141). Of the 26 women who used supplements for 10 or more years, 4 took a mean dosage of less than 400 mg/day, 12 took a mean dosage of 400 to 700 mg/day, and 10 took a mean dosage of more than 700 mg/day. However, use of supplements for fewer than 10 years had no statistical effect on the overall incidence of lens opacities (45).

References

1. Jacob RA. Vitamin C. In: Shils ME, Olson JA, Shike M, Ross AC, eds. *Modern Nutrition in Health and Disease.* 9th ed. Baltimore, Md: Williams & Wilkins; 1999:467–483.
2. Institute of Medicine. *Dietary Reference Intakes: Vitamin C, Vitamin E, Selenium, and Carotenoids.* Washington, DC: National Academy Press; 2000.
3. Hathcock JN, Azzi A, Blumberg J, et al. Vitamins E and C are safe across a broad range of intakes. *Am J Clin Nutr.* 2005;81:736–745.
4. Bendich A, Langseth L. The health effects of vitamin C supplementation: a review. *J Am Coll Nutr.* 1995;14:124–136.
5. Curhan GC, Willett WC, Rimm EB, et al. A prospective study of the intake of vitamins C and B-6, and the risk of kidney stones in men. *J Urol.* 1996;155:1847–1851.
6. Johnston CS. Biomarkers for establishing a Tolerable Upper Intake Level for vitamin C. *Nutr Rev.* 1999;57:71–77.
7. Podmore ED, Griffiths HR, Herbert KE, et al. Vitamin C exhibits pro-oxidant properties. *Nature.* 1998;329:559.
8. Johnston CS, Luo B. Comparison of the absorption and excretion of three commercially available sources of vitamin C. *J Am Diet Assoc.* 1994;94:779–781.
9. Carr AC, Frei B. Toward a new recommended dietary allowance for vitamin C based on antioxidant and health effects in humans. *Am J Clin Nutr.* 1999;69:1086–1107.
10. Pennington JA. *Bowes & Church's Food Values of Portions Commonly Used.* 17th ed. Philadelphia, Pa: Lippincott; 1998.
11. Shane B. Vitamin C pharmacokinetics: it's deja vu all over again. *Am J Clin Nutr.* 1997;66:1061–1062.

12. Blanchard J, Tozer TN, Rowland M. Pharmacokinetic perspectives on megadoses of ascorbic acid. *Am J Clin Nutr.* 1997;66:1165–1171.

13. Weber P, Bendich A, Schalch W. Vitamin C and human health—a review of recent data relevant to human requirements. *Int J Vitam Nutr Res.* 1996;66:19–30.

14. Levine M, Dhariwal KR, Welch RW, et al. Determination of optimal vitamin C requirements in humans. *Am J Clin Nutr.* 1995;62(6 Suppl):S1347-S1356.

15. Hemila H. Vitamin C supplementation and the common cold—was Linus Pauling right or wrong? *Int J Vitam Nutr Res.* 1997;67:329–335.

16. Douglas RM, Hemila H, D'Souza R, et al. Vitamin C for preventing and treating the common cold. *Cochrane Database Syst Rev.* 2004;18:CD00980.

17. Audera C, Patulny RV, Sander BH, et al. Mega-dose vitamin C in treatment of the common cold: a randomised controlled trial. *Med J Aust.* 2001;175:359–362.

18. Peters EM, Goetzsche JM, Grobbelaar B, et al. Vitamin C supplementation reduces the incidence of postrace symptoms of upper-respiratory-tract infection in ultramarathon runners. *Am J Clin Nutr.* 1993;57:170–174.

19. Schwartz J, Weiss ST. Relationship between dietary vitamin C intake and pulmonary function in the First National Health and Nutrition Examination Survey (NHANES I). *Am J Clin Nutr.* 1994;59:110–114.

20. Bielory L, Gandhi R. Asthma and vitamin C. *Ann Allergy.* 1994;73:89–96.

21. Hunt C, Chakravorty NK, Annan G, et al. The clinical effects of vitamin C supplementation in elderly hospitalized patients with acute respiratory infections. *Int J Vitam Nutr Res.* 1994;64:212–219.

22. Nieman DC, Henson DA, Butterworth DE, et al. Vitamin C supplementation does not alter the immune response to 2.5 hours of running. *Int J Sport Nutr.* 1997;7:173–184.

23. Peters EM, Anderson R, Theron AJ. Attenuation of increase in circulating cortisol and enhancement of the acute phase protein response in vitamin C-supplemented ultra-marathoners. *Int J Sports Med.* 2001;22:120–126.

24. Huang HY, Helzlsouer KJ, Appel LJ, et al. The effects of vitamin C and vitamin E on oxidative DNA damage: results from a randomized controlled trial. *Cancer Epidemiol Biomarkers Prev.* 2000;9:647–652.

25. Morris CD, Carson S. Routine vitamin supplementation to prevent cardiovascular disease: a summary of the evidence for the U.S. Preventive Services Task Force. *Ann Intern Med.* 2003;139:56–70.

26. Osganian SK, Stampfer MJ, Rimm E, et al. Vitamin C and risk of coronary heart disease in women. *J Am Coll Cardiol.* 2003;42:246–252.

27. Lee DH, Folsom AR, Harnack L, et al. Does supplemental vitamin C increase cardiovascular disease risk in women with diabetes? *Am J Clin Nutr.* 2004;80:1194–1200.

28. Salonen RM, Nyyssonen K, Kaikkonen J, et al. Six-year effect of combined vitamin C and E supplementation on atherosclerotic progression: the Antioxidant Supplementation in Atherosclerosis Prevention (ASAP) Study. *Circulation.* 2003;107: 947–953.

29. Engler MM, Engler MB, Malloy MJ, et al. Antioxidant vitamins C and E improve endothelial function in children with hyperlipidemia: Endothelial Assessment of Risk from Lipids in Youth (EARLY) trial. *Circulation.* 2003;108:1059–1063.

30. Collins R, Peto R, Armitage J. The MRC/BHF Heart Protection Study: preliminary results. *Int J Clin Pract.* 2002;56:53–56.

31. Ness AR, Powles JW, Khaw KT. Vitamin C and cardiovascular disease: a systematic review. *J Cardiovasc Risk.* 1996;3:513–521.

32. Nyyssonen K, Parviainen MT, Salonen R, et al. Vitamin C deficiency and risk of myocardial infarction: prospective population study of men from eastern Finland. *BMJ.* 1997;314:634–638.

33. Gale CR, Martyn CN, Winter PD, et al. Vitamin C and risk of death from stroke and coronary heart disease in a cohort of elderly people. *BMJ.* 1995;310:1563–1566.

34. Simon JA. Vitamin C and cardiovascular disease: a review. *J Am Coll Nutr.* 1992;11: 107–125.

35. Ness AR, Chee D, Elliott P. Vitamin C and blood pressure—an overview. *J Hum Hypertens.* 1997;11:343–350.

36. Fotherby MD, Williams JC, Forster LA, et al. Effect of vitamin C on ambulatory blood pressure and plasma lipids in older persons. *J Hypertens.* 2000;18:411–415.

37. Kim MK, Sasaki S, Sasazuki S, et al. Lack of long-term effect of vitamin C supplementation on blood pressure. *Hypertension.* 2002;40:797–803.

38. Block G, Mangels AR, Norkus EP, et al. Ascorbic acid status and subsequent diastolic and systolic blood pressure. *Hypertension.* 2001;37:261–267.

39. Mullan BA, Young IS, Fee H, et al. Ascorbic acid reduces blood pressure and arterial stiffness in type 2 diabetes. *Hypertension.* 2002;40:804–809.

40. Ocke MC, Kromhout D, Menotti A, et al. Average intake of antioxidant (pro)vitamins and subsequent cancer mortality in the 16 cohorts of the Seven Countries Study. *Int J Cancer.* 1995;61:480–484.

41. Blot WJ, Li JY, Taylor PR, et al. Nutrition intervention trials in Linxian, China: supplementation with specific vitamin/mineral combinations, cancer incidence, and disease-specific mortality in the general population. *J Natl Cancer Inst.* 1993;85:1483–1492.

42. Patterson RE, White E, Kristal AR, et al. Vitamin supplements and cancer risk: the epidemiologic evidence. *Cancer Causes Control.* 1997;8:786–802.

43. Jacobs EJ, Henion AK, Briggs PJ, et al. Vitamin C and vitamin E supplement use and bladder cancer mortality in a large cohort of US men and women. *Am J Epidemiol.* 2002;156:1002–1010.

44. Hankinson SE, Stampfer MJ, Seddon JM, et al. Nutrient intake and cataract extraction in women: a prospective study. *BMJ.* 1992;305:335–339.

45. Jacques PF, Taylor A, Hankinson SE, et al. Long-term vitamin C supplement use and prevalence of early age-related lens opacities. *Am J Clin Nutr.* 1997;66:911–916.

Vitamin D

Vitamin D, considered both a hormone and vitamin, functions primarily to maintain calcium homeostasis. Vitamin D is produced endogenously when ultraviolet light reacts with 7-dehydrocholesterol in the skin to produce cholecalciferol or vitamin D3. In the liver, vitamin D3 is hydroxylated to 25-hydroxy vitamin D3, the most abundant form of vitamin D in the body. This compound is further hydroxylated in the kidneys to produce the active form, 1, 25-dihydroxy vitamin D3. (Two other equivalent terms for 1,25-dihydroxy vitamin D3 are 1, 25-dihydroxy cholecalciferol and/or 1, 25(OH)$_2$D3.) When serum calcium levels decrease, the activated vitamin D increases calcium and phosphorus absorption in the intestine, increases resorption of calcium in the kidneys, and stimulates bone mineral release (1,2). Defects in vitamin D metabolism, lack of sun exposure, insufficient dietary intake, or a combination of these can result in rickets (children) or osteomalacia (adults). Vitamin D deficiency is fairly common among the elderly population, specifically those who are homebound or institutionalized (3–5).

Media and Marketing Claims	Efficacy
Improves bone health when taken with calcium	↑
Improves calcium status	↑
Reduces risk for falls	↑
Reduces risk of colorectal cancer	↔
Reduces risk for breast cancer	NR

Safety

- The Tolerable Upper Intake Level (UL) for adults is 2,000 IU vitamin D (50 µg) (6).
- People who use many supplements containing vitamin D and who consume high intakes of fish or fortified milk may be at risk for vitamin D toxicity (6).
- Excessive intakes of vitamin D are associated with hypercalcemia, hypercalciuria, and calcification of bone and soft tissues including the kidney (kidney stones), lungs, and the tympanic membrane of the ear, which can result in deafness (7).

Drug/Supplement Interactions

- Calcipotriene used for psoriasis is a vitamin D analog and can contribute to hypercalcemia if combined with oral vitamin D supplements.
- Estrogen therapy may increase blood levels of vitamin D and enhance calcium absorption.
- Vitamin D may decrease the effectiveness of verapamil (calcium-channel blocker for hypertension).
- The following drugs may increase risk of bone loss by interfering with the absorption and activity of vitamin D: anticonvulsant drugs, bile acid sequestrants (for hypercholesterolemia), cimetidine (antacid), corticosteroids (anti-inflammatory), heparin (anticoagulant), isoniazid (antibiotic), mineral oil, neomycin (antibacterial).

Key Points

- Vitamin D is necessary for bone health. When taken with calcium, vitamin D seems to favorably modulate bone health toward increases in bone mineral density (BMD).

- Vitamin D is necessary for efficient calcium absorption. Inadequate dietary vitamin D, insufficient exposure to sunlight, impaired activation of vitamin D, or defects in vitamin D metabolism interfere with calcium absorption. It is estimated that only 10% of dietary calcium is absorbed when vitamin D is deficient (8). More research is needed to determine the strength of the causal relationships between the two nutrients.

- Fracture rates have decreased substantially with combined therapy with calcium and vitamin D, but it is not clear which is the principal active agent or whether, in fact, the combination is optimal for fracture prevention (1). A meta-analysis for hip fracture risk and nonvertebral fracture risk in the elderly supports the role of supplemental vitamin D at a level of 700 to 800 IU/day (9).

- According to a recent meta-analysis, vitamin D supplementation in the elderly has also been associated with a reduction in the incidence/number of falls (10).

- Epidemiological studies have shown an inconsistent relationship between dietary vitamin D and reduced colorectal cancer risk. There seems to be a significant interaction between calcium and vitamin D. Among those with adequate vitamin D status, calcium supplementation may reduce risk and serum vitamin D levels may only be shown to be protective among those taking calcium supplements (11). The Women's Health Initiative trial showed no reduction in risk for colorectal cancer among those receiving 200 IU vitamin D daily for 7 years as compared with placebo (12). However, there was a significant trend for a protective effect of supplementation among a subsample of postmenopausal women who demonstrated low serum vitamin D levels prior to vitamin D supplementation.

- In vitro and animal data suggest that vitamin D may reduce the risk of certain cancers, including mammary tumors. Vitamin D analogues are currently being tested in laboratory studies and in patients with advanced cancer including breast and colorectal cancers. Mechanisms of potential cancer-protective activity include regulation of intestinal epithelial growth factors, cytokine response to inflammation, modulation of cell cycle, induction of apoptosis, and promotion of cellular differentiation (13).

- Vitamin D status may be compromised in elderly, institutionalized patients, and individuals with malabsorption disorders (as in liver failure, celiac disease, Crohn's disease, and Whipple's disease). If sun exposure and dietary vitamin D intakes are low, such individuals may require supplemental vitamin D to help meet the Adequate Intake (AI).

Food Sources

Food sources of vitamin D are limited. Egg yolks, liver, fish oils, fatty fish, fortified milk (100 IU/cup), and fortified breakfast cereals (40 to 80 IU/serving) are the best sources (7,14). The vitamin D content of fortified milk has been reported to vary (15). Estimates of US dietary intake of vitamin D are not available due to variability of vitamin D in fortified foods and because US surveys have not measured vitamin D intake (6).

Dosage Information/Bioavailability

The AI for vitamin D is 200 IU (5 µg) for adults younger than 50 years, 400 IU (10 µg) for adults ages 51 to 70 years, and 600 IU (15 µg) for adults 70 years and older (6) (1 µg = 40 IU). Vitamin D3 (cholecalciferol) or vitamin D2 (ergocalciferol) supplements are sold in single preparations or multivitamin/mineral supplements, usually providing 200 to 400 IU (5 to 10 µg). In general, vitamin D3 supplements increase blood levels of vitamin D3 and 25-hydroxy vitamin D (measure of vitamin D status) (16). In one study, vitamin D3 supplements increased serum 25-hydroxy vitamin D levels more than vitamin D2 supplements (17).

Relevant Research

Vitamin D Deficiency

- Reports suggest that vitamin D deficiency may be more prevalent than previously estimated (18). In a study of 290 hospitalized patients, 57% had serum levels less than 40 nmol/L, with 27% having levels less than 20 nmol/L. Of importance, 43% of adults who reported adequate dietary intake (> 400 IU/day) still demonstrated suboptimal serum levels of 25-hydroxyvitamin D (19). According to data from NHANES III, 46.6% of African-American females of child-bearing age, but only 4.7% of white women in this age group, had deficient serum levels of vitamin D, indicating that skin color is an important factor in identifying at-risk populations related to reduced endogenous vitamin D production (20).

Vitamin D (Alone or With Calcium) and Bone Health

- A meta-analysis of randomized, controlled clinical trials assessing the role of vitamin D in fracture prevention concluded that, "oral vitamin D supplementation between 700 and 800 IU/d appears to reduce the risk of hip and any nonvertebral fractures in ambulatory and institutionalized elderly persons. An oral vitamin D dose of 400 IU is not sufficient for fracture prevention." This analysis included 7 trials that had at least 1 year follow-up and in which all subjects (n = 9,820) were older than 60 years (9).

- A randomized, double-blind, placebo-controlled study of 120 peri- and post-menopausal Italian women between the ages of 45 and 55 years (mean BMI 27.9) receiving a placebo or a calcium/vitamin D supplement (500 mg calcium plus 200 IU vitamin D) showed that at the 30-month time point for measurement, BMD was significantly greater in the supplemented group as compared with placebo. In fact, those receiving the supplement showed an increase in BMD at an age when most adults lose bone mass, whereas mean BMD in the placebo group was reduced 0.4% per year during the 30-month study (21). Baseline vitamin D status was not reported, but dietary intake, as reported in food-frequency questionnaires, was stable during the course of the study.

- In a double-blind, placebo-controlled study, 389 men and women older than 65 years were randomly assigned to receive 500 mg calcium plus 700 IU (17.5 µg) vitamin D3 or a placebo daily for 3 years. There was a significant difference between the treatment and placebo groups in BMD at the femoral neck, spine, and total-body (assessed by dual-energy x-ray absorptiometry) after 1 year, but the difference remained significant only for total body BMD in the following 2 years. Of the 37 subjects who experienced nonvertebral fractures, significantly more were in the placebo group (n = 26) compared with the vitamin D and calcium–supplemented group (n = 11) (22).

♦ In a double-blind, placebo-controlled, prospective study, 2,578 free-living Dutch men and women older than 70 years were randomly assigned to receive 400 IU (10 μg) vitamin D3 or a placebo daily for a maximum of 3.5 years. Subjects had a mean dietary calcium intake of 868 mg/day. Vitamin D–supplemented subjects had higher mean serum 25-hydroxy vitamin D levels than the placebo group. However, there were no differences in incidence of hip fractures or other peripheral fractures (23).

♦ In a double-blind comparative study, 247 healthy postmenopausal women living in Boston were randomly assigned to receive 100 IU (2.5 μg) vitamin D3 or 700 IU (17.5 μg) vitamin D3 daily for 2 years. All women received 500 mg supplemental calcium as calcium citrate malate. Mean dietary intake of vitamin D for all subjects was 100 IU (2.5 μg). Femoral neck BMD decreased in both treatment groups, but the reduction was significantly less in the high-dose vitamin D–supplemented group than the group receiving the lesser dose. There were no changes in spinal and whole-body bone densities (assessed by dual-energy x-ray absorptiometry) between groups (24).

♦ In a double-blind, placebo-controlled trial, 249 healthy postmenopausal women were randomly assigned to receive 400 IU (10 μg) vitamin D3 or a placebo daily for 1 year. Usual dietary intake of vitamin D was 100 IU (2.5 μg) for both groups. All subjects received 377 mg supplemental calcium as calcium citrate malate. BMD was measured at 6-month intervals when serum 25-hydroxy vitamin D is highest (summer/fall) and lowest (winter/spring). Both groups had an increase in spinal BMD in the summer/fall. In both groups, spinal BMD decreased in the winter/spring, but the vitamin D–supplemented group had significantly less bone loss and a significant overall improvement in spinal BMD. During the winter/spring months, 25-hydroxy vitamin D levels were lower and parathyroid hormone levels were higher in the placebo group compared with the vitamin D group (25).

♦ In a meta-analysis, researchers evaluated randomized, controlled trials lasting at least 6 months to determine whether vitamin D plus calcium was more effective than no therapy or calcium supplementation alone in the management of corticosteroid-induced osteoporosis. Of nine trials, there was a moderate, significant benefit of vitamin D plus calcium compared with no therapy or calcium use alone (26).

♦ In a Norwegian cohort study, 1,144 frail, elderly nursing home residents (ages 77.1 to 92.4 years), were randomly assigned to 5 mL cod liver oil (with 2.2 μg/mL vitamin D3; n = 569) or 5 mL cod liver oil without vitamin D (extracted to contain only 0.15 μg/mL vitamin D3; n = 575) daily for a period of 2 years. All subjects had a life expectancy longer than 6 months and were not bedridden; 75% of them were women. One hundred ninety-seven women in the vitamin D group and 187 in the placebo remained in the study for 2 years. Just under 30% of the subjects in each group died during the study, and an additional 36% to 40% in each group dropped out or were excluded because they were prescribed calcium and/or vitamin D by their physician. Ninety-seven hip fractures and 146 nonvertebral fractures were reported. Vitamin D supplementation significantly increased serum levels of vitamin D but was not associated with a reduction in fracture risk (27). Because this study did not use calcium supplements and found no efficacy for vitamin D alone, this suggests that the decreased risk of fracture associated with vitamin D in other studies where vitamin D and calcium are taken concurrently is related to the vitamin's effects on calcium absorption.

◆ A 2-year double-blind, placebo-controlled, comparative trial evaluated risk of hip fracture in 610 elderly women (mean age 85 years). Subjects were randomly assigned to (*a*) a supplement containing 1,200 mg elemental tricalcium phosphate and 800 IU of vitamin D3 (n = 199), (*b*) calcium (1,200 mg tricalcium phosphate) plus vitamin D3 (400 IU twice daily), taken as separate supplements daily (n = 190), or (*c*) placebo (n = 194). Dietary intake of both calcium and vitamin D in this study population was assessed to be very low (mean dietary calcium intake = 557 mg/day; mean dietary intake of vitamin D intake = 40.8 IU/day). Serum vitamin D levels increased in both groups that took supplements as compared with both baseline and placebo ($P = .0001$). Compared with the placebo group, the groups taking supplements also had stable femoral neck BMD and reduced risk for hip fracture(hip fracture rates were 6.9% in the treated groups and 11.1% in the placebo group). There was no significant difference in clinical response biomarkers between those assigned to the combined supplement and the group taking separate calcium and vitamin D supplements (28).

◆ In a randomized, controlled, open-label trial, 3,314 women older than 70 years and identified as at-risk for fracture were randomly assigned in a 3:2 ratio control:intervention by medical practice site to (*a*) calcium (1,000 mg) and vitamin D3 (800 IU) plus educational brochure, or (*b*) educational brochure alone. The educational brochure included information on how to reduce risk for a fall and how to increase dietary vitamin D and calcium intake. The median follow-up time was 25 months. Only 149 confirmed fractures were identified. This study showed no significant differences in fracture rates, delay in time until fracture event, or fall rates across the two groups (29). The study was limited by the lack of a placebo group and by the overall low fracture rate, which is not clearly explained.

◆ A population-based, voluntary participation study evaluated Danish adults older than 66 years (mean age 74 years), 80% of whom demonstrated reduced (< 50 nM) serum vitamin D levels. Subjects were offered either 1,000 mg calcium plus 400 IU vitamin D daily (n = 2,426) or education focused on improving the subject's living environment so as to reduce fracture risk (n = 2,532). The education included a home safety inspection by a community nurse and dietary evaluation. A third group was offered both supplementation and the environmental education program (n = 2,531), and 2,116 subjects were not provided with supplement or education (control group). After 3 years, the rate of fractures in women was three times the rate in men ($P \leq .0001$). Fracture rates were significantly less in the calcium/vitamin D supplemented group (RR = 0.78; 95% CI = 0.63–0.96), as well as the environmental education group (RR = 0.82; 95% CI = 0.67–1.00) and the group receiving supplement and education (RR = 0.73; 95% CI = 0.58–0.93), as compared to placebo (30).

♦ The double-blind, placebo-controlled RECORD study (Randomised Evaluation of Calcium or vitamin D) evaluated the efficacy of supplemental vitamin D and calcium in 5,292 elderly subjects (mean age 77 years) who had had a low trauma osteoporotic fracture within the previous decade. Most of the subjects were women. Subjects were randomly assigned to (*a*) 800 IU vitamin D3, (*b*) 1,000 mg calcium, (*c*) 800 IU vitamin D3 plus 1,000 mg calcium, or (*d*) placebo daily for 24 to 62 months (31). The 698 fractures that occurred during the study were equally distributed across treatment groups, indicating no clinical efficacy for any of the supplements. The null findings of this research possibly may be (*a*) explained by the advanced age of the study population, (*b*) a result of low compliance (only 54.5% were taking supplements at the 24-month measurement), or (*c*) the result of a well-nourished study population (no dietary or serum vitamin D levels were included in the analysis).

♦ In a subanalysis from data collected in the context of a large randomized, controlled, double-blind study testing the effect of calcium and vitamin D supplementation on bone loss in 145 elderly subjects, vitamin D supplementation was associated with a significantly decreased loss in teeth during a 5-year period. Subjects were eligible if they had previously completed clinical oral exams at the beginning and end of the parent study. Tooth loss was assessed by clinical tooth count during periodontal exam as well as self-report questionnaire (32).

Vitamin D and Calcium Absorption

♦ Calcium absorption is enhanced when serum 25-hydroxyvitamin D levels are within normal limits. Two randomized, crossover studies were conducted to quantify calcium absorption with and without repletion of vitamin D. In the first study 34 postmenopausal women (mean age 56 years) were given 20 μg vitamin D as 25OHD-Calderol (Organon, West Orange, NJ) every other day for 3 weeks prior to taking 500 mg calcium with 200 IU vitamin D (either Os-Cal or Citracal, as randomly assigned) as part of a low calcium breakfast. In the second study, 34 postmenopausal women (14 subjects participated in both studies) were given 500 mg calcium with 200 IU vitamin D. This study did not have a pretreatment period of taking vitamin D only (33). In the first study, where all subjects were provided pretreatment with vitamin D, mean serum vitamin D levels increased to 86.5 nmol/L. In the second study, where subjects were not given vitamin D supplementation prior to calcium loading, mean serum vitamin D levels were 50.2 nmol/L. The area under the curve for calcium absorption was significantly higher in those pretreated with vitamin D as compared with those who were not, a difference indicating a 65% increase in calcium absorption related to presupplementation with vitamin D and an increase that was demonstrated regardless of the calcium supplement to which subjects were randomly assigned (Os-Cal or Citracal). The difference existed even though the nontreated group demonstrated normal serum values. This paper indicates that current levels of intake to achieve serum vitamin D levels more than 40 nmol/L may be sub-optimal in terms of increasing calcium uptake and reducing fracture rates or optimizing bone health.

Vitamin D and Risk of Falling

♦ In a study of vitamin D supplementation and fall risk, investigators assessed fall outcomes as well as improvements in parathyroid hormone (PTH) and body sway as potential indicators of fall risk in the elderly. Subjects (mean age 74 years) were randomly assigned to receive 1,200 mg calcium or 1,200 mg calcium combined with 800 IU vitamin D daily for 8 weeks (34). As compared with calcium alone, the combined supplement resulted in significant reduction in body sway, reduction in PTH of 18%, and a significant reduction in number of falls. A follow-up study conducted by the same research group comparing similar outcomes after 12 weeks of supplementation showed that among the 122 elderly subjects, the combined supplement treatment resulted in a significant 49% reduction in fall incidence (35).

♦ A meta-analysis of double-blind randomized, controlled trials of vitamin D in health-stable older populations (mean age 70 years) and fall risk showed a greater than 20% reduced risk of falls was associated with daily vitamin D supplementation in both institutionalized and free-living subjects. The analysis included 5 well-designed trials that were randomized, placebo-controlled and had a consistent definition of falls ("unintentional coming to rest on the ground, floor or other lower level"). A total of 1,237 subjects (81% women) were included in the 5 trials. Treatments varied and included between 400 and 800 IU vitamin D daily, with or without added calcium (1,200 mg/day), and lasted between 2 months and 3 years (10). The authors suggest that vitamin D may protect against falls by improving muscle function or reducing body sway.

Vitamin D and Cancer

♦ The Women's Health Initiative (WHI) randomized, controlled, double-blind clinical trial assessed the role of daily calcium (100 mg elemental calcium as calcium carbonate) plus 200 IU vitamin D supplementation on colorectal cancer occurrence. In this cohort of 36,282 postmenopausal women, supplementation was not associated with a significant reduction in colorectal cancer as compared with placebo during 7 years of follow-up (12). In a nested case-control analysis that included the assessment of serum vitamin D levels among 612 WHI participants, lower serum vitamin D levels were associated with a significant trend toward higher colorectal cancer risk.

♦ In the Nurses' Health prospective cohort study (n = 84,448 women), there was an inverse association between intake of total vitamin D from foods and supplements (mean daily intake of highest vitamin D quintile = 728 IU [18.3 µg], vs lowest quintile = 55 IU [1.4 µg]) and risk of colorectal cancer during 12 years. Calcium intake was not associated with a lower risk of colorectal cancer. The authors concluded that factors other than vitamin D in multivitamin supplements may account for this protective effect (36).

◆ In the Health Professionals' Follow-Up Study, a prospective cohort study (n = 47,935 men), there was an inverse relationship between intake of supplemental vitamin D from multivitamins and colon cancer risk, but not with dietary vitamin D. The authors postulated that the reduction in risk could be attributed to multivitamin use rather than vitamin D alone. Further research comparing supplemental vitamin D with placebo or dietary approaches to increasing vitamin D intake are warranted (37).

◆ In a prospective case-control study, 95,000 women who had never been diagnosed with cancer were assessed for vitamin D status between 1964 and 1972. By 1991, 2,131 women developed breast cancer. A random sample of 96 women older than 55 years with cancer were matched to control subjects. Prior to diagnosis, serum 1, 25 dihydroxy-vitamin D levels were measured in all subjects. The researchers chose to measure 1, 25 dihydroxy-vitamin D because this form has been recognized as a modulator of cell proliferation and differentiation in laboratory studies. (*Note*: This measure has little value in detecting vitamin D deficiency.) There was no relationship between breast cancer incidence and prediagnostic serum vitamin D levels (38).

References

1. Jones G, Strugnell SA, DeLuca HF. Current understanding of the molecular actions of vitamin D. *Physiol Rev.* 1998;78:1193–1231.
2. Reid IR. The roles of calcium and vitamin D in the prevention of osteoporosis. *Endocrinol Metab Clin North Am.* 1998;27:389–398.
3. Compston JE. Vitamin D deficiency: time for action. Evidence supports routine supplementation for elderly people and others at risk. *BMJ.* 1998;317:1466–1467.
4. Gloth FM III, Gundberg CM, Hollis BW, et al. Vitamin D deficiency in homebound elderly persons. *JAMA.* 1995;274:1683–1686.
5. Jacques PF, Felson DT, Tucker KL, et al. Plasma 25-hydroxy vitamin D and its determinants in an elderly population sample. *Am J Clin Nutr.* 1997;66:929–936.
6. Institute of Medicine. *Dietary Reference Intakes for Calcium, Phosphorus, Magnesium, Vitamin D, and Fluoride.* Washington, DC: National Academy Press; 1997.
7. Linder MC. Nutrition and metabolism of Vitamins. In: Linder MC, ed. *Nutritional Biochemistry and Metabolism with Clinical Applications.* 2nd ed. New York, NY: Elsevier; 1991:111–189.
8. Fife RS, Sledge GW Jr, Proctor C. Effects of vitamin D_3 on proliferation of cancer cells in vitro. *Cancer Lett.* 1997;120:65–69.
9. Bischoff-Ferrari HA, Willett WC, Wong JB, et al. Fracture prevention with vitamin D supplementation: a meta-analysis of randomized controlled trials. *JAMA.* 2005;293:2257–2264.
10. Bischoff-Ferrari HA, Dawson-Hughes B, Willett WC, et al. Effect of Vitamin D on falls: a meta-analysis. *JAMA.* 2004;291:1999–2006.

11. Grau MV, Baron JA, Sandler RS, et al. Vitamin D, calcium supplementation, and colorectal adenomas: results of a randomized trial. *J Natl Cancer Inst.* 2003;95:1765–1771.

12. Wactawski-Wende J, Kotchen JM, Anderson GL, et al. Calcium plus vitamin D supplementation and risk for colorectal cancer. *New Eng J Med.* 2006;354:684–696.

13. Harris DM, Go VL. Vitamin D and colon carcinogenesis. *J Nutr.* 2004;134(2 Suppl): S3463–S3471.

14. Pennington JA. *Bowes and Church's Food Values of Portions Commonly Used.* 17th ed. Philadelphia, Pa: Lippincott; 1998.

15. Holick MF, Shao Q, Liu WW, et al. The vitamin D content of fortified milk and infant formula. *N Engl J Med.* 1992;326:1178–1181.

16. Barger-Lux MJ, Heaney RP, Dowell S, et al. Vitamin D and its major metabolites: serum levels after graded oral dosing in healthy men. *Osteoporos Int.* 1998;8:222–230.

17. Trang HM, Cole DE, Rubin LA, et al. Evidence that vitamin D_3 increases serum 25-hydroxy vitamin D more efficiently than does vitamin D_2. *Am J Clin Nutr.* 1998;68:854–858.

18. Hanley DA, Davison KS. Vitamin D insufficiency in North America. *J Nutr.* 2005;135: 332–337.

19. Thomas MK, Lloyd-Jones DM, Thadhani RI, et al. Hypovitaminosis D in medical inpatients. *N Engl J Med.* 1998;338:777–783.

20. Nesby-O'Dell S, Scanlon KS, Cogswell ME, et al. Hypovitaminosis D prevalence and determinants among African American and white women of reproductive age: third National Health and Nutrition Examination Survey, 1988–1994. *Am J Clin Nutr.* 2002;76:187–192.

21. Di Daniele N, Carbonelli MG, Candeloro N, et al. Effect of supplementation of calcium and vitamin D on bone mineral density and bone mineral content in peri-and post-menopausal women: a double-blind, randomized, controlled trial. *Pharmacol Res.* 2004;50:637–641.

22. Dawson-Hughes B, Harris SS, Krall EA, et al. Effect of calcium and vitamin D supplementation on bone density in men and women 65 years of age or older. *N Engl J Med.* 1997;337:670–676.

23. Lips P, Graafmans WC, Ooms ME, et al. Vitamin D supplementation and fracture incidence in elderly persons. A randomized, placebo-controlled clinical trial. *Ann Intern Med.* 1996;124:400–406.

24. Dawson-Hughes B, Harris SS, Krall EA, et al. Rates of bone loss in postmenopausal women randomly assigned to one of two dosages of vitamin D. *Am J Clin Nutr.* 1995;61:1140–1145.

25. Dawson-Hughes B, Dallal GE, Krall EA, et al. Effect of vitamin D supplementation on wintertime and overall bone loss in healthy postmenopausal women. *Ann Intern Med.* 1991;115:505–512.

26. Amin S, LaValley MP, Simms RW, et al. The role of vitamin D in corticosteroid-induced osteoporosis: a meta-analytic approach. *Arthritis Rheum.* 1999;42:1740–1751.

27. Meyer H, Smedshaug GB, Kvaavik E, et al. Can vitamin D supplementation reduce the risk fracture in the elderly? A randomized controlled trial. *J Bone Miner Res.* 2002;17: 709–715.

28. Chapuy MC, Pamphile R, Paris E, et al. Combined calcium and vitamin D3 supplementation in elderly women: confirmation of reversal of secondary hyperparathyroidism and hip fracture risk: the Decalyos II study. *Osteoporos Int.* 2002;13:257–264.
29. Porthouse J, Cockayne S, King C, et al. Randomised controlled trial of calcium and supplementation with cholecalciferol (vitamin D3) for prevention of fractures in primary care. *BMJ.* 2005;330:1003.
30. Larsen ER, Mosekilde L, Foldspang A. Vitamin D and calcium supplementation prevents osteoporotic fractures in elderly community dwelling residents: a pragmatic population-based 3-year intervention study. *J Bone Miner Res.* 2004;19:370–378.
31. The RECORD Trial Group. Oral vitamin D3 and calcium for secondary prevention of low-trauma fractures in elderly people (Randomised Evaluation of Calcium Or vitamin D, RECORD): a randomised placebo-controlled trial. *Lancet.* 2005;365:1621–1628.
32. Krall EA, Wehler C, Garcia RI, et al. Calcium and vitamin D supplements reduce tooth loss in the elderly. *Am J Med.* 2001;111:452–456.
33. Heaney RP, Dowell MS, Hale CA, et al. Calcium absorption varies within the reference range for serum 25-hydroxyvitamin D. *J Am Coll Nutr.* 2003;22:142–146.
34. Pfeifer M, Begerow B, Minne HW, et al. Effects of a short term vitamin D and calcium supplementation on body sway and secondary hyperparathyroidism in elderly women. *J Bone Miner Res.* 2000;15:1113–1118.
35. Bischoff HA, Stahelin HB, Dick W, et al. Effects of vitamin D and calcium supplementation on falls: a randomized controlled trial. *J Bone Mineral Res.* 2003;18:343–351.
36. Martinez ME, Giovannucci EL, Colditz GA, et al. Calcium, vitamin D, and the occurrence of colorectal cancer among women. *J Natl Cancer Inst.* 1996;88:1375–1382.
37. Kearney J, Giovannucci E, Rimm EB, et al. Calcium, vitamin D, and dairy foods and the occurrence of colon cancer in men. *Am J Epidemiol.* 1996;143:907–917.
38. Hiatt RA, Krieger N, Lobaugh B, et al. Prediagnostic serum vitamin D and breast cancer. *J Natl Cancer Inst.* 1998;90:461–463.

Vitamin E

Vitamin E is an essential fat-soluble vitamin. The term *vitamin E* is the generic description for all tocopherol (alpha, beta, gamma, delta) and tocotrienol derivatives having the biologic activity of alpha tocopherol. There are eight naturally occurring vitamin E compounds in plants and numerous stereoisomers of synthetic vitamin E. However, according to the Food and Nutrition Board's 2000 report on antioxidants, vitamin E is only defined as alpha tocopherol. Alpha tocopherol is the most abundant and active of all the forms. It is also the primary form found in animal tissue, most concentrated in the plasma, liver, and adipose tissue. In foods, alpha and gamma tocopherols are generally the only isomers that have vitamin E activity (1–3).

Vitamin E deficiency is rare in healthy people but may occur in individuals with genetic abnormalities, fat malabsorption syndromes, cystic fibrosis, pancreatic insufficiency, short bowel syndrome, chronic steatorrhea, or patients receiving total parenteral nutrition (TPN) with inadequate vitamin E. Deficiency symptoms include peripheral neuropathy, hemolytic anemia, skeletal myopathy, ataxia, and retinopathy (1–3).

The main function of vitamin E is as a biologic antioxidant protecting cellular membranes from oxidative damage from peroxyl, hydroxyl, and superoxide radicals. In this role, it is critical in preventing the oxidation and peroxidation of polyunsaturated fatty acids (PUFAs) in and on the plasma membranes of cells. Several other functions of vitamin E have been identified in experimental studies that explain how the vitamin may be involved in protecting against heart disease. In vitro studies show that vitamin E inhibits low-density lipoprotein (LDL) oxidation. Oxidation of LDL is believed to contribute to cardiovascular disease. Vitamin E also inhibits protein kinase C activity (involved in smooth muscle cell proliferation and differentiation), thrombin formation (a hormone that stimulates aggregation), and intercellular and vascular adhesion molecules. Vitamin E also seems to enhance the expression of the rate-limiting enzymes cytosolic phopholipase A_2 and cyclooxygenase-1. This results in the release of prostacyclin, a potent vasodilator and inhibitor of platelet aggregation in humans (1–3).

Vitamin E supplements have become popular among the public because of several in vitro and some clinical studies suggesting that vitamin E in doses higher than achievable from the diet may have beneficial effects in cardiovascular disease, cancer, immune response, and other conditions related to oxidative stress. However, recent research does not show health benefits; instead it suggests that risk of cardiovascular events may increase with supplemental vitamin E at doses more than 250 IUs/day.

Media and Marketing Claims	Efficacy
Prevents heart disease	↓?
Prevents bladder cancer, prostrate cancer	↑?
Improves immune response	↑?
Improves cognition in individuals with Alzheimer's disease or dementia	↓?
Improves respiratory function	NR
Prevents cataracts	↔
Improves blood glucose control in diabetes	↔
Enhances exercise performance	NR

Safety

- The Tolerable Upper Intake Level (UL) for adults is 1,000 mg of any form of supplemental alpha tocopherol (equivalent to 1,500 IU natural, 1,100 IU synthetic vitamin E) (3).

- Using data from several randomized controlled vitamin E intervention trials, researchers assessed the dose-related morbidity and mortality associated with vitamin

E supplementation. The analysis included 135,967 participant data sets from 19 clinical trials (4). Dosage of vitamin E ranged from 16.5 to 2,000 IU/day, with 400 IU being the most frequent level of supplementation. Pooled all-cause mortality was significantly higher as doses of vitamin E increased above 250 IU/day. Study interpretation was somewhat limited by the fact that ill persons were included in several of the studies; however, this analysis suggests that supplementation more than 250 IU/day should not be encouraged until more is known about the safety of use, particularly long-term or among ill populations.

♦ In the ATBC Cancer Prevention Study, vitamin E supplements were associated with an increase in the number of deaths from hemorrhagic stroke in male smokers, although risk of ischemic stroke was lower and risk of total stroke death was unaffected by vitamin E (5).

♦ Daily dosages of 100 to 3,200 IU (66 to 2,112 mg) vitamin E for up to 5 years did not result in any short- or long-term toxicity in healthy volunteers, smokers, or in individuals with angina pectoris, diabetes, epilepsy, Parkinson's disease, tardive dyskinesia, or vascular disease (6).

♦ Use of high-dose vitamin E may be contraindicated in subjects with vitamin K–associated blood coagulation disorders or vitamin K deficiency (3,7). However, in one study, 800 to 1,200 IU (528 to 792 mg) doses of vitamin E did not influence prothrombin times in patients on warfarin therapy (8). Another small study reported that 900 IU (594 mg) daily for 12 weeks resulted in no changes in coagulation activity or laboratory values for kidney, liver, or thyroid function (9).

♦ In a double-blind, placebo-controlled trial supplementing 800 mg alpha tocopherol for 30 days to elderly subjects (> 65 years) showed no adverse effects (10).

Drug/Supplement Interactions

♦ Vitamin E may have an additive effect when combined with anticoagulant drugs (warfarin, heparin, aspirin) and other blood-thinning dietary supplements (eg, fish oil, ginkgo, garlic).

♦ The following may interfere with vitamin E absorption: bile acid sequestrants such as colestipol (for hypercholesterolemia), isoniazid (antibiotic), or mineral oil.

♦ Vitamin E may enhance the effects and reduce the dosage needed of cyclosporine (immune suppressant used to prevent transplant rejection).

♦ Vitamin E may potentially reduce cardiotoxicity associated with doxorubicin (chemotherapeutic drug).

♦ Vitamin E may increase blood levels of griseofulvin (antifungal for ringworm).

♦ Vitamin E may reduce efficacy of select chemotherapy agents such as cyclophosphamide, busulfan, thiotepa, and doxorubicin.

Key Points _____

♦ Evidence from controlled intervention trials suggests that supplemental vitamin E does not reduce the risk for cardiovascular disease and evidence from the HOPE long-term supplementation trial with 400 IU vitamin E suggests there may be an increased risk for cardiovascular hospitalization (11).

♦ The American Heart Association consensus statement on vitamin E recognizes the benefits of vitamin E supplementation as promising, but not proven (12). The statement was published in 1999 and has not been updated since the newer evidence indicating a lack of efficacy has been published in the past few years.

♦ Observational studies of vitamin E supplements and recent experimental trials do not support a protective role for vitamin E against cancer. If vitamin E is protective against cancer, it may be that the protection is derived from the synergistic effects of the vitamin in combination with other cancer-protective nutrients and phytochemicals found in foods.

♦ There is limited preliminary evidence that high-dose vitamin E supplements improve some immune function parameters in elderly subjects. The elderly population should be encouraged to consume vitamin E–rich plant foods and to consider low to moderate dose supplementation (50 to 200 IU) if diet is inadequate. More research is needed before specific recommendations can be made to this population.

♦ Preliminary evidence suggests that high doses of vitamin E may slow progression of Alzheimer's disease and reduce tardive dyskinesia, which requires further study.

♦ There is a paucity of evidence that dietary vitamin E is associated with improved lung function in elderly subjects. Results from the ATBC study are not suggestive of a benefit of vitamin E supplements in male smokers with chronic obstructive pulmonary disease. More research is needed to determine the potential role of vitamin E in lung function.

♦ According to observational studies, reduced incidence of cataracts is associated with reported vitamin E supplement use and with higher plasma concentrations of vitamin E. Clinical intervention trials are limited, but generally do not support a protective effect. More studies are needed to determine the potential role of vitamin E in cataract formation.

♦ Preliminary studies have shown improved metabolic parameters of patients with diabetes taking high doses of vitamin E. Additional controlled research is needed before recommendations can be made for this population.

♦ Although some studies reported that vitamin E supplements reduced oxidative damage from exercise, the overall effect on exercise performance has not been ergogenic. However, preliminary research under high-altitude conditions suggests a potential benefit with vitamin E supplements and requires further study.

Food Sources

The tocopherol content of the diet varies depending on time of harvest of vitamin E–containing plants, processing, storage, and food preparation techniques. Nearly two thirds of the vitamin E is lost during production of commercial oils. Furthermore, removing the germ from wheat and bleaching also destroys vitamin E. The mean daily intake for vitamin E in the United States is estimated at 7 to 11 mg for men and 7 mg for women; intake is primarily from vegetable and seed oils used in salad oils and margarine. Coconut and fish oils are poor sources (some fish oil supplements add vitamin E) (1,2).

Food	Alpha tocopherol, mg/serving
Wheat germ oil (1 Tbsp)	27.0
Kernels, sunflower seed (1 oz)	14.0
Oil, sunflower (1 Tbsp)	7.0
Hazelnuts/filberts (1 oz)	6.8
Oil, cottonseed (1 Tbsp)	5.3
Wheat germ (2 Tbsp)	4.9
Papaya (1)	3.4
Cereals, fortified (1 cup)	3.0–30.0
Peanut butter (2 Tbsp)	3.0
Oil, canola (1 Tbsp)	2.9
Avocado (1)	2.3
Mango (1)	2.3
Nuts, Brazil (1 oz)	2.2
Mustard greens (½ cup)	1.4
Broccoli (½ cup)	1.3
Butter (1 Tbsp)	0.2

Source: Data are from reference 13.

Dosage Information/Bioavailability

Vitamin E is available in single preparations, in antioxidant "cocktails," or in multivitamin/mineral supplements in doses ranging from 10 to 800 IU. Mixed tocopherol and tocotrienol supplements are also available. Both natural and synthetic forms of vitamin E are sold in the free form or bound to succinate or acetate. Natural vitamin E is derived from plant raw materials after several chemical processing steps and is designated on labels as *d*-alpha-tocopherol (or RRR-alpha-tocopherol). Synthetic vitamin E is designated as *d,l*-alpha-tocopherol (or *all-rac*-alpha-tocopherol). To date, most of the studies examining the benefits of vitamin E supplements have used the synthetic *d,l*-alpha-tocopherol form. (The RRR- and *all-rac*-alpha-tocopherol are the correct terms for *d* and *d,l*-alpha-tocopherol, respectively, even though the *d* and *d,l* designations are sometimes used on supplement labels.)

Several studies have shown that the natural form is absorbed more efficiently and is more biologically active than synthetic vitamin E (1,14,15). The absorption rate of dietary alpha tocopherol ranges from 50% to 70%. However, absorption decreases to less than 10% with pharmacologic doses (200 mg) (2). There is a dose-dependent increase in serum, erythrocyte, and platelet vitamin E levels with vitamin E supplementation (1).

The 1989 RDA was originally given in RRR-alpha-tocopherol equivalents (TE) expressed as milligrams (15). However, the new DRIs for vitamin E are based on alpha tocopherol only and do not include amounts obtained from the other seven naturally occurring forms historically called vitamin E (beta, gamma, delta, and the four tocotrienols). These other forms are not counted as contributing to requirements for vitamin E because they are not converted to alpha tocopherol in humans and are not easily recognized by the alpha tocopherol transfer protein in the liver. The new RDA for vitamin E is 15 mg/day (22 IU) of alpha tocopherol for women and men (3).

Supplement labels typically express vitamin E in International Units (IU), even though the DRIs are stated in milligrams. To determine the number of milligrams of alpha tocopherol in a supplement or food expressed in IUs, use the following conversion factors (3):

- If the form of vitamin E is "natural" (*d*-alpha-tocopherol or RRR-alpha-tocopherol), multiply IU by 0.67. For example, 30 IU of natural vitamin E = 20 mg alpha tocopherol (30 × 0.67).

- If the form of vitamin E is "synthetic" (*d,l*-alpha-tocopherol or *all-rac*-alpha-tocopherol) multiply IU by 0.45. For example, 30 IU of synthetic vitamin E = 13.5 mg alpha tocopherol (30 × 0.45).

Evidence suggests that supplementation with alpha tocopherol can negatively effect levels of gamma and delta tocopherols, which are also important to health (16). In this study 400 IU/day was associated with a 58% reduction in serum gamma tocopherol and a significant reduction in the number of subjects with detectable delta tocopherol as compared with placebo.

Relevant Research

Vitamin E and Cardiovascular Disease

- Epidemiological studies generally show an inverse relationship between vitamin E intake from food or supplements and coronary heart disease (17,18). Three large, prospective epidemiology studies (the Nurses' Health Study, the Health Professional's Follow Up Study, and the Established Populations for Epidemiologic Studies of the Elderly) reported that subjects who had used vitamin E supplements (> 100 IU [≈ 66 mg] for 2 or more years) had approximately 40% lower rates of coronary heart disease (1,19–21).

- In a well-publicized review analysis of seven randomized controlled clinical trials regarding the role of vitamin E supplementation in reducing cardiovascular disease risk, six of the seven studies indicated no significant relationship between vitamin E supplementation and cardiovascular disease (22). Studies cited included Linxian, China, ATBC, CHAOS, GISSI-P, HOPE, and HPS, which were conducted from 1993 through 2002. Outcomes assessed included nonfatal stroke, nonfatal myocardial infarction, or cardiovascular death. Although the higher incidence of hemorrhagic stroke in the vitamin E groups overall (136 vs 110 in placebo groups) received significant media attention, this differences was not statistically significant (odds ratio = 1.0).

◆ A meta-analysis published in *Lancet* in 2003 included seven studies, each with more than 1,000 subjects and vitamin E dosages ranging from 50 to 800 IU daily for 1.4 to 12 years of follow-up (23). A total of 81,788 patients were included in the analysis. Supplementation with vitamin E was not associated with reduced cardiovascular events or improved cardiovascular mortality to overall improved mortality as was initially hypothesized.

◆ Analysis of the effect of daily long-term vitamin E (400 IU) supplementation on cardiovascular events in the Heart Outcomes Prevention Evaluation (HOPE) study participants also showed no efficacy for longer-term vitamin E supplementation. In this analysis, relative risk for major cardiovascular events was 1.04. Of concern, long-term supplementation was associated with a significant increased relative risk for heart failure and hospitalizations for heart failure, and this finding was duplicated in the HOPE-TOO study (24).

◆ A subanalysis of subjects with renal insufficiency (n = 993) participating in the HOPE study showed that supplementation with 400 IU vitaman E/day vs placebo did not significantly reduce the risk of cardiovascular events or proteinuria (25).

◆ The Antioxidant Supplementation in Atherosclerosis Prevention (ASAP Trial) was initiated in the late 1990s to test the hypothesis that daily supplementation with vitamin E (136 IU) and 500 mg vitamin C would significantly reduce atherosclerosis in men and postmenopausal women, including both smokers and nonsmokers (n = 520) (26). All had elevated serum total cholesterol levels on enrollment. At the 3-year time point, men showed a beneficial effect in terms of carotid atherosclerosis, whereas women did not. The 6-year evaluation using carotid artery intima-media thickness as measured by ultrasound showed supplementation reduced progression of disease in all subjects by a mean of 26%, with a mean decrease in slope among men of 33% (as compared with placebo) and a mean 14% decrease in slope in women; the decrease in slope for women was nonsignificant. Efficacy tended to be higher in those with lower baseline ascorbic acid levels and less initial plaque buildup.

◆ In a study designed to test the use of vitamins C and E in improving endothelial function in hyperlipidemic children, a randomized, placebo-controlled design was used. Fifteen children with familial disease were recruited and randomly assigned to either 500 mg vitamin C plus 400 IU vitamin E or placebo for 6 weeks concurrent with the NCEP Step II diet, which was initiated 4.5 months before supplementation started and continued during supplementation. This study suggested a significant difference in flow-mediated dilation of the brachial artery with antioxidant use as compared with placebo, despite no significant improvements in inflammatory or oxidative stress biomarkers (27). Although pilot in nature, these findings support the need for further research as to the application of antioxidant supplementation in children with high risk disease.

◆ The Heart Protection Study (HPS) was initiated among 20,536 at-risk adults to determine the efficacy of statin or statins plus or minus antioxidants or placebo in modulating cardiovascular morbidity and mortality (28) using a muticenter, randomized, double-blind, placebo-controlled trial design. Although statins were proven to be highly effective in reducing total mortality (–12%) and CHD events (–24%), there was no significant benefit associated with daily supplementation with 250 mg vitamin C, 650 mg E, and 20 mg beta carotene.

◆ A meta-analysis pooling the four randomized trials (see subsequent trial descriptions for details of these studies) completed in Europe and America (total number of subjects = 51,000) reported no effect of vitamin E on cardiovascular or ischemic heart disease mortality and nonfatal myocardial infarction (29).

◆ In a double-blind, placebo-controlled study conducted in 19 countries (HOPE study), 2,545 women and 6,996 men (age > 55 years) at high risk for cardiovascular events were randomly assigned to receive 400 IU (268 mg) per day of natural source vitamin E or a placebo. After 4.5 years, vitamin E had no effect on total mortality, cardiovascular death, myocardial infarction, or stroke. There were also no significant differences between groups in secondary cardiovascular outcomes (unstable angina, congestive heart failure, revascularization or amputation, diabetes complications, or cancer) (11).

◆ In a double-blind, placebo-controlled trial, 27,271 Finnish male smokers from the Alpha Tocopherol Beta Carotene (ATBC) cancer prevention study (age 50 to 69 years) with no history of myocardial infarction (MI) were randomly assigned to receive 50 mg alpha tocopherol, 20 mg beta carotene, both supplements, or a placebo for 5 to 8 years. The following variables were controlled in the statistical analysis: smoking, age, blood pressure, alcohol intake, BMI, activity level, diet, history of angina and diabetes, and serum concentrations of vitamin E and beta carotene. Neither supplement affected the incidence of nonfatal MI. There was an insignificant 8% decrease in the incidence of fatal coronary disease with vitamin E supplementation. The authors concluded that: "Supplementation with a small dose of vitamin E has only a marginal effect on the incidence of fatal coronary heart disease in male smokers with no history of MI, but no influence on nonfatal MI" (30). In addition, follow-up ATBC studies showed no cardiovascular benefit with supplemental vitamin E in 1,862 male subjects with a history of MI (31) and in 1,795 male subjects with angina.

◆ In a double-blind, placebo-controlled study (Cambridge Heart Antioxidant Study [CHAOS]), 2,002 patients with angiographically proven atherosclerosis were randomly assigned to receive alpha tocopherol (800 IU [≈ 528 mg] for 546 patients, 400 IU [≈ 264 mg] for remainder) or a placebo daily for a median of 510 days. Plasma alpha tocopherol concentrations increased in vitamin E–supplemented subjects, but not in placebo subjects. In vitamin E–supplemented subjects, there was a significant 77% reduction in the risk of nonfatal MI compared with the placebo (14 vs 41 incidents). However, there was an nonsignificant excess of cardiovascular deaths in the vitamin E group (27 vs 23). The authors concluded: "In patients with symptomatic coronary atherosclerosis, alpha-tocopherol treatment substantially reduces the risk of nonfatal MI, with beneficial effects apparent after 1 year of treatment. The effect of alpha-tocopherol treatment on cardiovascular deaths requires further study" (32).

♦ In a short-term, double-blind, placebo-controlled study, 40 men with mildly elevated cholesterol were randomly assigned to receive 80 mg alpha tocopherol plus 140 mg tocotrienol or a single supplement of 80 mg alpha tocopherol for 6 weeks. There were no significant differences between groups in LDL or HDL cholesterol, triglycerides, lipoprotein A, or lipid peroxide concentrations (33).

Vitamin E and Cancer

♦ The HOPE study conducted to assess the relationship between supplemental vitamin E and cancer or cardiovascular events included longer term extension data from 3,994 subjects (11). This randomized, placebo-controlled trial used a dosage of 400 IU vitamin E daily for a mean follow-up of 7 years. Cancer incidence was not associated with vitamin E supplementation nor was cancer mortality.

♦ Earlier evidence showed a 32% reduction in prostate cancer risk with vitamin E supplementation. Analysis of serum levels of alpha tocopherol and gamma tocopherol among the 29,133 Finnish males (ATBC study) participating suggested that gamma tocopherol status was not significantly associated with a reduced risk for prostate cancer, although the P for trend was .05 with alpha tocopherol supplementation. This may indicate either an increase in the requirement or utilization of vitamin E in male smokers who are at increased risk for prostate cancer (34).

♦ The Cancer Prevention Study II also provided an opportunity to assess the role of vitamin E in prostate cancer (35). Self-reported data on vitamin E use was available from 1982 through 1999, including 4,281 diagnosed prostate cancer cases. Multivariant adjusted analysis indicated no protective effect of vitamin E supplementation at a frequency of more than 4 times weekly, nor was supplementation associated with earlier stage disease as might be suggested. This lack of effect was also evidenced for smokers.

♦ In a multicenter, double-blind, placebo-controlled trial of antioxidant supplementation for the prevention of head and neck cancer, 540 patients with early-stage disease who previously received radiation therapy were randomly assigned to daily beta carotene (30 mg) plus vitamin E (400 IU) or placebo for continuous therapy lasting 3 years (36). After study initiation, the beta carotene supplement was discontinued, but alpha tocopherol supplementation continued for up to a median of 52 months (unclear how blinding was sustained with this change in protocol). In the end, supplementation was associated with an increased risk for second primary cancers (HR = 2.88) and recurrence (HR = 1.86). Although the authors suggest events were significantly reduced after the discontinuation of supplementation, this is unclear in that the confidence intervals included 1.0 and the number of events reported after discontinuation was relatively small (as it was likely the study was not powered in terms of sample size to answer this second hypothesis).

♦ The US Cancer Prevention Study II that included 991,522 patients followed prospectively for 16 years tested the hypothesis that regular vitamin E supplementation was protective against bladder cancer. In this cohort, daily self-reported vitamin E supplementation for more than 10 years' duration was associated with a 40% reduction in risk for bladder cancer (RR = 0.60; 95% CI = 0.37–0.96) (37). Of interest, shorter duration of use was not effective in reducing risk. This data speak to the biological nature of carcinogenesis, supporting the notion that this is a multidecade process.

♦ In an observational study (American Cancer Society's Cancer Prevention Study II cohort), 711,891 men and women completed a health questionnaire in 1982 and were followed for 14 years for mortality. During that time, 4,404 deaths from colorectal cancer occurred. After adjustment for risk factors of colorectal cancer, regular use of vitamin E or C supplements was not associated with a decreased risk (38).

♦ In a double-blind, placebo-controlled study, 29,133 male smokers in the ATBC Cancer Prevention Study were randomly assigned to receive 50 mg alpha tocopherol, 20 mg beta carotene, both, or a placebo daily for 5 to 8 years. During that time 135 subjects developed colorectal cancers that were histologically confirmed. Colorectal cancer incidence was lower in the vitamin E group, but this difference did not reach statistical significance (39). A follow-up data analysis published in 2003, which included additional cases, showed no significant association between alpha tocopherol supplementation and colorectal cancer (40).

♦ In the ATBC study, vitamin E supplements were associated with significantly fewer incident cases of prostate cancer (99 vs 151 cases). There was an insignificant reduction in colorectal cancers (68 vs 81 cases) and an insignificant increased risk in stomach cancer (70 vs 56 cases) (41). Follow-up analyses of patients who developed prostate cancer showed no significant associations between baseline serum alpha tocopherol, dietary vitamin E, or vitamin E supplementation and prostate cancer (40,42).

♦ In the double-blind, placebo-controlled ATBC study, 2,132 men were identified as having atrophic gastritis. Of these subjects, 1,344 had upper gastrointestinal endoscopy after a median of 5.1 years of supplementation with vitamin E, beta carotene, both, or a placebo. Neither supplement had any association with the end-of-trial prevalence of gastric neoplasia after adjustment for other possible risk factors. This effect was not modified by baseline serum or dietary intake of vitamins or presence of *Helicobacter pylori* infection (43).

♦ In the ATBC study, 409 male smokers ages 55 to 74 years were examined for oral mucosal lesions. There were no significant differences among the study groups either in prevalence of oral mucosal lesions or in the cells of unkeratinized epithelium (44).

Vitamin E and Immunity in the Elderly

◆ Daily multivitamin-minerals and vitamin E supplements were used in a randomized 2 × 2 factorial design studying the role of supplementation in reducing acute respiratory infections in the elderly (45). Six hundred fifty-two elderly independently living subjects residing in the Netherlands were recruited for the study. Vitamin E supplementation was at a dosage of 200 mg/day for approximately 18 months. Multivitamin-mineral supplementation did not modulate respiratory infection rates, nor did daily vitamin E. Severity of infections was also not reduced with vitamin E supplementation and in fact was increased. These data suggest that routine vitamin E supplementation among well nourished elderly is not indicated. Efforts to identify individuals with vitamin E–deficient diets or serum levels should be made as depleted subjects may be more responsive in terms of improved immune function and infection-related events/outcomes.

◆ In a randomized, placebo-controlled study of individuals residing in nursing homes, where deficient diets are more commonly identified due to age, diagnosis, and/or health status, 617 residents were randomly assigned to 200 IU of vitamin E or placebo daily. Vitamin E supplementation showed no clinical efficacy in terms of incidence or number of days of lower respiratory infections. However, vitamin E supplementation was associated with a nonsignificant reduced incidence of common cold ($P = .06$) (46). In addition, among subjects who were compliant (based on serial measures of plasma vitamin E every 3 months) with the daily vitamin E supplementation, a protective effect for vitamin E was observed with regard to acquiring one or more respiratory infections during the 1-year intervention period (RR = 0.88; 95% CI = 0.75–0.99).

◆ In a double-blind, placebo-controlled study, 161 healthy elderly subjects (ages 65 to 80 years) were randomly assigned to receive either vitamin E (either 50 or 100 mg) or a placebo daily for 6 months. Cellular immune responsiveness (CIR) was measured in vivo by delayed-type hypersensitivity (DTH) skin tests and in vitro by measuring the peripheral mononuclear cell production of interleukin 2 (IL-2), interferon-gamma (a T helper cell type 1 cytokine), interleukin-4 (a typical T helper cell type 2 cytokine) after stimulation with phytohemagglutinin. Both DTH scores and IL-2 production showed a trend toward increased responsiveness with increasing doses of vitamin E, but this trend was not significant. In a subgroup analysis, elderly subjects who were apparently healthy but had a low DTH response or were less physically active at baseline had an enhanced DTH response after a 6-month supplementation with 100 mg vitamin E compared with use of a placebo. However, this difference was not significant when adjusted for multiple comparisons. No effect of 100 mg vitamin E was observed on T helper cell type 1 and type 2 cytokine production. The authors concluded that before vitamin E supplement use is widely recommended, new clinical trials should be conducted to assess whether vitamin E, possibly via an improvement of cellular immune responsiveness, is effective in reducing the morbidity of infectious diseases (47).

◆ In a double-blind, placebo-controlled study, 88 healthy subjects older than 65 years were randomly assigned to one of four groups for 235 days: (*a*) 60 mg vitamin E, (*b*) 200 mg vitamin E, (*c*) 800 mg vitamin E, or (*d*) a placebo. All subjects had normal serum vitamin E concentrations at the baseline. DTH skin response; antibody response to hepatitis B, tetanus and diphtheria, and pneumococcal vaccines; and autoantibodies to DNA and thyroglobulin were assessed before and after supplementation. Supplementation with vitamin E for 4 months improved certain clinically relevant indexes of cell-mediated immunity. Subjects taking 200 mg had a 65% increase in DTH and a 6-fold increase in antibody titer to hepatitis B compared with placebo (17% and 3-fold, respectively), 60 mg (41% and 3-fold, respectively), 800 mg (49% and 2.5-fold, respectively). The subjects taking 200 mg also had a significant increase in antibody titer to tetanus vaccine. Subjects with the highest tertile of serum alpha tocopherol concentrations after supplementation had significantly higher antibody response to hepatitis B and DTH. All findings were significant. Vitamin E had no effect on antibody titer to diphtheria and did not change immunoglobulin levels or T and B cell levels. There were no adverse effects observed (48).

◆ In a double-blind, placebo-controlled trial, 83 healthy subjects older than 65 years were randomly assigned to receive 100 mg alpha tocopherol or a placebo daily for 3 months. Cellular immune responsiveness was measured by the in vitro response of peripheral blood mononuclear cells (PBMC) to the mitogens concanavalin A and phytohemagglutinin. Additionally, the humoral immune response was tested by measuring immunoglobulin antibody concentrations (IgG4 and IgA) against common antigens. Vitamin E supplementation was associated with a significant 51% increase in plasma levels of alpha tocopherol compared with no change in the placebo group. No significant changes were observed in cellular immune responsiveness in either group. There was no effect of vitamin E on immunoglobulin levels. However, in the control group, there was a small but significant increase in certain immunoglobulin levels against antigens. The authors concluded that 100 mg of vitamin E did not seem to have a beneficial effect on the overall immune response in elderly subjects (49).

Vitamin E and Neuropsychiatric Disorders

◆ In a double-blind, placebo-controlled study (Alzheimer's Disease Cooperative Study), 341 patients with Alzheimer's disease were randomly assigned to receive one of four treatments daily for 2 years: (*a*) 2,000 IU (1,320 mg) alpha tocopherol; (*b*) 10 mg selegiline (selective monoamine oidase inhibitor); (*c*) both alpha tocopherol and selegiline; or (*d*) a placebo. The primary outcome was the time to the occurrence of any of the following: death, institutionalization, loss of the ability to perform basic activities of daily living, or severe dementia. Despite randomization, the baseline score on the Mini-Mental State Examination was higher in the placebo group than in any of the other three groups, and this variable was predictive of the primary outcome. In the unadjusted analyses, there were no significant differences in the outcomes among the four groups. After adjustment, there were significant delays in the time to the primary outcome for patients treated with vitamin E (670 days), selegiline (655 days), and combination therapy (585 days), compared with the placebo (440 days) (50).

◆ A study of plasma levels of vitamin E in patients with dementia (including 43 with dementia, 15 with Alzheimer's disease, and 28 with senile dementia) and matched control subjects, showed that plasma vitamin E was not significantly associated with diagnosis of dementia (51). Dementia was verified using standardized Mini-Mental State Examination cognitive measurement tools.

◆ A retrospective chart review was conducted using data from the medical records of 130 patients who attended a Memory Disorder Clinic and whose medical records indicated they were taking 1,000 IU vitamin E with 5 mg donepezil daily for the treatment of Alzheimer's disease (a treatment approach that was commonly recommended at the clinic) for a minimum of 12 months (52). Patients were selected based on diagnosed dementia and Alzheimer's disease using standardized measurement instruments, including the Mini-Mental State Examination. Overall, there was a favorable response; however, the study lacked a placebo group, and optimally the study should be repeated using a 2 × 2 factorial design or a crossover approach with an adequate washout between treatments.

◆ In a double-blind, placebo-controlled study, 35 patients with tardive dyskinesia (TD) (29 diagnosed with schizophrenia, 6 diagnosed with mood disorder) were randomly assigned to receive 1,600 IU (1,056 mg) alpha tocopherol or a placebo for 2 months. Patients were assessed using the Abnormal Involuntary Movement Scale (AIMS) and Brief Psychiatric Rating Scale. In a subgroup of 23 patients, instrumental measurements of dyskinesia were assessed. There was a significant reduction of dyskinesia in the vitamin E group, but not the placebo group, on both the AIMS and the instrumental assessments. The overall reduction in AIMS was 24% in the vitamin E group. Of the vitamin E–treated subjects, there was a greater reduction in mean AIMS score (35%) in a subgroup of patients with TD for 5 years or less compared with the reduction (11%) in patients with TD for more than 5 years. No changes in Parkinsonism (tremor, muscle rigidity) were observed (53).

Vitamin E and Pulmonary Function

◆ In an observational study, dietary intakes of vitamin E and C and lung function were assessed in 178 elderly subjects (ages 70 to 96 years) selected on the basis of reported respiratory symptoms. After adjustment for age, gender, height, smoking, total energy intake, and vitamin C intake, vitamin E intake was significantly associated with FEV_1 (forced expiratory volume in 1 second) and forced vital capacity (FVC). For every extra milligram increase in vitamin E in the daily diet, FEV_1 increased by an estimated 42 mL and FVC by an estimated 54 mL (54).

◆ In the ATBC study, 50 mg/day alpha tocopherol did not influence symptoms of chronic obstructive pulmonary disorders in middle-aged male smokers, but there was a reported beneficial effect of dietary intake of fruits and vegetables rich in vitamin E and beta carotene (55). In addition, results from the ATBC study did not report a reduction in lung cancer with vitamin E supplements (56).

Vitamin E and Cataracts/Age-Related Maculopathy

◆ A randomized, placebo-controlled trial of 500 IU vitamin E in soy oil or placebo taken daily for 4 years by patients with early or no indication of cataracts showed that vitamin E supplementation and placebo group subjects demonstrated similar rates of cataract incidence over time (57). Posterior subscapsular cataracts were slightly more frequent in the placebo group but did not reach statistical significance (P = .08). Patients completed cataract extraction surgery at similar rates as well. In a separate analysis from this same study, early age-related macular degeneration was identified at similar rates over the same 4-year intervention period regardless of treatment assignment (500 IU vitamin E or placebo daily) (58).

◆ In a prospective study (Nurses' Health Study cohort), 478 nondiabetic women ages 53 to 73 years were given several food frequency questionnaires over the course of 13 to 15 years. The prevalence of nuclear lens opacities was significantly less with increasing duration of use of vitamin C, E, and multivitamins. However, only vitamin C supplement use remained significantly associated with nuclear opacities after mutual adjustment for use of vitamin E or multivitamin. Plasma vitamins C and E were also inversely related to prevalence of age-related nuclear lens opacities (59).

◆ In a prospective epidemiological study (Beaver Dam Eye Study), nuclear opacity was assessed in 1,354 subjects (ages 43 to 84 years) using lens photographs taken at the baseline and at 5-year follow-up. After 5 years, 246 subjects developed a nuclear cataract in at least one eye. Antioxidant intakes were assessed using a food frequency questionnaire at baseline (assessing intake during the previous year and 10 years before baseline). Median intake of vitamin E was 3.7 mg in the lowest quintile and was 28.3 mg in the highest quintile. In the overall group, nuclear cataracts were not significantly related to intake of vitamin E or C. However, these vitamins were inversely associated with opacities in subjects who had other risk factors for cataracts. Lutein was the only carotenoid associated with a significant reduction in cataract incidence (60). In a subgroup of the Beaver Dam Eye Study, serum tocopherols (alpha plus gamma) were inversely related to the incidence of cataracts (after adjusting for age, smoking, serum cholesterol, heavy drinking, adiposity, and dietary linoleic acid intake) (61).

◆ In a prospective epidemiological study (Longitudinal Study of Cataract), dietary intake, use of vitamin supplements, and plasma levels of vitamin E were assessed in 764 male and female subjects (mean age 64 years; 47% had nuclear opacities in at least one eye) at baseline and at yearly follow-up visits for 4 years. The risk of nuclear opacification at follow-up was decreased by 31% in regular users of multivitamin supplements, by 57% in vitamin E supplement users, and by 42% in subjects with higher plasma levels of vitamin E. The authors concluded: "Because these data are based on observational studies only, the results are suggestive but inconclusive" (62).

◆ In a random sample of 1,828 participants from the ATBC study, supplementation with 50 mg alpha tocopherol per day was not associated with the end-of-trial prevalence of nuclear, cortical, or posterior subscapsular cataract when adjusted for possible confounders. The authors concluded that supplementation with alpha tocopherol or beta carotene for 5 to 8 years does not influence cataract prevalence among middle-aged, male smokers (63).

Vitamin E and Diabetes

◆ An epidemiological analysis of data from participants enrolled in the Atherosclerotic Risk in Communities Study evaluated the association between established diabetic retinopathy and intake of vitamins C and E (64). In this study no association was seen for overall intake of vitamin E and retinopathy; however, separate analysis for those taking vitamin E supplements (of varying doses) for more than 3 years showed a 50% reduction in risk for those taking vitamin E (RR = 0.5; 95% CI = 0.2–0.8). Further research in this population is warranted, particularly with an a priori hypothesis, given the effect size can now be estimated for sample size estimates.

◆ The HOPE and MICRO-HOPE substudy tested the hypothesis that vitamin E modulates cardiovascular and microvascular health in patients with type 2 diabetes (24). A total of 3,654 patients were enrolled in this 2 × 2 factorial design and randomly assigned to (*a*) 400 IU vitamin E, (*b*) ramipril, (*c*) a combination of vitamin E and ramipril, or (*d*) placebo. Vitamin E had no effect on cardiovascular-related disease in individuals with type 2 diabetes.

◆ In a double-blind, placebo-controlled, crossover study, 20 elderly, nonobese subjects with normal glucose tolerance were randomly assigned to receive 900 mg vitamin E or a placebo daily for 4 months each. After each study period, subjects underwent a euglycemic hyperinsulinemic glucose clamp. All subjects were eating a weight-maintenance diet providing 250 or more grams of carbohydrate and 13.8 mg (± 0.6 mg) vitamin E per day. (The authors did not provide data on diet administration or compliance.) In each subject, the pattern of daily vitamin E intake (assessed by dietary records) was accounted for in the statistical analysis. Vitamin E supplementation was related to a significant improvement in whole-body glucose disposal compared with the placebo. Net changes in plasma vitamin E were significantly correlated with net changes in insulin-stimulated glucose disposal. Plasma triglycerides and free fatty acids were significantly reduced with vitamin E supplementation. The authors concluded that vitamin E supplements may be useful in improving insulin action in the elderly, but "further studies will need to clarify the safety and the exact pharmacological mechanisms by which such results may be achieved" (65).

Vitamin E and Exercise Performance

◆ A study of seven trained cyclists used a four-tiered supplementation approach with placebo plus placebo, followed by 1 g vitamin C plus placebo, followed by 200 IU vitamin E and 1 g vitamin C, and, finally, by 400 IU vitamin E plus placebo (66). Subjects were then tested at 70% VO_{2max} workloads using the cycle ergometer. Only vitamin E supplementation was associated with reduced oxidative damage as measured by malondialdehyde (MDA) levels. Vitamin C supplementation increased MDA levels in both the resting and exercise state as compared with placebo, but sample size was too small to test the statistical significance.

♦ In a double-blind study of repeated bouts of resistance exercise, the hypothesis tested was that vitamin E supplementation of 1,200 IU after each repeat bout of exercise would improve recovery in men who are not resistance-trained (67). Nine subjects received vitamin E and nine subjects received a placebo for a period of 3 weeks. After 3 weeks of supplementation, subjects completed three separate resistance training sessions, each separated by a 3-day recovery period. No difference in muscle soreness, performance, or plasma MDA levels (a marker of oxidative stress) were shown between vitamin E and placebo groups.

♦ Vitamin E efficacy in controlling exercise-related oxidative stress was tested in the context of eccentric exercise (in which muscles are stretched as they try to contract, such as skiing or running downhill) where supplementation was provided to both young and older males (68). Thirty-two subjects participated in this 12-week supplementation trial using 1,000 IU vitamin E daily or placebo. A downhill race for 45 minutes at 75% VO_{2max} was completed at baseline and after 12 weeks. Vitamin E supplementation was associated with reduced peak serum creatine kinase levels (indicating reduced muscle damage) in the young, but not older males. It was also associated with reduced resting and postexercise levels of isoprostanes, a measure of lipid peroxidation that has been associated with heart disease risk.

♦ In a double-blind, placebo-controlled study, nine young (ages 22 to 29 years) and 12 older (ages 55 to 74 years) sedentary men were randomly assigned to receive 800 IU ($\approx$ 528 mg) alpha tocopherol or a placebo daily for 48 days. After 48 days, there was a significant increase in vitamin E concentrations in plasma and skeletal muscle (assessed by biopsy). Subjects then performed a bout of eccentric exercise at 75% of their maximum heart rate by running on a treadmill with a downward incline for 45 minutes. All vitamin E–treated subjects excreted significantly less urinary thiobarbituric acid adducts (marker of oxidative damage) after exercise than did placebo subjects at 12 days postexercise (35% and 18% more than baseline in young and old subjects, respectively) (69).

♦ In a double-blind, placebo-controlled study, 13 mountaineers were given 400 mg vitamin E daily (divided into two doses) or a placebo for 4 weeks at the start of an expedition in Nepal. For 4 weeks before the climb, all subjects were given a vitamin/mineral supplement without vitamin E. Erythrocyte filterability, blood viscosity, and three blood coagulation factors were measured at the baseline (base camp at 1,500 meters) and twice at high altitude (4,300 meters) after supplementation. Both groups experienced a marked increase in hematocrit levels during the ascent because of an increase in erythrocytes and leukocytes. The erythrocyte filterability did not change in the vitamin E group but showed a significant impairment in the control group. The placebo group had a significantly higher blood viscosity compared with subjects taking vitamin E supplements. In the placebo group, but not in the vitamin

E group, the protein C activity (a vitamin K–dependent coagulation factor) decreased significantly. The authors concluded: "All the parameters investigated indicate that an extended stay at high altitude in combination with physical exertion can impair the flow characteristics of blood. Supplementation with vitamin E appears to be a suitable prophylactic measure" (70).

References

1. Weber P, Bendich A, Machlin LJ. Vitamin E and human health: rationale for determining recommended intake levels. *Nutrition.* 1997;13:450–460.
2. Traber MG. Vitamin E. In: Shils ME, Olson JA, Shike M, et al, eds. *Modern Nutrition in Health and Disease.* 9th ed. Baltimore, Md: Williams & Wilkins; 1999:347–362.
3. Institute of Medicine. *Dietary Reference Intakes: Vitamin C, Vitamin E, Selenium, and Carotenoids.* Washington, DC: National Academy Press; 2000.
4. Miller ER 3rd, Pastor-Barriuso R, Dalal D, et al. Meta-analysis: high-dosage vitamin E supplementation may increase all-cause mortality. *Ann Intern Med.* 2005;142:37–46.
5. Leppala JM, Virtamo J, Fogelholm, et al. Controlled trial of alpha-tocopherol and beta-carotene supplements on stroke incidence and mortality in male smokers. *Arterioscler Thromb Vasc Biol.* 2000;20:230–235.
6. Bendich A. Safety issues regarding the use of vitamin supplements. *Ann N Y Acad Sci.* 1992;669:300–310.
7. Diplock AT. Safety of antioxidant vitamins and beta-carotene. *Am J Clin Nutr.* 1995;62(6 Suppl):S1510-S1516.
8. Kim JM, White RH. Effect of vitamin E on the anticoagulant response to warfarin. *Am J Cardiol.* 1996;77:545–546.
9. Kitagawa M, Mino M. Effects of elevated d-alpha (RRR)-tocopherol dosage in man. *J Nutr Sci Vitaminol (Tokyo).* 1989;35:133–142.
10. Meydani SN, Meydani M, Rall LC, et al. Assessment of the safety of high-dose, short-term supplementation with vitamin E in healthy older adults. *Am J Clin Nutr.* 1994;60:704–709.
11. Lonn E, Bosch J, Yusuf S, et al. Effects of long-term vitamin E supplementation on cardiovascular events and cancer: A randomized controlled trial. *JAMA.* 2005;293:1338–1347
12. Tribble DL. AHA Science Advisory. Antioxidant consumption and risk of coronary heart disease: emphasis on vitamin C, vitamin E, and beta-carotene: a statement for healthcare professionals from the American Heart Association. *Circulation.* 1999;99:591–595.
13. Pennington JA. *Bowes & Church's Food Values of Portions Commonly Used.* 17th ed. Philadelphia, Pa: Lippincott; 1998.
14. Ferslew KE, Acuff RV, Daigneault EA, et al. Pharmacokinetics and bioavailability of the RRR and all racemic stereoisomers of alpha-tocopherol in humans after single oral administration. *J Clin Pharmacol.* 1993;33:84–88.
15. National Research Council. *Recommended Dietary Allowances.* 10th ed. Washington, DC: National Academy Press; 1989.

16. Huang HY, Appel LJ. Supplementation of diets with alpha-tocopherol reduces serum concentrations of gamma- and delta-tocopherol in humans. *J Nutr.* 2003;133:3137–3140.

17. Rexrode KM, Manson JE. Antioxidant and coronary heart disease: observational studies. *J Cardiovasc Risk.* 1996;3:363–367.

18. Kushi LH, Folsom AR, Prineas RJ, et al. Dietary antioxidant vitamins and death from coronary heart disease in postmenopausal women. *N Engl J Med.* 1996;334:1156–1162.

19. Stampfer MJ, Rimm EB. Epidemiologic evidence for vitamin E in prevention of cardiovascular disease. *Am J Clin Nutr.* 1995;62(6 Suppl):S1365-S1369.

20. Stampfer MJ, Hennekens CH, Manson JE, et al. Vitamin E consumption and the risk of coronary disease in women. *N Engl J Med.* 1993;328:1444–1449.

21. Losonczy KG, Harris TB, Havlik RJ. Vitamin E and vitamin C supplement use and risk of all-cause and coronary heart disease mortality in older persons: the Established Populations for Epidemiologic Studies of the Elderly. *Am J Clin Nutr.* 1996;64:190–196.

22. Eidelman RS, Hollar D, Hebert PR, et al. Randomized trials of vitamin E in the treatment and prevention of cardiovascular disease. *Arch Intern Med.* 2004;164:1552–1556.

23. Vivekananthan DP, Penn MS, Sapp SK, et al. Use of antioxidant vitamins for the prevention of cardiovascular disease: meta-analysis of randomised trials. *Lancet.* 2003;361:2017–2023.

24. Lonn E, Yusuf S, Hoogwerf B, et al. Effects of vitamin E on cardiovascular and microvascular outcomes in high-risk patients with diabetes: results of the HOPE study and MICRO-HOPE substudy. *Diabetes Care.* 2002;25:1919–1927.

25. Mann JF, Lonn EM, Yi Q, et al. Effects of vitamin E on cardiovascular outcomes in people with mild to moderate renal insufficiency: results of the HOPE study. *Kidney Int.* 2004;65:1375–1380.

26. Salonen RM, Nyyssonen K, Kaikkonen J, et al. Six-year effect of combined vitamin C and E supplementation on atherosclerotic progression: the Antioxidant Supplementation in Atherosclerosis Prevention (ASAP) Study. *Circulation.* 2003;107:947–953.

27. Engler MM, Engler MB, Malloy MJ, et al. Antioxidant vitamins C and E improve endothelial function in children with hyperlipidemia: Endothelial Assessment of Risk from Lipids in Youth (EARLY) Trial. *Circulation.* 2003;108:1059–1063.

28. Heart Protection Study Collaborative Group. MRC/BHF Heart Protection Study of antioxidant vitamin supplementation in 20,536 high-risk individuals: a randomised placebo-controlled trial. *Lancet.* 2002;360:23–33.

29. Dagenais GR, Marchioli R, Yusuf S, et al. Beta-carotene, vitamin C, and vitamin E and cardiovascular diseases. *Curr Cardiol Rep.* 2000;2:293–299.

30. Virtamo J, Rapola JM, Ripatti S, et al. Effect of vitamin E and beta carotene on the incidence of primary nonfatal myocardial infarction and fatal coronary heart disease. *Arch Intern Med.* 1998;158:668–675.

31. Rapola JM, Virtamo J, Ripatti S, et al. Randomized trial of alpha-tocopherol and beta-carotene supplements on incidence of major coronary events in men with previous myocardial infarction. *Lancet.* 1997;349:1715–1720.

32. Stephens NG, Parsons A, Schofield PM, et al. Randomised controlled trial of vitamin E in patients with coronary disease: Cambridge Heart Antioxidant Study. *Lancet.* 1996;347:781–786.

33. Mensink RP, van Houwelingen AC, Kromhout D, et al. A vitamin E concentrate rich in tocotrienols had no effect on serum lipids, lipoproteins, or platelet function in men with mildly elevated serum lipid concentrations. *Am J Clin Nutr.* 1999;69:213–219.

34. Weinstein SJ, Wright ME, Pietinen P, et al. Serum alpha-tocopherol and gamma-tocopherol in relation to prostate cancer risk in a prospective study. *J Natl Cancer Inst.* 2005;97:396–399.

35. Rodriguez C, Jacobs EJ, Mondul AM, et al. Vitamin E supplements and risk of prostate cancer in U.S. men. *J Cancer Epidemiol Biomarkers Prev.* 2004;13:378–382.

36. Bairati I, Meyer F, Gelinas M, et al. A randomized trial of antioxidant vitamins to prevent second primary cancers in head and neck cancer patients. *J Natl Cancer Inst.* 2005;97:481–488.

37. Jacobs EJ, Henion AK, Briggs PJ, et al. Vitamin C and vitamin E supplement use and bladder cancer mortality in a large cohort of US men and women. *Am J Epidemiol.* 2002;156:1002–1010.

38. Jacobs EJ, Connell CJ, Patel AV, et al. Vitamin C and vitamin E supplement use and colorectal cancer mortality in a large American Cancer Society cohort. *J Cancer Epidemiol Biomarkers Prev.* 2001;10:17–23.

39. Albanes D, Malila N, Taylor PR, et al. Effects of supplemental alpha-tocopherol and beta-carotene on colorectal cancer: results from a controlled trial (Finland). *Cancer Causes Control.* 2000;11:197–205.

40. Virtamo J, Pietinen P, Huttunen JK, et al. Incidence of cancer and mortality following alpha-tocopherol and beta-carotene supplementation: a postintervention follow-up. *JAMA.* 2003;290:476–485.

41. Albanes D, Heinonen OP, Huttunen JK, et al. Effects of alpha-tocopherol and beta-carotene supplements on cancer incidence in the Alpha-Tocopherol Beta-Carotene Cancer Prevention Study. *Am J Clin Nutr.* 1995;62(6 Suppl):S1427–S1430.

42. Hartman TJ, Albanes D, Pietinen P, et al. The association between baseline vitamin E, selenium, and prostate cancer in the alpha-tocopherol, beta-carotene cancer prevention study. *Cancer Epidemiol Biomarkers Prev.* 1998;7:335–340.

43. Varis K, Taylor PR, Sipponen P, et al. Gastric cancer and premalignant lesions in atrophic gastritis: a controlled trial on the effect of supplementation with alpha-tocopherol and beta-carotene. The Helsinki Gastritis Study Group. *Scand J Gastroenterol.* 1998;33:294–300.

44. Liede K, Hietanen J, Saxen L, et al. Long-term supplementation with alpha-tocopherol and beta-carotene and prevalence of oral mucosal lesions in smokers. *Oral Dis.* 1998;4:78–83.

45. Graat JM, Schouten EG, Kok FJ. Effect of daily vitamin E and multivitamin-mineral supplementation on acute respiratory tract infections in elderly persons: a randomized controlled trial. *JAMA.* 2002;288:715–721.

46. Meydani SN, Leka LS, Fine BC, et al. Vitamin E and respiratory tract infections in elderly nursing home residents. *JAMA* [erratum in *JAMA.* 2004;292:1305]. 2004;2929:828–836.

47. Pallast EG, Schouten EG, de Waart FG, et al. Effect of 50- and 100-mg vitamin E supplements on cellular immune function in noninstitutionalized elderly persons. *Am J Clin Nutr.* 1999;69:1273–1281.

48. Meydani SN, Meydani M, Blumberg JB, et al. Vitamin E supplementation and in vivo immune response in healthy elderly subjects. A randomized controlled trial. *JAMA.* 1997;277:1380–1386.

49. de Waart FG, Portengen L, Doekes G, et al. Effects of three months of vitamin E supplementation on indices of the cellular and humoral immune response in elderly subjects. *Br J Nutr.* 1997;78:761–774.

50. Sano M, Ernesto C, Thomas RG, et al. A controlled trial of selegiline, alpha-tocopherol, or both as treatment for Alzheimer's disease. The Alzheimer's Disease Cooperative Study. *N Engl J Med.* 1997;336:1216–1222.

51. Charlton KE, Rabinowitz TL, Geffen LN, et al. Lowered plasma vitamin C, but not vitamin E, concentrations in dementia patients. *J Nutr Health Aging.* 2004;8:99–107.

52. Klatte ET, Scharre DW, Nagaraja HN, et al. Combination therapy of donepezil and vitamin E in Alzheimer disease. *Alzheimer Dis Assoc Disord.* 2003;17:113–116.

53. Lohr JB, Caligiuri MP. A double-blind, placebo-controlled study of vitamin E treatment of tardive dyskinesia. *J Clin Psychiatry.* 1996;57:167–173.

54. Dow L, Tracey M, Villar A, et al. Does dietary intake of vitamins C and E influence lung function in older people? *Am J Respir Crit Care Med.* 1996;154:1401–1404.

55. Rautalahti M, Virtamo J, Haukka J, et al. The effect of alpha-tocopherol and beta-carotene supplementation on COPD symptoms. *Am J Respir Crit Care Med.* 1997;156: 1447–1452.

56. Albanes D, Heinonen OP, Taylor PR, et al. Alpha-Tocopherol and beta-carotene supplements and lung cancer incidence in the alpha-tocopherol, beta-carotene cancer prevention study: effects of base-line characteristics and study compliance. *J Natl Cancer Inst.* 1996;88:1560–1570.

57. McNeil JJ, Robman L, Tikellis G, et al. Vitamin E supplementation and cataract: randomized controlled trial. *Ophthalmology.* 2004;111:75–84.

58. Taylor HR, Tikellis G, Robman LD, et al. Vitamin E supplementation and macular degeneration: randomized controlled trial. *BMJ.* 2002;325:11–16.

59. Jacques PF, Chylack LT, Hankinson SE, et al. Long-term nutrient intake and early age-related nuclear opacities. *Arch Ophthalmol.* 2001;119:1009–1019.

60. Lyle BJ, Mares-Perlman JA, Klein BE, et al. Antioxidant intake and risk of incident age-related nuclear cataracts in the Beaver Dam Eye Study. *Am J Epidemiol.* 1999;149: 801–809.

61. Lyle BJ, Mares-Perlman JA, Klein BE, et al. Serum carotenoids and tocopherols and incidence of age-related nuclear cataract. *Am J Clin Nutr.* 1999;69:272–277.

62. Leske MC, Chylack LT, He Q, et al. Antioxidant vitamins and nuclear opacities: the longitudinal study of cataract. *Ophthalmology.* 1998;105:831–836.

63. Teikari JM, Virtamo J, Rautalahti M, et al. Long-term supplementation with alpha-tocopherol and beta-carotene and age-related cataract. *Acta Ophthalmol Scand.* 1997;75:634–640.

64. Millen AE, Klein R, Folsom AR, et al. Relation between intake of vitamin C and E and risk of diabetic retinopathy in the Atherosclerosis Risk Communities Study. *Am J Clin Nutr.* 2004;79:865–873.

65. Paolisso G, Di Maro G, Galzerano D, et al. Pharmacological doses of vitamin E and insulin action in elderly subjects. *Am J Clin Nutr.* 1994;59:1291–1296.

66. Bryant RJ, Ryder J, Martino P, et al. Effects of vitamin E and C Supplementation either alone or in combination on exercise-induced lipid peroxidation in trained cyclists. *J Strength Cond Res.* 2003;17:792–800.
67. Avery NG, Kaiser JL, Sharman MJ, et al. Effects of vitamin E supplementation on recovery from repeated bouts of resistance exercise. *J Strength Cond Res.* 2003;17: 801–809.
68. Sacheck JM, Milbury PE, Cannon JG, et al. Effect of vitamin E and eccentric exercise on selected biomarkers of oxidative stress in young and elderly men. *Free Radic Biol Med.* 2003;34:1575–1588.
69. Meydani M, Evans WJ, Handelman G, et al. Protective effect of vitamin E on exercise-induced oxidative damage in young and older adults. *Am J Physiol.* 1993;264(5 Pt 2): R992–R998.
70. Simon-Schnass I, Korniszewski L. The influence of vitamin E on rheological parameters in high altitude mountaineers. *Int J Vitam Nutr Res.* 1990;60:26–34.

Vitamin K

Vitamin K is a fat-soluble vitamin and is found in two forms in nature. Vitamin K1 (phylloquinone) is found in plants. Vitamin K2 (menaquinone) is found in foods of animal origin and is synthesized by several different types of bacteria. There is a synthetic form known as vitamin K3 (menadione). The "K" comes from the German word *koagulation,* because coagulation is one of its essential roles. Vitamin K is essential for the synthesis of multiple proteins required for the normal coagulation of blood and is also plays a large role in hemostasis (1). As a cofactor to the carboxylase that generates gamma-carboxyglutamic acid, vitamin K goes through a reduction-oxidation cycle that allows for its reuse. This is important because the body stores very little vitamin K. Individuals with clotting problems are prescribed coumarin-based oral anticoagulants, such as warfarin (Coumadin), to inhibit coagulation by acting as a vitamin K antagonist.

In the last decade, vitamin K has been recognized for its important role in maintaining bone health. Three vitamin K–dependent proteins have been isolated from bone tissue: osteocalcin, matrix gla protein, and anticoagulant protein S. Clinical trials have demonstrated that pharmacological doses of vitamin K2 can decrease loss of bone density and decrease fracture rates (2). In one clinical trial, physiological doses of vitamin K1 decreased loss of bone density in postmenopausal women (3).

Media and Marketing Claims	Efficacy
Prevents and treats hypoprothrombinemia	NR
Prevents excessive blood thinning associated with warfarin use	↑
Improves bone density	NR

Safety

Vitamin K is considered safe at recommended dosages. The AI is 90 µg for women and 120 µg for men. No Tolerable Upper Intake Limit (UL) has been set, and deficiencies are rare except in newborns, who require a single dose of supplementation at birth. Full-term newborns are given a 1 mg injection at birth; premature infants should receive a reduced dose of 0.5 mg, and infants under 2 pounds at birth should receive only 0.3 mg/kg.

Drug/Supplement Interactions

Vitamin K may interact with aspirin, antibiotics, anticoagulant/antiplatelet drugs, doxorubicin, laxatives, weight-loss medications, anti-seizure medications, and warfarin. Individuals should consult a physician before beginning a vitamin K regimen.

Key Points

- ◆ Vitamin K is effective at preventing and treating hypoprothrombinemia (abnormally high thrombin content of the blood, which often leads to intravascular coagulation) (4).

- ◆ Vitamin K supplementation is prescribed when it is necessary to reverse the anticoagulant effects of warfarin.

- ◆ While there have been positive reports of vitamin K2 reducing loss of bone density and reducing fractures (5), another study found it ineffective in preventing osteoporosis in postmenopausal women when used alone (6). One study has reported that vitamin K1 reduces bone loss in postmenopausal women (3).

- ◆ Researchers have determined that the function of osteocalcin, protein found in bone that contributes to bone density, is dependent on vitamin K nutriture (7).

Food Sources

Food	Vitamin K, µg/serving
Kale, cooked (½ cup)	531
Collards, frozen (½ cup cooked)	530
Spinach, frozen (½ cup cooked)	514
Turnip greens, cooked (½ cup)	265
Brussels sprouts, cooked (½ cup)	150
Broccoli, cooked (½ cup)	110
Leaf lettuce, green (1 cup)	97.2
Cabbage, cooked (½ cup)	36
Asparagus, boiled (4 spears)	30.4

Source: Data are from reference 8.

Dosage Information/Bioavailability

Vitamin K is available in topical cream, capsule, tablet, softgel, and injection. There are no standard recommendations for vitamin K supplementation; however, the Adequate Intake (AIs) are: adolescents, 75 µg; men, 120 µg; women, 90 µg; pregnant women, 90 µg; lactating women, 90 µg (9).

Relevant Research

Vitamin K and Coagulation

- Hypoprothrombinemia can be caused by a vitamin K deficiency. Researchers noted that patients receiving high dose interleukin-2 therapy frequently developed hypoprothrombinemia. Investigators theorized that the increased prothrombin time was caused by a deficiency of clotting factors synthesized by the liver and that vitamin K replacement could prevent the hypoprothrombinemia. In a prospective study of 16 patients (9 control group, 7 treatment group) on interleukin-2 therapy, none of the vitamin K–treated patients developed hypoprothrombinemia. In three of the nine control subjects prothrombin time increased significantly (10). More studies are warranted to determine if prophylactic vitamin K supplementation is effective for other medical treatments of this nature.

- Although warfarin-associated elevations in clotting time can be medically managed either more passively by withholding warfarin until levels come down to appropriate range, they can also be treated using vitamin K supplementation to produce a more immediate response in patients at greater risk for hemorrhagic events related to elevated clotting times. The following studies describe the role of vitamin K supplementation in warfarin-associated coagulopathy.

- A multicenter, double-blind, placebo-controlled, randomized trial of the treatment of warfarin-associated coagulopathy with oral vitamin K included 92 subjects with INRs (International Normalized Ratio For Prothrombin Activity) between 4.5 and 10 (normal goal for therapy is between 2 and 3). Subjects were randomly assigned, half received a placebo, and half took 1 mg/day of oral vitamin K. Each group temporarily discontinued warfarin treatment (time not reported). In the treatment group, a significantly greater number of subjects showed the target reduction in INR at day 1 after treatment as compared with "respondent" subjects in the control group. The treatment group also had fewer bleeding episodes during the 3-month follow-up period than the control group (11).

- In a multicenter, randomized, open-label, controlled trial investigating the effectiveness of oral vitamin K vs subcutaneous vitamin K for the treatment of warfarin-induced coagulopathy, 51 patients subjects with INR between 4.5 and 10 were recruited. Twenty-six subjects were assigned to the oral vitamin K group and 25 were assigned to the subcutaneous vitamin K group. Both groups were removed from there usual warfarin treatment for 1 day prior to supplementation. INR was tested at baseline and 1 day after treatment. A significant number of subjects in the oral vitamin K group demonstrated normal therapeutic INR levels the day after treatment when compared with the subcutaneous group (12). This study provides more support for oral vitamin K when treating warfarin-associated coagulopathy.

Vitamin K and Osteoporosis

♦ Associations between vitamin K intake, apo E genotype, bone mineral density (BMD), and hip fracture, vitamin K intake were assessed in 335 men and 553 women (mean age 75 years) participating in the Framingham Heart Study. This sample population was comprised of subjects who had complete diet data (collected using a food-frequency questionnaire) and complete bone mineral density and follow-up fracture data. Results showed that women in the highest quartile of reported vitamin K intake had a significantly lower relative risk of developing a hip fracture as compared with the lowest quartile (13). However, BMD was not associated with dietary vitamin K intake in men or women. Apo E genotype did not seem to modulate any of the associations between dietary vitamin K intake and bone health in this study population, despite subjects with apo E2 allele having the highest serum phylloquinone concentrations in this and other research studies. (13).

♦ In a randomized controlled study to investigate the effect of vitamin K2 on BMD compared with vitamin D3 and estrogen-progestin replacement therapy (hormone replacement therapy [HRT]), 72 healthy postmenopausal women were assigned to one of four treatment groups: (*a*) untreated control group, (*b*) hormonal replacement therapy with conjugated equine estrogen at dose of 0.625 mg/day, (*c*) 1.0 g/day vitamin D3, or (*d*) 45 mg/day vitamin K2. BMD was analyzed by dual energy x-ray absorptiometry at baseline and after 6 and 12 months of treatment. A combination of vitamin K2 and vitamin D3 supplementation reduced BMD loss compared with placebo, whereas HRT increased BMD during the 1-year treatment (6).

♦ In a randomized controlled study (unblinded) to investigate the efficacy of vitamin K2 and D3 in BMD, 172 postmenopausal women with osteopenia or osteoporosis were given (*a*) 45 mg vitamin K2, (*b*) 1 μg vitamin D3, (*c*) a combination of vitamins K2 and D3, or (*d*) a controlled diet plan (milk with meals) for 2 years. BMD was evaluated by dual energy x-ray absorptiometry at baseline and every 6 months. Bone metabolism and blood coagulation factors were also evaluated. Vitamin K2 supplementation was associated with a greater increase in BMD than control (diet) at 18 and 24 months, but not prior to 18 months. The combination therapy of both vitamins had significant positive effects on bone mineral density at all time points, including a 5.88% increase in BMD above baseline at 6 months, 5.85% at 12 months, 5.01% at 18 months, and 4.92% at 24 months. Vitamin K2 alone had very little effect on bone mineralization or coagulation activity (14).

References

1. Vitamin K. Oregon State University Linus Pauling Institute Micronutrient Information Center. Available at: http://lpi.oregonstate.edu/infocenter/vitamins/vitaminK. Accessed May 26, 2005.
2. Weber P. Vitamin K and bone health. *Nutrition.* 2001;17:880–887.

3. Braam LA, Knapen MH, Geusens P, et al. Vitamin K1 supplementation retards bone loss in postmenopausal women between 50 and 60 years of age. *Calcif Tissue Int.* 2003;73:21–26.

4. McKevoy GK, ed. *AHFS Drug Information.* Bethesda, Md: American Society of Health-System Pharmacists; 1998.

5. Shiraki M, Shiraki Y, Aoki C, et al. Vitamin K_2 (menatetrenone) effectively prevents fractures and sustains lumbar bone mineral density in osteoporosis. *J Bone Miner Res.* 2000;15:515–521.

6. Iwamoto I, Kosha S, Noguchi S, et al. A longitudinal study of the effect of vitamin K_2 on bone mineral density in postmenopausal women: a comparative study with vitamin D_3 and estrogen-progestin therapy. *Maturitas.* 1999;31:161–164.

7. Binkley NC, Kreuger DC, Kawahara TN, et al. A high phylloquinone intake is required to achieve maximal osteocalcin gamma-carboxylation. *Am J Clin Nutr.* 2002;76:1055–1060.

8. USDA National Nutrient Database for Standard Reference, Release 18. Available at: http://www.nal.usda.gov/fnic/foodcomp/search/index.html. Accessed May 8, 2006.

9. Institute of Medicine. *Dietary Reference Intakes for Vitamin A, Vitamin K, Arsenic, Boron, Chromium, Copper, Iodine, Iron, Manganese, Molybdenum, Nickel, Silicon, Vanadium, and Zinc.* Washington, DC: National Academy Press; 2000.

10. Birchfield GR, Rodgers GM, Girodias KW, et al. Hypoprothrombinemia associated with interleukin-2 therapy: correction with vitamin K. *J Immunother.* 1992;11:71–75.

11. Crowther MA, Julian J, McCarty D, et al. Treatment of warfarin-associated coagulopathy with oral vitamin K: a randomized trial. *Lancet.* 2000;356:1551–1553.

12. Crowther MA, Douketis JD, Schnurr T, et al. Oral vitamin K lowers the international normalized ratio more rapidly than subcutaneous vitamin K in the treatment of warfarin-associated coagulopathy. *Ann Intern Med.* 2002;137:251–254.

13. Booth SL, Tucker KL, Chen H, et al. Dietary vitamin K intakes are associated with hip fracture but not with bone mineral density in elderly men and women. *Am J Clin Nutr.* 2000;71:1201–1208.

14. Ushiroyama T, Ikeda A, Ueki M. Effect of continuous combined therapy with vitamin K_2 and vitamin D_3 on bone mineral density and coagulofibrinolysis function in postmenopausal women. *Maturitas.* 2002;41:211–221.

Wheat Grass and Barley Grass

Wheat and barley are grains that have been farmed for centuries for use in breads and cereals. Wheat grass (also known as intermediate wheat grass or sprouted wheat) is a relative of wheat that is grown for hay or planted on pastures where cattle, sheep, or horses graze. More recently, the freshly sprouted young leaves of wheat or barley grasses have been crushed to make a beverage or dried into tablets and powders. The dried extract of young barley leaves is widely used in Japan as a supplement. Both of these grasses, like other leafy vegetables, contain vitamins, minerals, and other phytochemicals important in human health (1–3).

Note: Wheat grass and barley grass are not related to, and should not be confused with, wheat germ.

Media and Marketing Claims	Efficacy
Acts as an antioxidant	NR
Enhances immunity	NR
A nutrient-dense food	↓
Reduces cholesterol	NR

Safety

There are no studies testing the safety of supplementing the diet with liquid or dried juices of wheat or barley grasses.

Drug/Supplement Interactions

Theoretically, vitamin K content of wheat grass or barley grass may interfere with blood-thinning medications (eg, warfarin [Coumadin]).

Key Points

♦ Extracts from wheat and barley grasses have demonstrated antioxidant and antimutagenic properties in vitro. This effect may be due to the chlorophyll as well as beta carotene and alpha tocopherol content. Chlorophyll is also present in similar amounts in many green vegetables (leaf lettuce, spinach, broccoli, etc) that also have been shown to possess antimutagenic activity in vitro. Animal and human studies are needed to determine whether the in vitro antioxidant activity of wheat or barley grasses also occurs in vivo (4).

♦ One laboratory study reported that wheat and barley grasses and the green algae *Chlorella* were potent stimulators of macrophages in vitro. Controlled clinical trials are needed to determine the effects of wheat or barley grass extracts on immune function and oxidative DNA damage in humans.

♦ The liquid or dried extracts of wheat or barley grasses, like any dried extract of a plant, provide a concentrated source of certain nutrients in a small volume (2 to 4 teaspoons). However, the contribution of these grasses to the overall vitamin and mineral content of the diet is relatively small (*see* Dosage Information/ Bioavailability). In addition, pills and powders do not provide the fiber found in whole vegetables. It is also not known whether processing the extracts alters the content or bioavailability of phytochemicals in wheat and barley grasses.

♦ There is currently no evidence from well-controlled clinical trials demonstrating a cholesterol-reducing effect of wheat or barley grasses.

Food Sources

Fresh-squeezed wheat grass or barley grass juice (available at health-food stores and juice bars)

Dosage Information/Bioavailability

Fresh wheat or barley grass juices are available at many health food stores and juice bars. The extract is dried to form tablets or powders, usually in doses equivalent to 2 to 9 g (usually 2 to 3 teaspoons of powder). Several supplements combine different ingredients such as wheat and barley grass, algae *(Spirulina, Chlorella),* kelp, brown rice extract, bee pollen, probiotics, and other herbs.

Nutritional analysis of 10 g (dry weight) of wheat grass indicates that it provides 39 kcal, 1.5 g protein, 8.5 g carbohydrate, less than 1 g fat, less than 1 g fiber, 1.2 RE beta carotene, 0.04 mg thiamin, 0.02 mg riboflavin, 0.61 mg niacin, 0 µg vitamin B-12, 0.01 mg vitamin E, 7.6 µg folate, 0.4 mg iron, 16 mg magnesium, 6 mg calcium, 33 mg potassium, 8.5 µg selenium, and 0.33 mg zinc (5).

Nutrient analysis provided by one manufacturer's combination of dried wheat and barley grasses (10 g) reportedly contains 1.6 g protein, 7.4 g carbohydrate, 0.08 g fat, 180 RE beta carotene, 0.08 mg thiamin, 0.12 mg riboflavin, 2.0 µg vitamin B-12, 100 mg calcium, and 1.6 mg iron.

Relevant Research

Wheat and Barley Grasses and Immunity and In Vitro Antioxidant Activity

- ◆ In an in vitro study, a flavonoid isolated from freeze-dried young barley leaves (2"-*O*-glycosylisovitexin [2"-*O*-GIV]) demonstrated antioxidant activity almost equivalent to that of alpha tocopherol. In other in vitro studies, 2"-*O*-GIV demonstrated antioxidant activity against glyoxal (potent mutagenic compound) formation from the oxidation of three fatty acid ethyl esters and against malonaldehyde and acetaldehyde formation in lipid peroxidation systems (3,6,7).

- ◆ In an in vitro study, green barley enhanced macrophage activity. When a commercial combination of dried plant extracts (young barley, wheat grass, *Chlorella* [a green algae], and *Laminaria* [kelp]) was tested, there was a greater effect on macrophage activity. An in vitro mutagenicity assay demonstrated that the combination of dried plant extracts inhibited bacterial mutation induced by a chemical procarcinogen alfla-toxin B$_1$ and the binding of this carcinogen to calf thymus DNA (8).

- ◆ A randomized, double-blind, placebo-controlled study conducted among 23 patients with ulcerative colitis provided preliminary evidence that daily wheat grass juice for 1 month resulted in a 4-fold reduction in gastrointestinal bleeds and bowel movements and improved global health assessment. It is unclear how the wheat grass juice placebo was developed to allow for blinding as wheat grass supplements have distinctive flavor and smell (9).

References

1. Becker R, Wagoner P, Hanners GD, et al. Compositional, nutritional, and function evaluation of intermediate wheatgrass *(Thinopyrum intermedium)*. *J Food Processing and Preservation.* 1991;15:63–77.
2. Osawa T, Katsuzaki H, Hagiwara Y, et al. A novel antioxidant isolated from young green barley leaves. *J Agric Food Chem.* 1992;40:1135–1138.
3. Nishiyama T, Hagiwara Y, Hagiwara H, et al. Inhibitory effect of 2"-O-glycosyl isovitexin on alpha-tocopherol on genotoxic glycoxal formation in lipid peroxidation system. *Food Chem Toxicol.* 1994;32:1047–1051.
4. Lai CN, Butler MA, Matney TS. Antimutagenic activities of common vegetables and their chlorophyll content. *Mutat Res.* 1980;77:245–250.
5. US Department of Agriculture. Agricultural Research Service. Nutrient Data Laboratory. Available at: http://www.ars.usda.gov/main/site_main.htm?modecode= 12354500. Accessed December 12, 2005.
6. Miyake T, Shibamoto T. Inhibition of malonaldehyde and acetaldehyde formation from blood plasma oxidation by naturally occurring antioxidants. *J Agric Food Chem.* 1998;46:3694–3697.
7. Kitta K, Hagiwara Y, Shibamoto T. Antioxidant activity of an isoflavonoid, 2"-O-glycosylisovitexin isolated from green barley leaves. *J Agric Food Chem.* 1992;40:1843–1845.
8. Lau BHS, Lau EW. Edible plant extracts modulate macrophage activity and bacterial mutagenesis. *Int Clin Nutr Rev.* 1992;12:147–155.
9. Ben-Arye E, Golden E, Wengrower D, et al. Wheat grass juice in the treatment of active distal ulcerative colitis a randomized double-blind placebo-controlled trial. *Scand J Gastroenterol.* 2002;4:444–9.

Whey Protein

Whey protein is a generic term that refers to various types of whey, including whey protein concentrates and isolates. Whey protein, a natural byproduct of cheese and casein production, is the yellow-green liquid that separates from the curd. Whey contains nearly 100% of the milk carbohydrate (lactose) and 20% of the total milk protein. Beta lactoglobulin and alpha lactalbumin make up about 70% to 80% of the protein in whey. Other constituents in the protein include rennet whey, bovine serum albumin, lactoferrin, immunoglobulins, cysteine, phospholipoproteins, and several enzymes (1).

Media and Marketing Claims	Efficacy
Builds muscle and improves exercise performance	↔
Improves immunity in individuals with HIV	NR
Acts as an anticancer agent	NR

Safety

- There are no long-term studies of whey protein supplementation in humans.

- Many products recommend consuming whey protein in amounts two to three times the Recommended Dietary Allowance for protein (0.8 g/kg). Individuals with hepatic encephalopathy and renal diseases should be cautioned against ingesting excess protein from protein supplements.

- Whey protein should be avoided by those diagnosed with allergies or severe sensitivities to milk or milk proteins. Individuals with lactose intolerance should not use whey protein concentrate because it does contain lactose. In contrast, whey protein isolate has insignificant quantities of lactose.

Drug/Supplement Interactions

No reported adverse interactions.

Key Points

- Although whey protein increased weight gain and improved nitrogen retention in injured or starving animals when compared with a diet of equivalent free amino acids, the effects must be examined more closely in humans. More evidence is needed to determine the effect of whey protein supplementation on muscle mass, and whether it does indeed have greater benefits on muscle anabolism than any other source of high-quality protein.

- Preliminary trials suggest that whey protein supplementation may increase muscle strength in some, but not all, laboratory measures of strength. These results need to be examined further in controlled trials with larger numbers of subjects.

- Whey protein seems to increase the glutathione levels of immune cells in animal studies and in small studies in humans, and thus may be beneficial to patients with HIV or cancer. However, controlled trials in large numbers of subjects are needed to determine if supplementation with whey protein improves the clinical outcomes in these patients.

- Whey protein has a similar protein quality (as measured by amino acid scores and protein digestibility) to other dietary protein sources, including nonfat and low-fat dairy, eggs, and lean meats.

- There is currently insufficient evidence to suggest that whey protein supplementation is indicated or contraindicated for cancer prevention.

Food Sources

Cow's milk (milk proteins are 20% whey and 80% casein)

Dosage Information/Bioavailability

Whey protein is sold as a powder. Whey protein products are sold in the pure form, hydrolyzed form, or with additional supplements such as creatine, glutamine, branched-chain amino acids (BCAA), and flavor enhancers. Some products recommend taking 25 to 50 g whey protein with a source of high-glycemic carbohydrate immediately after exercise, and an additional 25 g between meals and prior to bedtime (total whey protein intake = 100 to 125 g). The biological value of whey protein depends on the processing technique. Heat and mechanical processing may reduce the biological value of proteins (1).

Relevant Research

Whey Protein and Weight Gain

- Thermally injured guinea pigs (n = 45) fed diets containing whey protein (via gastrostomy feeding tube) maintained body weight and nitrogen retention better than the same diet containing corresponding free amino acids as the nitrogen source (2).

Whey Protein and Exercise Performance

- In a randomized, placebo-controlled trial, healthy young males and females (n = 23) were randomly assigned to consume 300 mL of beverage 1 hour after completing heavy resistance-training exercises. Seven subjects were assigned to placebo, seven to casein, and nine to whey proteins. Outcome was assessed using net muscle protein balance as determined from muscle biopsy samples as well as blood concentrations of free amino acids pre- and postexercise. Protein consumption resulted in net positive protein balance postexercise; whey protein resulted in improved leucine balance as compared with casein; and both protein solutions resulted in net positive phenylalanine concentrations (3).

- A double-blind, placebo-controlled, randomized trial was conducted among 44 healthy men (mean age 22 years, age range 18 to 35 years) to determine whether intake of a beverage supplement containing whey protein, creatine, and carbohydrate along with strength training promoted a significant increase in fat free mass, muscle strength, or anaerobic performance after 10 weeks of intervention. Forty-one subjects completed the study, and dropout rate was equal across groups. Both the supplement group and the control group showed an increase in fat-free mass with training, and there was no statistical difference between groups in terms of the increase. Similarly, supplementation was not associated with significant differences in repetition maximum strength, external work (leg press), or anaerobic capacity across the two groups. Both groups showed an improvement in each of these measures from baseline to end of study (4).

- In a double-blind, placebo-controlled study, 20 healthy young adults were randomly assigned to receive a whey protein concentrate (Immunocal, 10 g dose, twice daily) or an equivalent amount of casein placebo for 3 months. Muscular performance was assessed at baseline and at the end of the study by whole-leg isokinetic cycle testing (peak power and work capacity during a 30-second cycling sprint). Lymphocyte glutathione was used as a marker of tissue glutathione. (Glutathione is considered a major intracellular antioxidant, the synthesis of which is dependent on cysteine availability. Whey protein is a cysteine donor.) At baseline, there were no significant differences between groups (eg, body composition, height, weight, glutathione levels, or performance on muscular tests). Peak power and 30-second work capacity increased significantly in the whey protein group, but did not change in the placebo group. Additionally, lymphocyte glutathione increased in the whey protein group, but not in the placebo group. Body weight did not change significantly in either group, but the whey group had a decrease in percentage body fat (5).

♦ In a double-blind, placebo-controlled study, 36 male subjects were randomly assigned to receive one of three treatments during 6 weeks of resistance training: (*a*) whey protein (1.2 g/kg/day), (*b*) 1.2 g whey protein plus creatine monohydrate (0.1 g/kg/day), or a placebo (maltodextrin; 1.2 g/kg/day). Measures included lean tissue mass by dual energy x-ray absorptiometry, bench press and squat strength (one-repetition maximum), and knee extension/flexion peak torque. Lean tissue mass increased to a greater extent with training in the whey-creatine group compared with the other groups, and in the whey group compared with the placebo group. Bench press strength increased significantly more for the whey-creatine group compared with the whey and placebo groups. Knee extension peak torque increased significantly with training for the whey-creatine and whey groups, but not for the placebo group. Subjects who supplemented with creatine and/or whey protein had similar increases in squat strength and knee flexion peak torque compared with subjects who received the placebo (6).

Whey Protein and HIV/Immunity

♦ The role of long-term whey protein supplementation on plasma glutathione levels in individuals with HIV was tested in a 6-month randomized, double-blind clinical trial (7). Thirty subjects were randomly assigned to 45 g whey protein as either Protectamin or Immunocal for 1 week. Supplements were similar in protein, carbohydrate, and fat content, as well as trace elements; no vitamins were provided in the supplements. Each supplement was flavored with vanilla for blinding and administered three times daily in 5-g doses mixed with milk, yogurt, or buttermilk. After the initial week of supplementation, subjects were told which supplement they were receiving. Eighteen subjects continued on Protectamin for 6 months. Baseline glutathione levels (which are responsive to glutathione in the diet) were substantially less than plasma values measured in healthy blood donors. After 2 weeks of whey protein supplementation, glutathione levels increased regardless of product used; however, the 44% increase in glutathione in the Protectamin group was significant while the 24.5% increase in the Immunocal group was not. With continued supplementation for 6 months, glutathione levels remained at the increased level. The increased glutathione levels were not associated with any improvement in body weight, T-cell counts, or clinical status. Efforts to test these supplements in the context of improved disease outcomes are warranted.

♦ In a preliminary study of three individuals with HIV, a progressive daily dose of whey protein (8 to 39 g) during 3 months increased levels of the antioxidant glutathione in mononuclear cells. Subjects also experienced an increase in body weight. The whey protein in this study replaced other protein sources in the diet, keeping the total protein intake constant (8).

♦ In a 6-month study, aging mice fed a diet enriched with whey protein had increased liver and heart glutathione concentration and longer lifespans than casein diet–fed and Purina-fed mice (9).

Whey Protein and Cancer

♦ In an animal study, rats were fed whey, casein, meat, or soy protein–based diets and then injected with dimethylhydrazine to induce colon cancer. Whey and casein diets were more protective against the development and incidence of intestinal tumors than meat or soy protein diets (10).

♦ A review article discussed animal studies demonstrating that whey protein diets increase tissue glutathione concentrations (11). A follow-up review article presented animal data showing that whey protein concentrates have anticancer activity. The author of this article suggested that "this non-toxic intervention, which is not based on the principles of current cancer chemotherapy, will hopefully attract the attention of laboratory and clinical oncologists" (12).

References

1. Smithers GW, Ballard FJ, Copeland AD, et al. New opportunities from the isolation and utilization of whey proteins. *J Dairy Sci.* 1996;79:1454–1459.
2. Trocki O, Mochizuki H, Dominioni L, et al. Intact protein versus free amino acids in the nutrition support of thermally injured animals. *JPEN.* 1986;10:139–145.
3. Tipton KD, Elliott TA, Cree MG,, et al. Ingestion of casein and whey proteins result in muscle anabolism after resistance exercise. *Med Sci Sports Exerc.* 2004;36:2073–2081.
4. Chromiak JA, Smedley B, Carpenter W, et al. Effect of a 10-week strength training program and recovery drink on body composition, muscular strength and endurance, and anaerobic power and capacity. *Nutrition.* 2004;20:420–427.
5. Lands LC, Grey VL, Smountas AA. Effect of supplementation with a cysteine donor on muscular performance. *J Appl Physiol.* 1999;87:1381–1385.
6. Burke DG, Chilibeck PD, Davidson KS, et al. The effect of whey protein supplementation with and without creatine monohydrate combined with resistance training on lean tissue mass and muscle strength. *Int J Sport Nutr Exerc Metab.* 2001;11:349–364.
7. Micke P, Beeh KM, Buhl R. Effects of long-term supplementation with whey proteins on plasma glutathione levels of HIV-infected patients. *Eur J Nutr.* 2002;41:12–18.
8. Bounous G, Baruchel S, Falutz J, et al. Whey proteins as a food supplement in HIV-seropositive individuals. *Clin Invest Med.* 1993;16:204–209.

9. Bounous G, Gervais F, Amer V, et al. The influence of dietary whey protein on tissue glutathione and the diseases of aging. *Clin Invest Med.* 1989;12:343–349.

10. McIntosh GH, Regester GO, Le Leu RK, et al. Dairy proteins protect against dimethyl-hydrazine-induced intestinal cancers in rats. *J Nutr.* 1995;125:809–816.

11. Bounous G, Batist G, Gold P. Whey proteins in cancer prevention. *Cancer Lett.* 1991;57:91–94.

12. Bounous G. Whey protein concentrate (WPC) and glutathione modulation in cancer treatment. *Anticancer Res.* 2000;20:4785–4792.

Wild Yam *(Dioscorea villosa)*

As far back as the Mayans, people have been using the root of this climbing vine to treat pain. In the 18th century, herbalists began to prescribe wild yam to treat menstrual pain and problems related to childbirth. Some women currently take wild yam because they falsely believe that it is a natural source of progesterone. Wild yam does contain diosgenin (1,2), which can be converted into progesterone in the laboratory. However, the transformation is not possible in the human body. Wild yam has been used to treat a variety of ailments, but there are no scientific data to support its use.

Media and Marketing Claims	Efficacy
Treats menopausal symptoms	NR

Safety

- There have been no substantial reports of adverse reactions in clinical trials using either oral or topical preparations.
- Large doses of wild yam tincture have been reported to cause vomiting (3).

Drug/Supplement Interactions

None are known at this time.

Key Points

- A randomized study investigating the effects of topical applications of wild yam on menopausal symptoms found no significant differences between wild yam and placebo in weight changes, blood pressure, hormonal measures, or menopausal symptoms (4).
- There is no evidence that wild yam has any specific health benefits in humans.

Food Sources

None

Dosage Information/Bioavailability

Wild yam is available as a cream, gel, liquid, capsule, tincture, and tablet. There is no standard dosage.

Relevant Research

Wild Yam and Menopause

♦ In a double-blind, randomized, placebo-controlled, crossover study to investigate the safety and efficacy of the topical use of wild yam extract in the management of menopausal symptoms, 50 healthy, overweight (mean BMI 27.3) women, ages 45 to 60 years who reported menopausal symptoms and had not taken any hormone-containing therapy for the previous 6 weeks were randomly assigned to apply a wild yam extract cream (BioGest, AquaConnexions, Melbourne, Australia) or placebo to arms, legs, and abdomen twice daily for 3 months. No washout period was implemented between treatments. Only 23 subjects completed the 6 months of therapy. The high dropout rate was attributed by the investigators to "unrelieved symptoms" (19 dropouts were in the BioGest group and 9 in the placebo group). Effectiveness was determined by evaluation of symptom diaries maintained by subjects, including episodes of flushing and Likert-type scores for severity of menopausal symptoms (breast soreness, mood, libido, and energy levels). Blood and saliva samples were also collected at baseline and at the end of each 3 month period for lipid profile analysis and hormone status. No statistical difference was found in serum lipids, and serum hormone levels, including FSH, did not differ significantly between groups or compared with baseline. Flushing was significantly reduced from baseline, regardless of treatment group assignment, whereas night sweats were reduced significantly from baseline only among those on placebo (4).

♦ To assess the hormonal activities of 20 natural products and nutraceuticals, in vitro BT-474 breast carcinoma cells were used to detect biological activity. Cells were exposed to products in various dilutions, and supernatants were analyzed for expression of estrogen-responsive or androgen/progestin-responsive gene products by a modified ELISA technique. Wild yam root exhibited antiestrogenic activity, as did dong quai. Proestrogenic effects were found for grape seed and chamomile extracts (5).

References

1. Benghuzzi H, Tucci M, Eckie R, et al. The effects of sustained delivery of diosgenin on the adrenal gland of female rats. *Biomed Sci Instrum.* 2003;39:335–340.

2. Accatino L, Pizzaro M, Solis N, et al. Effects of diosgenin, a plant-derived steroid, on bile secretion and hepatocellular cholestasis induced by estrogens in the rat. *Hepatology.* 1998;28:129–140.

3. McGuffin M, Hobbs C, Upton R, et al, eds. *American Herbal Products Association's Botanical Safety Handbook.* Boca Raton, Fla: CRC Press; 1997.

4. Komesaroff PA, Black CV, Cable V, et al. Effects of wild yam extract on menopausal symptoms, lipids, and sex hormones in healthy menopausal women. *Climacteric.* 2001;4:144–150.

5. Rosenberg Zand RS, Jenkins DJ, Diamandis EP. Effects of natural products and nutraceuticals on steroid hormone-related gene expression. *Clinica Chimica Acta.* 2001;312:213–219.

Yohimbine/Yohimbe

Yohimbine is the major alkaloid in the bark of the yohimbe *(Pausinystalia yohimbe)* tree indigenous to West Africa. The bark is made up of 6% alkaloids, 10% to 15% of which are yohimbine. Yohimbine is an alpha 2-adrenergic antagonist that stimulates norepinephrine release. The bark is traditionally used as an aphrodisiac in Africa. Yohimbine, as a prescription drug, has been studied for its potential role in the treatment of sexual disorders and weight control (1).

Media and Marketing Claims	Efficacy
Increases sexual function	↓?
Aids in weight loss	NR
Builds muscle	NR

Safety

♦ There are no long-term studies evaluating the safety of yohimbine/yohimbe.

♦ Case reports have associated yohimbine ingestion (4 to 20 mg) with side effects including nervousness, insomnia, anxiety, urinary frequency, dizziness, tremors, headache, tachycardia, hypotension, hypertension, nausea and vomiting, bronchospasm, and lupus-like syndrome (1–5).

♦ Yohimbine/yohimbe is contraindicated in individuals with high or low blood pressure, bipolar disorder, existing liver and kidney disease, as well as individuals on tricyclic antidepressants (2,6).

♦ Yohimbe bark is not approved for use in Germany, a country that regulates herbal preparations, because of insufficient proof of efficacy and the "unforeseeable correlation between risk and benefit" (6).

- Low-tyramine diet is advisable with yohimbe use due to altered blood pressure.
- Medical supervision is advised.

Drug/Supplement Interactions

- There is a potential for toxic effects when yohimbine/yohimbe is combined with phenothiazines (for mental disorders), monoamine oxidase inhibitors, naloxone, antihypertensive drugs, sympathomimetic drugs, tricyclic antidepressants, or antidiabetes drugs.
- Yohimbine/yohimbe should not be used in combination with blood pressure medications because blood pressure control may be altered.

Key Points

- Clinical evidence supporting use of yohimbine/yohimbe as an aphrodisiac is lacking. A meta-analysis concluded that prescription yohimbine does seem to have a therapeutic benefit over placebo for erectile dysfunction. In the only study of women with hypoactive sexual desire, yohimbine had no benefit.
- There is insufficient evidence on the efficacy and safety of yohimbine/yohimbe to support its use in weight loss.
- Although yohimbine (in the form of the herbal supplement yohimbe bark) is marketed to body builders and athletes, there is currently a lack of research to support its use to enhance sport performance and muscle-building.

Dosage Information/Bioavailability

Yohimbine or yohimbine hydrochloride is available in tablet, capsule, and tincture form, with manufacturers recommending 10 to 20 mg/day divided into four doses. It is also available as a prescription drug. One study by FDA scientists found commercial products contained yohimbine but also contained undeclared diluents and were devoid of other alkaloids normally found in the tree bark (7). In one study of young males, 10 mg yohimbine hydrochloride increased peak plasma levels of yohimbine within 10 to 45 minutes after oral intake (8). Bioavailability ranged from 7% to 87%, with a mean value of 33%.

Relevant Research

Yohimbine and Sexual Function

- In a meta-analysis of seven controlled trials examining yohimbine therapy for erectile dysfunction, yohimbine was found to be superior to a placebo. The methodological quality of the studies was rated to be satisfactory. Despite other case reports of adverse effects, there were few serious adverse reactions reported in these seven trials (9).

- In a placebo-controlled, crossover design study, nine women with clinically diagnosed hypoactive sexual desire were assigned in random order to two treatment phases starting at the beginning of menses and continuing for 1 month each: (*a*) a placebo, or (*b*) 5.4 mg yohimbine three times daily. Daily logs of mood and sexual activity, and trimonthly blood drawings were obtained during an initial baseline month, followed by the two treatment cycles. When compared with healthy control subjects, subjects with hypoactive sexual desire had an insignificant trend toward lower plasma levels of 3-methyl-4-hydroxyphenylglycol (MHPG), the major metabolite of norepinephrine, at the baseline. Yohimbine treatment caused a sustained increase in plasma MHPG similar to previously reported levels in men. However, in this study, it had no therapeutic effect on improving sexual desire (10).

- In a double-blind, placebo-controlled trial, 86 men with erectile dysfunction without clearly detectable organic or psychological causes were given 30 mg yohimbine hydrochloride divided into three doses per day or a placebo for 8 weeks. Efficacy was determined by subjective criteria (self-evaluation of sexual desire, sexual satisfaction, frequency of intercourse, and quality of erection) and by objective criteria (improvement in penile rigidity). There were no statistical differences on subjective or objective measures alone. However, when objective responders and subjective responders were combined, yohimbine was significantly more effective than the placebo (71% vs 45%). Seven percent of the patients rated tolerability of yohimbine as fair or poor (11). The authors did not describe the adverse effects subjects experienced during treatment.

- In a double-blind, placebo-controlled, crossover study, 29 men with impotence of mixed etiology (organic or psychogenic) were given two 25-day treatments in random order: (*a*) 36 mg yohimbine hydrochloride/day, or (*b*) a placebo. Treatments were separated by a 14-day washout period. Erectile function, ejaculation, interest in sex, physical examination findings, blood pressure, pulse rate, weight, and audiovisual sexual stimulation test were evaluated before and after treatment. Yohimbine was no more effective than the placebo in treating mixed-type impotence in this study (12).

- In a double-blind, placebo-controlled, partial crossover study, 63 men with clinically diagnosed psychogenic impotence were randomly assigned to receive 15 mg yohimbine daily in conjunction with the antidepressant trazodone or a placebo for 8 weeks each. Erectile function, ejaculation, interest in sex, and sexual thoughts were investigated at the end of drug treatment and at 3- and 6-month follow-ups. Fifty-five patients (87%) completed the whole trial. Significantly improved clinical results were obtained in 71% of the patients who took the combination of yohimbine and trazodone compared with the placebo. However, the experimental design makes it impossible to attribute the effects to yohimbine, trazodone, or a combination of both (13).

- According to one review article, a study of intravenous yohimbine (0.30 mg/kg) administration to young, healthy volunteers reported no beneficial effects on penile circumference or sexual drive (1).

Yohimbine and Weight Loss

- In a double-blind, placebo-controlled, randomized study, 20 obese female outpatients were put on a low-energy diet (1,000 kcal/day) for 3 weeks (day 1 to 21). After this period, subjects continued on the diet for 3 more weeks (day 22 to 42) while taking 20 mg yohimbine divided into four doses or a placebo daily. Weight reduction did not differ between groups in the first 3 weeks of diet alone. During the second 3 weeks (day 22 to 42), subjects in the diet plus yohimbine group had a significant increase in mean weight loss compared with the placebo (3.55 kg vs 2.21 kg). Yohimbine had no effect on lipolysis as estimated by plasma glycerol levels measured at baseline and at the end of each 3-week period. At day 42, exercise energy expenditure (EEE) and resting energy expenditure (REE) were significantly lower in the placebo group than on day 0 and day 21. In yohimbine-supplemented subjects, REE, but not EEE, was significantly lower at day 42 compared with day 21. The authors speculated that the effect on EEE may account for the weight loss associated with yohimbine (14).

◆ In a placebo-controlled crossover study, 14 healthy, normal-weight males were given an acute dose of 0.2 mg/kg of oral yohimbine (mean dose for 70-kg subject = 14 mg) after an overnight fast or 1 hour after a standard 400-kcal breakfast. Blood samples were taken 45, 60, 75, 90, and 105 minutes after yohimbine ingestion. There was a 1-week washout period between treatments. Yohimbine increased fat mobilization as measured by plasma glycerol levels and plasma nonesterified fatty acids concentrations in fasting subjects, while the effect was not apparent 1 hour after a meal. Yohimbine had no significant effects on heart rate or blood pressure. In a second controlled experiment of eight fasting male subjects, the lipid mobilizing action of yohimbine was reinforced during and after 30 minutes of aerobic exercise on a cycle ergometer. Plasma norepinephrine concentrations increased 40% to 50% after yohimbine intake but were not associated with autonomic symptoms (15).

References

1. Riley AJ. Yohimbine in the treatment of erectile disorder. *Br J Clin Pract.* 1994;48: 133–136.
2. De Smet PA, Smeets OS. Potential risks of health food products containing yohimbe extracts. *BMJ.* 1994;309:958.
3. Sandler B, Aronson P. Yohimbine-induced cutaneous drug eruption, progressive renal failure, and lupus-like syndrome. *Urology.* 1993;41:343–345.
4. Landis E, Shore E. Yohimbine-induced bronchospasm. *Chest.* 1989;96:1424.
5. Price LH, Charney DS, Heninger GR. Three cases of manic symptoms following yohimbine ingestion. *Am J Psychiatry.* 1984;141:1267–1268.
6. Blumenthal M, ed. *The Complete German Commission E Monographs Therapeutic Guide to Herbal Medicines.* Boston, Mass: Integrative Medicine Communications; 1998.
7. Betz JM, White DK, der Marderosian AH. Gas chromatography determination of yohimbine in commercial yohimbe products. *J AOAC Int.* 1995;78:1189–1194.
8. Guthrie SK, Hariharan M, Grunhaus LJ. Yohimbine bioavailability in humans. *Eur J Clin Pharmacol.* 1990;39:409–411.
9. Ernst E, Pittler MH. Yohimbine for erectile dysfunction: a systematic review and meta-analysis of randomized clinical trials. *J Urol.* 1998:159:433–436.
10. Piletz JE, Segraves KB, Feng YZ, et al. Plasma MHPG response to yohimbine treatment in women with hypoactive sexual desire. *J Sex Marital Ther.* 1998;24:43–54.

11. Vogt HJ, Brandl P, Kockott G, et al. Double-blind, placebo-controlled safety and efficacy trial with yohimbine hydrochloride in the treatment of nonorganic erectile dysfunction. *Int J Impot Res.* 1997;9:155–161.

12. Kunelius P, Hakkinen J, Lukkarinen O. Is high-dose yohimbine hydrochloride effective in the treatment of mixed-type impotence? A prospective, randomized, controlled double-blind crossover study. *Urology.* 1997;49:441–444.

13. Montorsi F, Strambi LF, Guazzoni G, et al. Effect of yohimbine-trazodone on psychogenic impotence: a randomized, double-blind, placebo-controlled study. *Urology.* 1994;44:732–736.

14. Kucio C, Jonderko K, Piskorska D. Does yohimbine act as a slimming drug? *Isr J Med Sci.* 1991;27:550–556.

15. Galitzky J, Taouis M, Berlan M, et al. Alpha 2-antagonist compounds and lipid mobilization: evidence for a lipid mobilizing effect of oral yohimbine in healthy male volunteers. *Eur J Clin Invest.* 1988;18:587–594.

Zinc

Zinc, a trace mineral, is part of more than 200 enzymes involved in carbohydrate metabolism, protein synthesis and catabolism, carbon dioxide transport, the synthesis of nucleic acid and heme, and gene expression. The highest concentrations are located in bone, muscle, integumental tissue (skin, hair, nails), retina, pancreas, and male reproductive organs. Needed for the antioxidant enzyme superoxide dismutase, zinc is thought to play a protective role against damage from superoxide anions (1).

Although overt zinc deficiency is rare, symptoms of zinc depletion are diverse due to zinc's numerous roles in metabolic processes. Clinical signs of deficiency may include impaired growth, alopecia, diarrhea, delayed sexual maturity, impotence, eye and skin lesions, and anorexia. Individuals most susceptible to inadequate zinc intake and deficiency include the elderly, individuals with HIV, people with alcoholism, pregnant and lactating women, individuals with diabetes, people with malabsorption disorders (Crohn's disease, short-bowel syndrome), trauma patients, and female athletes (1,2).

Media and Marketing Claims	Efficacy
Treats colds	↔
Reduces risk for macular degeneration	↔
Improves athletic performance	NR
Treats acne	NR
Enhances male fertility	NR
Improves immune function	↑?

Safety

- The Tolerable Upper Intake Level (UL) for zinc is 40 mg/day for adults, based on the adverse effects of higher amounts on copper status (2).

- Zinc supplementation in the Health Professionals' Follow-up Study conducted among more than 46,000 males showed a 2.3-fold increased risk for developing prostate cancer among men who regularly consumed supplements with more than 100 mg zinc per day (3).

- Chronic intake of doses ranging 100 to 300 mg zinc per day are associated with copper deficiency with symptoms of anemia and neutropenia, impaired immune function, and an adverse effect on the ratio of LDL to HDL cholesterol. Some of these effects are also seen with 15-mg to 100-mg doses (4).

- Sideroblastic anemia, leukopenia, and neutropenia, headache, and fatigue were reported in a 17-year-old male who had been taking 300 mg zinc/day for 2 years as a remedy for his acne. All symptoms resolved 17 months after discontinuing zinc (5).

- Chronic ingestion of doses more than the UL may impair immune function, induce copper deficiency, and negatively affect cholesterol levels.

- Acute ingestion of high doses of zinc may cause nausea and vomiting.

Drug/Supplement Interactions

- Zinc supplements interfere with copper absorption.

- Zinc and iron may interfere with the absorption of one another.

- Zinc and penicillin bind, interfering with the absorption of both.

- Zinc may reduce the absorption of tetracycline (antibiotic).

- Zinc may bind with warfarin (anticoagulant), thus reducing efficacy.

- Zinc may increase toxicity of cisplatin.

- Caution with potassium-sparing diuretics because zinc levels can be elevated; whereas thiazide diuretics increase zinc excretion.

- A high-calcium diet and supplement providing approximately 1,200 mg calcium decreased zinc absorption by 2 mg/day in postmenopausal women during a 36-day controlled study. Zinc as part of a calcium supplement can offset the effects of calcium on zinc absorption (6). In contrast, another study using the same zinc balance methodology reported that calcium had no effect on zinc absorption (7).

- The following drugs may decrease zinc status: angiotensin-converting enzyme inhibitors for hypertension (captopril, enalapril); aspirin; oral contraceptives; thiazide diuretics.

Key Points

- A supplement providing the RDA for zinc may be necessary when dietary intake is not adequate. However, individuals using zinc supplements should not consume more than the UL (40 mg/day for adults) to avoid potential problems including copper deficiency resulting in anemia, elevated cholesterol, and impaired immune function.

- Studies are conflicting regarding the potential benefit of zinc lozenges on cold symptoms. Some researchers have suggested that the variability of dosage, formulation, and administration of zinc among studies is responsible for the equivocal results. In addition, zinc studies only measured subjective reports of cold symptoms. Further research will need to test immune function and confirm the existence of rhinovirus using microbiological tests.

- Preliminary research suggests that diets rich in zinc may provide a mild protective effect against macular degeneration. Research from the 2001 Age-Related Eye Disease Study reported that zinc supplements (80 mg) plus antioxidants and copper slowed the progression of advanced age-related macular degeneration (AMD) only in a subgroup of subjects at high risk. Individuals with AMD should discuss zinc supplementation with their physician, because this high dose is more than the UL.

- A few small studies testing the effect of zinc supplementation on immune markers in athletes have provided conflicting results. Also, there is a lack of substantial evidence to suggest that zinc has an ergogenic effect in exercise performance.

- Preliminary research in the 1970s and 1980s suggested some benefit of taking high doses of zinc to treat acne. No further studies have verified these results. Furthermore, the dosages used are associated with potentially dangerous side effects.

- Although zinc content in the semen of infertile men seems to be lower than in fertile men, and short-term zinc-deficient diets are associated with decreased semen volume, there are currently no well-controlled studies beyond animal data demonstrating that zinc supplementation improves fertility in humans. However, it may be advisable for infertile men to take a multivitamin providing the RDA for zinc if dietary intake is inadequate.

- Although zinc deficiency negatively affects the immune response and the elderly tend to have lower plasma zinc levels (1), more controlled research is required to determine the effect of zinc supplements on immunity in the elderly. Reviews of the role of zinc in immunity and immune function of the elderly suggest that zinc supplementation improves immune function, particularly in those who are zinc deficient (8,9). Data from trials in children suggest that supplemental zinc may have a role in reducing infections in small for gestational age children and at-risk children in developing countries, but additional studies are needed.

Food Sources

Meats, eggs, seafood, whole grains, nuts, and legumes are good sources of zinc. The median daily intake of zinc in the United States is approximately 9 mg for women and 13 mg for men (2). Phytic acid in plants binds with zinc, reducing the intestinal absorption of zinc from these foods. Protein digestibility also influences zinc absorption. In general, zinc uptake is higher from a diet rich in animal protein than a diet rich in plant proteins such as soy (2). Processing of whole grains results in the loss of almost 80% of the total zinc (1).

Food	Zinc, mg/serving
Beef, ground, broiled (3.5 oz)	5.36
Wheat germ, toasted (2 Tbsp)	3.22
Beans, garbanzo (1 cup)	2.51
Seeds, sunflower (1 oz)	1.50
Chicken, light meat (3.5 oz)	1.23
Rice, brown (1 cup)	1.23
Milk, nonfat (1 cup)	0.98
Egg (1)	0.53
Codfish (3 oz)	0.49

Source: Data are from reference 10.

Dosage Information/Bioavailability

Zinc is sold in lozenges and tablets bound to gluconate, citrate, sulfate, glycerate, acetate, or picolinate. Several studies have used zinc sulfate or gluconate dosages ranging from 50 to 100 mg elemental zinc per day—these dosages exceed the RDA. Bioavailability of zinc supplements is variable. One study found that excipients in some lozenges such as citrate, mannitol, and sorbitol inhibited the ionization of zinc to free Zn^{2+}, whereas glycine did not interfere with ionization to free zinc (11).

An in vitro study using blue vs brown irides cultured with zinc shows that zinc uptake is significant higher in brown irides and is directly related to the higher melanin content which binds zinc. The study implies that zinc supplementation levels for the prevention of age-related macular degeneration may require variable dosing depending on the iris color of the patient (12).

The Institute of Medicine released Dietary Reference Intakes (DRIs) for zinc in 2001. The new adult RDA for zinc is 8 mg for women, 11 mg for men, 11 mg during pregnancy, and 12 mg during lactation (2). Although no vegetarian RDA was specified, the requirement for dietary zinc may be as much as 50% greater for vegetarians, especially for strict vegetarians who consume mainly grains and legumes (dietary phytate:zinc molar ratio > 15:1). For people with alcoholism, the daily zinc requirement exceeds the RDA, but an exact amount was not specified in the Institute of Medicine report (2).

Relevant Research

Zinc and the Common Cold

- ♦ A meta-analysis of six randomized, placebo-controlled, double-blind clinical trials reported no statistical benefit of using zinc lozenges to reduce rhinovirus duration. The studies included in the analysis used zinc gluconate or acetate ranging from 4.3

to 23.7 mg taken every 2 hours while subjects were awake. However, when a study with a low dose of zinc (4.3 mg) was excluded, the analysis did suggest a benefit with zinc treatment. The authors criticized many of the studies for poor blinding because many subjects correctly identified the active treatment, which may have resulted in a false treatment effect. They concluded: "The evidence for effectiveness of zinc salt lozenges in reducing the duration of common colds is still lacking" (13).

♦ Two additional analyses of randomized, controlled trials of zinc for the common cold reported that evidence that zinc treats cold symptoms is inconclusive (14,15).

♦ Zincum gluconium nasal gel (Zemulose) was compared with placebo nasal gel for the treatment of common cold among healthy adults. Eighty people participated and were randomly assigned to receive nasal gel containing 2.1 mg elemental zinc or placebo four times/day for a maximum of 10 days. Subjects and investigators were blinded to the intervention, but final analysis indicated that even after 1 day of treatment subjects correctly guessed which treatment they were taking ($P = .01$) based on clinical response. Thirty-five percent of subjects in the zinc group and 34% of subjects in the control group had confirmed rhinovirus (culture or PCR analysis). The primary outcome—time until cold symptoms resolved—was significantly shorter in the zinc supplemented group by a median of 1.7 days (16).

♦ A retrospective chart review was used to tests the hypothesis that children using zinc lozenges had shorter duration of colds (17). Children residing at the Heritage Center before 1998 had no access to zinc lozenges. In 1999 use was encouraged through the health care staff and by the year 2000 prophylactic use was promoted. The investigators reviewed medical records of all subjects with documented colds to ascertain the duration prior to zinc availability. This duration was then compared with duration of colds among those receiving zinc (four lozenges per day). Antibiotic use was also compared. The results showed that the frequency of colds was significantly less among those receiving prophylactic treatment with zinc (0.9% of zinc users vs 1.7% of those not using zinc). Cold duration was also significantly reduced with zinc supplementation (7.5 vs 9.0 days). Antibiotic use was also reduced with 3% of cold sufferers requiring antibiotic therapy in the zinc group and 39.3% of the control group. The researchers conclude that zinc lozenges can significantly reduce frequency of colds when used prophylactically and reduce duration as well as antibiotic requirements in those diagnosed with a cold.

♦ In a double-blind, placebo-controlled trial, 50 subjects recruited within 24 hours of developing symptoms for the common cold were randomly assigned to receive 12.8 mg zinc (as zinc acetate) or a placebo every 2 to 3 hours awake as long as symptoms remained. Subjective symptom scores (sore throat, nasal discharge, congestion, sneezing, cough, scratchy throat, hoarseness, muscle ache, fever, and headache) were recorded daily for 12 days. Plasma zinc and proinflammatory cytokines were measured on day 1 and after subjects were well. Compared with the placebo, the zinc group had shorter mean overall duration of symptoms (4.5 vs 8.1 days) and significantly decreased severity scores for all symptoms. There were no significant differences between groups on cytokine levels (18).

- In a double-blind, placebo-controlled trial, 249 students (grades 1 to 12) were randomly assigned to take zinc gluconate glycine (ZGG) lozenges (10 mg elemental zinc, five or six times per day) or a placebo within the first 24 hours of developing a cold. There was no difference in time to resolution of cold symptoms between groups. Compared with the placebo group, the zinc group experienced significantly more adverse effects, including bad taste, nausea, diarrhea, and mouth discomfort. The authors concluded: "ZGG lozenges were not effective in treating cold symptoms in children and adolescents" (19).

- In a double-blind, placebo-controlled study, 100 patients who developed symptoms of the common cold were randomly assigned to receive 13.3 mg zinc as zinc gluconate lozenges (one lozenge every 2 hours awake) or a placebo for as long as symptoms lasted. Time to complete resolution of symptoms was significantly shorter with zinc than the placebo (4.4 vs 7.6 days). The zinc-supplemented group had fewer days of coughing, headache, hoarseness, nasal congestion and drainage, and sore throat. There were no differences between groups in fever, muscle ache, scratchy throat, or sneezing. The zinc group had significantly more side effects (nausea, bad taste). Because of the lack of dramatic clinical benefit, the authors concluded that patients must decide whether the possible benefits of zinc gluconate on cold symptoms outweigh the adverse effects (20).

- An article reviewing eight controlled trials with zinc lozenges found that zinc seemed to have efficacy in four studies and was ineffective in the others. The authors suggested the discrepancies may be caused by inadequate placebo control, and differences in lozenge formulation and dosage. They noted that zinc gluconate lozenges seem to be effective when taken immediately after the onset of symptoms (21).

- One proposed explanation for the mechanism of action behind zinc is that the mineral may bind with proteins of critical nerve endings in the respiratory tract and surface proteins of the human rhinovirus, thereby interrupting virus infection (22).

Zinc and Age-Related Macular Degeneration (AMD)

- In a double-blind, placebo-controlled, multicenter study (Age-Related Eye Disease Study), 3,640 subjects ages 55 to 80 years with AMD (with at least one eye with the best-corrected vision of 20/32 or better) were randomly assigned to receive one of four treatments daily: (*a*) antioxidants (500 mg vitamin C, 400 IU vitamin E, 15 mg beta carotene); (*b*) 80 mg zinc (as zinc oxide) and 2 mg copper (added to correct for copper deficiency associated with high dose zinc); (*c*) antioxidants plus zinc and copper; or (*d*) a placebo. Subjects were followed for a mean of 6.3 years. Almost two thirds of the subjects chose to take a multivitamin/mineral supplement in addition to their treatment. Compared with those using the placebo, subjects taking antioxidants plus zinc had a significant odds reduction (28%) for the development of advanced AMD. Risk decreased 25% subjects taking zinc alone and 20% for antioxidants alone. Reduction in risk increased for all three treatments when 1,063 subjects with a low risk of developing advanced AMD were excluded. There was a significant reduction in moderate visual acuity loss only in subjects assigned to antioxidants plus zinc. None of the supplements had any effect on the progression of cataract. There were no significant adverse effects associated with any of the treatments (23).

◆ In a 2-year, double-blind, placebo-controlled study, 112 patients with age-related macular degeneration, exudative lesions in one eye and a 20/40 or better visual acuity, and macular degeneration without lesion in the second eye were studied. Subjects were randomly assigned to receive 200 mg zinc sulfate (80 mg elemental zinc) or a placebo daily. Mean serum zinc increased significantly in the treatment group, whereas there was no effect on serum copper, hemoglobin, and red blood cell count. Zinc had no short-term effect on the course of macular degeneration as measured by visual acuity, contrast sensitivity, color discrimination, and retinal grating acuity (24).

◆ In a double-blind, placebo-controlled trial, 151 patients with bilateral drusen (hyaline deposits beneath retinal pigment epithelium) or age-related macular degeneration were randomly assigned to receive 200 mg zinc sulfate (80 mg elemental zinc) for 24 months. There was a significantly lower incidence of visual loss in zinc-treated subjects at 12 to 24 months. The authors concluded: "Because of the pilot nature of the study and the possible toxic effects and complications of oral zinc administration, widespread use of zinc in macular degeneration is not now warranted" (25).

Zinc and Exercise Performance

◆ An unblinded study among 30 teenage subjects randomly assigned to one of three groups [(*a*) 3 mg zinc/kg/day and no exercise, (*b*) wrestling and exercise for 90 to 120 minutes five times per week, (*c*) the same exercise plus the 3 mg zinc/kg/day (26)] showed that zinc supplementation was associated with increase lymphocyte count and hemoglobin levels as compared with the control group at 4 weeks. However, the author also reports there was not significant change in these parameters over time, suggesting the difference across groups at the end of the study was small. Only the abstract was available for review and it is questionable why these specific measures were reported/measured and not others.

◆ In a nonrandomized, double-blind, placebo-controlled, crossover study, 16 healthy female subjects received 135 mg zinc (formulation not specified) or a placebo for 14 days each. Muscle strength and endurance was measured with an isokinetic, one-leg exercise test before and after both treatments. Zinc supplements significantly increased dynamic isokinetic strength and isometric endurance (27).

Zinc and Acne

◆ In the 1970s and 1980s, several trials investigated the effects of zinc sulfate on acne vulgaris. One placebo-controlled study of 52 subjects found that zinc sulfate offered a small benefit in reducing pustules but not on comedones, papules, infiltrates, or cysts (28). Another double-blind, parallel-group study compared zinc sulfate/citrate complex to tetracycline and found the antibiotic to be significantly more effective than zinc in the treatment of moderate to severe acne (29). In contrast, two double-blind, placebo-controlled studies showed significant improvement in acne with 400 to 600 mg zinc sulfate ($\approx$ 160 to 240 mg elemental zinc) during 12 weeks (30,31). Reported adverse events associated with these high doses of zinc included nausea, vomiting, and abdominal pain. No further research has been completed since 1989.

Zinc and Male Fertility

♦ Zinc is necessary for growth, sexual maturation, and reproduction. Infertile men have been reported to have reduced seminal and serum zinc levels compared with fertile men (32–34).

♦ In a randomized, controlled-feeding, crossover study, 11 male subjects living on a metabolic ward were fed a diet composed of a mixture of semisynthetic formula and conventional foods supplemented with zinc sulfate to supply a total of 1.4, 2.5, 3.4, 4.4, or 10.4 mg zinc/day. After an equilibration period of 28 days (10.4 mg zinc per day), all treatments were presented for 35 days each, the first four in random order and the fifth last. Compared with when they were consuming 10.4 mg zinc, subjects consuming 1.4 mg zinc had decreased semen volumes and serum testosterone concentrations, and no change in seminal zinc concentrations. The authors concluded that these measures are sensitive to short-term zinc depletion in young men (35).

Zinc and Immunity

♦ In a double-blind, placebo-controlled, partial crossover study, 63 elderly subjects were given 15 or 100 mg zinc as zinc acetate capsules or a placebo daily for 12 months. All subjects were also given a multivitamin/mineral supplement without zinc. Blood samples and immune functions were assessed at 0, 3, 6, 12, and 16 months. Dietary zinc intake was consistently less than recommended intakes during the study. Natural killer cell activity was transiently enhanced by the 100-mg dose after 3 months. Delayed dermal hypersensitivity and lymphocyte proliferation responses to two mitogens were significantly increased in the placebo group than either zinc treatment. The authors concluded: "Zinc had a beneficial effect on one measure of cellular immune function while simultaneously having an adverse effect on another measure" (36).

♦ Zinc supplementation was investigated for efficacy against respiratory illness and related mortality in small-for-gestational-age infants (37). The low–birth-weight infants all demonstrated reduced cord blood zinc levels. The 1,154 infants received one of four oral treatments (5 mL each) in a randomized, blinded design: (*a*) riboflavin (0.5 mg/day); (*b*) riboflavin and zinc (5 mg/day); (*c*) riboflavin, folate (60 μmol/day), calcium (180 mg/day), phosphorus (90 mg/day), and iron (10 mg/day); or (*d*) riboflavin, folate, calcium, phosphorus, iron, and zinc. Supplementation continued from age 30 to age 284 days. Home visits were made 6 days/week to assess health status and provide supplements. Only the zinc supplementation was associated with lower mortality (groups *b* and *d* combined vs groups *a* and *c* combined) (hazard ratio = 0.32; 95% CI = 0.12–0.89).

References

1. King JC, Keen CL. Zinc. In: Shils ME, Olson JA, Shike M, et al, eds. *Modern Nutrition in Health and Disease.* 9th ed. Philadelphia, Pa: Lea & Febiger; 1999:223–239.
2. Institute of Medicine. *Dietary Reference Intakes for Vitamin A, Vitamin K, Arsenic, Boron, Chromium, Copper, Iodine, Iron, Manganese, Molybdenum, Nickel, Silicon, Vanadium, and Zinc.* Washington, DC: National Academy Press, 2002.
3. Leitzmann MF, Sampfer MJ, Wu K, et al. Zinc supplement use and risk for prostate cancer. *J Natl Cancer Inst.* 2003;95:1004–1007.
4. Fosmire GJ. Zinc toxicity. *Am J Clin Nutr.* 1990;51:225–227.
5. Porea TJ, Belmont JW, Mahoney DH. Zinc-induced anemia and neutropenia in an adolescent. *J Pediatr.* 2000;136:688–690.
6. Wood RJ, Zheng JJ. High dietary calcium intakes reduce zinc absorption and balance in humans. *Am J Clin Nutr.* 1997;65:1803–1809.
7. McKenna AA, Ilich JZ, Andon MB. Zinc balance in adolescent females consuming a low- or high-calcium diet. *Am J Clin Nutr.* 1997;65:1460–1464.
8. Ferencik M, Ebringer L. Modulatory effects of selenium and zinc on the immune system. *Folia Microbiol.* 2003;48:417–426.
9. Bogden JD. Influence of zinc on immunity in the elderly *J Nutr Health Aging.* 2004;8: 48–54.
10. Pennington JA. *Bowes and Church's Food Values of Portions Commonly Used.* 17th ed. Philadelphia, Pa: Lippincott-Raven Publishers; 1998.
11. Zarembo JE, Godfrey JC, Godfrey NJ. Zinc (II) in saliva: determination of concentrations produced by different formulations of zinc gluconate lozenges containing common excipients. *J Pharm Sci.* 1992;81:128–130.
12. Kokkinou D, Kasper HU, Batrz-Schmidt KU, et al. The pigmentation of human iris influences the uptake and storing of zinc. *Pigment Cell Res.* 2004;17:515–518.
13. Jackson JL, Peterson C, Lesho E. A meta-analysis of zinc salts lozenges and the common cold. *Arch Intern Med.* 1997;157:2373–2376.
14. Jackson JL, Lesho E, Peterson C. Zinc and the common cold: a meta-analysis revisited. *J Nutr.* 2000;130(5 Suppl):S1512–S1515.
15. Marshall I. Zinc for the common cold. *Cochrane Database Syst Rev.* 2000;2:CD001364.
16. Mossad SB. Effect of zincum gluconicum nasal gel on the duration and symptom severity of the common cold in otherwise healthy adults. *QJM.* 2003;96:35–43.
17. McElroy BH, Miller SP. Effectiveness of zinc gluconate glycine lozenges (Cold-Eeze) against the common cold in school-aged subjects: a retrospective chart review. *Am J Ther.* 2002;9:472–475.
18. Prasad AS, Fitzgerald JT, Bao B, et al. Duration of symptoms and plasma cytokine levels in patients with the common cold treated with zinc acetate. A randomized, double-blind, placebo-controlled trial. *Ann Intern Med.* 2000;133:245–252.
19. Macknin ML, Piedmonte M, Calendine C, et al. Zinc gluconate lozenges for treating the common cold in children: a randomized controlled trial. *JAMA.* 1998;279:1962–1967.
20. Mossad SB, Macknin ML, Medendorp SV, et al. Zinc gluconate lozenges for treating the common cold. A randomized, double-blind, placebo-controlled study. *Ann Intern Med.* 1996;125:81–88.

21. Garland ML, Hagmeyer KO. The role of zinc lozenges in the treatment of the common cold. *Ann Pharmacother.* 1998;32:63–69.
22. Novick SG, Godfrey JC, Pollack RL, et al. Zinc-induced suppression of inflammation in the respiratory tract, caused by infection with human rhinovirus and other irritants. *Med Hypotheses.* 1997;49:347–357.
23. Age-Related Eye Disease Study Research Group. A randomized, placebo-controlled, clinical trial of high-dose supplementation with vitamins C and E, beta-carotene, and zinc for age-related macular degeneration and vision loss: AREDS report no. 8. *Arch Ophthalmol.* 2001;119:1417–1436.
24. Stur M, Tittl M, Reitner A, et al. Oral zinc and the second eye in age-related macular degeneration. *Invest Ophthalmol Vis Sci.* 1996;37:1225–1235.
25. Newsome DA, Swartz M, Leone NC, et al. Oral zinc in macular degeneration. *Arch Ophthalmol.* 1988;106:192–198.
26. Kilic M, Baltaci AK, Gunay M. Effect of zinc supplementation on hematological parameters in athletes. *Biol Trace Elem Res.* 2004;100:31–38.
27. Krotkiewski M, Gudmundsson M, Backstrom P, et al. Zinc and muscle strength and endurance. *Acta Physiol Scand.* 1982;116:309–311.
28. Weimar VM, Puhl SC, Smith WH, et al. Zinc sulfate in acne vulgaris. *Arch Dermatol.* 1978;114:1776–1778.
29. Cunliffe WJ, Burke B, Dodman B, et al. A double-blind trial of a zinc sulfate/citrate complex and tetracycline in the treatment of acne vulgaris. *Br J Dermatol.* 1979;101:321–325.
30. Verma KC, Saini AS, Dhamija SK. Oral zinc sulfate therapy in acne vulgaris: a double-blind trial. *Acta Derm Venereol.* 1980;60:337–340.
31. Hillstrom L, Pettersson L, Hellbe L, et al. Comparison of oral treatment with zinc sulfate and placebo in acne vulgaris. *Br J Dermatol.* 1977;97:679–684.
32. Mohan H, Verma J, Singh I. Inter-relationship of zinc levels in serum and semen in oligospermic infertile patients and fertile males. *Indian J Pathol Microbiol.* 1997;40:451–455.
33. Kvist U, Bjorndahl L, Kjellberg S. Sperm nuclear zinc, chromatin stability, and male fertility. *Scanning Microsc.* 1987;1:1241–1247.
34. Chia SE, Ong CN, Chua LH, et al. Comparison of zinc concentrations in blood and seminal plasma and the various sperm parameters between fertile and infertile men. *J Androl.* 2000;21:53–57.
35. Hunt CD, Johnson PE, Herbel J, et al. Effects of dietary zinc depletion on seminal volume and zinc loss, serum testosterone concentrations, and sperm morphology in young men. *Am J Clin Nutr.* 1992;56:148–157.
36. Bodgen JD, Oleske JM, Lavenhar MA, et al. Effects of one year of supplementation with zinc and other micronutrients on cellular immunity in the elderly. *J Am Coll Nutr.* 1990;9:214–225.
37. Sazawal S, Black RE, Menon VP, et al. Zinc supplementation in infants born small for gestational age reduces mortality: a prospective, randomized, controlled trial. *Pediatrics.* 2001;108:1280–1286.

Appendixes

Appendix A

Government Regulation of Dietary Supplements

Revised by Leila G. Saldanha, PhD, RD

This appendix recounts the development of legislation and government bodies that regulate the dietary supplements industry. It also discusses quality control and the issues that health professionals face in recommending use of supplements. The Food and Drug Administration (FDA) Dietary Supplement Labeling Guide provides an overview of federal regulations and is recommended reading for dietetics professionals who want to learn more on this topic (1).

History of Dietary Supplement Regulation

Dietary supplements were first regulated as foods under the Federal Food Drug and Cosmetic Act of 1938 (FDAC) (2) prior to passage of the Dietary Supplement Health and Education Act of 1994 (DSHEA) (3). In 1941, the US Food and Drug Administration (FDA) defined foods for special dietary uses to include supplementing the diet with vitamins, minerals, or other dietary substances. Thirty years later, the agency sought to regulate the dosage and quantity of vitamins and minerals in dietary supplements. However, a 1974 court decision and the Rogers-Proxmire Vitamin Amendments passed in 1976 prevented implementation of these regulations (4).

In 1993, FDA published the work of its Dietary Supplements Task Force as an Advance Notice of Proposed Rulemaking (ANPR), which again suggested limiting the dosage of vitamins and minerals permitted in supplements and declared that some supplements were unapproved food additives or drugs. This ANPR led to public debate on the role of dietary supplements in promoting health and the need for consumers to have access to current and accurate information about supplements. The controversy over the FDA's proposal of a stricter regulatory approach coupled with lobbying by consumer advocacy and the supplement industry groups contributed to the passage of the Dietary Supplement Health Education Act of 1994 (DSHEA) (4,5).

Dietary Supplement Health Education Act

When Congress signed DSHEA into law in October 1994, dietary supplements became a separate regulatory category for the first time (5). This law authorized the FDA to regulate supplements as a subset of food and prohibited their regulation as drugs or food additives. DSHEA (5) made substantial changes that affected the supplement industry, consumers, and health professionals by providing:

- A definition of dietary supplement
- A new framework for addressing safety
- Guidelines for third-party literature (pamphlets, books, handouts) provided at the point of sale
- Appropriate use of statements of nutritional support
- Ingredient and nutrition information labeling standards
- FDA authority to establish Good Manufacturing Practices (GMPs) for dietary supplements
- The formation of the Presidential Commission on Dietary Supplements Labels to review and make recommendations on supplement labeling
- The establishment of the Office of Dietary Supplements (ODS) under the National Institutes of Health (NIH) to facilitate and conduct research exploring the role of dietary supplements in health and disease

Definition of Dietary Supplement in DSHEA

Under DSHEA, a *dietary supplement* is defined as (*a*) a product intended to supplement the diet that contains at least one of the following: a vitamin, a mineral, an herb or other botanical, or an amino acid; or (*b*) a dietary substance for use to supplement the diet by increasing the total dietary intake; or (*c*) a concentrate, metabolite, constituent, extract, or combination of any of the previously described ingredients. Dietary supplements may be in the form of a tablet, capsule, powder, softgel, gelcap, or liquid. They must be labeled as a dietary supplement, and they cannot be represented for use as a conventional food or sole item of a meal or diet (5).

Product Safety

Under DSHEA, dietary supplement manufacturers are responsible for providing safe and properly labeled products (5). However, the FDA bears the burden of proof for showing that a supplement is unsafe or mislabeled before it can restrict or ban a product. Dietary supplements, like conventional foods, are not subject to premarket approval by the FDA. However, some ingredients used in supplements that do not meet the definition of a dietary supplement, such as food additives, must meet regulatory requirements for that category. Food additives must undergo studies to demonstrate safety before they are approved for use by FDA and allowed on the market.

When a supplement poses a safety issue, the FDA can choose to issue a public warning or request a product recall, instead of taking formal legal action. In 1997, for example, the discovery that a plantain product was contaminated with digitalis resulted in a prompt recall. The same year, after investigating more than 800 adverse events, the agency issued a warning on consuming ephedra and proposed new rules to limit the amount of ephedrine alkaloids permitted in products and to require warning labels. In the years that followed, the FDA took further actions to restrict the sale of ephedra, but it was challenged on most these decisions. In February 2004, FDA issued a final rule that deemed products containing ephedra to be illegal "because these dietary supplements present an unreasonable risk of illness or injury . . . including heart attack, stroke, and death, and that these risks are unreasonable in light of any benefits that may result from the use of these products." This action [was] taken under the DSHEA (6). Current warnings and safety information about dietary supplements are posted on the FDA's Center for Food Safety and Applied Nutrition (CFSAN) Web site (7).

Ingredients that meet the DSHEA definition of a dietary supplement are exempt from regulations for food additives. Ingredients marketed before October 1994 are grandfathered under DSHEA (ie, they are recognized as safe and do not require FDA approval). For new dietary supplement ingredients (ie, those introduced to the market after October 1994), manufacturers are required to provide the FDA with evidence that the ingredients are "reasonably expected to be safe" at the recommended level of use. This evidence must be submitted at least 75 days before marketing. The FDA does not formally approve such ingredients but has the opportunity to reject them. Because there is no authoritative list of dietary ingredients that were marketed in dietary supplements before October 1994, manufacturers are responsible for determining whether an ingredient is a new dietary ingredient. If the manufacturer claims that the ingredient is not new, it must document that a dietary supplement containing the dietary ingredient was marketed before October 15, 1994 (8).

DSHEA Requirements for Literature

Before the passage of DSHEA, the FDA considered all books, reprints of articles, or other materials displayed next to a product in a store or shipped with a product as "labeling." In contrast, DSHEA now allows "third party" literature, such as reprints, scientific abstracts and articles, book chapters, and other publications used in connection with a sale, to be exempt from labeling regulations if the publication meets all of the following requirements (5):

- Is not false or misleading
- Does not promote a supplement brand
- Is reprinted in its entirety without any added information
- Presents a balanced view of available scientific information
- Is displayed with other similar materials, separate from supplement products
- Is not attached to any other product promotional materials

In practice, however, the FDA does not have adequate resources to fully monitor and enforce these regulations.

Labeling Standards

Dietary supplement labels can carry a variety of claims (5). These claims are grouped under three broad categories: structure/function claims, health claims, and nutrient content claims.

The regulatory requirements differ for each category of claims. In particular, there are variances in the level and amount of scientific substantiation required and whether or not FDA approval to make the claim is required.

Statements of Nutritional Support

Under DSHEA (5), supplement labels may carry "statements of nutritional support." Such statements are generally referred to as *structure/function claims*. Nutritional support statements describe the link between a nutrient and a deficiency, the effect of an ingredient on the body's structure or function, or its effect on well-being. Examples of permissible structure function statements include: "Helps maintain healthy intestinal flora," "Helps maintain cardiovascular health," "Promotes relaxation," and "Builds strong bones." To make these claims, supplement labels must carry the disclaimer: *"This statement has not been evaluated by the Food and Drug Administration. This product is not intended to diagnose, treat, cure, or prevent any disease."*

Manufacturers must be able to substantiate that the structure/function claims are truthful and not misleading, but they are not required to provide this substantiation to the FDA. In addition, if manufacturers make this type of claim, they must notify the FDA of the statements within 30 days after marketing commences. Although the FDA does not approve structure/function claims, it can object to them.

Health Claims

The Nutrition Labeling and Education Act (NLEA) of 1990 gave the FDA the authority to authorize health claims in food and supplement labeling. Health claims describe a link between specific nutrients or substances in food and a particular disease or health-related condition. Such claims must be based on significant scientific agreement. The FDA Modernization Act of 1997 (FDAMA) provided an additional mechanism for manufacturers to use health claims based on authoritative statements by certain scientific bodies. These health claims are authorized by the agency only after a comprehensive review of scientific evidence. The FDA has approved several health claims, which are listed on the CFSAN Web site (9), along with the requirements a product must meet to make them.

The underlying legal framework for the NLEA health claims system has been challenged, and the courts have ruled that it is a violation of the First Amendment for the FDA to ban certain statements that may truthfully describe the current evidence, even if "significant scientific agreement" on the subject had not been reached (10). The courts have required FDA to consider whether some qualified claims should be permitted as long as the statements are truthful and not misleading when appropriately qualified to indicate the level of scientific support for the claim. As part of the 2003 Consumer Health Information for Better Nutrition Initiative, the FDA announced a proposed framework for regulating qualified health claims (11). Under this framework, FDA has permitted several qualified health claims; these are listed on the CFSAN Web site (12), along with the requirements a product must meet to make them.

In November 2005, FDA held a public meeting to present research findings and implications of these findings on consumer perceptions of health claims. Research findings focused on whether consumers were able to differentiate among the different types of claims (ie unqualified health claims, qualified health claims, and structure/function claims). Also discussed was how these claims could be structured so that they are not misleading to consumers. The findings revealed a wide range of conclusions on how the public perceives each type of claim both independently and relative to other claims using only words and with graphic images (13). The agenda and transcript from this November meeting can be downloaded from the FDA Web site.

Nutrient Content Claims

DSHEA (5) requires that all supplement labels carry the name of each ingredient and the total quantity of all dietary ingredients (excluding inert ingredients). The words *dietary supplement* must appear as part of the product name, or, alternatively, the term *dietary* can be replaced by a descriptive phrase, such as *multivitamin and mineral supplement.* For botanical products, the part of the plant from which the ingredient is derived must be identified. A product is considered "misbranded" if the quality, purity, strength, and identity are misrepresented or if any other statements on the label are false and misleading.

FDA Rules for Supplement Labels

In September 1997, the FDA published final rules for supplement labels that took effect March 1999 (14). Chapter 1 in FDA's Dietary Supplement Labeling Guide provides guidance on general labeling of dietary supplements (15). The rules require all supplements to carry a "Supplement Facts" panel listing the following information:

- An appropriate serving size is listed.

- Information given includes quantity and percent Daily Values (DV) for 14 nutrients and any other added vitamins or minerals when present at significant levels.

- For products with no established Reference Daily Intakes (RDIs), the amount per serving must be stated (eg, 300 mg omega-3 fatty acids).

- If a product contains a proprietary blend, the total amount of the blend must be stated, although the individual amounts of each ingredient do not have to be labeled.

- Below the Supplement Facts panel, ingredients must be listed by common name in descending order by weight. "Other ingredients" such as fillers, excipients, artificial colors or flavors, sweeteners, or binders (eg, gelatin, water, lactose, starch, cellulose) must also be listed.

- In addition, labels must include directions for use and the name and place of business of the manufacturer, packager, or distributor.

- The final rules also mandate that the phrase *high potency* can only be used on products that contain 100% or more of the established RDI for that vitamin or mineral. Only nutrient content claims, or their synonyms, that are specifically defined in regulations may be used. For example, *antioxidant* can only be used with descriptors such as "good source" and "high" if scientific evidence has demonstrated that the nutrient inactivates free radicals or prevents free radical–initiated reactions in the body (as has been shown for vitamins C and E) (16).

Role of the Federal Trade Commission

Although DSHEA does not directly address the advertising of dietary supplements, the Federal Trade Commission (FTC) is responsible for monitoring claims in advertising, including print and broadcast advertisements, infomercials, and catalogs, as well as direct marketing materials. In November 1998, the FTC issued a guide for the supplement industry to clarify long-standing FTC policies and enforcement practices for dietary supplement advertising (17).

Establishment of Good Manufacturing Practices

DSHEA authorized the FDA to establish Good Manufacturing Practices (GMPs) specifically for dietary supplements, modeled after GMPs for conventional foods (5). Enforced by the FDA, GMPs are a set of standard procedures for a number of manufacturing components, such as production and processing controls, equipment, plant conditions, sanitation, record-keeping, and employee qualifications. Currently, supplement manufacturers must follow food GMPs, which do not address the unique aspects of supplement manufacturing.

In 1995, in response to DSHEA, the supplement industry submitted a draft of GMPs specifically for dietary supplements to FDA. The proposed GMPs are stricter than food GMPs but not as rigorous as drug GMPs. The stated goals of the proposed draft are to ensure that supplements (*a*) are safe, not adulterated or misbranded; (*b*) contain the identity and provide the quantity of dietary ingredients stated in the label; and (*c*) meet quality specifications that the supplement is represented to meet.

In 1997, the FDA published the dietary supplement GMPs submitted by the supplement industry as an advance notice of proposed rule making, along with a set of questions about appropriate GMPs (18). In 2003, a proposed rule was issued. FDA has reviewed comments received in response to this March 2003 *Federal Register* notice, and has drafted a final rule. (A timeline of FDA activities related to dietary supplements CGMPs [Current GMPs] is available on the CFSAN Web site [19].) When final supplement GMPs are adopted, this rule should offer more assurance that all supplement manufacturers are using quality control procedures and are providing reliable products. Some supplement manufacturers have already begun using proposed dietary supplement CGMPs, although this practice is not yet legally required.

Office of Dietary Supplements

DSHEA mandated the formation of the ODS to explore the role of dietary supplements in improving health care in the United States (5). ODS is responsible for coordinating research on supplements at the NIH, organizing symposia, and compiling research on supplements into two databases: the International Bibliographic Information on Dietary Supplements (IBIDS) and Computer Access to Research on Dietary Supplements (CARDS). IBIDS is a database of published, international scientific literature about dietary supplements, including vitamins, minerals, and botanicals. It was developed to assist the public, health professionals, and researchers in locating credible, scientific literature on dietary supplements (20). CARDS provides information about current federally supported research on dietary supplements and individual nutrients supported (21). ODS also publishes fact sheets on dietary supplements and the *Annual Bibliography of Significant Advances in Dietary Supplement Research,* which each year highlights 25 exemplary papers on dietary supplements (22).

ODS funds clinical trials on dietary supplements and has initiated a number of programs, such as the Botanical Research Centers Program, Analytical Methods and Reference Materials Program, and the Evidence-Based Review Program. In 2002, Congress authorized the Analytical Methods and Reference Materials Program to develop and disseminate validated analytical methods and reference materials for the most commonly used botanicals and other dietary supplements. These efforts will play an important role in enforcing the quality and safety of dietary supplements. Updates on the activities of ODS can be accessed on its Web site (23).

National Center for Complementary and Alternative Medicine

The National Center for Complementary and Alternative Medicine (NCCAM), which was established by Congress as part of the NIH in 1998, also supports research on dietary supplements and other alternative therapies. NCCAM programs are listed on the center's Web site (24).

Quality Control

Industry Self-Regulation

Because the current food GMPs do not address the specific concerns of supplement manufacturing, many companies set their own standards to ensure quality products. For instance, some pharmaceutical companies also sell dietary supplements, and therefore already follow drug GMPs. The quality control regulations for these GMPs are much stricter than the regulations for food GMPs that currently apply to dietary supplements. In addition, some manufacturers hire independent auditors to conduct spot checks and provide feedback about manufacturing processes.

A number of third-party voluntary quality assurance programs have been developed to help build consumer confidence in the quality of dietary supplements. These programs include:

◆ ConsumerLab.com (25)

◆ NSF International's Dietary Supplement Certification Program (26)

◆ United States Pharmacopoeia (USP) Dietary Supplement Verification Program (27)

◆ National Nutritional Foods Association (NNFA) GMP Certification Program (28)

Choosing Quality Dietary Supplements

The law requires products to have the proper identity and potency, but some supplement manufacturers purchase and use supplement ingredients without adequately testing for purity or identity before packaging. Although there are no set rules or guarantees for selecting supplements, the following tips may be useful:

◆ Check the manufacturer name—nationally known food and supplement companies often have stricter quality control procedures in place, and may be more likely to provide reliable products.

◆ Contact the company—ask to speak to a technical expert about how products are made, quality control procedures, and GMPs. Companies should be willing to provide answers to the following questions:

> ▶ Has the particular product been used in any clinical studies published in peer-reviewed journals? Can the company share the scientific studies to substantiate the structure/function statements or health claims? (Obtain citations and ask the representative to send copies of the published articles.)

> ▶ Does the company complete an analysis on the final product (not just ingredients) to guarantee the contents in the package match those stated on the label?

> ▶ Is the product tested for content uniformity?

> ▶ Does the product meet any existing standards for disintegration and dissolution, or other tests of bioavailability?

◆ Review the label—it should contain accurate and appropriate information. If statements are unclear or the label makes outrageous claims, the manufacturer is not following DSHEA. If a company does not abide by DSHEA in this regard, it is possible that the manufacturer is also lax in quality control procedures.

Summary

DSHEA marked a major change in the regulation of the supplement industry. Under this act, dietary supplements are regulated similarly to food even though they may have drug-like actions. Although supplements are legally required to be safe and unadulterated, the 1994 law puts the burden of proof on the FDA to demonstrate that a product is unsafe or misbranded. Unfortunately, the agency lacks the resources to fully monitor and enforce industry compliance with the safety and labeling regulations. Therefore, although most products may be relatively safe, health professionals must be informed and educated about regulations, efficacy, and potential safety concerns.

References

1. US Food and Drug Administration Center for Food Safety and Applied Nutrition. Guidance for Industry. A Dietary Supplement Labeling Guide. Available at: http://www.cfsan.fda.gov/~dms/dslg-toc.html. Accessed July 6, 2005.
2. Food, Drug, and Cosmetic Act of 1938. Pub L No. 75-717, 52 Stat 1040 (1938).
3. Rogers & Proxmire Vitamins Amendments. Pub L No. 94-278, 90 Stat 410 (1976).

4. US Food and Drug Administration Center for Food Safety and Applied Nutrition. Dietary Supplement Health and Education Act of 1994. Available at: http://www.cfsan.fda.gov/~dms/dietsupp.html. Accessed August 18, 2005.

5. Dietary Supplement Health and Education Act of 1994 (DSHEA). Pub L No. 103-417 108 Stat (1994).

6. FDA Final Rule. Declaring dietary supplements containing ephedrine alkaloids adulterated because they present an unreasonable risk. *Federal Register.* February 11, 2004; 69:6787–6854.

7. US Food and Drug Administration Center for Food Safety and Applied Nutrition. Dietary Supplements: Warnings and Safety Information. Available at: http://www.cfsan.fda.gov/~dms/ds-warn.html. Accessed February 9, 2006.

8. US Food and Drug Administration Center for Food Safety and Applied Nutrition. New Dietary Ingredients in Dietary Supplements. Available at: http://www.cfsan.fda.gov/~dms/ds-ingrd.html. Accessed February 9, 2006.

9. US Food and Drug Administration Center for Food Safety and Applied Nutrition. A Food Labeling Guide: Appendix C. September 1994. Available at: http://www.cfsan.fda.gov/~dms/flg-6c.html. Accessed February 9, 2006.

10. Food Labeling: health claims and label statements for dietary supplements; strategy for implementation of Pearson court decision. *Federal Register.* December 1, 1999;64: 67289–67291.

11. US Food and Drug Administration Center for Food Safety and Applied Nutrition. Consumer Health Information for Better Nutrition Initiative: Task Force Report. July 10, 2003. Available at: http://www.cfsan.fda.gov/~dms/nuttftoc.html. Accessed February 9, 2006.

12. US Food and Drug Administration Center for Food Safety and Applied Nutrition. Qualified Health Claims Subject to Enforcement Discretion. Available at: http://www.cfsan.fda.gov/~dms/qhc-sum.html. Accessed February 9, 2006.

13. US Food and Drug Administration Center for Food Safety and Applied Nutrition. Public Meeting on Assessing Consumer Perceptions of Health Claims. Available at: http://www.cfsan.fda.gov/~dms/qhctran.html. Accessed March 24, 2006.

14. FDA Final Rule. Food labeling; statement of identity, nutrition labeling and ingredient labeling of dietary supplements; compliance policy guide, revocation; final rules. *Federal Register.* September 23, 1997;62:49826–49858.

15. US Food and Drug Administration Center for Food Safety and Applied Nutrition. Guidance for Industry. A Dietary Supplement Labeling Guide. Chapter 1: General dietary supplement labeling. April 2005. Available at: http://www.cfsan.fda.gov/~dms/dslg-1.html. Accessed February 9, 2006.

16. FDA Final Rule. Food labeling; nutrient content claims: definition for "high potency" and definition of "antioxidant" for use in nutrient content claims for dietary supplements and conventional foods. *Federal Register.* September 23, 1997;62:49868–49881.

17. Federal Trade Commission. Dietary Supplements: An Advertising Guide for Industry. Available at: http://www.ftc.gov/bcp/conline/pubs/buspubs/dietsupp.htm. Accessed February 9, 2006.

18. FDA Advance Notice of Proposed Rulemaking. Current good manufacturing practice in manufacturing, packing, or holding dietary supplements. *Federal Register.* February 6, 1997;62:5700–5709.

19. US Food and Drug Administration Center for Food Safety and Applied Nutrition. Dietary Supplements: Industry Information and Regulations. Available at: http://www.cfsan.fda.gov/~dms/ds-ind.html #GMPS. Accessed February 9, 2006.

20. National Institutes of Health. Office of Dietary Supplements. International Bibliographic Information on Dietary Supplements (IBIDS) Database. Available at: http://ods.od.nih.gov/Health_Information/IBIDS.aspx. Accessed February 9, 2006.

21. National Institutes of Health. Office of Dietary Supplements. Computer Access to Research on Dietary Supplements (CARDS) Database. Available at: http://ods.od.nih. gov/research/cards_database.aspx. Accessed February 9, 2006.

22. National Institutes of Health. Office of Dietary Supplements. Annual Bibliographies of Significant Advances in Dietary Supplement Research. Available at: http://ods.od.nih. gov/Research/Annual_Bibliographies.aspx. Accessed February 9, 2006.

23. National Institutes of Health. Office of Dietary Supplements Web site. Available at: http://dietary-supplements.info.nih.gov. Accessed February 9, 2006.

24. National Institutes of Health. National Center for Complementary and Alternative Medicine Web site. Available at: http://nccam.nih.gov. Accessed February 9, 2006.

25. ConsumerLab.com. Available at: http://www.consumerlab.com. Accessed February 9, 2006.

26. NSF International. Dietary Supplements, Functional Food and Beverages. Available at: http://www.nsf.org/business/dietary_supplements. Accessed February 9, 2006.

27. US Pharmacopoeia Web site. Available at: http://www.usp.org. Accessed February 9, 2006.

28. National Nutritional Foods Association (NNFA). NNFA GMP Certification Program. Available at: http://www.nnfa.org/site/PageServer?pagename=ic_gmp. Accessed March 24, 2006.

Appendix B

Ethical Issues and Dietary Supplements

Lisa K. Fieber, MS, RD, and Samuel L. Fieber, JD
Revised by Nancy Cotugna, DrPH, RD

Dietary supplement use is widespread in the United States: approximately 34% of the population consumes vitamins and/or minerals daily, and 6% report daily use of a nonvitamin nonmineral supplement (1). Ethical issues will continue to be an area of concern in the dietary supplement arena as long as controversy and conflict surround this topic. Lack of definitive scientific evidence regarding safety and efficacy of many supplements make this subject a challenging one for health professionals. Registered dietitians (RDs) are often called on to use their professional judgment when navigating areas of practice where information is often equivocal, and predicaments arise as to how to responsibly advise clients. Both ethical and legal considerations need to be recognized. This appendix provides information and resources in this area; however, it is not meant to be a complete guide to ethical considerations nor a substitute for qualified legal advice. Questions about ethical considerations can be directed to the American Dietetic Association (ADA) House of Delegates Governance team (800/877-1600 or ethics@eatright.org).

Ethical Standards

Most organizations for health professionals offer codes of ethical conduct. When dealing with dietary supplements, ethical conduct is of particular concern because some therapies may be risky, and because the sale of supplements by health professionals may raise the question of a conflict of interest.

The ADA/Commission on Dietetic Registration (CDR) Code of Ethics (2) serves as the foundation of ethical guidance for RDs. Principle 12 states, "The dietetics practitioner is alert to situations that might cause a conflict of interest or have the appearance of conflict. The dietetics practitioner provides full disclosure when a real or potential conflict of interest arises" (2). Since the publication of the code in 1999, the organization has also published an Ethics Opinion designed to help practitioners apply the code on issues of conflicts of interest in dietetics research, presentations, and publications (3).

Legal and Regulatory Issues

Health professionals must comply with the law when performing professional duties such as providing advice or recommendations about supplements. State laws that regulate allied health professions, including RDs, often define scopes of practice. RDs should become familiar with the licensure laws in their state and take care to stay within practice boundaries regarding the diagnosis or treatment of disease. Forty-three states, the District of Columbia, and Puerto Rico have laws that regulate RDs or nutritionists. The CDR Web site provides the most current information on laws regulating RDs and links to state licensure agencies (4). Practicing medicine without a license is a felony in many states. To avoid any allegations of this type, the RD must become familiar with state laws defining the practice of medicine and proceed with caution when advising clients about dietary supplements.

The ADA's practice paper on dietary supplements provides legal and ethical perspectives on the topic (5). ADA, in conjunction with the American Pharmaceutical Association, has also published *A Healthcare Professional's Guide to Evaluation of Dietary Supplements,* which includes sections on regulatory, legal, and ethical issues (6).

Health professionals should keep abreast of current regulatory developments related to dietary supplements. This can be done by periodically checking the Food and Drug Administration (FDA) Web site (www.fda.gov). Health professionals are responsible for reporting adverse effects to the FDA and misleading advertising to the Federal Trade Commission.

ADA Resources

ADA has a number of position papers and other publications that serve as valuable resources for practitioners seeking insights into the challenges of dealing with dietary supplements in practice. The "Guidelines Regarding the Recommendation and Sale of Dietary Supplements" published in the *Journal of the American Dietetic Association* (7) provides direction to professionals who are thinking about recommending or selling dietary supplements.

The ADA Taskforce on Complementary and Alternative Medicine has developed dietary supplement competencies. One of these compentencies states that registered dietitians should be able to identify the legal, ethical, and moral issues surrounding dietary supplements, including scope of practice issues, and describe practice implications of dietary supplement legislation and regulation (8).

ADA position papers on food and nutrition misinformation, food fortification, functional foods, and dietary supplements also address ethical issues. The complete text of these papers can be found on the ADA Web site (9).

The ADA's Standards of Practice in Nutrition Care and Updated Standards of Professional Performance (10) define an RD's responsibility for providing quality services in all areas of practice. These standards describe expected minimum levels of performance in the areas of competence and accountability. The standards clearly require adherence to the code of ethics.

Conclusion

Health professionals are responsible for promoting the well being and protecting the health of the public. Responsibly advising clients about dietary supplements will continue to be a challenge, but it can be managed by being familiar with state laws pertaining to dietetics practice, abiding by professional codes of conduct, and continually updating one's knowledge base in this ever-changing and expanding area. It is always a good idea to apply medicine's underlying principles of beneficence (maximizing good), nonmaleficence (doing no harm), and respect for others. Because dietary supplements are commonly used as self-care treatments, the concerns about the risks for consumers related to the safety and efficacy of the products are real. Inappropriate use of dietary supplements can have serious adverse health effects including fatalities. A qualified ethical practitioner is essential to ensure that the health of the client is not jeopardized by use of these products and to minimize risks and maximize benefits (11).

References

1. Millen AE, Dodd KW, Subar AF. Use of vitamin, mineral, nonvitamin and nonmineral supplements in the United states: The 1987, 1992, and 2000 National Health Interview Survey results. 2004. *J Am Diet Assoc.* 2004;104:942–950.
2. Code of ethics for the profession of dietetics. The American Dietetic Association. *J Am Diet Assoc.* 1999;99:109–113.
3. Woteki CE. Ethics opinion: conflicts of interest in presentations and publications and dietetics research. *J Am Diet Assoc.* 2006;106:27–31.
4. Commission on Dietetic Registration Web site. Available at: http://www.cdrnet.org. Accessed February 9, 2006.
5. American Dietetic Association practice paper: dietary supplements. *J Am Diet Assoc.* 2005;102:460–470.
6. American Dietetic Association and American Pharmaceutical Association. A Healthcare Professional's Guide to Evaluating Dietary Supplements. Available at: http://www.eatright.org/DietarySupplementsText.pdf. Accessed February 9, 2006.
7. Thomson C. Diekman C, Fragakis AS, Meerschaert C, Holler H, Devlin C. Guidelines regarding the recommendation and sale of dietary supplements. *J Am Diet Assoc.* 2002;102:1158–1164.
8. Touger-Decker R, Thomson C. Complementary and alternative medicine: competencies for dietetics professionals. *J Am Diet Assoc.* 2003;103:1464–1469.
9. American Dietetic Association Web site. Available at: http://www.eatright.org. Accessed February 9, 2006.
10. American Dietetic Association: Standards of practice in nutrition care and updated standards of professional performance. *J Am Diet Assoc.* 2005;105:641–645.
11. World Health Organization. Guidelines on Developing Consumer Information on Proper Use of Traditional, Complementary, and Alternative Medicine. Available at: http://www.who.int/medicines/library/trm/Consumer.pdf. Accessed July 8, 2005.

Appendix C

Dietary Intake Tables

Table C.1: Dietary Reference Intakes (DRIs): Recommended Intakes for Individuals, Vitamins
Food and Nutrition Board, Institute of Medicine, The National Academies

Life Stage Group	Vitamin A (µg/d)[a]	Vitamin C (mg/d)	Vitamin D (µg/d)[b,c]	Vitamin E (mg/d)[d]	Vitamin K (µg/d)	Thiamin (mg/d)	Riboflavin (mg/d)	Niacin (mg/d)[e]	Vitamin B_6 (mg/d)	Folate (µg/d)[f]	Vitamin B_{12} (µg/d)	Pantothenic Acid (mg/d)	Biotin (µg/d)	Choline (mg/d)[g]
Infants														
0–6 mo	400*	40*	5*	4*	2.0*	0.2*	0.3*	2*	0.1*	65*	0.4*	1.7*	5*	125*
7–12 mo	500*	50*	5*	5*	2.5*	0.3*	0.4*	4*	0.3*	80*	0.5*	1.8*	6*	150*
Children														
1–3 y	300	15	5*	6	30*	0.5	0.5	6	0.5	150	0.9	2*	8*	200*
4–8 y	400	25	5*	7	55*	0.6	0.6	8	0.6	200	1.2	3*	12*	250*
Males														
9–13 y	600	45	5*	11	60*	0.9	0.9	12	1.0	300	1.8	4*	20*	375*
14–18 y	900	75	5*	15	75*	1.2	1.3	16	1.3	400	2.4	5*	25*	550*
19–30 y	900	90	5*	15	120*	1.2	1.3	16	1.3	400	2.4	5*	30*	550*
31–50 y	900	90	5*	15	120*	1.2	1.3	16	1.3	400	2.4	5*	30*	550*
51–70 y	900	90	10*	15	120*	1.2	1.3	16	1.7	400	2.4[h]	5*	30*	550*
>70 y	900	90	15*	15	120*	1.2	1.3	16	1.7	400	2.4[h]	5*	30*	550*
Females														
9–13 y	600	45	5*	11	60*	0.9	0.9	12	1.0	300	1.8	4*	20*	375*
14–18 y	700	65	5*	15	75*	1.0	1.0	14	1.2	400[i]	2.4	5*	25*	400*
19–30 y	700	75	5*	15	90*	1.1	1.1	14	1.3	400[i]	2.4	5*	30*	425*
31–50 y	700	75	5*	15	90*	1.1	1.1	14	1.3	400[i]	2.4	5*	30*	425*
51–70 y	700	75	10*	15	90*	1.1	1.1	14	1.5	400	2.4[h]	5*	30*	425*
>70 y	700	75	15*	15	90*	1.1	1.1	14	1.5	400	2.4[h]	5*	30*	425*
Pregnancy														
≤ 18 y	750	80	5*	15	75*	1.4	1.4	18	1.9	600[j]	2.6	6*	30*	450*
19–30 y	770	85	5*	15	90*	1.4	1.4	18	1.9	600[j]	2.6	6*	30*	450*
31–50 y	770	85	5*	15	90*	1.4	1.4	18	1.9	600[j]	2.6	6*	30*	450*
Lactation														
≤ 18 y	1,200	115	5*	19	75*	1.4	1.6	17	2.0	500	2.8	7*	35*	550*
19–30 y	1,300	120	5*	19	90*	1.4	1.6	17	2.0	500	2.8	7*	35*	550*
31–50 y	1,300	120	5*	19	90*	1.4	1.6	17	2.0	500	2.8	7*	35*	550*

NOTE: This table (taken from the DRI reports, see www.nap.edu) presents Recommended Dietary Allowances (RDAs) in **bold type** and Adequate Intakes (AIs) in ordinary type followed by an asterisk (*). RDAs and AIs may both be used as goals for individual intake. RDAs are set to meet the needs of almost all (97 to 98 percent) individuals in a group. For healthy breastfed infants, the AI is the mean intake. The AI for other life stage and gender groups is believed to cover needs of all individuals in the group, but lack of data or uncertainty in the data prevent stating with confidence the percentage of individuals covered by this intake.

[a] As retinol activity equivalents (RAEs). 1 RAE = 1 mg retinol, 12 mg b-carotene, 24 mg a-carotene, or 24 mg b-cryptoxanthin. To calculate RAEs from REs of provitamin A carotenoids in foods, divide the REs by 2. For preformed vitamin A in foods or supplements and for provitamin A carotenoids in supplements, 1 RE = 1 RAE.

[b] calciferol. 1 µg calciferol = 40 IU vitamin D.

[c] In the absence of adequate exposure to sunlight.

[d] As a-tocopherol. a-Tocopherol includes RRR-a-tocopherol, the only form of a-tocopherol that occurs naturally in foods, and the 2R-stereoisomeric forms of a-tocopherol (RRR-, RSR-, RRS-, and RSS-a-tocopherol) that occur in fortified foods and supplements. It does not include the 2S-stereoisomeric forms of a-tocopherol (SRR-, SSR-, SRS-, and SSS-a-tocopherol), also found in fortified foods and supplements.

[e] As niacin equivalents (NE). 1 mg of niacin = 60 mg of tryptophan; 0–6 months = preformed niacin (not NE).

[f] As dietary folate equivalents (DFE). 1 DFE = 1 µg food folate = 0.6 µg of folic acid from fortified food or as a supplement consumed with food = 0.5 µg of a supplement taken on an empty stomach.

[g] Although AIs have been set for choline, there are few data to assess whether a dietary supply of choline is needed at all stages of the life cycle, and it may be that the choline requirement can be met by endogenous synthesis at some of these stages.

[h] Because 10 to 30 percent of older people may malabsorb food-bound B_{12}, it is advisable for those older than 50 years to meet their RDA mainly by consuming foods fortified with B_{12} or a supplement containing B_{12}.

[i] In view of evidence linking folate intake with neural tube defects in the fetus, it is recommended that all women capable of becoming pregnant consume 400 µg from supplements or fortified foods in addition to intake of food folate from a varied diet.

[j] It is assumed that women will continue consuming 400 µg from supplements or fortified food until their pregnancy is confirmed and they enter prenatal care, which ordinarily occurs after the end of the periconceptional period—the critical time for formation of the neural tube.

Reprinted with permission. Copyright 2001 by the National Academy of Sciences. Courtesy of the National Academy Press, Washington, DC.

Table C.2: Dietary Reference Intakes (DRIs): Recommended Intakes for Individuals, Elements

Food and Nutrition Board, Institute of Medicine, National Academies

Life Stage Group	Calcium (mg/d)	Chromium (µg/d)	Copper (µg/d)	Fluoride (mg/d)	Iodine (µg/d)	Iron (mg/d)	Magnesium (mg/d)	Manganese (mg/d)	Molybdenum (µg/d)	Phosphorus (mg/d)	Selenium (µg/d)	Zinc (mg/d)
Infants												
0–6 mo	210*	0.2*	200*	0.01*	110*	0.27*	30*	0.003*	2*	100*	15*	2*
7–12 mo	270*	5.5*	220*	0.5*	130*	11	75*	0.6*	3*	275*	20*	3
Children												
1–3 y	500*	11*	340	0.7*	90	7	80	1.2*	17	460	20	3
4–8 y	800*	15*	440	1*	90	10	130	1.5*	22	500	30	5
Males												
9–13 y	1,300*	25*	700	2*	120	8	240	1.9*	34	1,250	40	8
14–18 y	1,300*	35*	890	3*	150	11	410	2.2*	43	1,250	55	11
19–30 y	1,000*	35*	900	4*	150	8	400	2.3*	45	700	55	11
31–50 y	1,000*	35*	900	4*	150	8	420	2.3*	45	700	55	11
51–70 y	1,200*	30*	900	4*	150	8	420	2.3*	45	700	55	11
>70 y	1,200*	30*	900	4*	150	8	420	2.3*	45	700	55	11
Females												
9–13 y	1,300*	21*	700	2*	120	8	240	1.6*	34	1,250	40	8
14–18 y	1,300*	24*	890	3*	150	15	360	1.6*	43	1,250	55	9
19–30 y	1,000*	25*	900	3*	150	18	310	1.8*	45	700	55	8
31–50 y	1,000*	25*	900	3*	150	18	320	1.8*	45	700	55	8
51–70 y	1,200*	20*	900	3*	150	8	320	1.8*	45	700	55	8
>70 y	1,200*	20*	900	3*	150	8	320	1.8*	45	700	55	8
Pregnancy												
≤18 y	1,300*	29*	1,000	3*	220	27	400	2.0*	50	1,250	60	12
19–30 y	1,000*	30*	1,000	3*	220	27	350	2.0*	50	700	60	11
31–50 y	1,000*	30*	1,000	3*	220	27	360	2.0*	50	700	60	11

Lactation

≤ 18 y	1,300*	44*	1,300	3*	290	10	360	2.6*	50	1,250	70	13
19–30 y	1,000*	45*	1,300	3*	290	9	310	2.6*	50	700	70	12
31–50 y	1,000*	45*	1,300	3*	290	9	320	2.6*	50	700	70	12

Table C.3: Dietary Reference Intakes (DRIs): Tolerable Upper Intake Levels (UL^a), Vitamins

Food and Nutrition Board, Institute of Medicine, National Academies

Life Stage Group	Vitamin A (μg/d)^b	Vitamin C (mg/d)	Vitamin D (μg/d)	Vitamin E (mg/d)^{c,d}	Vitamin K	Thiamin	Ribo-flavin	Niacin (mg/d)^d	Vitamin B$_6$ (mg/d)^d	Folate (μg/d)^d	Vitamin B$_{12}$	Pantothenic Acid	Biotin	Choline (g/d)	Carote-noids^e
Infants															
0–6 mo	600	ND^f	25	ND	ND	ND	ND	ND	ND	ND	ND	ND	ND	ND	ND
7–12 mo	600	ND	25	ND	ND	ND	ND	ND	ND	ND	ND	ND	ND	ND	ND
Children															
1–3 y	600	400	50	200	ND	ND	ND	10	30	300	ND	ND	ND	1.0	ND
4–8 y	900	650	50	300	ND	ND	ND	15	40	400	ND	ND	ND	1.0	ND
Males,															
Females															
9–13 y	1,700	1,200	50	600	ND	ND	ND	20	60	600	ND	ND	ND	2.0	ND
14–18 y	2,800	1,800	50	800	ND	ND	ND	30	80	800	ND	ND	ND	3.0	ND
19–70 y	3,000	2,000	50	1,000	ND	ND	ND	35	100	1,000	ND	ND	ND	3.5	ND
>70 y	3,000	2,000	50	1,000	ND	ND	ND	35	100	1,000	ND	ND	ND	3.5	ND
Pregnancy															
≤18 y	2,800	1,800	50	800	ND	ND	ND	30	80	800	ND	ND	ND	3.0	ND
19–50 y	3,000	2,000	50	1,000	ND	ND	ND	35	100	1,000	ND	ND	ND	3.5	ND
Lactation															
≤18 y	2,800	1,800	50	800	ND	ND	ND	30	80	800	ND	ND	ND	3.0	ND
19–50 y	3,000	2,000	50	1,000	ND	ND	ND	35	100	1,000	ND	ND	ND	3.5	ND

^{a}UL = The maximum level of daily nutrient intake that is likely to pose no risk of adverse effects. Unless otherwise specified, the UL represents total intake from food, water, and supplements. Due to lack of suitable data, ULs could not be established for vitamin K, thiamin, riboflavin, vitamin B$_{12}$, pantothenic acid, biotin, or carotenoids. In the absence of ULs, extra caution may be warranted in consuming levels above recommended intakes.

^{b}As preformed vitamin A only.

^{c}As α-tocopherol; applies to any form of supplemental α-tocopherol.

^{d}The ULs for vitamin E, niacin, and folate apply to synthetic forms obtained from supplements, fortified foods, or a combination of the two.

^{e}β-Carotene supplements are advised only to serve as a provitamin A source for individuals at risk of vitamin A deficiency.

^{f}ND = Not determinable due to lack of data of adverse effects in this age group and concern with regard to lack of ability to handle excess amounts. Source of intake should be from food only to prevent high levels of intake.

Reprinted with permission from *Dietary Reference Intakes for Calcium, Phosphorous, Magnesium, Vitamin D, and Fluoride* (1997); *Dietary Reference Intakes for Thiamin, Riboflavin, Niacin, Vitamin B$_6$, Folate, Vitamin B$_{12}$, Pantothenic Acid, Biotin, and Choline* (1998); *Dietary Reference Intakes for Vitamin C, Vitamin E, Selenium, and Carotenoids* (2000); and *Dietary Reference Intakes for Vitamin A, Vitamin K, Arsenic, Boron, Chromium, Copper, Iodine, Iron, Manganese, Molybdenum, Nickel, Silicon, Vanadium, and Zinc* (2001). Copyright 2001 by the National Academy of Sciences. Courtesy of the National Academy Press, Washington, DC.

Table C.4: Dietary Reference Intakes (DRIs): Tolerable Upper Intake Levels (UL[a]), Elements

Food and Nutrition Board, Institute of Medicine, National Academies

Life Stage Group	Arsenic[b]	Boron (mg/d)	Calcium (g/d)	Chromium	Copper (µg/d)	Fluoride (mg/d)	Iodine (µg/d)	Iron (mg/d)	Magnesium (mg/d)[c]	Manganese (mg/d)	Molybdenum (µg/d)	Nickel (mg/d)	Phosphorus (g/d)	Selenium (µg/d)	Silicon[d]	Vanadium (mg/d)[e]	Zinc (mg/d)
Infants																	
0–6 mo	ND[f]	ND	ND	ND	ND	0.7	ND	40	ND	ND	ND	ND	ND	45	ND	ND	4
7–12 mo	ND	ND	ND	ND	ND	0.9	ND	40	ND	ND	ND	ND	ND	60	ND	ND	5
Children																	
1–3 y	ND	3	2.5	ND	1,000	1.3	200	40	65	2	300	0.2	3	90	ND	ND	7
4–8 y	ND	6	2.5	ND	3,000	2.2	300	40	110	3	600	0.3	3	150	ND	ND	12
Males, Females																	
9–13 y	ND	11	2.5	ND	5,000	10	600	40	350	6	1,100	0.6	4	280	ND	ND	23
14–18 y	ND	17	2.5	ND	8,000	10	900	45	350	9	1,700	1.0	4	400	ND	ND	34
19–70 y	ND	20	2.5	ND	10,000	10	1,100	45	350	11	2,000	1.0	4	400	ND	1.8	40
>70 y	ND	20	2.5	ND	10,000	10	1,100	45	350	11	2,000	1.0	3	400	ND	1.8	40
Pregnancy																	
≤18 y	ND	17	2.5	ND	8,000	10	900	45	350	9	1,700	1.0	3.5	400	ND	ND	34
19–50 y	ND	20	2.5	ND	10,000	10	1,100	45	350	11	2,000	1.0	3.5	400	ND	ND	40
Lactation																	
≤18 y	ND	17	2.5	ND	8,000	10	900	45	350	9	1,700	1.0	4	400	ND	ND	34
19–50 y	ND	20	2.5	ND	10,000	10	1,100	45	350	11	2,000	1.0	4	400	ND	ND	40

[a]UL = The maximum level of daily nutrient intake that is likely to pose no risk of adverse effects. Unless otherwise specified, the UL represents total intake from food, water, and supplements. Due to lack of suitable data, ULs could not be established for arsenic, chromium, and silicon. In the absence of ULs, extra caution may be warranted in consuming levels above recommended intakes.

[b]Although the UL was not determined for arsenic, there is no justification for adding arsenic to food or supplements.

[c]The ULs for magnesium represent intake from a pharmacological agent only and do not include intake from food and water.

[d]Although silicon has not been shown to cause adverse effects in humans, there is no justification for adding silicon to supplements.

[e]Although vanadium in food has not been shown to cause adverse effects in humans, there is no justification for adding vanadium to food and vanadium supplements should be used with caution. The UL is based on adverse effects in laboratory animals and this data could be used to set a UL for adults but not children and adolescents.

[f]ND = Not determinable due to lack of data of adverse effects in this age group and concern with regard to lack of ability to handle excess amounts. Source of intake should be from food only to prevent high levels of intake.

Reprinted with permission from *Dietary Reference Intakes for Calcium, Phosphorous, Magnesium, Vitamin D, and Fluoride* (1997); *Dietary Reference Intakes for Thiamin, Riboflavin, Niacin, Vitamin B₆ Folate, Vitamin B₁₂, Pantothenic Acid, Biotin, and Choline* (1998); *Dietary Reference Intakes for Vitamin C, Vitamin E, Selenium, and Carotenoids* (2000); and *Dietary Reference Intakes for Vitamin A, Vitamin K, Arsenic, Boron, Chromium, Copper, Iodine, Iron, Manganese, Molybdenum, Nickel, Silicon, Vanadium, and Zinc* (2001). Copyright 2001 by the National Academy of Sciences. Courtesy of the National Academy Press, Washington, DC.

Appendix D

Additional Resources

Organizations and Government Institutes

American Botanical Council
6200 Manor Rd
Austin, TX 78723
Phone: 800/373-7105 (to place orders);
512/926-4900
Web site: http://www.herbalgram.org

American Dietetic Association
120 South Riverside Plaza, Suite 2000
Chicago, IL 60606-6995
Phone: 800/877-1600
Web site: http://www.eatright.org

Center for Food Safety and Applied Nutrition
US Food and Drug Administration
5100 Paint Branch Parkway
College Park, MD 20740-3835
Phone: 888/723-3366
Web site: http://www.cfsan.fda.gov
Includes links to general information on dietary supplements (http://vm.cfsan.fda.gov/~dms/supplmnt.html); information on dietary supplement regulations (http://www.cfsan.fda.gov/~dms/ds-labl.html); and warnings about certain dietary supplements (http://www.cfsan.fda.gov/~dms/ds-warn.html).

Center for Science in the Public Interest
1875 Connecticut Ave NW, Suite 300
Washington, DC 20009
Phone: 202/332-9110
E-mail: cspi@cspinet.org
Web site: http://www.cspinet.org

Council for Responsible Nutrition
1828 L St NW, Suite 900
Washington, DC 20036-5409
Phone: 202/776-7929
Web site: http://www.crnusa.org
Trade organization for supplement industry.

Food and Nutrition Board
Institute of Medicine
500 Fifth St NW
Washington, DC 20001
Phone: 202/334-2352
Web site: http://www.iom.edu/
CMS/3788.aspx

Food and Nutrition Information Center
Agricultural Research Service, USDA
National Agricultural Library, Room 105
10301 Baltimore Ave
Beltsville, MD 20705-2351
Phone: 301-504-5719
Web site: http://www.nal.usda/fnic

Herb Research Foundation
4140 15th St
Boulder, CO 80304
Phone: 303/449-2265
Web site: http://www.herbs.org

International Food Information Council
1100 Connecticut Ave NW, Suite 430
Washington, DC 20036
Phone: 202/296-6540
E-mail: foodinfo@ific.org
Web site: http://www.ific.org

National Center for Complementary and Alternative Medicine
National Institutes of Health
9000 Rockville Pike
Bethesda, MD 20892
Phone: 888/644-6226
E-mail: info@nccam.nih.gov
Web site: http://nccam.nih.gov

Office of Dietary Supplements
National Institutes of Health
6100 Executive Blvd
Room 3B01, MSC 7517
Bethesda, MD 20892-7517
Phone: 301/435-2920
E-mail: ods@nih.gov
Web site: http://ods.od.nih.gov

Organizations Providing Independent Certification for Dietary Supplements

ConsumerLab.com
333 Mamaroneck Ave
White Plains, NY 10605
Phone: 914/722-9149
E-mail: info@consumerlab.com
Web site: http://www.consumerlab.com

NSF International
PO Box 130140
789 Dixboro Road
Ann Arbor, MI 48113-0140
Phone: 800/NSF-MARK
E-mail: info@nsf.org
Web site: http://www.nsf.org

US Pharmacopoeia (USP)
12601 Twinbrook Parkway
Rockville, MD 20852
Phone: 800/227-8772
E-mail: custsvc@usp.org
Web site: http://www.usp.org

Journals

Alternative Medicine Review: A Journal of Clinical Therapeutics
Thorne Research, Inc
PO Box 25
Dover, ID 83825
Phone: 208/263-1337
E-mail: info@thorne.com
Web site: http://www.thorne.com/index/mod/amr/a/amr

Alternative Therapies in Health and Medicine
InnoVision Communications
PO Box 627
Holmes, PA 19043-9650
Phone: 303/440-7402
Web site: http://www.alternative-therapies.com/at/login/index.jsp

Journal of Dietary Supplements
Haworth Press, Inc.
10 Alice St
Binghamton, NY 13904
Phone: 800/429-6784
E-mail: getinfo@haworthpress.com
Web site: http://www.haworthpressinc.com

Journal of the American Dietetic Association
120 South Riverside Plaza, Suite 2000
Chicago, IL 60606-6995
Phone: 800/654-2452
Web site: http://www.adajournal.org

Journal of the American Medical Association
Subscriber Services Center
PO Box 10946
Chicago, IL 60610-0946
Phone: 800/262-2350
E-mail: ama-subs@ama-assn.org
Web site: http://jama.ama-assn.org

Scientific Review of Alternative Medicine
Commission for Scientific Medicine and
    Mental Health
PO Box 741
Amherst, NY 14226
Phone: 716/636-4869
E-mail: Editorial@sram.org
Web site: http://www.sram.org

Newsletters

HerbalGram
(Joint effort of the American Botanical
    Council and the Herb Research
    Foundation)
6200 Manor Rd
Austin, TX 78723
Phone: 512/926-4900
E-mail: abc@herbalgram.org
Web site: http://www.herbalgram.org

Nutrition Action Healthletter
Center for Science in the Public Interest
1875 Connecticut Ave NW, Suite 300
Washington, DC 20009
Phone: 202/332-9110
E-mail: circ@cspinet.org
Web site: http://www.cspinet.org/nah

Nutrition Business Journal
4452 Park Blvd, Suite 306
San Diego, CA 92116
Phone: 619/295-7685
E-mail: info@nutritionbusiness.com
Web site: http://www.nutritionbusiness.com

Nutrition in Complementary Care, A Dietetic Practice Group of the American Dietetic Association, quarterly newsletter
Phone: 800/877-1600 (American Dietetic
Association, for subscriptions)
Web site: http://www.
    complementarynutrition.org

SCAN's Pulse
(Newsletter for Sports, Cardiovascular,
    and Wellness Nutritionists (SCAN)
    Dietetic Practice Group)
SCAN Office
PO Box 8088
Chicago, IL 60680-8088
Phone: 800/877-1600 (American Dietetic
    Association, for subscriptions); or
    800/249-2857 (SCAN office)
Web site: http://scandpg.org

Tufts University Health and Nutrition Letter
PO Box 420235
Palm Coast, FL 32142-0235
Phone: 800/274-7581
Web site: http://healthletter.tufts.edu

University of California Berkeley Wellness Letter
Subscription Dept
PO Box 420148
Palm Coast, FL 32142
Phone: 800/829-9170

Scientific Research Databases

Agency for Healthcare Research Quality
US Department of Health and Human
    Services
Web site: http://www.ahrq.gov

Dr. James Duke's Phytochemical and Ethnobotanical Databases
Web site: http://www.ars-grin.gov/duke

Herb Research Foundation
Web site: http://www.herbs.org

International Bibliographic Information on Dietary Supplements (IBIDS)
Web site: http://ods.od.nih.gov/databases/ibids.html

NAPRALERT—Natural Products Alert Database
Web site: http://www.napralert.org

National Center for Complementary and Alternative Medicine
Web site: http://nccam.nih.gov

Natural Standard
Web site: http://www.naturalstandard.com

Pharmacist's Letter/Natural Medicine Database
Web site: http://www.naturaldatabase.com

PubMed/Medline
Web site: http://www.ncbi.nlm.nih.gov/pubmed
The National Library of Medicine's bibliographic database.

Supplement Watch
Web site: http://www.supplementwatch.com

Resources on Health Fraud

National Council Against Health Fraud
119 Foster St
Peabody, MA 01960
Phone: 978/532-9383
Web site: http://www.ncahf.org

Quackwatch
Web site: http://www.quackwatch.com

Reporting Adverse Effects of Dietary Supplements

Food and Drug Administration
Health care professionals can report to 800/FDA-1088 or http://www.fda.gov/medwatch/report/hcp.htm. Consumers can report to 800/FDA-1088 or http://

www.fda.gov/medwatch/report/consumer/consumer.htm

Books

Bibliography of Significant Advances in Dietary Supplement Research. Bethesda, Md: National Institutes of Health, Office of Dietary Supplements; 2002, 2003, 2004.

Blumenthal M, Brinckmann J, Dinda K, et al. *The American Botanical Council's ABC Clinical Guide to Herbs.* Austin, Tex: American Botanical Council; 2003.

Brinker F. *Herb Contraindications and Drug Interactions.* 3rd ed. Sandy, Ore: Eclectic Medical Publications; 2001.

Coates PM, Blackman MR, Cragg GM, Levine M, Moss J, White JD. *Encyclopedia of Dietary Supplements.* New York, NY: Marcel Dekker; 2004.

Gruenwald J. *PDR for Herbal Medicines.* 3rd ed. Montvale, NJ: Medical Economics; 2004.

Jacksch F, Roman M. *Handbook of Analytical Methods for Dietary Supplements.* Washington, DC: APhA Publications; 2005.

Jellin JM, Gregory P, Batz F, et al. *Pharmacist's Letter/Prescriber's Letter Natural Medicines Comprehensive Database.* Updated annually. Stockton, Calif: Therapeutic Research Faculty.

MacWilliam L. *Comparative Guide to Nutritional Supplements.* 3rd ed. Vernon, British Columbia, Canada: Northern Dimensions Publishing; 2003.

Mahady GB, Hong Sang Fong H, Farnsworth NR. *Botanical Dietary Supplements: Quality, Safety, and Efficacy.* Lisse, The Netherlands: Swets & Zeitlinger; 2001.

Webb Goeffrey P. *Dietary Supplements and Functional Foods.* Oxford, UK: Blackwell Publishing; 2006.

Appendix E

Dietary Supplement Intake Assessment: Questions to Ask Clients

As part of any nutrition assessment, health professionals should ask clients questions about dietary supplement intake. The following questions are designed to gather information that will help clients make informed decisions about supplement use. Ask your clients to bring supplement packages to an appointment to help answer these questions.

Note: For questions marked with an asterisk, ask the question for each supplement taken and check labels.

- ◆ What supplements do you use? (Be sure to explain that supplements include vitamins and minerals, herbals, amino acids, protein, fiber, fatty acids, etc.)
- ◆ What are your main reasons for taking this supplement?* (Suggest reasons, such as to prevent a disease, to help treat a disease or condition, general health, energy, weight loss, pregnancy, mood, muscle-building, etc.)
- ◆ How long have you used this supplement?*
- ◆ How long do you plan on using it?*
- ◆ How often do you take this supplement?*
- ◆ What brand of supplement do you take?
- ◆ What form of supplement do you take?*
- ◆ How much of the supplement do you take?*
- ◆ Do you ever take more than the dose shown on the label?*
- ◆ How much money do you spend on supplements? Does this cost make it hard to afford food?
- ◆ Have you had any changes in your health or medical condition since you started taking this supplement?*
- ◆ Since you started using this supplement, have you had any bad reactions?* (Give examples of adverse effects, such as rash, stomach problems, mood changes, or nervousness.)
- ◆ Are you allergic to any foods, insects, plants, or flowers? Are any of your supplements made from things that give you allergies? (To answer the second question, it

may be necessary to read supplement labels. For example, if a patient has an allergy to bee stings or honey, he or she may react to bee pollen supplements.)

◆ What other drugs do you take? (Ask about both prescription and over-the-counter medications.)

◆ Do you drink alcohol or drinks with caffeine (coffee, tea, cola)? Do you drink these when you take supplements?

INDEX

abdominal fat, branched chain amino acids (BCAA) and, 61

Acacia greggi, 93, 94

acetyl L-carnitine, Alzheimer's disease and, 87–88

acidophilus/*Lactobacillus acidophilus* (LA), 2–10
  atopic disease and, 8
  cancer and, 7–8
  cholesterol and, 7
  dosage information/bioavailability, 4
  drug/supplement interactions, 3
  food sources, 4
  irritable bowel syndrome and, 5–6
  key points, 3–4
  media and marketing claims, 2
  safety, 2
  vaginal yeast infections and, 6–7

acne
  vitamin A and, 521, 531
  zinc and, 632–633

acquired immunodeficiency syndrome (AIDS). *See also* human immunodeficiency virus (HIV); immune function
  arginine and, 33–34
  carnitine and, 89–90
  cobalamin and, 563
  coenzyme Q10 and, 120
  colostrum/bovine colostrum and diarrhea related to, 126

Agency for Healthcare Research Quality, 660

age-related macular degeneration. *See* macular degeneration

aging. *See* elderly

AIDS. *See* acquired immunodeficiency syndrome (AIDS)

alanine, 10–14
  dosage information/bioavailability, 11
  drug/supplement interactions, 10
  exercise and, 13
  food sources, 11
  key points, 10–11
  liver function and, 12–13
  media and marketing claims, 10
  safety, 10

allergic rhinitis
  lactobacillus acidophilus and, 7
  methylsulfonylmethane (MSM) and, 376

aloe vera, 14–18
  blood lipid control and, 16–17

diabetes and, 17
  dosage information/bioavailability, 15–16
  drug/supplement interactions, 15
  gastrointestinal health and, 16
  key points, 15
  media and marketing claims, 14
  safety, 14
  wound healing and, 17

alpha-linolenic acid, 176, 188

alpha-lipoic acid (ALA), 18–23
  cardiovascular disease and, 22
  cognition/dementia and, 22
  diabetes and, 20–21
  dosage information/bioavailability, 20
  drug/supplement interactions, 19
  food sources, 20
  human immunodeficiency virus (HIV) and, 22
  key points, 19–20
  liver disease and, 22
  media and marketing claims, 19
  safety, 19

Alternative Medicine Review, 659

Alternative Therapies in Health and Medicine, 659

Alzheimer's disease. *See also* dementia; memory
  choline and, 328–329
  ginkgo and, 239–241
  melatonin and, 369
  phosphatidylserine and, 402
  vitamin E and, 599–600

American Botanical Council, 658

American Dietetic Association (ADA), 649–650, 658, 659

American Heart Association (AHA) recommendations on fish oil, 175

Anabolic Steroid Control Act (2004), 24

Analytical Methods and Reference Materials Program, 645

androstenediol and androstenedione, 23–26
  dosage information/bioavailability, 25
  drug/supplement interactions, 25
  key points, 25
  media and marketing claims, 24
  safety, 24–25

anemia, iron-deficiency, and iron supplements, 316, 318

anemia of chronic disease, and iron supplements, 318

Angelica sinensis. See dong quai *(Angelica sinensis)*

Annual Bibliography of Significant Advances in Dietary Supplement Research, 645

anorexia in the elderly, branched chain amino acids
    (BCAA) and, 62
antioxidants. *See also* vitamin A/beta carotene; vitamin C;
    vitamin E
    cat's claw, 95
    grape seed extract, 276
    green tea extract, 280
    wheat grass/barley grass, 614
anxiety
    5-hydroxy-tryptophan (5-HTP) and, 300–301
    kava and, 323–324
    valerian and, 512
appetite, 5-hydroxy-tryptophan (5-HTP) and, 301–302
arginine (L-arginine), 26–36
    acquired immunodeficiency syndrome (AIDS) and,
        33–34
    breast cancer and, 32
    cancer and, 32
    cardiovascular disease and, 29
    colorectal cancer and, 32
    dosage information/bioavailability, 29
    for the elderly, 32
    erectile dysfunction and, 34
    exercise hormones and, 29
    food sources, 28
    key points, 27–28
    media and marketing claims, 27
    necrotizing enterocolitis in newborns, 34
    ornithine and, 32, 33
    safety, 27
    wound healing and, 33
arthritis. *See also* osteoarthritis; rheumatoid arthritis
    glucosamine hydrochloride and chondroitin
        combinations and, 258–260
    methylsulfonylmethane (MSM) and, 376
    niacin and, 548–549
    pantothenic acid and, 397–398
ascorbic acid. *See* vitamin C
aspartic acid/asparagine, 36–39
    dosage information/bioavailability, 37
    drug/supplement interactions, 37
    exercise and, 38
    food sources, 37
    and hepatic encephalopathy, 38
    key points, 37
    media and marketing claims, 36
    safety, 36–37
assessment of dietary supplement intake, questions for,
    662–663
asthma
    acidophilus and, 7
    lycopene and, 342–343
    pau d'arco and, 399
    pyridoxine and, 555–556
    selenium and, 470
    vitamin C and, 571
atherosclerosis. *See also* blood lipids; cardiovascular
    disease; cholesterol

fish oil and, 175, 177–178
    garlic and, 226–227
    lycopene and, 343
athletic performance. *See* exercise/athletic performance
atopic dermatitis, gamma-linolenic acid and, 215
atopic disease, acidophilus and, 8
attention deficit/hyperactivity disorder, fish oil and, 184
autism, pyridoxine and, 556

barberry, 271
barley grass. *See* wheat grass/barley grass
BCAA. *See* branched chain amino acids (BCAA)
bee pollen, 39–42
    dosage information/bioavailability, 40–41
    food sources, 40
    key points, 40
    media and marketing claims, 40
    memory and, 41
    premenstrual syndrome and, 41
    prostatitis and, 41–42
benign prostatic hypertrophy
    phytosterols and, 406–407
    pygeum and, 420–421
    saw palmetto and, 460–461
berberine, 271
beta carotene, 405. *See also* vitamin A/beta carotene
beta-sitosterol, 404, 405
bipolar disorder, fish oil and, 184
bitter melon *(Momordica charantia),* 42–46
    blood glucose control and, 44
    blood lipids and, 44–45
    cancer and, 45
    dosage information/bioavailability, 44
    drug/supplement interactions, 43
    food sources, 44
    immunity in human immunodeficiency virus (HIV)
        and, 45
    key points, 43–44
    media and marketing claims, 43
    safety, 43
black cohosh *(Cimicifuga racemosa),* 46–51
    dong quai and, 159
    dosage information/bioavailability, 48
    drug/supplement interactions, 48
    media and marketing claims, 47
    menopause and, 49–50
    premenstrual syndrome and, 50
    safety, 47–48
black currant oil *(Ribes nigrum),* 210, 212, 217
black tea, 278, 279
blood clotting
    shark cartilage and, 477
    vitamin K and, 610–611
blood glucose. *See also* diabetes
    alanine and hypoglycemia, 11–12
    bitter melon and, 44
    fenugreek and, 167–168
    fish oil and, 179–180

fructo-oligosaccharides (FOS) and, 208–209
    ginger and, 232
blood lipids. *See also* atherosclerosis; cardiovascular
        disease; cholesterol
    acidophilus and, 3
    aloe vera and, 16–17
    bitter melon and, 44–45
    fenugreek and, 168
    fish oil and, 175, 177–180
    pantothenic acid and, 397
    phytosterols and, 406
    pyruvate and, 427
    red yeast rice and dyslipidemia associated with HIV,
        434
blood pressure
    calcium and, 74–76
    fish oil and, 175, 180–181
    garlic and, 227
    green tea extract and, 280–282
    magnesium and, 353–354
    potassium and, 416–418
    royal jelly and, 440
    vitamin C and, 574–575
blue-green algae. *See* spirulina/blue-green algae
body building, boron and, 55
body composition/body mass. *See also* muscle mass
    boron and, 55
    branched chain amino acids (BCAA) and abdominal
        fat, 61
    chromium and, 111–112
    colostrum/bovine colostrum and, 127
    conjugated linoleic acid (CLA) and, 131–133
    creatine and, 144–145
    dehydroepiandrosterone (DHEA) and, 155
    gamma-oryzanol and, 221
    β-hydroxy β-methylbutyrate (HMB) and, 306
bone health/bone mineral density. *See also* osteoporosis
    boron and, 54–55
    calcium and, 73–74
    lysine and, 348–348
    soy protein and, 494–494
    vitamin D and, 581–584
    vitamin K and, 611
borage oil, 210, 212, 217
boron, 52–57
    body building and, 55
    bone health and, 54–55
    cancer prevention and, 56
    cognitive function and, 55
    dosage information/bioavailability, 54
    drug/supplement interactions, 53
    estrogen therapy and, 54
    food sources, 53–54
    key points, 53
    media and marketing claims, 52
    osteoarthritis and, 55
    prostate cancer and, 56
    safety, 52–53

Botanical Research Centers Program, 645
bovine colostrum. *See* colostrum/bovine colostrum
bovine spongiform encephalopathy (BSE)
    colostrum/bovine colostrum and, 124
    phosphatidylserine and, 400–401
bowel function. *See* constipation; diarrhea;
        gastrointestinal disorders/health
branched chain amino acids (BCAA), 57–63
    abdominal fat and, 61
    anorexia in the elderly and, 62
    dosage information/bioavailability, 59
    drug/supplement interactions, 58
    exercise performance and, 59–60
    food sources, 59
    hepatic encephalopathy and, 61
    key points, 58–59
    media and marketing claims, 57
    safety, 58
breast cancer
    arginine and, 32
    black cohosh and, 47
    dehydroepiandrosterone (DHEA) and, 153–154
    vitamin A/beta carotene and, 524
breast tenderness, red clover and, 429–430
bromelain, 63–69
    antibiotic activity and, 67
    cancer and, 67–68
    dosage information/bioavailability, 64–65
    drug/supplement interactions, 64
    food sources, 64
    inflammation/joint pain and, 66–67
    key points, 64
    media and marketing claims, 63
    platelet aggregation and, 67
    safety, 63
    sinusitis/bronchitis infections and, 65–66
bronchitis, bromelain and, 65–66. *See also* respiratory
        illness/infection

cachexia. *See* wasting/cachexia
calcium, 69–81
    bone health and, 73–74, 581–584
    colon cancer and, 76–77
    dosage information/bioavailability, 72
    drug/supplement interactions, 70–71
    food sources, 72
    hypertension and, 74–76
    key points, 71
    lysine and absorption of, 347–348
    media and marketing claims, 69
    premenstrual syndrome (PMS) and, 78–79
    safety, 70
    vitamin D and absorption of, 584–585
    weight control and, 77–78
campesterol, 404
cancer. *See also* breast cancer; cancer prevention;
        chemotherapy; colon cancer; lung cancer; pancreatic
        cancer; prostate cancer

cancer (*continued*)
  acidophilus and, 7–8
  arginine and, 32
  bitter melon and, 45
  bromelain and, 67–68
  carnitine and fatigue in, 86–87
  coenzyme Q_{10} and, 120
  conjugated linoleic acid (CLA) and, 133
  dehydroepiandrosterone (DHEA) and, 153–154
  fenugreek and, 168–169
  fish oil and, 184–185
  flaxseed and, 192
  folate/folic acid and, 200–202
  gamma-linolenic acid and, 217
  garlic and, 228–229
  ginseng and, 252
  grape seed extract and, 276
  green tea extract and, 280–282
  β-hydroxy β-methylbutyrate (HMB) and wasting in, 306
  indole-3-carbinol (I-3C) and, 312–314
  melatonin and, 372
  milk thistle and, 380–381
  noni juice and, 389, 390
  pau d'arco and, 399
  resveratrol and, 436
  selenium and, 465–467
  shark cartilage and, 476–477
  soy protein and isoflavones and, 488–490
  spirulina/blue-green algae and, 502–503
  turmeric and, 507–508
  vitamin A/beta carotene and, 523–526
  vitamin C and, 575–576
  vitamin D and, 585–586
  vitamin E and, 596–597
  whey protein and, 619
cancer cachexia/wasting
  fish oil and, 184
  β-hydroxy β-methylbutyrate (HMB) and, 306
cancer prevention
  acidophilus and, 3–4
  boron and, 56
  licorice and, 333
  lutein and, 338
  lycopene and, 342
cardiac elasticity, garlic and, 227
cardiovascular disease. *See also* atherosclerosis; blood
    lipids; blood pressure; cholesterol
  alpha-lipoic acid (ALA) and, 22
  arginine and, 29
  carnitine and, 84–86
  chromium and, 110–111
  cobalamin and, 563–564
  coenzyme Q10 and, 117, 118–119
  conjugated linoleic acid (CLA) and, 133–134
  creatine and congestive heart failure, 146
  dehydroepiandrosterone (DHEA) and, 153
  fenugreek and, 168

fish oil and, 178–179
flaxseed and, 191
folate/folic acid and, 199–200
gamma-linolenic acid and, 216–217
garlic and, 226–228
grape seed extract and, 276
green tea extract and, 280–282
hawthorn and, 294
licorice root and prevention of, 334
magnesium and, 352–353
niacin and, 546–547
pyridoxine and, 554–555
resveratrol and, 436
royal jelly and, 440
selenium and, 467–468
shark cartilage and, 477
soy protein and isoflavones and, 485–488
vitamin A/beta carotene and, 526–528
vitamin C and, 572–574
vitamin E and, 593–596
CARDS (Computer Access to Research on Dietary
    Supplements), 644–645
carnitine, 81–92, 344
  cardiovascular disorders and, 84–86
  dosage information/bioavailability, 84
  drug/supplement interactions, 82–83
  exercise performance and, 86
  fatigue and, 86–87
  food sources, 84
  immune function/AIDS and, 89–90
  key points, 83
  male infertility and, 89
  media and marketing claims, 82
  safety, 82
  thyroid function and, 88–89
  weight loss and, 90
carotenoids, 518, 523
carpal tunnel syndrome, pyridoxine and, 553
cataracts
  lutein and age-related, 337–338
  riboflavin and, 543
  thiamin and, 539
  vitamin C and, 576
  vitamin E and, 600–601
cat's claw (*Uncaria tomentosa*), 92–95
  antioxidant, 95
  dosage information/bioavailability, 93–94
  drug/supplement interactions, 93
  key points, 93
  media and marketing claims, 92
  osteoarthritis and, 94
  rheumatoid arthritis and, 94
  safety, 93
Center for Food Safety and Applied Nutrition (CFSAN),
    641, 642, 658
Center for Science in the Public Interest, 658
chemotherapy
  ginger for nausea related to, 235

glutamine and mucositis from, 265–266
Chinese bitter melon. *See* bitter melon *(Momordica charantia)*
chitosan, 96–101
    cholesterol and, 99–100
    dental plaque formation and, 100
    dosage information/bioavailability, 97
    drug/supplement interactions, 97
    food sources, 97
    key points, 97
    media and marketing claims, 96
    safety, 96
    weight loss and, 97–98
chloasma, grape seed extract and, 277
cholecalciferol, 578, 581
cholesterol. *See also* atherosclerosis; blood lipids; cardiovascular disease; hyperlipidemia
    acidophilus and, 7
    chitosan and, 99–100
    fenugreek and, 168
    fructo-oligosaccharides (FOS) and, 208–209
    gamma-oryzanol and, 221
    garlic and, 226–227
    guggulu and, 291–292
    pantothenic acid and, 397
    policosanol and, 408, 410–412
    red yeast rice and, 433–434
    spirulina/blue-green algae and, 502
Cholestin, 432. *See also* red yeast rice
choline. *See* lecithin/choline
chondroitin sulfate, 101–105. *See also* glucosamine
    arthritis and, 103–104, 258–260
    dosage information/bioavailability, 102
    drug/supplement interactions, 102
    key points, 102
    media and marketing claims, 101
    safety, 101
choroideremia, lutein and, 337
chromium, 105–114
    cardiovascular disease and, 110–111
    corticosteroids and, 107
    diabetes and, 109–110
    dosage information/bioavailability, 108–109
    drug/supplement interactions, 106–107
    food sources, 107–108
    key points, 107
    media and marketing claims, 105
    obesity and, 111
    safety, 106
    strength training and body mass and, 111–112
chronic fatigue syndrome, carnitine and, 86–87
chronic venous insufficiency, horse chestnut and, 296–297
circadian rhythms, melatonin and, 366
circulation, garlic and, 227–228
cirrhosis. *See also* liver health/liver disease
    choline and prevention of, 329
    milk thistle and, 378–379

citrulline, 26
CLA. *See* conjugated linoleic acid (CLA)
coagulation. *See* blood clotting/coagulation
cobalamin. *See* vitamin B-12 (cobalamin)
coenzyme Q_{10}, 115–123
    cancer and, 120
    cardiovascular disease and, 117, 118–119
    dosage information/bioavailability, 117
    drug/supplement interactions, 116
    exercise performance and, 119–120
    food sources, 117
    HIV/AIDS, immunity, and, 120
    key points, 116–117
    media and marketing claims, 115
    migraines and, 121
    neurodegenerative disease and, 120–121
    safety, 115–116
cognition. *See also* Alzheimer's disease; dementia; memory
    alpha-lipoic acid (ALA) and, 22
    boron and, 55
    folate/folic acid and, 202–203
    ginseng and, 250
    iron and, 318–319
    phosphatidylserine and, 402
    pyridoxine and, 556–557
colds. *See* common cold; respiratory illness/infection
colitis, ulcerative, and fish oil, 182
colon cancer
    arginine and, 32
    calcium and, 76–77
    fructo-oligosaccharides (FOS) and, 208
colostrum/bovine colostrum, 123–129
    AIDS-related diarrhea and, 126
    athletic performance and, 127
    body weight and, 127
    dosage information/bioavailability, 125
    drug/supplement interactions, 124–125
    food sources, 125
    gastrointestinal disorders and, 125–126
    key points, 125
    media and marketing claims, 124
    NSAID-induced gut injury and, 126
    safety, 124
common cold. *See also* respiratory illness/infection
    echinacea and, 162–164
    vitamin C and, 570–571
    zinc and, 629–631
Computer Access to Research on Dietary Supplements (CARDS), 644–645
congestive heart failure, creatine and, 146. *See also* cardiovascular disease
conjugated linoleic acid (CLA), 129–136
    body composition/obesity and, 131–133
    cancer and, 133
    cardiovascular disease and, 133–134
    diabetes and, 134
    dosage information/bioavailability, 131

conjugated linoleic acid (*continued*)
  drug/supplement interactions, 130
  food sources, 130–131
  immunity and, 133
  key points, 130
  media and marketing claims, 129
  safety, 129
constipation
  flaxseed and, 193
  magnesium and, 358
  senna and, 473–474
ConsumerLab.com, 645, 659
coronary heart disease. *See* cardiovascular disease
Council for Responsible Nutrition, 658
cranberry extract, 136–140
  dosage information/bioavailability, 137–138
  drug/supplement interactions, 137
  food sources, 137
  key points, 137
  media and marketing claims, 136
  safety, 137
  urinary tract infections and, 138–139
creatine, 140–148
  body composition and, 144–145
  congestive heart failure and, 146
  dosage information/bioavailability, 143
  drug/supplement interactions, 141
  elderly and, 145
  food sources, 142–143
  high-intensity exercise and, 143–144
  key points, 142
  media and marketing claims, 140
  muscle strength and, 145
  muscular disease and, 145
  safety, 140–141
Crohn's disease, fish oil and, 182
Curcuma longa/curcumin. *See* turmeric *(Curcuma longa)*

dehydroepiandrosterone (DHEA), 148–157
  aging and, 151–152
  ban in sports, 149
  body composition and, 155
  cancer and, 153
  cardiovascular disease and, 153
  dosage information/bioavailability, 150–151
  drug/supplement interactions, 149
  HIV infection and, 154–155
  immunity and, 152
  key points, 150
  libido and, 151–152
  lupus and, 154
  media and marketing claims, 148
  memory and, 151–152
  menopausal symptoms and, 155
  mood and, 151–152
  safety, 149
dementia. *See also* Alzheimer's disease
  alpha-lipoic acid (ALA) and, 22

  ginkgo and, 239–241
  thiamin and, 537–538
dental plaque formation, chitosan and, 100
depression
  fish oil and, 183–184
  5-hydroxy-tryptophan (5-HTP) and, 300
  S-adenosylmethionine and, 447–448
  St John's wort and, 454–457
dermatitis
  aloe vera and, 17
  gamma-linolenic acid and, 215
DHA. *See* docosahexaenoic acid (DHA)
DHEA. *See* dehydroepiandrosterone (DHEA)
diabetes. *See also* blood glucose
  aloe vera and, 17
  alpha-lipoic acid (ALA) and, 20
  chromium and, 109–110
  cobalamin and, 564
  conjugated linoleic acid (CLA) and, 134
  fish oil and, 179–180
  gamma-linolenic acid and, 216
  ginger and, 232
  ginseng and, 251–252
  magnesium and, 354
  niacin and, 547–548
  pau d'arco and, 399
  soy protein and isoflavones and, 494–495
  vanadium and, 516–517
  vitamin E and, 602
diarrhea
  acidophilus and, 5
  colostrum/bovine colostrum and AIDS-related, 126
  goldenseal and infectious, 273–274
Dietary Reference Intake tables, 652–657
Dietary Supplement Health and Education Act of 1994
    (DSHEA), 639–645
dietary supplements. *See also* ethical issues; government
    regulation of dietary supplements; industry self-
    regulation of dietary supplements
  definition of, 640
  industry sales, xiii
  intake assessment questions, 662–663
dihe, 499
Dioscorea villosa. *See* wild yam *(Dioscorea villosa)*
docosahexaenoic acid (DHA), 173, 174, 176, 177. *See also*
    fish oil
dong quai *(Angelica sinensis)*, 157–160
  black cohosh and, 159
  dosage information/bioavailability, 159
  drug/supplement interactions, 158
  key points, 158
  media and marketing claims, 158
  menopause and, 159
  premenstrual syndrome (PMS) and, 159
  safety, 158
drug tests, goldenseal and, 274
DSHEA. *See* Dietary Supplement Health and Education
    Act of 1994 (DSHEA)

dyslipidemia. *See* blood lipids; cholesterol
dyspepsia. *See also* gastrointestinal disorders/health
   licorice root and, 332
   turmeric and, 506

echinacea, 160–165
   common cold/respiratory infection and, 162–164
   dosage information/bioavailability, 161
   drug/supplement interactions, 161
   immunity and, 162
   key points, 161
   media and marketing claims, 160
   safety, 160–161
eczema
   acidophilus and, 4, 8
   gamma-linolenic acid and, 215
   licorice root and, 332–333
eicosapentaenoic acid (EPA), 173, 174, 176, 177. *See also* fish oil
elderly
   arginine and ornithine and, 32
   branched chain amino acids (BCAA) and anorexia in, 62
   cobalamin and dementia in, 562–563
   creatine and, 145
   dehydroepiandrosterone (DHEA) and, 151–152
   phosphatidylserine and cognitive function in, 402
   pyridoxine and cognition in, 556–557
   thiamin and, 537–538
   vitamin E and immunity in, 598–599
encephalopathy. *See also* bovine spongiform encephalopathy (BSE)
   branched chain amino acids (BCAA) and, 61
   L-aspartate and, 38
   thiamin and, 537–538
eosinophilia-myalgia syndrome, banning of L-tryptophan and, 298
EPA. *See* eicosapentaenoic acid (EPA)
Ephedra sinica, 640–641. *See also* ma huang *(Ephedra sinica)*
erectile dysfunction
   arginine and, 34
   ginseng and, 250–251
   yohimbine and, 623–624
ethical issues, 649–651
evening primrose oil *(Oenothera biennis)*, 210, 211, 212, 216–217
Evidence-Based Review Program, 645
exercise/athletic performance
   alanine and, 13
   arginine and ornithine and, 29
   aspartic acid and asparagine and, 38
   boron and bodybuilding, 55
   branched chain amino acids (BCAA) and, 59–60
   carnitine and, 86
   choline and, 328
   coenzyme Q_{10} and, 119–120
   colostrum and, 127
   creatine and, 143–145
   dehydroepiandrosterone (DHEA) ban and, 149
   ginseng and, 248–249
   glycerol and, 270
   magnesium and, 356–358
   N-acetylcysteine and, 386
   pantothenic acid and, 397
   potassium and cramping from, 418
   pyruvate and, 425–427
   selenium and, 469
   sodium bicarbonate and, 480–481
   thiamin and, 537
   vitamin C and, 572
   vitamin E and, 602–604
   whey protein and, 617–618
   zinc and, 632
eye health. *See also specific conditions*
   vitamin A/beta carotene and, 530

falling, vitamin D and risk of, 585
fatigue
   carnitine and, 86–87
   royal jelly and, 440–441
Federal Trade Commission, 644, 650
Femal, 438, 441. *See also* royal jelly
fenugreek *(Trigonella foenum-graecum)*, 166–169
   blood cholesterol levels and, 168
   blood glucose control and, 167–168
   cancer and, 168–169
   coronary artery disease and, 168
   dosage information/bioavailability, 167
   drug/supplement interactions, 167
   food sources, 167
   key points, 167
   media and marketing claims, 166
   safety, 166–167
fertility, male. *See* male fertility
feverfew *(Tanacetum parthenium)*, 169–172
   dosage information/bioavailability, 171
   drug/supplement interactions, 170
   key points, 170
   media and marketing claims, 170
   migraines and, 171–172
   safety, 170
fibromyalgia
   5-hydroxy-tryptophan (5-HTP) and, 301
   S-adenosylmethionine and, 446–447
fish oil, 172–187
   attention deficit/hyperactivity disorder and, 184
   blood lipids/atherosclerosis and, 175, 177–178
   blood pressure and, 175, 180–181
   cancer and, 184–185
   cancer cachexia and, 184
   cardiovascular morbidity or mortality and, 178–179
   diabetes and, 179–180
   dosage information/bioavailability, 177
   drug/supplement interactions, 174
   food sources, 176–177

fish oil (*continued*)
  inflammatory bowel disease and, 182
  key points, 175–176
  media and marketing claims, 173
  mental illness and, 183–184
  psoriasis and, 182–183
  rheumatoid arthritis and, 181–182
  safety, 173–174
flaxseed, 188–195
  α–linolenic acid (n-3), 188
  cancer and, 192
  cardiovascular disease and, 191
  constipation and, 193
  dosage information/bioavailability, 190–191
  drug/supplement interactions, 189
  food sources, 190
  inflammatory disorders and, 192–193
  key points, 189–190
  lignans, 188
  lupus and, 191–192
  media and marketing claims, 188
  safety, 189
folate/folic acid, 195–205
  cancer and, 200–202
  cardiovascular disease, homocysteine levels, and, 199–200
  cognitive impairment and, 202–203
  dosage information/bioavailability, 198
  drug/supplement interactions, 196
  food sources, 197–198
  key points, 197
  media and marketing claims, 195
  neural tube defects and, 198–199
  safety, 195–196
Food and Drug Administration. *See also* Dietary Supplement Health and Education Act of 1994 (DSHEA)
  Center for Food Safety and Applied Nutrition (CFSAN), 641, 642, 658
  Dietary Supplement Labeling Guide, 639, 643
  FDA Modernization Act of 1997 (FDAMA), 642
  Good Manufacturing Practices (GMPs), 644
  health claims and, 642–643
  health fraud reporting/MedWatch, xv, 661
  product safety and, 640–641
  supplement label rules, 643
  Web site, 650
Food and Nutrition Board, 658
Food and Nutrition Information Center, 658
Food, Drug and Cosmetic Act, 24, 639
fructo-oligosaccharides (FOS), 205–210
  blood glucose and cholesterol and, 208–209
  colon cancer and, 208
  dosage information/bioavailability, 207
  drug/supplement interactions, 206
  food sources, 206–207
  gastrointestinal health and, 207–208
  key points, 206

  media and marketing claims, 205
  safety, 205–206
function claims, 642

gamma-linolenic acid, 210–219
  cancer and, 217
  cardiovascular disease and, 216–217
  diabetes and, 216
  dosage information/bioavailability, 212–213
  drug/supplement interactions, 211
  food sources, 212
  key points, 211–212
  mastalgia and, 213–214
  media and marketing claims, 210–211
  menopause and, 213–214
  PMS and, 213–214
  rheumatoid arthritis and, 214–215
  safety, 211
  skin disorders and, 215–216
gamma-oryzanol, 219–222. *See also* phytosterols
  cholesterol and, 221
  dosage/information/bioavailability, 221
  food sources, 221
  key points, 220
  media and marketing claims, 220
  muscle mass and, 221
  safety, 220
Garcinia cambogia. See hydroxycitric acid (*Garcinia cambogia*)
garlic, 222–232
  atherogenesis, cholesterol, and, 226–227
  blood pressure and, 227
  cancer and, 228–229
  cardiac elasticity and, 227
  circulation and platelet function and, 227–228
  dosage information/bioavailability, 225
  drug/supplement interactions, 223–224
  food sources, 225
  immune function and, 229
  key points, 224–225
  media and marketing claims, 223
  safety, 223
gastrointestinal cancer, vitamin A/beta carotene and, 525
gastrointestinal disorders/health. *See also* constipation; diarrhea; dyspepsia; nausea
  acidophilus and, 4–5
  aloe vera gel and, 16
  colostrum/bovine colostrum and, 125–126
  fructo-oligosaccharides and, 207–208
  pancreatin and, 393
  spirulina/blue-green algae and, 503
genistein, 428
ginger (*Zingiber officinale*), 232–236
  dosage information/bioavailability, 233
  drug/supplement interactions, 232
  food sources, 233
  key points, 233
  media and marketing claims, 232

morning sickness and, 233–235
nausea and, 235
safety, 232
Ginkgo biloba, 236–245
Alzheimer's disease/dementia and, 239–241
dosage information/bioavailability, 239
drug/supplement interactions, 238
key points, 238–239
media and marketing claims, 237
memory in healthy people and, 241–242
mountain sickness and, 243
peripheral vascular disease and, 242
safety, 237–238
tinnitus and, 243
ginseng, 245–254
cancer and, 252
diabetes and, 251–252
dosage information/bioavailability, 248
drug/supplement interactions, 246–247
exercise performance and, 248–249
food sources, 248
key points, 247–248
media and marketing claims, 246
mood and cognitive function and, 250
safety, 246
sexual function and, 250–251
glucosamine, 254–260
arthritis and, 256–260
dosage information/bioavailability, 256
key points, 255–256
media and marketing claims, 255
safety, 255
glutamine, 262–267
dosage information/bioavailability, 263
food sources, 263
glycogen stores and, 264
HIV wasting and, 265
immunity and, during exercise training, 263–264
key points, 262–263
media and marketing claims, 262
mucositis from chemotherapy and, 265–266
safety, 262
glycerol, 267–271
dosage information/bioavailability, 269
exercise performance and, 270
food sources, 269
hydration and, 267, 269
key points, 268
media and marketing claims, 268
safety, 268
thermoregulation and, 269–270
glycyrrhizin, 331. *See also* licorice root
goldenseal *(Hydrastis canadensis),* 271–274
antibiotic activity, 273
dosage information/bioavailability, 272–273
drug/supplement interactions, 272
infectious diarrhea and, 273–274
key points, 272

media and marketing claims, 271
safety, 272
urinary drug tests and, 274
goldthread *(Coptis chinensis),* 271
Good Manufacturing Practices (GMPs), 644
government regulation of dietary supplements, 639–648
and professional ethics, 650
grape seed extract, 275–277
antioxidant activity, 276
cancer and, 276
cardiovascular health and, 276
chloasma and, 277
dosage information/bioavailability, 276
food sources, 276
key points, 275–276
media and marketing claims, 275
safety, 275
green tea extract, 278–286
antioxidant activity, 280
cancer and, 280–282
cardiovascular disease and, 282–284
dosage information/bioavailability, 280
drug/supplement interactions, 279
food sources, 280
hypertension and, 284
key points, 279
media and marketing claims, 278
safety, 278–279
weight control and, 284
guarana, 287–289
dosage information/bioavailability, 288
drug/supplement interactions, 288
food sources, 288
key points, 288
media and marketing claims, 287
safety, 287–288
weight loss and, 288–289
guggul/guggulipids, 289–292
dosage information/bioavailability, 291
drug/supplement interactions, 290
hypercholesterolemia and, 291–292
hypothyroidism and, 291
key points, 290
media and marketing claims, 290
safety, 290

hawthorn, 292–295
cardiovascular disease and, 294
dosage information/bioavailability, 293
drug/supplement interactions, 293
key points, 293
media and marketing claims, 293
safety, 293
HCA. *See* hydroxycitric acid *(Garcinia cambogia)*
headache. *See* migraines; tension headache
A Healthcare Professional's Guide to Evaluation of Dietary Supplements, 650
health claims, for dietary supplements, 642–643

heart disease. *See* cardiovascular disease

heme iron, 315

hepatic encephalopathy
 branched chain amino acids (BCAA) and, 61
 L-aspartate and, 38

hepatitis, milk thistle and, 379–380

HerbalGram, 660

Herb Research Foundation, 658, 660

Herpes simplex virus, lysine and, 346–347

HIV. *See* human immunodeficiency virus (HIV)

HMB (β-hydroxy β-methylbutyrate). *See* β-hydroxy β-methylbutyrate (HMB)

horse chestnut, 295–297
 chronic venous insufficiency and, 296–297
 dosage information/bioavailability, 296
 drug/supplement interactions, 296
 key points, 296
 media and marketing claims, 295
 safety, 295

hot flashes. *See also* menopause
 gamma-linolenic acid and, 213–214
 red clover and, 430

human immunodeficiency virus (HIV). *See also* acquired immunodeficiency syndrome (AIDS); immune function
 alpha-lipoic acid (ALA) and, 22
 bitter melon and, 45
 cobalamin and, 563
 coenzyme Q$_{10}$ and, 120
 dehydroepiandrosterone (DHEA) and, 154–155
 dyslipidemia associated with, red yeast rice and, 434
 glutamine and, 265
 β-hydroxy β-methylbutyrate (HMB) and wasting in, 306
 N-acetylcysteine and, 385–386
 selenium and, 468
 whey protein and, 618–619

Hydrastis canadensis. See goldenseal *(Hydrastis canadensis)*

hydration, glycerol and, 267, 269

5-hydroxy-tryptophan (5-HTP), 298–303
 anxiety-related disorders and, 300–301
 appetite and, 301–302
 depression and, 300
 dosage information/bioavailability, 299–300
 drug/supplement interactions, 299
 fibromyalgia and, 301
 key points, 299
 media and marketing claims, 298
 safety, 298

β-hydroxy β-methylbutyrate (HMB), 303–307
 creatine and, 143
 dosage information/bioavailability, 304
 food sources, 304
 key points, 304
 media and marketing claims, 303
 safety, 303

strength, body composition, muscle damage and, 305–306
 wasting in HIV or cancer and, 306

hydroxycitric acid *(Garcinia cambogia),* 307–311
 dosage information/bioavailability, 308
 food sources, 308
 key points, 308
 media and marketing claims, 308
 safety, 308
 weight control and, 309–310

hypercholesterolemia. *See* blood lipids; cholesterol

Hypericum perforatum. See St John's Wort *(Hypericum perforatum)*

hyperlipidemia. *See also* blood lipids; cardiovascular disease; cholesterol
 acidophilus and, 3
 pantothenic acid and, 397
 phytosterols and, 406

hypertension. *See also* blood pressure
 calcium and, 74–76
 garlic and, 227
 green tea extract and, 280–282
 vitamin C and, 574–575

hyperthyroidism, carnitine and, 88–89

hypoglycemia, alanine and, 11–12

hypothyroidism, guggul and, 291

IBIDS, 644, 661

immune function. *See also* specific immune diseases
 acidophilus and, 2
 bitter melon and, 45
 carnitine and, 89–90
 coenzyme Q10 and, 120
 conjugated linoleic acid (CLA) and, 133
 dehydroepiandrosterone (DHEA) and, 152–153
 echinacea and, 162
 garlic and, 229
 glutamine and, 263, 264
 pancreatin and, 393–394
 pau d'arco and, 399
 royal jelly and, 439–440
 selenium and, 468–469
 spirulina/blue-green algae and, 502
 vitamin A/beta carotene and, 528–530
 vitamin C and, 571–572
 vitamin E and, 598–599
 whey protein and, 618–619
 zinc and, 633

impotence, male. *See* erectile dysfunction

indole-3-carbinol (I-3C), 311–314
 cancer and, 312–314
 drug/supplement interactions, 311
 key points, 312
 media and marketing claims, 311
 safety, 311

indole-3-methanol. *See* indole-3-carbinol (I-3C)

industry self-regulation of dietary supplements, 645

inflammation. *See also specific conditions/diseases*
  bromelain and, 66–67
  flaxseed and, 192–193
inflammatory bowel disease, fish oil and, 182
influenza virus, N-acetylcysteine and, 384–385
ingredients, choosing quality, 645–646
insomnia. *See* sleep
intermittent claudication
  garlic and, 227–228
  policosanol and, 412
International Bibliographic Information on Dietary
    Supplements (IBIDS), 644, 661
International Food Information Council, 659
International Olympic Committee, creatine use and, 141
iron, 315–320
  absorption, 317–318
  anemia of chronic disease and, 318
  cognitive function and, 318–319
  dosage information/bioavailability, 317–318
  drug/supplement interactions, 316
  food sources, 316–317
  iron-deficiency anemia and, 316, 318
  key points, 316
  media and marketing claims, 315
  safety, 315–316
irritable bowel syndrome
  acidophilus and, 3, 5–6
  fructo-oligosaccharides and, 207–208
isoflavones. *See* soy protein and isoflavones

jet lag, melatonin and, 370–371
joint pain, bromelain and, 66–67. *See also* arthritis
Journal of Dietary Supplements, 659
Journal of the American Dietetic Association, 659
Journal of the American Medical Association, 660

kava *(Piper methysticum)*, 320–325
  anxiety and, 323–324
  dosage information/bioavailability, 322
  drug/supplement interactions, 321–322
  food sources, 322
  key points, 322
  media and marketing claims, 320
  safety, 320–321
  sleep disturbance and, 324

labeling standards for dietary supplements, 641–644
lactation, caution regarding supplement use during, xv
Lactobacillus acidophilus (LA). *See*
    acidophilus/*Lactobacillus acidophilus* (LA)
lactose intolerance, acidophilus and, 4
L-arginine. *See* arginine (L-arginine)
L-aspartate. *See* aspartic acid/asparagine
laxatives. *See* constipation
lecithin/choline, 325–330
  dosage information/bioavailability, 328
  exercise and, 328

food sources, 327
key points, 326–327
liver health and, 329
media and marketing claims, 326
neurological disorders and, 328–329
safety, 326
legal issues, 639–648
leucine, 57, 58, 59. *See also* branched chain amino acids
    (BCAA)
leukemia, anti-carcinogenic effects of ajoene and, 229
libido. *See also* sexual function
  dehydroepiandrosterone (DHEA) and, 151–152
  ginseng and, 250–251
licorice root, 330–335
  cancer prevention and, 333
  cardiovascular disease prevention and, 334
  drug/supplement interactions, 331
  dyspepsia and, 332
  eczema and, 332–333
  food sources, 332
  key points, 331–332
  media and marketing claims, 331
  safety, 331
lignans, 188
lipases, 390, 392
lipoic acid. *See also* alpha-lipoic acid (ALA)
  thiamin and, 534
liver health/liver disease
  alanine and, 12–13
  alpha-lipoic acid (ALA) and, 22
  branched chain amino acids (BCAA) and hepatic
      encephalopathy, 61
  choline and, 329
  L-aspartate and hepatic encephalopathy, 38
  milk thistle and, 378–379, 380–381
  S-adenosylmethionine and, 448–449
lung cancer
  vitamin A/beta carotene and, 524–525
  vitamin E and, 600–601
lung function. *See* pulmonary function
lupus
  dehydroepiandrosterone (DHEA) and, 154
  flaxseed and, 191–192
lutein, 335–339, 518
  age-related cataracts and, 337–338
  age-related macular degeneration and, 337
  cancer prevention and, 338
  dosage information/bioavailability, 336–337
  drug/supplement interactions, 335
  food sources, 336
  key points, 335–336
  media and marketing claims, 335
  retinitis pigmentosa and, 338
  safety, 335
lycopene, 340–344, 406, 518
  atherosclerosis prevention and, 343
  cancer prevention and, 342

lycopene (*continued*)
    dosage information/bioavailability, 341
    exercise-induced asthma and, 342–343
    food sources, 341
    key points, 340–341
    media and marketing claims, 340
    prostate cancer and, 341–342
    safety, 340
lysine, 344–348
    calcium metabolism/bone health and, 347–348
    dosage information/bioavailability, 346
    drug/supplement interactions, 345
    food sources, 345–346
    Herpes simplex virus and, 346–347
    key points, 345
    media and marketing claims, 344
    safety, 345

macular degeneration/maculopathy
    lutein and, 337
    vitamin E and, 600–601
    zinc and, 631–632
magnesium, 349–360
    blood pressure and, 353–354
    bowel function and, 358
    cardiovascular disease and, 352–353
    diabetes and, 354
    dosage information/bioavailability, 351–352
    drug/supplement interactions, 350
    exercise performance and, 356–358
    food sources, 351
    key points, 350–351
    media and marketing claims, 349
    migraine and, 354–356
    premenstrual syndrome and, 356
    safety, 349
ma huang (*Ephedra sinica*), 360–366, 640–641
    dosage information/bioavailability, 363
    drug/supplement interactions, 362
    key points, 362–363
    media and marketing claims, 361
    safety, 361–362
    weight loss and, 364–365
male fertility
    carnitine and, 89
    zinc and, 633
mastalgia, gamma-linolenic acid and, 213–214
Medline, xiii, 661
MedWatch, xv, 661
melasma, grape seed extract and, 277
melatonin, 366–375
    cancer and, 372
    dosage information/bioavailability, 368–369
    drug/supplement interactions, 367
    food sources, 368
    jet lag and, 370–371
    key points, 367–368
    media and marketing claims, 366

    migraine and, 372–373
    night shift work and, 370–371
    safety, 366–367
    sleep and, 369–370
memory. *See also* Alzheimer's disease; cognition;
    dementia
    bee pollen and, 41
    dehydroepiandrosterone (DHEA) and, 151–152
    ginkgo and, 241–242
Menhaden oil, 173–174
menopause
    black cohosh and, 49–50
    dehydroepiandrosterone (DHEA) and, 155
    dong quai and, 159
    gamma-linolenic acid and, 213–214
    red clover and, 430
    soy protein and isoflavones and, 490–492
    wild yam and, 620
mental illness. *See specific types*
methylsulfonylmethane (MSM), 375–377
    allergic rhinitis and, 376
    arthritis and, 376
    dosage information/bioavailability, 376
    food sources, 376
    key points, 375–376
    media and marketing claims, 375
    safety, 375
migraines
    coenzyme Q10 and, 121
    feverfew and, 171–172
    magnesium and, 354–356
    melatonin and, 372–373
    riboflavin and, 542
milk thistle (*Silybum marianum*), 377–382
    cancer and, 380–381
    cirrhosis of the liver and, 378–379
    dosage information/bioavailability, 378
    drug/supplement interactions, 377–378
    hepatitis and, 379–380
    key points, 378
    liver health and, 380
    media and marketing claims, 377
    safety, 377
minerals. *See* boron; calcium; chromium; magnesium;
    potassium; selenium; vanadium; zinc
Momordica charantia. See bitter melon (*Momordica*
    charantia)
mood. *See also* anxiety; depression
    dehydroepiandrosterone (DHEA) and, 151–152
    ginseng and, 250
    phosphatidylserine and, 403
Morinda citrifolia. See noni juice
morning sickness, ginger and, 233–235
mountain sickness, *Ginkgo biloba* and, 243
mouth ulcers, thiamin and, 538–539
MSM. *See* methylsulfonylmethane (MSM)
mucositis, glutamine and, 265–266
muscle cramping, potassium and, 418

muscle mass. *See also* body composition/body mass
 gamma-oryzanol and, 221
 vanadium and, 517
muscle strength. *See also* exercise/athletic performance
 chromium and, 111–112
 creatine and, 145
 vanadium and, 517
muscular disease, creatine and, 145
myotonic dystrophy type 2, creatine and, 145

N-acetylcysteine (NAC), 382–388
 dosage information/bioavailability, 384
 drug/supplement interactions, 383
 exercise and, 386
 food sources, 384
 HIV and, 385–386
 influenza virus and respiratory illness and, 384–385
 key points, 383–384
 media and marketing claims, 383
 polycystic ovary syndrome and, 386
 safety, 383
NAPRALERT—Natural Products Alert Database, 661
National Center for Complementary and Alternative
 Medicine (NCCAM), 645, 659, 661
National Council Against Health Fraud, 661
National Nutritional Foods Association (NNFA) GMP
 Certification Program, 645
Natural Standard (Web site), 661
nausea, ginger and, 235
necrotizing enterocolitis, arginine and, 34
neural tube defects, folate/folic acid and, 198–199
neurological disorders. *See also specific disorders*
 choline and, 328–329
 coenzyme Q_{10} and, 120–121
 vitamin E and, 599–600
neuromuscular disease, creatine and, 145
niacin. *See* vitamin B-3 (niacin)
Niaspan, 545, 546, 547
nicotinamide, 545, 549
nicotinic acid therapy, 545
night shift work, melatonin and, 370–371
nonheme iron, 315
noni juice, 388–390
 dosage information/bioavailability, 389–390
 food sources, 389
 key points, 389
 media and marketing claims, 389
 safety, 389
NSF International, 645, 659
Nutrition Action Healthletter, 660
Nutrition Business Journal, 660
Nutrition in Complementary Care Newsletter, 660
Nutrition Labeling and Education Act (NLEA) of 1990,
 642

obesity. *See also* weight control/weight loss
 chromium and, 111
 conjugated linoleic acid (CLA) and, 131–133

Office of Dietary Supplements, xiii–xiv, 644–645, 659
oral cancer, vitamin A/beta carotene and, 525–526
ornithine, 26, 29, 32, 33
oryzanol, 219
osteoarthritis. *See also* arthritis
 boron and, 55
 cat's claw and, 94
 chondroitin sulfate and, 103–104
 glucosamine sulfate and, 256–258
 S-adenosylmethionine and, 444–446
osteoporosis. *See also* bone health/bone mineral density
 calcium and, 73–74
 red clover and, 431
 soy protein and isoflavones and, 492–494
 vitamin K and, 611
overtraining syndrome, glutamine and, 263

pancreatic cancer, pancreatin and, 394
pancreatin, 390–395
 dosage information/bioavailability, 392–393
 drug/supplement interactions, 391
 food sources, 392
 gastrointestinal disorders and, 393
 immunity and, 393–394
 key points, 391–392
 media and marketing claims, 391
 pancreatic cancer and, 394
 safety, 391
panic attacks, 5-hydroxy-tryptophan (5-HTP) and,
 300
pantothenic acid, 395–398
 arthritis and, 397–398
 cholesterol and, 397
 dosage information/bioavailability, 396–397
 exercise performance and, 397
 food sources, 396
 key points, 396
 media and marketing claims, 395
 safety, 395
 thiamin and, 534
Parkinson's disease
 choline and, 329
 coenzyme Q_{10} and, 120–121
pau d'arco, 398–400
 dosage information/bioavailability, 399
 drug/supplement interactions, 399
 key points, 399
 media and marketing claims, 399
 safety, 399
peripheral vascular disease, ginkgo and, 242
Pharmacist's Letter/Natural Medicine Database, 661
phosphatidylserine (PS), 400–404
 acute stress response/mood enhancement and, 403
 cognitive function in the aging population and, 402
 dosage information/bioavailability, 401
 drug/supplement interactions, 401
 food sources, 401
 media and marketing claims, 400

phosphatidylserine (PS) (*continued*)
    physical stress and, 402–403
    safety, 400–401
phytosterols, 404–408. *See also* gamma-oryzanol
    benign prostatic hypertrophy and, 406–407
    dosage information/bioavailability, 405–406
    drug/supplement interactions, 404
    hyperlipidemia and, 406
    key points, 405
    media and marketing claims, 404
    safety, 404
Piper methysticum. See kava (*Piper methysticum*)
plant sterols and stanols. *See* phytosterols
platelet aggregation/function
    bromelain and, 67
    garlic and, 227–228
PMS. *See* premenstrual syndrome (PMS)
policosanol, 408–413
    dosage information/bioavailability, 410
    drug/supplement interactions, 409
    hypercholesterolemia and, 408, 410–412
    intermittent claudication and, 412
    key points, 409
    media and marketing claims, 408
    safety, 409
pollen. *See* bee pollen
polycystic ovary syndrome, N-acetylcysteine and, 386
potassium, 414–419
    blood pressure and, 416–418
    dosage information/bioavailability, 416
    drug/supplement interactions, 415
    exercise-associated muscle cramping and, 418
    food sources, 416
    key points, 415–416
    media and marketing claims, 414
    safety, 414–415
pregnancy
    caution regarding supplement use in, xv
    ginger and morning sickness in, 233–235
premenstrual syndrome (PMS)
    bee pollen and, 41
    black cohosh and, 50
    calcium and, 71, 78–79
    dong quai and, 159
    gamma-linolenic acid and, 213–214
    magnesium and, 356
    pyridoxine and, 553–554
    royal jelly and, 441
prostate cancer
    boron and, 56
    lycopene and, 341–342
    saw palmetto and, 461
prostatitis, bee pollen and, 41–42
PS. *See* phosphatidylserine (PS)
psoriasis
    fish oil and, 182–183
    shark cartilage and, 477–478

PubMed/Medline, xiii, 661
pulmonary function. *See also* asthma; respiratory
        illness/infection
    vitamin C and, 571
    vitamin E and, 600–601
purple cone flower. *See* echinacea
pygeum, 419–422
    benign prostatic hyperplasia and, 420–421
    dosage information/bioavailability, 420
    key points, 420
    media and marketing claims, 419
    safety, 419
pyridoxine. *See* vitamin B-6 (pyridoxine)
pyruvate, 422–428
    blood lipids and, 427
    dosage information/bioavailability, 423–424
    exercise endurance and, 425–427
    food sources, 423
    key points, 423
    media and marketing claims, 422
    safety, 423
    weight loss and, 424–425

Quackwatch, 661
quality control, 645–646

red clover, 428–432
    breast tenderness and, 429–430
    dosage information/bioavailability, 429
    drug/supplement interactions, 428
    key points, 429
    media and marketing claims, 428
    menopause and, 430
    osteoporosis and, 431
    safety, 428
red yeast rice, 432–434
    dosage information/bioavailability, 433
    drug/supplement interactions, 432
    dyslipidemia associated with HIV and, 434
    food sources, 433
    hypercholesterolemia and, 433–434
    key points, 433
    media and marketing claims, 432
    safety, 432
regulations. *See* government regulation of dietary
        supplements; industry self-regulation of dietary
        supplements
Remifemin, 46, 48–49
renal function in diabetes, soy and, 494–495
respiratory illness/infection. *See also* common cold;
        pulmonary function
    bromelain and sinusitis/bronchitis, 65–66
    echinacea and, 162–164
    N-acetylcysteine and, 384–385
resveratrol, 435–437
    cancer and, 436
    coronary heart disease and, 436

dosage information/bioavailability, 436
drug/supplement interactions, 435
food sources, 436
key points, 435
media and marketing claims, 435
safety, 435
retinitis pigmentosa, lutein and, 338
retinol. *See* vitamin A/beta carotene
rheumatoid arthritis. *See also* arthritis
cat's claw and, 94
fish oil and, 181–182
selenium and, 469
rhinitis, allergic
lactobacillus acidophilus and, 7
methylsulfonylmethane (MSM) and, 376
riboflavin. *See* vitamin B-2 (riboflavin)
Rogers-Proxmire Vitamin Amendments, 639
royal jelly, 438–442
antibacterial properties, 439–449
blood pressure and, 440
cardiovascular disease and, 440
dosage information/bioavailability, 439
fatigue and, 440–441
immunity and, 439–440
key points, 439
media and marketing claims, 438
premenstrual syndrome and, 441
safety, 438

S-adenosylmethionine (SAM-e), 442–451
depression and, 447–448
dosage information/bioavailability, 444
drug/supplement interactions, 443
fibromyalgia and, 446–447
key points, 443–444
liver function and, 448–449
media and marketing claims, 442
osteoarthritis and, 444–446
safety, 442–443
safety, xv. *See also* Dietary Supplement Health Education
Act of 1994 (DSHEA); *under specific supplements*
St John's wort *(Hypericum perforatum)*, 451–458
depression and, 454–457
dosage information/bioavailability, 454
drug/supplement interactions, 452–453
key points, 453
media and marketing claims, 452
safety, 452
SAM-e. *See* S-adenosylmethionine (SAM-e)
saw palmetto *(Serenoa repens)*, 459–462
benign prostatic hyperplasia and, 460–461
dosage information/bioavailability, 460
drug/supplement interactions, 459
key points, 460
media and marketing claims, 459
prostate cancer and, 461
safety, 459

SCAN's Pulse, 660
schizophrenia, fish oil and, 184
Scientific Review of Alternative Medicine, 660
selenium, 462–472
asthma and, 470
cancer and, 465–467
cardiovascular disease and, 467–468
dosage information/bioavailability, 465
drug/supplement interactions, 463–464
exercise and, 469
food sources, 465
immunity and, 468–469
key points, 464–465
media and marketing claims, 463
rheumatoid arthritis and, 469
safety, 463
senna, 472–474
constipation and, 473–474
dosage information/bioavailability, 473
drug/supplement interactions, 473
key points, 473
media and marketing claims, 472
safety, 472
Serenoa repens. See saw palmetto *(Serenoa repens)*
sexual function. *See also* libido
arginine and erectile dysfunction, 34
ginseng and, 250–251
yohimbine and, 623–624
shark cartilage, 474–478
angiogenesis and, 476–477
blood clotting and, 477
cancer and, 476–477
dosage information/bioavailability, 476
key points, 475–476
media and marketing claims, 475
psoriasis and, 477–478
safety, 475
Silybum marianum. See milk thistle *(Silybum marianum)*
silymarin. *See* milk thistle *(Silybum marianum)*
sinusitis, bromelain and, 65–66. *See also* respiratory
illness/infection
sitostanol, 404
skin, health of. *See also specific disorders*
gamma-linolenic acid and, 215–216
vitamin A/beta carotene and, 531
skin cancer
ajoene and, 229
vitamin A/beta carotene and, 526
sleep
cobalamin and, 563
5-hydroxy-tryptophan (5-HTP) and, 300–301
kava and, 324
melatonin and, 369–370
valerian and, 511–512
sodium bicarbonate, 479–482
dosage information/bioavailability, 480
exercise performance and, 480–481

sodium bicarbonate (*continued*)
    food sources, 480
    key points, 479
    media and marketing claims, 479
    safety, 479
soy protein and isoflavones, 482–499
    cancer and, 488–490
    cardiovascular disease and, 485–488
    diabetes and, 494–495
    dosage information/bioavailability, 485
    drug/supplement interactions, 483
    food sources, 484–485
    key points, 483–484
    media and marketing claims, 482
    menopause and, 490–492
    osteoporosis and, 492–494
    safety, 483
spirulina/blue-green algae, 499–504
    cancer and, 502–503
    cholesterol and, 502
    dosage information/bioavailability, 501
    food sources, 501
    gastrointestinal health and, 503
    immunity and, 502
    key points, 500–501
    media and marketing claims, 499
    safety, 500
statements of nutritional support, 642
strength training, chromium for, 111–112. *See also*
        muscle strength
stroke, glycerol and, 267
structure/function claims, 642
Supplement Facts panel, 643
Supplement Watch, 661
systemic inflammatory response syndrome (SIRS),
        selenium and, 468–469

tea. *See* black tea; green tea extract
tension headache, 5-hydroxy-tryptophan (5-HTP) and,
        300–301
thermoregulation, glycerol and, 269–270
thiamin. *See* vitamin B-1 (thiamin)
thyroid function
    carnitine and hyperthyroidism, 88–89
    guggul and hypothyroidism, 291
tinnitus, ginkgo and, 243
tocopherol, 588
Trigonella foenum-graecum. See fenugreek (*Trigonella
        foenum-graecum*)
Tufts University Health and Nutrition Newsletter, 660
turmeric (*Curcuma longa*), 505–508
    anterior uveitis and, 506–507
    cancer and, 507–508
    dosage information/bioavailability, 506
    drug/supplement interactions, 505
    dyspepsia and, 506
    food sources, 505–506
    key points, 505

    media and marketing claims, 505
    safety, 505

ubiquinone, 115. *See also* coenzyme Q_{10}
ulcerative colitis, and fish oil, 182
Uncaria tomentosa. See cat's claw (*Uncaria tomentosa*)
University of California Berkeley Wellness Letter, 660
urinary tract infections (UTIs), cranberry extract and,
        138–139
US Pharmacopoeia (USP), 659
uveitis, turmeric and, 506–507

Vaccinium macrocarpon. See cranberry extract
valerian (*Valeriana officinalis*), 508–512
    anxiety and, 512
    dosage information/bioavailability, 510
    drug/supplement interactions, 509–510
    key points, 510
    media and marketing claims, 509
    safety, 509
    sleep and, 511–512
valine, 57, 59. *See also* branched chain amino acids
        (BCAA)
vanadium, 514–518
    diabetes and, 516–517
    dosage information/bioavailability, 515–516
    drug/supplement interactions, 515
    food sources, 515
    key points, 515
    media and marketing claims, 514
    muscle mass/muscle strength and, 517
    safety, 514–515
vanadyl sulfate. *See* vanadium
vitamin A/beta carotene, 518–534
    breast cancer and, 524
    cancer and, 523–524
    cardiovascular disease, 536–528
    dosage information/bioavailability, 522–523
    drug/supplement interactions, 520
    eye health and, 530
    food sources, 522
    gastrointestinal cancers and, 525
    immunity and, 528–530
    key points, 521
    lung cancer and, 524–525
    media and marketing claims, 519
    oral cancer and, 525–526
    plasma carotenoids and, 523
    safety, 519–520
    skin cancer and, 526
    skin health and, 531
vitamin B-1 (thiamin), 534–540
    cataracts and, 539
    dementia and, 537–538
    dosage information/bioavailability, 536–537
    drug/supplement interactions, 535
    for the elderly, 537–538
    encephalopathy and, 537–538

exercise and, 537
food sources, 536
key points, 535–536
media and marketing claims, 535
mouth ulcers and, 538–539
safety, 535
vitamin B-2 (riboflavin), 540–543
cataracts and, 543
dosage information/bioavailability, 541
drug/supplement interactions, 540
food sources, 541
key points, 541
media and marketing claims, 540
migraines and, 542
safety, 540
vitamin B-3 (niacin), 543–550
arthritis and, 548–549
cardiovascular disease and, 546–547
diabetes and, 547–548
dosage information/bioavailability, 546
drug/supplement interactions, 544–545
food sources, 545–546
key points, 545
media and marketing claims, 544
safety, 544
thiamin and, 534
vitamin B-6 (pyridoxine), 550–558
asthma and, 555–556
autism and, 556
cardiovascular disease and, 554–555
carpal tunnel syndrome and, 553
cognition in the elderly and, 556–557
dosage information/bioavailability, 552–553
drug/supplement interactions, 551
food sources, 552
key points, 551–552
media and marketing claims, 550
premenstrual syndrome and, 553–554
safety, 550–551
vitamin B-12 (cobalamin), 558–566
cardiovascular disease and, 563–564
dementia in the elderly and, 562–563
diabetes and, 564
dosage information/bioavailability, 561–562
drug/supplement interactions, 560
food sources, 561
HIV/AIDS and, 563
key points, 560–561
media and marketing claims, 559
safety, 559
sleep disorders and, 563
vitamin C, 566–578
asthma and, 571
cancer and, 575–576
cardiovascular disease and, 572–574
cataracts and, 576
common cold and, 570–571
dosage information/bioavailability, 569–570

drug/supplement interactions, 567–568
exercise-induced oxidative stress and, 572
food sources, 569
hypertension and, 574–575
immune function and, 571–572
key points, 568–569
media and marketing claims, 566
pulmonary function and, 571
safety, 567
vitamin D, 578–588
bone health and, 581–584
calcium absorption and, 584–585
cancer and, 585–586
dosage information/bioavailability, 581
drug/supplement interactions, 579
food sources, 580
key points, 579–580
media and marketing claims, 579
risk of falling and, 585
safety, 579
vitamin E, 588–608
cancer and, 596–597
cardiovascular disease and, 593–596
cataracts/age-related maculopathy and, 601–602
diabetes and, 602
dosage information/bioavailability, 592–593
drug/supplement interactions, 590
exercise performance and, 602–604
food sources, 592
immunity in the elderly and, 598–599
key points, 591
media and marketing claims, 589
neuropsychiatric disorders and, 599–600
pulmonary function and, 600–601
safety, 589–590
selenium and, 462, 469
vitamin K, 608–612
coagulation and, 610–611
dosage information/bioavailability, 610
drug/supplement interactions, 609
food sources, 609
key points, 609
media and marketing claims, 608
osteoporosis and, 611
safety, 609

wasting/cachexia
branched chain amino acids (BCAA) and anorexia in
the elderly, 62
fish oil and, 184
glutamine, 265
β-hydroxy β-methylbutyrate (HMB) and, 306
weight control/weight loss. *See also* body
composition/body mass; obesity
calcium and, 77–78
carnitine (*L-Carnitine*) and, 90
chitosan and, 97–98
chromium and, 111

weight control/weight loss (*continued*)
  conjugated linoleic acid (CLA) and, 131–133
  ephedrine (synthetic) and, 364–365
  green tea extract and, 284
  guarana and, 288–289
  hydroxycitric acid and, 309–310
  pyruvate and, 424–425
  yohimbine and, 624–625
weight gain, whey protein and, 617. *See also*
    wasting/cachexia
weight loss. *See* obesity; wasting/cachexia; weight
    control/weight loss
wheat grass/barley grass, 612–615
  antioxidant activity, 614
  drug/supplement interactions, 613
  food sources, 614
  immunity and, 614
  key points, 613
  media and marketing claims, 613
  safety, 613
whey protein, 615–620
  cancer and, 619
  dosage information/bioavailability, 617
  exercise performance and, 617–618
  food sources, 616
  HIV/immunity and, 618–619
  key points, 616
  media and marketing claims, 615
  safety, 616
  weight gain and, 617
wild yam (*Dioscorea villosa*), 620–622
  dosage information/bioavailability, 621
  key points, 620
  media and marketing claims, 620
  menopause and, 621
  safety, 620
wound healing
  aloe vera (topical) and, 17
  arginine and ornithine and, 33

yeast infections, acidophilus and, 6–7
yohimbine/yohimbe, 622–626
  dosage information/bioavailability, 623
  drug/supplement interactions, 623
  key points, 623
  media and marketing claims, 622
  safety, 622–623
  sexual function and, 623–624
  weight loss and, 624–625

zinc, 626–635
  acne and, 632–633
  age-related macular degeneration and, 631–632
  common cold and, 629–631
  dosage information/bioavailability, 629
  drug/supplement interactions, 627
  exercise performance and, 632
  food sources, 628–629
  immunity and, 633
  key points, 628
  male fertility and, 633
  media and marketing claims, 626
  safety, 627
Zingiber officinale. *See* ginger (*Zingiber officinale*)